Essentials of Anesthesia & Critical Care

Essentials of Anesthesia & Critical Care

SECOND EDITION

As per the Competency Based Medical Education Curriculum (NMC)

Anshul Jain MD
Professor and Head
Department of Anesthesiology and Critical Care
Maharani Laxmi Bai Medical College
Director, MLB Government Paramedical Institute
Jhansi, Uttar Pradesh, India

Pradeep Bhatia MD FICCM FICA
Professor and Head
Department of Anesthesiology and Critical Care
All India Institute of Medical Sciences
Jodhpur, Rajasthan, India
Editor-in-Chief: Journal of Anaesthesiology Clinical Pharmacology (JOACP)

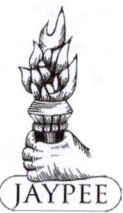

JAYPEE BROTHERS MEDICAL PUBLISHERS
The Health Sciences Publisher
New Delhi | London

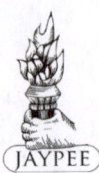

Jaypee Brothers Medical Publishers (P) Ltd.

Headquarters
Jaypee Brothers Medical Publishers (P) Ltd
EMCA House
23/23-B, Ansari Road, Daryaganj
New Delhi - 110 002, India
Landline: +91-11-23272143, +91-11-23272703
+91-11-23282021, +91-11-23245672
Email: jaypee@jaypeebrothers.com

Corporate Office
Jaypee Brothers Medical Publishers (P) Ltd
4838/24, Ansari Road, Daryaganj
New Delhi 110 002, India
Phone: +91-11-43574357
Fax: +91-11-43574314
Email: jaypee@jaypeebrothers.com

Overseas Office
J.P. Medical Ltd
83 Victoria Street, London
SW1H 0HW (UK)
Phone: +44 20 3170 8910
Fax: +44 (0)20 3008 6180
Email: info@jpmedpub.com

Website: www.jaypeebrothers.com

Website: www.jaypeedigital.com

© 2024, Jaypee Brothers Medical Publishers

The views and opinions expressed in this book are solely those of the original contributor(s)/author(s) and do not necessarily represent those of editor(s) and publisher of the book.

All rights reserved. No part of this publication may be reproduced, stored or transmitted in any form or by any means, electronic, mechanical, photocopying, recording or otherwise, without the prior permission in writing of the publishers.

All brand names and product names used in this book are trade names, service marks, trademarks or registered trademarks of their respective owners. The publisher is not associated with any product or vendor mentioned in this book.

Medical knowledge and practice change constantly. This book is designed to provide accurate, authoritative information about the subject matter in question. However, readers are advised to check the most current information available on procedures included and check information from the manufacturer of each product to be administered, to verify the recommended dose, formula, method and duration of administration, adverse effects and contraindications. It is the responsibility of the practitioner to take all appropriate safety precautions. Neither the publisher nor the author(s)/editor(s) assume any liability for any injury and/or damage to persons or property arising from or related to use of material in this book.

This book is sold on the understanding that the publisher is not engaged in providing professional medical services. If such advice or services are required, the services of a competent medical professional should be sought.

Every effort has been made where necessary to contact holders of copyright to obtain permission to reproduce copyright material. If any have been inadvertently overlooked, the publisher will be pleased to make the necessary arrangements at the first opportunity.

Inquiries for bulk sales may be solicited at: jaypee@jaypeebrothers.com

Essentials of Anesthesia & Critical Care

First Edition: 2015
Second Edition: **2024**

ISBN: 978-93-5696-292-7

Printed in India by Rajkamal Electric Press, Kundli, Haryana.

Dedication

This work is lovingly dedicated to my late mother, Smt Saroj Jain, whose teachings and life profoundly shaped my journey. Her wisdom paved the path I walk upon, and her spirit continues to guide and inspire me. Even in her passing, she selflessly contributed to the education of future medical professionals by donating her body to a medical college. This act of generosity embodies the essence of her being—a continuous source of knowledge and inspiration, not just to me but to many others. Her legacy lives on through the countless students who will learn and grow from her gift. This dedication is a small token of my immense gratitude and enduring love.

—*Anshul Jain*

This book is dedicated to students who wish to pursue their careers in the field of anesthesia and allied sub-specialties.

—*Pradeep Bhatia*

CONTRIBUTORS

UNIT CONTRIBUTORS

Practice and Management in ICU
Mohan Gurjar MD PDCC (Critical Care)
Professor
Department of Critical Care Medicine
Sanjay Gandhi Postgraduate Institute of Medical Sciences
Lucknow, Uttar Pradesh, India

Pain Management
Manish Kumar Singh MD PDCC (Pain Management)
Associate Professor
Department of Anesthesiology and Critical Care
King's George Medical University
Lucknow, Uttar Pradesh, India

CHAPTER CONTRIBUTORS

Advaith A Chetan
Registrar
Department of Critical Care Medicine
Chandramma Dayananda Sagar Institute of Medical Education and Research
Harohalli, Karnataka, India

Akashdeep
Assistant Professor
Department of Anesthesiology and Critical Care
MLB Medical College
Jhansi, Uttar Pradesh, India

Ankur Sharma
Additional Professor
Department of Anesthesiology
All India Institute of Medical Sciences
Jodhpur, Rajasthan, India

Apurva Abhinandan Mittal
Professor
Department of Anesthesiology
SN Medical College
Agra, Uttar Pradesh, India

Ashok Mittal
Associate Professor
Department of Anesthesiology and Critical Care
MLB Medical College
Jhansi, Uttar Pradesh, India

Avtar Singh
Professor, Department of Anesthesiology
Shyam Shah Medical College
Rewa, Madhya Pradesh, India

Bhanuprakash Bhaskar
Specialist, Department of Critical Care Medicine
Medeor Hospital
Dubai, United Arab Emirates

Bharat Paliwal
Additional Professor
Department of Anesthesiology
All India Institute of Medical Sciences
Jodhpur, Rajasthan, India

Brijendra Verma
Assistant Professor
Department of Anesthesiology and Critical Care
MLB Medical College
Jhansi, Uttar Pradesh, India

Chris Leslie Lemos
Assistant Professor
Department of Neuroanesthesia
NSCB Medical College
Jabalpur, Madhya Pradesh, India

Darshana Rathod
Assistant Professor
Department of Anesthesiology
All India Institute of Medical Sciences
Jodhpur, Rajasthan, India

Fahad Suhail
Assistant Professor
Department of Anesthesiology and Critical Care
MLB Medical College
Jhansi, Uttar Pradesh, India

Gautham Raju
Consultant, Department of Critical Care Medicine
Manipal Hospital
Bengaluru, Karnataka, India

Ghansham Biyani
Associate Professor
Department of Anesthesiology
All India Institute of Medical Sciences
Mangalagiri, Andhra Pradesh, India

Contributors

Jitendra Agarwal
Professor, Department of Anesthesiology
Gajra Raja Medical College
Gwalior, Madhya Pradesh, India

Kamlesh Kumari
Associate Professor, Department of Anesthesiology
All India Institute of Medical Sciences
Jodhpur, Rajasthan, India

Keshav Goyal
Additional Professor
Department of Neuroanesthesia
All India Institute of Medical Sciences
New Delhi, India

Manbir Kaur
Assistant Professor
Department of Anesthesiology
All India Institute of Medical Sciences
Jodhpur, Rajasthan, India

Manu Varma MK
Consultant
Department of Critical Care Medicine
Narayana Health City
Bengaluru, Karnataka, India

Pooja Bihani
Assistant Professor, Department of Anesthesiology
SN Medical College
Jodhpur, Rajasthan, India

Pooja Chaubey
Assistant Professor
Department of Anesthesiology and Critical Care
MLB Medical College
Jhansi, Uttar Pradesh, India

Priyanka Sethi
Additional Professor
Department of Anesthesiology
All India Institute of Medical Sciences
Jodhpur, Rajasthan, India

Rajasekhar Metta
Assistant Professor
Department of Anesthesiology
All India Institute of Medical Sciences
Mangalagiri, Andhra Pradesh, India

Rakesh Kumar
Additional Professor, Department of Anesthesiology
All India Institute of Medical Sciences
Jodhpur, Rajasthan, India

Reena
Assistant Professor, Department of Anesthesiology
Institute of Medical Sciences
Banaras Hindu University
Varanasi, Uttar Pradesh, India

Rupali Patnaik
Associate Professor
Department of Critical Care Medicine
Institute of Medical Sciences and Sum Hospital
Bhubaneswar, Odisha, India

Sachin Maheshwari
Senior Consultant
Department of Anesthesiology
Yashoda Hospital
Ghaziabad, Uttar Pradesh, India

Sachin Wali
Senior Resident
Department of Critical Care Medicine
Sanjay Gandhi Postgraduate Institute of Medical Sciences
Lucknow, Uttar Pradesh, India

Sadik Mohammed
Additional Professor
Department of Anesthesiology
All India Institute of Medical Sciences
Jodhpur, Rajasthan, India

Sagarika Panda
Associate Professor
Department of Critical Care Medicine
Institute of Medical Sciences and Sum Hospital
Bhubaneswar, Odisha, India

Sandeep Sahu
Additional Professor
Department of Anesthesiology
Sanjay Gandhi Postgraduate Institute of Medical Sciences
Lucknow, Uttar Pradesh, India

Sarvesh Singh
Professor
Department of Anesthesiology
Bhagat Phool Singh Women's Medical College
Rohtak, Haryana, India

Saurabh Nanda
Senior Consultant
Department of Anesthesiology and Critical Care
Medanta —The Medicity
Gurugram, Haryana, India

Shivali Pandey
Associate Professor
Department of Anesthesiology and Critical Care
MLB Medical College
Jhansi, Uttar Pradesh, India

Susmita Ghosh
Associate Professor
Department of Anesthesiology
Murshidabad Medical College
Murshidabad, West Bengal, India

Swati Chhabra
Additional Professor
Department of Anesthesiology
All India Institute of Medical Sciences
Jodhpur, Rajasthan, India

Tanvi M Meshram
Assistant Professor
Department of Anesthesiology
All India Institute of Medical Sciences
Jodhpur, Rajasthan, India

PREFACE TO THE SECOND EDITION

In the ever-evolving field of anesthesiology and critical care, continuous learning and adaptation are not just beneficial but essential. The first edition of *Essentials of Anesthesia and Critical Care* was embraced by students and educators alike for its comprehensive coverage, clear explanations, and student-friendly format. As the landscape of medical education and the demands of healthcare evolve, so must our resources.

With immense pride and a sense of responsibility towards the medical community, we present the second edition of this esteemed book. This fully revised edition not only adheres to the competencies listed by the National Medical Commission (NMC) but also expands its scope to cover all fundamental aspects of critical care. The updates in this edition are significant, aiming to provide a complete and thorough understanding of anesthesia and critical care for both undergraduate (MBBS) and postgraduate students.

Recognizing the importance of collaborative knowledge, this edition includes contributions from renowned anesthesia faculty across India. Their expertise and insights bring a richness to the content that is both diverse and comprehensive. These contributions ensure that the book remains current with the latest practices and innovations in the field.

Key features of this new edition include:
- Expanded content that covers the full spectrum of anesthesia and critical care, tailored to meet the educational needs of both MBBS and PG students.
- Inclusion of competencies as outlined by the National Medical Commission, ensuring that the material is relevant and up-to-date with current medical education standards.
- Enhanced focus on critical care, addressing the increasing importance and complexity of this area in modern healthcare.
- Contributions from a panel of distinguished anesthesia faculty from across India, providing a range of perspectives and expertise.
- Updated tables, line diagrams, and flowcharts for clearer understanding and quick reference.
- Additional mnemonics and key points, facilitating easier recall and retention of information.
- Comprehensive review questions at the end of each chapter, including updated questions from recent PGMEE and NEET examinations.

Our commitment is to equip the future generations of medical professionals with knowledge that is not only foundational but also forward-thinking. We believe this edition will serve as an indispensable resource for students preparing for their professional exams, PGMEE, NEET, or simply seeking a deeper understanding of anesthesiology and critical care.

Embarking on this journey with you, we hope this book continues to be a valuable companion in your educational endeavors and beyond.

Anshul Jain
Pradeep Bhatia

PREFACE TO THE FIRST EDITION

Anesthesia is a specialty that provides pain-free environment in every aspect of human illness. Anesthesia is an upcoming branch; being specialized, most of the basic things are out of reach of MBBS students. Though the subject is easy, but due to lack of lectures and related text materials most of the students find it difficult to understand the basics of this specialty.

Essentials of Anesthesia and Critical Care is written with the goal of providing a concise description of the Anesthesia and Critical Care that is must to know by MBBS students. The text is formatted in a student-friendly manner which will not only help the undergraduate students during their theory exams but also help in solving Postgraduate Medical Entrance Examination (PGMEE) questions. Questions asked in previous years' PGMEE have been denoted by "Q" as superscript in theory portion itself. Tables, line diagrams and flowcharts have been added in each and every chapter for quick and easy grasp of the respective topic. Various important aspects related to the topics have been incorporated as "Key Points" in separate boxes. Each chapter is followed by review questions that include previous years' PGMEE and National Eligibility-cum-Entrance Examination (NEET) based sample questions. Language has been kept very easy; and mnemonics have been added wherever necessary to help students retain information for long time. In a nutshell, it is a complete resource of anesthesia for undergraduate students. Be it professional exams, PGME examination or NEET examination, a student needs to look no further for anesthesia.

Anshul Jain
dranshulrachna@gmail.com

ACKNOWLEDGMENTS

To Bhagwan Mahavir and Ganesha whose blessings made our goal possible

Dr Anshul Jain is extremely grateful and obliged to::
- **Dr Narendra Singh Sengar** Principal, Maharani Laxmi Bai Medical College, Jhansi, Uttar Pradesh, India
- **Dr Rajeev Sinha** Professor Department, Surgery, Maharani Laxmi Bai Medical College, Jhansi, Uttar Pradesh, India
- **Dr Naveen Malhotra** Senior Professor and Head, Department of Cardiac Anesthesia, PGIMS, Rohtak, Haryana, India
- **Dr S Sharma** Professor, Department of Gynecology and Obstetrics, Maharani Laxmi Bai Medical College, Jhansi, Uttar Pradesh, India
- **Dr JP Purohit** Professor, Department of ENT, Maharani Laxmi Bai Medical College, Jhansi, Uttar Pradesh, India
- **Dr Anil Verma** Professor and Head, Department of Anesthesiology, GSVM, Kanpur, Uttar Pradesh
- **Dr Apurva Agarwal** Professor, Department of Anesthesiology, GSVM, Kanpur, Uttar Pradesh
- **Dr Roopesh Kumar** Professor, Department of Anesthesiology, Maharani Laxmi Bai Medical College, Jhansi, Uttar Pradesh, India

Dr Anshul Jain heartly acknowledge family members and friends for their support:
- I do not have words for my wife and co-editor, Dr Rachna Chaurasia who read this text as a reader and made it user-friendly.
- I am extremely thankful to Dr Vikas Chaurasia, Dr Gaurav Tiwari whose inspiration made the task possible.
- Thanks are also due for my family Dr DB Jain (Father), Ayusha Jain and Ankita Jain (Sisters), my daughter Riya and son Ansh whose innocence empowers me in every moment.

Dr Anshul Jain offers cordial thanks to the friends for their support and inspiration:
- Shri Andra Vamsi, IAS
- Shri Shailensh Kumar, IAS
- Dr Sachin Mahur, CMS, MLB Medical College, Jhansi, Uttar Pradesh
- Dr Nootan Agarwal, Professor, Department of Medicine, MLB Medical College, Jhansi, Uttar Pradesh
- Dr Suryaprakash, Professor, Department of Surgery, MLB Medical College, Jhansi, Uttar Pradesh
- Dr Neeraj Banoriya, Professor, Department of Surgery, MLB Medical College, Jhansi, Uttar Pradesh
- Dr Rajkumar Rajpoot, Professor, Department of Surgery, MLB Medical College, Jhansi, Uttar Pradesh
- Dr Dinesh Rajpoot, Lecturer, Neurosurgery)
- Dr Saurabh Agarwal, Professor and Head, Department of Orthopedics, MLB Medical College, Jhansi, Uttar Pradesh
- Dr Paras Gupta, Professor and Head, Department of Orthopedics, Government Medical College, Jalaun, Uttar Pradesh
- Dr Mayank Bansal, Assistant Professor, Department of Orthopedics
- Dr OS Chaurasia, Assistant Professor, Department of Pediatrics
- Dr Mayank Kumar Singh, Professor and Head, Department of Pathology, MLB Medical College, Jhansi, Uttar Pradesh
- Mr Amol Agarwal

Dr Pradeep Bhatia wants to acknowledge all the authors and co-authors of the chapters for their significant contributions in compiling the subject material in a presentable manner.

Acknowledgments

Special acknowledgments to our publishers:
Our gratitudes to Shri Jitendar P Vij (Group Chairman), Mr Ankit Vij (Managing Director), Mr MS Mani (Group President), Dr Madhu Choudhary (Director–Educational Publishing), Ms Pooja Bhandari (Director–Production (Books and Journals).

I would also like to thank Dr Upma Tomar (Development Editor) and her entire team who brought the book to its present shape.

Thanks are due to:
- Mr Rajesh Sharma (Production Coordinator)
- Ms Uma Adhikari (Typesetter)
- Ms Geeta Barik (Proofreader)
- Ms Neha (Cover Designer)
- Mr Nitin Bhardwaj (Graphic Designer) for speedy completion of this mega task.

Last but most important, we gratefully acknowledge to all the staff members of Aashirvad Diagnostic Centre, Jhansi, Uttar Pradesh, India, for their support, and all readers, who will act as a guide to improve and upgrade the content of the book.

CONTENTS

SECTION 1: ANESTHESIA

UNIT I: BASICS OF ANESTHESIA

Chapter 1: Introduction   3
- Role of an Anesthesiologist   3
- Intraoperative Anesthesia   3
- Emergency Medicine   6
- Critical Care Unit   7
- Pain Medicine   7

Chapter 2: History of Anesthesia   8
- Inhalation Anesthesia   8
- Local and Regional Anesthesia   8
- Intravenous Anesthesia   9
- Stages of Anesthesia   9
- Muscle Relaxants   9

Chapter 3: Career Opportunities in Anesthesia   12
- Overview of Anesthesiology as a Specialty   12

Chapter 4: Respiratory Physiology   16
- Anatomy   16
- Breathing Mechanics   20
- Lung Volumes   21
- Dead Space and Uneven Ventilation   23
- Ventilation-Perfusion Relationship   23
- Regulation of Respiration   24
- Measuring Lung Function   25
- Fitness for Anesthesia   26

Chapter 5: Oxygen and Carbon Dioxide Transport   28
- Oxygen Cascade   28
- Oxygen Transport   28
- Oxygen-Hemoglobin Dissociation Curve   29
- Carbon Dioxide Transport   30

Chapter 6: Operation Theater   33
- Location   33
- Number of Operation Theaters   33
- Design   33
- Layout   33
- Operation Room Asepsis   34

Chapter 7: Anesthesia Machine and Vaporizers   36
- Standards for an Anesthesia Machine   36
- Anatomy of an Anesthesia Machine   36
- Testing Anesthesia Machine   41
- Vaporizers   42
- Safety Features in an Anesthesia Machine   45

Chapter 8: Anesthesia Breathing System   47
- Properties of an Ideal Breathing System   47
- Classification of Breathing System   47
- Mapleson Systems   48
- Absorber Breathing System   53
- Carbon Dioxide Absorbent   54
- Other Oxygen Delivery Devices   56

Chapter 9: Airway Management   58
- Airway Assessment   58
- Equipment for Airway Management   60
- Techniques of Direct Laryngoscopy and Intubation   64
- Emergency Airway Management   67
- Rapid Sequence Induction and Intubation   68

Chapter 10: Preanesthetic Evaluation   71
- General Principles   71
- Implementation of Preanesthetic Assessment   71
- Steps of Assessment   71
- Effect of Pre-existing Drug Therapy on Anesthetic Management and Modifications Required   74
- Premedication   75

UNIT II: ANESTHESIA PHARMACOLOGY

Chapter 11: Inhalational Anesthetics   81
- Mechanism of Inhalational Anesthesia   81
- Minimum Alveolar Concentration   81
- General Principles of Inhalational Anesthesia   83

- Recovery From Inhalational Anesthesia 85
- Metabolism of Inhaled Anesthetics 85
- Organ System Effects and Toxicities 85
- Metabolic Effect 87
- Other Effects 87
- Individual Anesthetic Agents 87
- Agents no Longer Used 95
- Nonanesthetic Gases in Anesthesia 96

Chapter 12: Intravenous Anesthetics   99
- Barbiturates 99
- Thiopentone Thiopental 99
- Methohexitone 103
- Propofol 103
- Ketamine 106
- Benzodiazepines 110
- Flumazenil 113
- Etomidate 113
- Neuroleptanalgesia 114
- Droperidol 115
- Opioid Anesthetics 115
- Clinical Pharmacology of Important Agonists 119
- Agonist-Antagonist Opioids 120
- Opioid Antagonists 121
- α_2 Adrenergic Agonists 121

Chapter 13: Local Anesthetics   125
- Basic Pharmacology 125
- Mechanism of Action 125
- Clinical Pharmacology 127
- Factors Influencing Anesthetic Activity in Humans 127
- Choice of Local Anesthetics 128
- Pharmacokinetics 129
- Toxicity 130
- Local Anesthetic Failure 132
- Individual Agents 132
- Other Local Anesthetics not in Anesthesia Practice 135
- Novel Local Anesthetics 135
- Sterilization of Local Anesthesia 135

Chapter 14: Muscle Relaxants   138
- Mechanism of Action of Neuromuscular Blockers at the Neuromuscular Junction 138
- Depolarizing Muscle Relaxants 140
- Nondepolarizing Neuromuscular Blockers 144
- Clinical Uses 147
- Adverse Effects 147
- Factors Affecting Response to Neuromuscular Blockers 148
- Recovery from Neuromuscular Blockade 150
- Antagonism of Residual Neuromuscular Blockade 150
- Other Antagonists of Nondepolarizing Neuromuscular Blockers 151

Chapter 15: Additional Drugs in Anesthesia   154
- Sympathomimetics 154
- Antihypertensives 156
- Antiemetics 157

UNIT III: PERIOPERATIVE CARE

Chapter 16: Monitoring Under Anesthesia   161
- Clinical Monitoring 161
- Cardiovascular Monitoring 161
- Respiratory Monitoring 167
- Capnography 168
- Anesthetic Gas Analysis 169
- Blood Gas Analysis 169
- Intraoperative Spirometry and Airway Pressure Monitoring 170
- Neuromuscular Monitoring 170
- Temperature Monitoring 173
- Monitoring the Depth of Anesthesia 174
- Monitoring Blood Loss 174
- Monitoring Coagulation 175

Chapter 17: Perioperative Fluid Therapy and Blood Transfusion   178
- Fluid Compartments 178
- Intravenous Fluids 179
- Perioperative Fluid Therapy 182
- Blood Transfusion 184

Chapter 18: Blood Salvage Techniques   190
- Perioperative Blood Salvage 190

Chapter 19: Anesthesiologist as a Perioperative Physician   197

UNIT IV: REGIONAL ANESTHESIA: TECHNIQUES AND COMPLICATIONS

Chapter 20: Central Neuraxial Blockade   203
- Applied Anatomy 203
- Central Neuraxial Blockade 206
- Systemic Effects of Neuraxial Blockade 207
- Spinal Anesthesia 209
- Segmental Spinal Anesthesia 210
- Epidural Anesthesia 214
- Caudal Anesthesia 216

Chapter 21: Nerve Blocks   221
- Blocks of Head and Neck   221
- Local Anesthesia of the Airway   223
- Blocks of Upper Extremity   224
- Blocks of Thorax and Abdomen   227
- Blocks of Lower Extremity   228

UNIT V: ANESTHESIA AND ASSOCIATED DISEASES

Chapter 22: Anesthesia for Patients with Cardiovascular Disease   233
- Systemic Hypertension   233
- Ischemic Heart Disease   235
- Valvular Heart Disease   236
- Congenital Heart Disease   239

Chapter 23: Anesthesia for Patients with Respiratory Disease   241
- General Considerations   241
- Specific Disease   242

Chapter 24: Anesthesia for Patients with Hematological Disorders   245
- Anemia   245
- Sickle Cell Anemia   246
- Platelet Disorders   246
- Coagulation Factor Disorders   246

Chapter 25: Anesthesia for Patients with Hepatobiliary Disorders   250
- Effect of Anesthetic Agents on Hepatic Function   250
- Anesthetic Management   250
- Biliary Disorders   252

Chapter 26: Anesthesia for Patients with Neuropsychiatric Disease   254
- Epilepsy   254
- Cerebrovascular Disease   254
- Degenerative and Demyelinating Disease   255
- Psychiatric Disorders   256
- Anesthesia for Electroconvulsive Therapy   256

Chapter 27: Anesthesia for Patients with Musculoskeletal Disease   258
- Myasthenia Gravis   258
- Lambert-Eaton Myasthenic Syndrome   259
- Periodic Paralysis (Hyperkalemic and Hypokalemic)   259
- Muscular Dystrophies   259
- Metabolic Myopathies   260
- Malignant Hyperthermia   260

Chapter 28: Anesthesia For Patients with Endocrine Disease   263
- Diabetes Mellitus   263
- Thyroid Disorders   266
- Adrenal Gland   268
- Pheochromocytoma   268

Chapter 29: Anesthesia for Patients with Renal Disease   271
- Effect of Anesthetic Agent on Renal Physiology   271
- Effect of Renal Disease on Anesthetic Agents   271
- Preoperative Considerations   272
- Perioperative Considerations   272
- Postoperative Management   272

Chapter 30: Anesthesia for Obese Patients   274
- Classification   274
- Anesthetic Considerations   274

UNIT VI: ANESTHESIA PRACTICE

Chapter 31: Anesthesia for Difficult Airway   281
- Anesthetic Management   281
- Unanticipated Difficult Intubation   282
- Awake Fiberoptic Intubation   282

Chapter 32: Anesthesia for Ophthalmic Surgery   287
- Anatomy of Eye   287
- Ocular Physiology   287
- Anesthetic Management   288

Chapter 33: Anesthesia for Ear, Nose and Throat Surgery   291
- Ear Surgery   291
- Nasal Surgery   292
- Intraoral Surgery   292

Chapter 34: Anesthesia for Orthopedic Surgery   294
- Preoperative Evaluation   294
- Perioperative Complications   294
- Anesthetic Management of Different Procedures   295

Chapter 35: Anesthesia for Genitourinary Surgery   299
- Anesthetic Considerations   299

Chapter 36: Anesthesia for Laser Surgery   302
- Laser Hazards   302

Chapter 37: Anesthesia for Laparoscopy   304
- Physiological and Pathological Consequences of Pneumoperitoneum   304
- Alternatives to CO_2 Pneumoperitoneum   307

- Anesthetic Management 307
- Laparoscopy in Children and During Pregnancy 308

Chapter 38: Anesthesia for Neurosurgery 310
- Cerebral Physiology and Pharmacology 310
- Anesthetic Management 312
- Specific Conditions 314
- Intracranial Mass Lesions 315
- Posterior Fossa Procedures 316
- Intracranial Aneurysms and Arteriovenous Malformation 317
- Seizure Surgery 317
- Awake Craniotomy 318
- Transsphenoidal Surgery 318

Chapter 39: Anesthesia for Cardiothoracic Surgery 320
- Cardiopulmonary Bypass 320
- Anesthetic Management of Cardiac Surgery in Adults 322
- Off-pump Coronary Artery bypass Surgery 324
- Anesthesia for Thoracic Surgery 324
- Physiological Considerations 325
- Anesthetic Management of Lung Resection 327

Chapter 40: Geriatric Anesthesia 331
- Physiological Changes with Aging 331
- Anesthetic Management 333

Chapter 41: Obstetric Anesthesia 335
- Physiological Changes in Pregnancy and Their Anesthetic Implications 335
- Placental Transfer of Anesthetic Drugs 338
- Evaluation of the Fetus 338
- Role of Intrauterine Resuscitation 338
- Anesthesia for Spontaneous Vaginal Delivery 338
- Regional Techniques for Labor Analgesia 339
- Anesthesia for Cesarean Section 341
- Specific Conditions 343
- Anesthesia for Nonobstetric Surgery During Pregnancy 345
- Basic Life Support in Pregnancy 345
- Anesthesia for Manual Removal of Placenta 345

Chapter 42: Pediatric Anesthesia 347
- Anatomical and Physiological Differences 347
- Pharmacological Difference 349
- Anesthetic Considerations 350
- Anesthetic Management of Specific Disorders 351

Chapter 43: Anesthesia Outside Operating Room 354

Chapter 44: Anesthesia 357
- Anesthetic Management 357

Chapter 45: Hypotensive Anesthesia 359
- Methods for Inducing Hypotension 359
- Other Techniques to Reduce Intraoperative Bleeding 360

Chapter 46: Anesthesia for Organ Donation 362
- Types of Organ Donation 362
- Contraindications to Organ Donation 363
- Organ Preservation 363
- Pathological Changes after Circulatory Death 363
- Pathological Changes after Brain Death 364
- Anesthetic Management of Organ Donors in Operation Theater 364
- Crime and Laws Related to Organ Donation 365

UNIT VII: PAIN MANAGEMENT

Chapter 47: Basic Concepts of Pain 371
- Transmission of Pain 371
- Theories of Pain 371
- Classification of Pain 372
- Evaluation of Pain 373

Chapter 48: Postoperative Pain Management 375
- Assessment of Pain 375
- Methods of Postoperative Pain Management 375

Chapter 49: Chronic Pain and Palliation 379
- Assessment and Management 379
- Management According to Pain Types 379
- Combining Pain Management with Palliative Care 381
- Pain Management in Terminally Ill 381

SECTION 2: CRITICAL CARE

UNIT VIII: PRACTICE AND MANAGEMENT IN ICU

Chapter 50: Organization and Management of ICU 385
- Open Versus Closed Units 385
- ICU Operations 385
- Audits, Research Education and Quality Improvement 389

Chapter 51: Oxygen Therapy Devices — 391
- Historical Perspective *391*
- Indications of Oxygen Use *391*
- Oxygen Delivery Devices *392*
- Low-flow Devices *393*
- High-flow Devices *395*
- Noninvasive Ventilation *397*

Chapter 52: Principles of Mechanical Ventilation — 400

Chapter 53: Clinical Management in ICU — 412
- Assessment of Severity of Illness *412*
- Circulatory Shock *412*
- Respiratory Failure *416*
- Complications in Intensive Care Unit *417*

Chapter 54: Cardiopulmonary Resuscitation — 420
- Sudden Cardiac Arrest *420*
- Systematic Approach *420*
- Initial Assessment *422*
- Basic Life Support *422*
- Advanced Cardiovascular Life Support *425*
- Cardiac Arrest in Pregnancy *428*
- Drug Therapy *428*
- Monitoring During CPR *429*
- Terminating Resuscitative Efforts *429*
- Postcardiac Arrest Care *430*
- American Heart Association Updates in 2020 Guidelines *430*

Chapter 55: Acid–Base and Electrolyte Imbalance — 432
- Normal Acid–Base Homeostasis *432*
- Acid–Base Disturbances *432*
- Electrolyte Disturbances *437*

Chapter 56: Nutritional Support in Intensive Care Unit — 447
- Indication of Nutrition Support *447*
- Nutrition Requirement *448*

Chapter 57: Brain Death — 452
- Diagnostic Tests for Brain Death *453*
- Certification *454*

Chapter 58: Ethics Related to Anesthesia and Critical Care Practice — 455
- Basic Principles of Medical Ethics *455*

Index — *459*

COMPETENCY TABLE

ANESTHESIOLOGY (CODE: AS)

Number	COMPETENCY The student should be able to	Core (Y/N)	Suggested teaching learning method	Chapter No.
Topic: Anesthesiology as a Specialty	**Number of competencies: (04)**		**Number of procedures that require certification: (NIL)**	
AS1.1	Describe the evolution of anesthesiology as a modern specialty.	N	Lecture	1
AS1.2	Describe the roles of anesthesiologist in the medical profession (including as a perioperative physician, in the intensive care and high dependency units, in the management of acute and chronic pain, including labor analgesia, in the resuscitation of acutely ill).	N	Lecture	1 19
AS1.3	Enumerate and describe the principle of ethics as it relates to anesthesiology.	N	Lecture	58
AS1.4	Describe the prospects of anesthesiology as a career.	N	Lecture	3
Topic: Cardiopulmonary Resuscitation	**Number of competencies: (02)**		**Number of procedures that require certification: (NIL)**	
AS2.1	Enumerate the indications, describe the steps and demonstrate in a simulated environment, basic life support in adults, children and neonates.	N	DOAP session	54
AS2.2	Enumerate the indications, describe the steps and demonstrate in a simulated environment, advanced life support in adults and children.	N	DOAP session	54
Topic: Preoperative Evaluation and Medication	**Number of competencies: (06)**		**Number of procedures that require certification: (NIL)**	
AS3.1	Describe the principles of preoperative evaluation.	Y	Lecture, small group discussion	10
AS3.2	Elicit, present and document an appropriate history including medication history in a patient undergoing surgery as it pertains to a preoperative anesthetic evaluation.	Y	DOAP session, bedside clinic	10
AS3.3	Demonstrate and document an appropriate clinical examination in a patient undergoing general surgery.	Y	DOAP session, Bedside clinic	10
AS3.4	Choose and interpret appropriate testing for patients undergoing surgery.	Y	DOAP session, bedside clinic	10
AS3.5	Determine the readiness for general surgery in a patient based on the preoperative evaluation	Y	DOAP session, bedside clinic	10

Competency Table

Number	COMPETENCY The student should be able to	Core (Y/N)	Suggested teaching learning method	Chapter No.
AS3.6	Choose and write a prescription for appropriate premedication's for patients undergoing surgery	Y	DOAP session, bedside clinic	10
Topic: General Anesthesia	**Number of competencies: (07)**	**Number of procedures that require certification: (NIL)**		
AS4.1	Describe and discuss the pharmacology of drugs used in induction and maintenance of general anesthesia (including intravenous and inhalation induction agents, opiate and non-opiate analgesics, depolarizing and non-depolarizing muscle relaxants, anticholinesterases)	Y	Lecture, small group discussion	11–15
AS4.2	Describe the anatomy of the airway and its implications for general anesthesia	Y	Lecture, small group discussion	9
AS4.4	Observe and describe the principles and the steps/techniques in maintenance of vital organ functions in patients undergoing surgical procedures	Y	Lecture, small group discussion	31–42
AS4.5	Observe and describe the principles and the steps/techniques in monitoring patients during anesthesia	Y	Lecture, small group discussion	16 44
AS4.6	Observe and describe the principles and the steps/techniques involved in daycare anesthesia	Y	Lecture, small group discussion	44
AS4.7	Observe and describe the principles and the steps/techniques in maintenance of vital organ functions in patients undergoing surgical procedures	Y	Lecture, small group discussion	43
Topic: Regional Anesthesia	**Number of competencies: (06)**	**Number of procedures that require certification: (NIL)**		
AS5.1	Enumerate the indications for and describe the principles of regional anaesthesia (including spinal, epidural and combined)	Y	Lecture, small group discussion	20
AS5.2	Describe the correlative anatomy of the brachial plexus, subarachnoid and epidural spaces	Y	Lecture, small group discussion	21
AS5.3	Observe and describe the principles and steps/techniques involved in peripheral nerve blocks	Y	Lecture, small group discussion	21
AS5.4	Observe and describe the pharmacology and correct use of commonly used drugs and adjuvant agents in regional anesthesia	Y	Lecture, small group discussion	13, 19, 20
AS5.5	Observe and describe the principles and steps/techniques involved in caudal epidural in adults and children	Y	Lecture, small group discussion	20
AS5.6	Observe and describe the principles and steps/techniques involved in common blocks used in surgery (including brachial plexus blocks)	Y	Lecture, small group discussion	21
Topic: Post-anesthesia Recovery	**Number of competencies: (03)**	**Number of procedures that require certification: (NIL)**		
AS6.3	Describe the common complications encountered by patients in the recovery room, their recognition and principles of management	Y	Lecture, small group discussion	22–30

Competency Table

Number	COMPETENCY The student should be able to	Core (Y/N)	Suggested teaching learning method	Chapter No.
Topic: Intensive Care Management	**Number of competencies: (05)**		**Number of procedures that require certification: (NIL)**	
AS7.1	Visit, enumerate and describe the functions of an intensive care unit	Y	Lecture, small group discussion	50
AS7.2	Enumerate and describe the criteria for admission and discharge of a patient to an ICU	Y	Lecture, small group discussion	50
AS7.3	Observe and describe the management of an unconscious patient	Y	Lecture, small group discussion	53
AS7.4	Observe and describe the basic setup process of a ventilator	Y	Lecture, small group discussion	52
AS7.5	Observe and describe the principles of monitoring in an ICU	Y	Lecture, small group discussion	53
Topic: Pain and its Management	**Number of competencies: (05)**		**Number of procedures that require certification: (NIL)**	
AS8.1	Describe the anatomical correlates and physiologic principles of pain	Y	Lecture, small group discussion	47
AS8.2	Elicit and determine the level, quality and quantity of pain and its tolerance in patient or surrogate	Y	Lecture, small group discussion	47
AS8.3	Describe the pharmacology and use of drugs in the management of pain	Y	Lecture, small group discussion	48
AS8.4	Describe the principles of pain management in palliative care	Y	Lecture, small group discussion	49
AS8.5	Describe the principles of pain management in the terminally ill	Y	Lecture, small group discussion	49
Topic: Fluids	**Number of competencies: (04)**		**Number of procedures that require certification: (NIL)**	
AS9.3	Describe the principles of fluid therapy in the preoperative period	Y	Lecture, small group discussion	17
AS9.4	Enumerate blood products and describe the use of blood products in the preoperative period	Y	Lecture, small group discussion	17 18
Integration				
PY3.4	Describe the structure of neuromuscular junction and transmission of impulses	Y	Lecture, small group discussion	14
PY3.5	Discuss the action of neuromuscular blocking agents	Y	Lecture, small group discussion	14
PH1.15	Describe mechanism/s of action, types, doses, side effects, indications and contraindications of skeletal muscle relaxants	Y	Lecture	14
PH1.17	Describe the mechanism/s of action, types, doses, side effects, indications and contraindications of local anesthetics	Y	Lecture	13
PH1.18	Describe the mechanism/s of action, types, doses, side effects, indications and contraindications of general anesthetics, and pre-anesthetic medications	Y	Lecture	15

SECTION 1 ANESTHESIA

UNIT I
Basics of Anesthesia

Unit Outline

1. Introduction
2. History of Anesthesia
3. Career opportunities in Anesthesia
4. Respiratory Physiology
5. Oxygen and Carbon Dioxide Transport
6. Operation Theater
7. Anesthesia Machine and Vaporizers
8. Anesthesia Breathing System
9. Airway Management
10. Preanesthetic Evaluation

COMPETENCIES COVERED IN UNIT I

Competency Number	Competency Name	Chapter Number
AS1.1	Describe the evolution of anesthesiology as a modern specialty.	01
AS1.2	Describe the roles of anesthesiologist in the medical profession (including as a perioperative physician, in the intensive care and high dependency units, in the management of acute and chronic pain, including labour analgesia, in the resuscitation of acutely ill).	01
AS1.4	Describe the prospects of anesthesiology as a career.	03
AS4.2	Describe the anatomy of the airway and its implications for general anaesthesia.	09
AS3.1	Describe the principles of preoperative evaluation.	10
AS3.2	Elicit, present and document an appropriate history including medication history in a patient undergoing Surgery as it pertains to a preoperative anaesthetic evaluation.	10
AS3.3	Demonstrate and document an appropriate clinical examination in a patient undergoing general surgery.	10
AS3.4	Choose and interpret appropriate testing for patients undergoing surgery.	10
AS3.5	Determine the readiness for General Surgery in a patient based on the preoperative evaluation.	10
AS3.6	Choose and write a prescription for appropriate premedication's for patients undergoing surgery.	10

CHAPTER 1

Introduction

Anshul Jain, Pradeep Bhatia

Anesthesiology is the medical specialty concerned with the pharmacologic, physiologic, and clinical basis of anesthesia and related fields, including resuscitation, intensive respiratory care and the management of acute and chronic pain.

Despite anesthesiology being a superspecialty branch, most of the MBBS students lack its knowledge and importance in medical practice.

The goal of this book is to provide basic knowledge of the procedures and practices of the anesthesiology.

ROLE OF AN ANESTHESIOLOGIST

An anesthesiologist plays an important role in medical services, viz:

Intraoperative Anesthesia

Biggest role of an anesthesiologist is to provide anesthesia during surgical procedures. Thus, an anesthesiologist plays a pivotal role in deciding whether the patient would undergo surgery or not!

Emergency Medicine

From field care in disaster management to in hospital medical catastrophic events, an anesthesiologist provides his expertise for resuscitation and lifesaving procedures, in any ward at any time.

Critical Care

Patients requiring intensive care and mechanical ventilation get services of an anesthesiologist.

Pain Medicine

Latest addition to services rendered by an anesthesiologist. By their multimodality approach, an anesthesiologist provides variety of methods to control acute and/or chronic pain.

INTRAOPERATIVE ANESTHESIA

Commonly for a routine or emergency patient, an anesthesiologist comes into role when he or she is posted for surgery. Most (if not all) patients posted for surgery undergo preanesthetic check-up (PAC), this is the time where the patient first meets an anesthesiologist.

In PAC, all patients are examined thoroughly so as to detect any coexisting disease or disorder which can affect anesthetic management. Any special investigations, if required are ordered, and patients are classified according to American Society of Anesthesiologists (ASA) physical status classification **(Table 1.1)**.[1] Thus, an anesthesiologist plays a pivotal role in deciding whether the patient would undergo surgery or not!

In operation theater (OT) complex, patient is first kept in preoperative ward where he is examined again, after ensuring the fitness of patient for anesthesia and surgery, intravenous (IV) access is secured usually by IV cannula. He may receive premedication which usually included anxiolytics and antiemetics in preoperative ward **(Flowchart 1.1)**.

He is then shifted to OT where it is first confirmed that the correct patient is taken; by matching patients record number, name, age and type of surgical procedure that he has to undergo. This procedure called as "Time out" is thus meant for "correct patient correct surgery".

Afterwards monitors [blood pressure monitor, pulse oximeter, electrocardiography (ECG), etc.] are attached. A usual protocol is to attach

Table 1.1: American Society of Anesthesiologists (ASA) classification.

Category	Definition	Adult examples, including, but not limited to	Pediatric examples, including but not limited to	Obstetric examples including, but not limited to
ASA I	A normal healthy patient	Healthy, nonsmoking, no or minimal alcohol use	Healthy (no acute or chronic disease) normal BMI percentile for age	None
ASA II	A patient with mild systemic disease	Mild diseases only without substantive functional limitations. Current smoker, social alcohol drinker, pregnancy, obesity (30<BMI<40), well-controlled DM/HTN, mild lung disease.	Asymptomatic congenital cardiac disease, well controlled dysrhythmias, well controlled systemic disease like diabetes, abnormal BMI percentile for age, mild/moderate OSA, oncologic state in remission, autism with mild limitations.	Normal pregnancy*, well controlled gestational HTN, controlled preeclampsia without severe features, diet-controlled gestational DM.
ASA III	A patient with severe systemic disease	Substantive functional limitations; one or more moderate to severe diseases. Poorly controlled DM or HTN, COPD, morbid obesity (BMI ≥40), active hepatitis, alcohol dependence or abuse, implanted pacemaker, moderate reduction of ejection fraction, ESRD undergoing regularly scheduled dialysis, history (>3 months) of MI, CVA, TIA, or CAD/stents.	Uncorrected stable congenital cardiac abnormality, asthma with exacerbation, poorly controlled epilepsy, insulin dependent diabetes mellitus, morbid obesity, malnutrition, severe OSA, oncologic state, renal failure, symptomatic hydrocephalus, premature infant PCA <60 weeks, autism with severe limitations, metabolic disease, difficult airway, long term parenteral nutrition. Full term infants <6 weeks of age.	Preeclampsia with severe features, gestational DM with complications or high insulin requirements, a thrombophilic disease requiring anticoagulation.
ASA IV	A patient with severe systemic disease that is a constant threat to life	Recent (<3 months) MI, CVA, TIA or CAD/stents, ongoing cardiac ischemia or severe valve dysfunction, severe reduction of ejection fraction, shock, sepsis, DIC, ARD or ESRD not undergoing regularly scheduled dialysis	Symptomatic congenital cardiac abnormality, congestive heart failure, active sequelae of prematurity, acute hypoxic ischemic encephalopathy, shock, sepsis, severe trauma, severe respiratory distress, advanced oncologic state.	Preeclampsia with severe features complicated by HELLP or other adverse event, peripartum cardiomyopathy with EF <40, decompensated heart disease, acquired or congenital.

Contd...

Contd...

Category	Definition	Adult examples, including, but not limited to	Pediatric examples, including but not limited to	Obstetric examples including, but not limited to
ASA V	A moribund patient who is not expected to survive without the operation.	Ruptured abdominal/thoracic aneurysm, massive trauma, intracranial bleed with mass effect, ischemic bowel in the face of significant cardiac pathology or multiple organ/system dysfunction.	Massive trauma, intracranial hemorrhage with mass effect, patient requiring ECMO, respiratory failure or arrest, decompensated congestive heart failure, encephalopathy, ischemic bowel or multiple organ/system dysfunction.	Uterine rupture.
ASA VI	A declared braindead patient whose organs are being removed for donor purposes			

(BMI: body mass index; DM: diabetes mellitus; HTN: hypertension; OSA: obstructive sleep apnea; COPD: chronic obstructive pulmonary disease; ESRD: end-stage kidney disease; MI: myocardial infarction; CVA: cerebral vascular accident; TIA: transient ischemic attack; CAD: coronary artery disease; PCA: postconceptional age; DIC: disseminated intravascular coagulation; ARD: acute respiratory distress; HELLP: hemolysis, elevated liver enzymes and low platelets; ECMO: extracorporeal membrane oxygenation; EF: ejection fraction)

Note: *Although pregnancy is not a disease, the parturient's physiologic state is significantly altered from when the woman is not pregnant, hence the assignment of ASA 2 for a woman with uncomplicated pregnancy.
**The addition of "E" denotes Emergency surgery (An emergency is defined as existing when delay in treatment of the patient would lead to a significant increase in the threat to life or body part)

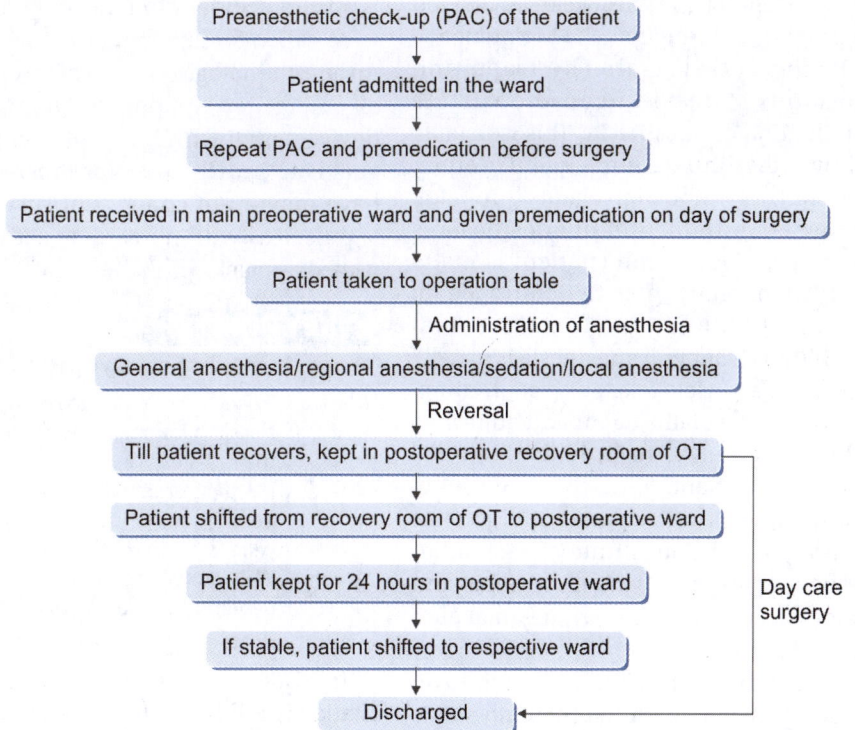

Flowchart 1.1: Procedure for patients posted for operation.

noninvasive monitors prior to anesthesia and invasive monitors (arterial line, central venous line, pulmonary artery catheterization, urinary catheter, etc.) after patient is anesthetized, however, this is not a rigid practice and exception includes serious patients, etc.

Now is the time for anesthetic procedure which can range from regional anesthesia (local infiltration, nerve blocks, central neuraxial blockade) to general anesthesia.

In regional anesthesia, patient remains awake, it is only the site of surgery (nerve blocks) or portion of body (spinal/epidural anesthesia) that is made insensitive to all sort of stimuli.

On the other hand in general anesthesia, patient is fully unconscious and is dissociated from the environment. Depending on the type of surgical procedure, his respiration can be spontaneous (patient controlled) or doctor controlled, i.e., by intermittent positive pressure ventilation (IPPV), later usually require muscle relaxants and placement of an airway device (endotracheal tube, laryngeal mask airway). General anesthesia can be divided into three stages: (1) Induction, (2) Maintenance and (3) Recovery/reversal. The transition from conscious state to unconscious state is called induction of anesthesia. This is usually achieved by either inhalational agents (ether, halothane, etc.) or IV induction agents (propofol, thiopentone, etc.). Induction of anesthesia is preceded by preoxygenation (patient is made to breath 100% oxygen) so as to denitrogenate the lungs, i.e., to fill the functional residual volume by 100% O_2. General anesthesia is usually "maintained" on a muscle relaxant (vecuronium, pancuronium, etc.), volatile agent and adjuvants like opioids. The aim is to provide "balance anesthesia" to the patient.

It must be noted that regional and general anesthesias are not the substitute of each other and same patient may receive both regional and general anesthesia simultaneously, regional after general or vice versa.

After completion of surgical procedure, depending on patient's condition (hemodynamic stability), he is reversed from unconscious state to conscious state, this is termed "reversal" in anesthetic practice. It is not necessary that the reversal takes place in OT, if patient's condition is critical, he may be shifted as such in CCU where he is then reversed. After reversal, if patient is stable, he can be shifted to postoperative ward. Postoperative ward is fully equipped ward to deal with any sort of emergencies. The goal is to vacate the OT for another patient without hampering the care of already operated patient.

EMERGENCY MEDICINE

An anesthesiologist is a vital element of core team of lifesaving medical staff for both in hospital and out hospital emergencies. If any patient of hospital suddenly underwent myocardial infarction (MI), this core team is called (announced internationally as code blue). Under such circumstances, an anesthesiologist manages airway and establish IV access. For out of hospital emergency medicine services, we can simulate a situation. Suppose there is a train accident in a nearby area and doctors were called for emergency help on accident site. An anesthesiologist is a part of core team; he carries all emergency equipment (laryngoscope, airway devices, etc.) with him. On accident site, main goal is to provide care for those patients which have maximum chances of survival. If patient is pulseless with no cardiac activity, then he is tagged as black.

KEY POINTS

Triage color coding during disaster management[2]

Black : Dead, to be shifted to mortuary
Red : Needing immediate resuscitation. Shift in the red area, i.e., main casualty hall
Yellow : Needing urgent medical attention and possible surgery after 4–6 hours. Shift in the yellow area, i.e., disaster room
Green : Walking wounded (non-urgent ambulatory) needing first aid and delayed treatment—in the green area, i.e., observation room.

In disaster situation, cardiopulmonary resuscitation (CPR) is not attempted as the time required for CPR (minimum 2 minutes) is enough to save many other patients. Patients who require urgent lifesaving care (e.g., as in tension pneumothorax) to save life are tagged red.

CRITICAL CARE UNIT

In most hospitals, an anesthesiologist is the In-charge of CCU. Patient input to CCU is from OT or postoperative ward and emergency wards (if patient condition deteriorates suddenly). In CCU an anesthesiologist takes care of ventilation, circulation, nutrition, etc. Mechanical ventilation may also be required in critically ill patients.

PAIN MEDICINE

These services are provided to patients suffering from chronic pain, cancer pain, etc.

Anesthesiologists are particularly suited to take care of such conditions because of their multimodal approach which includes not only analgesics but also local anesthetics, nerve blocking procedures, etc.

In the upcoming chapters, you will learn the details of these services.

 LAST-MINUTE REVISION

- *Time out*: Procedure carried out to ensure correct patient is taken for correct surgery.
- *Code blue in emergency*: If an admitted patient underwent any life-threatening catastrophic event, then paramedical staff announce code blue to ensure immediate service of concerned emergency doctor to the victim.
- A normal pregnant woman posted for surgery is classified as ASA II.
- A full term infant <6 weeks of age posted for surgery is classified as ASA III as per **ASA Physical Status Classification System.**

REFERENCES

1. ASA Physical Status Classification System available on https://www.asahq.org/standards-and-guidelines/asa-physical-status-classification-system. Accessed on 1st July 2022.
2. Koenig KL, Schultz CH. Koenig and Schultz's Disaster Medicine: Comprehensive Principles and Practices. Cambridge University Press, 2010.

REVIEW QUESTIONS

1. "Time out" in operation theater (OT) practice means:
   a. When all OT cases get operated
   b. When patient is postponed due to lack of time
   c. When patient is reverified with case sheet and OT list
   d. When surgeon is late and he is not allowed to operate
2. After an earthquake, a team goes for rescue mission, they apply black tag on few victims. What does this implicate?
   a. They are toxic
   b. They are dead
   c. They are very serious and require urgent intervention
   d. They are all right

ANSWERS

1. c   2. b

CHAPTER 2

History of Anesthesia

Anshul Jain, Shivali Pandey

INTRODUCTION

History of anesthetic practices dates back from ancient times as suggested by 2250 BC maiden record of Babylonanian clay tablets from Nippus. Yet the evolution of the specialty began in the mid-19th century and became firmly established only after 1960s.

Ancient civilizations had used opium poppy, coca leaves, mandrake root, and alcohol to abolish intraoperative pain. Regional anesthesia in ancient times consisted of compression of nerve trunks (nerve ischemia) or the application of cold (cryoanalgesia). The name anesthesia (*Greek* an, "without," and esthesia, "sensation") was suggested by Oliver Wendell Holmes.

INHALATION ANESTHESIA

As hypodermic needles were not available until 1855, the initial anesthetics were inhalational agents.

Ether (really diethyl ether), was originally prepared by Valerius Cordus, and was first used as an anesthetic agent in humans by Crawford W Long and William E Clark in 1842. However, they did not publicize this discovery. Four years later, in Boston, on October 16, 1846 (16th October is now celebrated as World Anesthesia Day), William TG Morton conducted the first public demonstration of general anesthesia using ether. That exhibition was a big success.

Chloroform was introduced into clinical practice by the Scottish obstetrician Sir James Simpson, who administered it, to relieve the pain of labor.

Joseph Priestley synthesized nitrous oxide in 1772, whereas Humphry Davy first noted

KEY POINTS

First labor analgesic: Chloroform
First volatile anesthetic: Ether
First anesthetic gas: Nitrous oxide

its analgesic properties in 1800. Nitrous oxide was least popular of the three early inhalation anesthetics because of its low potency and was overshadowed by the popularity of ether and chloroform. Reports of chloroform-related cardiac arrhythmias, respiratory depression, and hepatotoxicity eventually increased the popularity of ether. Ether remained the standard general anesthetic until the early 1960s. Current volatile agents halothane (developed in 1951; released in 1956), methoxyflurane (developed in 1958; released in 1960), enflurane (developed in 1963; released in 1973), and isoflurane (developed in 1965; released in 1981) were introduced later.

Newer agents, desflurane and sevoflurane were developed in 1990s.[1]

LOCAL AND REGIONAL ANESTHESIA

Cocaine was the first drug used as local anesthetic and credit goes to Carl Koller, who used topical cocaine for surgical anesthesia of the eye. Credit of first spinal anesthesia goes to August Bier, who in 1898 administered 3 mL of 0.5% cocaine intrathecally. He was also the first to describe intravenous regional anesthesia (Bier's Block) in 1908.

Subsequently introduced local anesthetics include dibucaine, tetracaine, lidocaine (1947), mepivacaine, prilocaine, bupivacaine (1963). Ropivacaine and levobupivacaine, an isomer of bupivacaine, are newer less cardiotoxic agents. Currently lidocaine[Q] and bupivacaine[Q] are most commonly used local anesthetics.

INTRAVENOUS ANESTHESIA

Intravenous anesthesia followed the invention of the hypodermic syringe and needle in 1855 by Alexander Wood.[2]

Barbiturates were synthesized in 1903 by Fischer and von Mering. The first barbiturate used for induction of anesthesia was barbital. Thiopental, synthesized in 1932 was first used clinically by John Lundy and Ralph Waters in 1934, and remains the most common induction agent for anesthesia. Ketamine was synthesized in 1962 by Stevens and first used clinically in 1965 by Corssen and Domino, it was the first IV agent associated with minimal cardiac and respiratory depression. The release of propofol and diisopropylphenol in 1989 was a major advance in outpatient anesthesia because of its short duration of action.

STAGES OF ANESTHESIA

In 1920, Guedel[Q] described four stages with ether anesthesia (**Fig. 2.1 and Table 2.1**).[3]

MUSCLE RELAXANTS

The use of curare by Harold Griffith and Enid Johnson in 1942 was a milestone in anesthesia. Curare greatly facilitated tracheal intubation and provided excellent abdominal relaxation for surgery. Subsequently other neuromuscular blocking agents (gallamine, decamethonium, metocurine, alcuronium, and pancuronium)—were soon introduced. Succinylcholine was synthesized by Bovet in 1949 and become a standard agent for facilitating tracheal intubation.[4]

Recently introduced agents include vecuronium, atracurium, pipecuronium, doxacurium, rocuronium, and cisatracurium.

There is still a huge scope of invention and researches in anesthesiology as still today there is no ideal anesthetic agent.

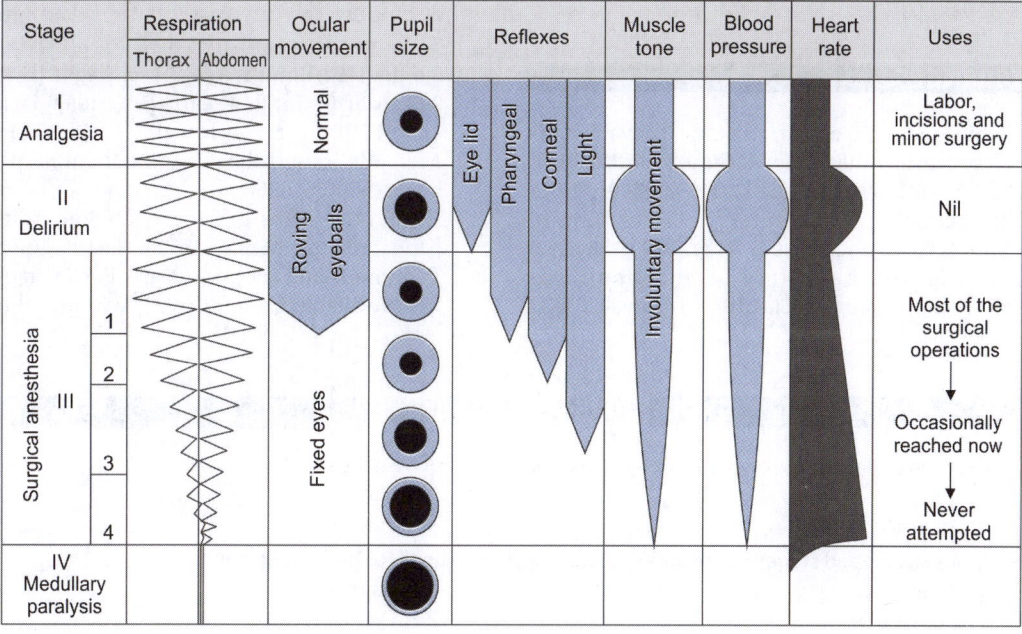

Fig. 2.1: Physiological changes during stages of general anesthesia.

Table 2.1: Stages of anesthesia.

Stages		Effects
Stage I		Beginning of ether inhalation to loss of consciousness
Stage II		Loss of consciousness to beginning of regular respiration (stage of excitement)
Stage III		Extends from onset of regular respiration to cessation of spontaneous breathing. This stage is further divided into four planes
	Plane I	Roving eyeballs. This plane ends when eyes become fixed
	Plane II	Loss of corneal and laryngeal reflexes
	Plane III	Pupil start dilating and light reflex is lost
	Plane IV	Intercostal paralysis and shallow abdominal respiration
Stage IV		Medullary paralysis—cessation of breathing to failure of circulation and death

Note: Under modern anesthesia, stage II is not seen.

LAST-MINUTE REVISION

- *First public demonstration of ether*: WTG Morton
- Chloroform was first used by Simson.
- *First spinal anesthesia given by*: August Bier
- Thiopentone was first used by John Lundy.
- Succinylcholine was synthesized by Bovet.
- Stages of anesthesia were given by Guedel, using ether as inducing agent.
- Stage II is called as stage of delirium or excitement, whereas most surgical procedures are carried out in stage III, plane II.

REFERENCES

1. Robinson DH, Toledo AH. Historical development of modern anesthesia. J Invest Surg. 2012; 25(3):141-9. doi: 10.3109/08941939.2012. 690328. PMID: 22583009.
2. Norn S, Kruse PR, Kruse E. Traek af injektionens historie [On the history of injection]. Dan Medicinhist Arbog. 2006;34:104-13. Danish. PMID: 17526154.
3. Siddiqui BA, Kim PY. Anesthesia Stages. [Updated 2022 Mar 9]. In: StatPearls [Internet]. Treasure Island (FL): StatPearls Publishing; 2022 Jan-. Available from: https://www.ncbi.nlm.nih.gov/books/NBK557596/
4. Hager HH, Burns B. Succinylcholine Chloride. [Updated 2022 May 4]. In: StatPearls [Internet]. Treasure Island (FL): StatPearls Publishing; 2022 Jan-. Available from: https://www.ncbi.nlm.nih.gov/books/NBK499984/

REVIEW QUESTIONS

1. Most surgical procedures are carried out in which stage of anesthesia:
   a. Stage I
   b. Stage II
   c. Stage III
   d. Stage IV
2. Guedel described stages of anesthesia, which agent he used for his descriptions:
   a. Chloroform
   b. Halothane
   c. Diethyl ether
   d. Cyclopropane

Chapter 2: History of Anesthesia

3. First agent used for labor analgesia:
   a. Ether
   b. Chloroform
   c. Trilene
   d. Nitrous oxide
4. Intravenous regional anesthesia was devised by:
   a. August Bier
   b. Griffith
   c. Carl Koller
   d. WTG Morton
5. Excitement seen in which of the following stages of anesthesia:
   a. Stage I
   b. Stage II
   c. Stage III
   d. Stage IV

ANSWERS

1. c   2. c   3. b   4. a   5. b

CHAPTER 3

Career Opportunities in Anesthesia

Swati Chhabra, Rakesh Kumar, Darshana Rathod

INTRODUCTION

Anesthesiologists are physicians with training in perioperative care, critical care medicine and pain management. Patient safety during the perioperative phase is the responsibility of anesthesiologists so much so that they are known as the 'Perioperative guardians of the patients.' Their primary role is to maintain the patient's physiology towards their baseline as they undergo surgical or diagnostic procedures, which many a time are a challenging, daunting, and unique task. Outside the realm of operating rooms and diagnostic suites, anesthesiologists are the intensivists or pain and palliative care physicians, each providing a specific opportunity in contributing to patient care.

OVERVIEW OF ANESTHESIOLOGY AS A SPECIALTY

Current policy is to make safe anesthesia accessible to all. As World Federation of Societies of Anaesthesiologists (WFSA) recommendation, 4–5 anesthesia providers per 1, 00,000 populations is a necessary aim for safe anesthesia delivery at a population level.[1] Some high-income countries, such as the United States, Sweden, and Australia, have more than 20 anesthetists per 1, 00,000 people while in India this count is around 1.27:1 lakh.[2] India is short of nearly 40,000 anesthesiologists.[3]

With the tremendous growth in knowledge, skills and innovation, anesthesia has now become one of the most advanced specialities in modern medicine. Anesthesiology is no longer just about inducing unconsciousness to relieve pain. It covers a wide range of services, from perioperative patient care to pain management, critical care, and palliative care.

During the COVID-19 pandemic, the role of the anesthesiologists was highlighted and acknowledged. They have been identified for their abilities as team players, consultants for critically ill patients, and medical managers, strategists, and leaders. The public has taken notice of the work performed by anesthesiologists. The anesthesiologist also made it to the cover of Time magazine's April 2020 issue and all this recognition has infused new energy into the specialty and the specialists.[4]

Eligibility to Pursue a Course to be an Anesthesiologist

The country offers three types of postgraduate anesthesia courses. A two-year diploma in anesthesiology (DA) and three-year MD and DNB Anesthesiology program is available. Medical graduates have to compete either National Eligibility Cum Entrance Test for Postgraduation (NEET-PG) or The Institute of National Importance Combined Entrance Test (INI-CET). After clearing the competitive exam, students can apply for MD/DNB/Diploma programs at various institutes in India.

Roles of the Anesthesiologist

Anesthesiologists are specialized trained physicians that make up most of any health institution's specialty. Anesthesiologists were the

frontline warriors in the fight against the COVID-19 campaign.[4] They are usually involved in patient care in a variety of settings, including:
- Operating rooms
- Medical care before and after surgery (perioperative physician)
- For patients undergoing procedures outside the operating theater, e.g., radiology, cath lab, etc.
- Intensive care unit
- Trauma and emergency department
- Resuscitation
- Pain and palliative care clinic
- Transportation of critically ill patients
- Teaching and research.

The urge for superspecialization has significantly increased in recent years since it offers an affiliation to major corporations and prominent government institutions, which in turn promotes academic brilliance, higher recognition, and employee happiness. To provide training in a variety of subspecialties like cardiac anesthesia, critical care, pediatric anesthesia, pain medicine, transplant anesthesia, oncoanesthesia, neuroanesthesia, and bariatric anesthesia. Top disciplines of superspecialization include pain medicine, critical care, and cardiac anesthesia.

Job Opportunities

Anesthesiology is the only medical specialty a candidate gets the job right on the day of completion of a postgraduate degree/diploma. One has a wide selection of professional options to choose from. Senior residents/lecturers in medical colleges, specialist doctors in government hospitals, consultants in corporate hospitals, freelancers in private nursing homes, or superspecialization based on personal interest are all numerous possibilities.[5]

Work-life Integration

It is the idea of managing your priorities in work and life rather than investing more in any of these areas. Doing so helps in progress and growth in the areas of work and life that are important to an individual **(Fig. 3.1)**. Awareness about

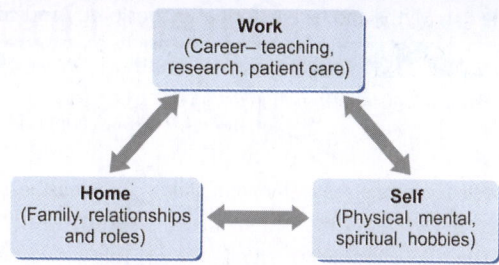

Fig. 3.1: Work-life integration.

this is making people choose a job that can easily integrate with their lifestyle choices and prospects.[6]

Anesthesiology is one such specialty where the professional roles, duties and hours are customizable depending on the type of job. For instance, anesthesiologists deal with emergencies and working hours can be long whereas the intensivists usually work in shifts and pain physicians have better flexible working hours. In teaching institutes, generally, there is a team that divides the work to maintain a better work-life balance.

Myths and Facts

The various myths and facts relating to anesthesiology as a specialty are discussed in **Table 3.1**.

Limitations

Like any other medical specialty, anesthesiology too does have its limitations, however, these are individualized in such a way that an aspect that one may perceive as a limitation, might be taken positively by someone else.

It is a dependent specialty. No patient would be admitted under you except for the pain physician and critical care unit. You might find the specialty nonrewarding as it is not appreciated as much as it deserves. Also, they don't receive personal feedback or gratitude from their patients.

This may not be the case anymore as nowadays, we are getting visibility and credit for our work in critical care, pain management and palliative care.

Table 3.1: Myths and facts about anesthesiology and critical care specialty.

Myths	Facts
Anesthesiologists are not involved in patient care	They play an important role when it comes to the perioperative management of patients. Their roles as intensivists and pain-palliative care physicians also involve direct patient care.
Anesthesiologists leave the operating room after surgery starts	The anesthesiologists monitor the functions of all body systems and optimize them. They anticipate and manage the critical events throughout the surgery.
Adverse events during surgery are because an overdose of anesthesia	This is a vague statement. Patient's general condition and comorbidities, type and duration of surgery, and events during the surgery (like bleeding, and vagal stimulation) are some of many factors which are responsible for adverse outcome
They just put the patient to sleep which anyone can do	They work in various departments, including research, pediatric anesthesia, neuroanesthesia, cardiac anesthesia, ambulatory anesthesia, obstetrics, critical care, pain medicine, etc. This needs extensive training and experience.

The anesthesiologists working in the operating rooms must introduce themselves to the patients before the surgery and discuss the complexities, comorbidities, different types of anesthesia, and postoperative course [including pain, postoperative nausea and vomiting (PONV) requirement of ICU/mechanical ventilation, etc.]

Many times anesthesiologists deal with high-risk patients and are responsible for their well-being in critical conditions. This might be stressful for them and a reason for their dissatisfaction with the job. Litigations (legal action) from the patients who believe they didn't get proper care, is another challenge for anesthesiologists, threatening job, and financial security.[7]

Scope Abroad

Currently, Indian postgraduate training is not recognized abroad. There are various other extra qualifications/training which needs to be acquired to get a job abroad. Among other countries, the United Kingdom, Ireland, USA, Canada, Australia and New Zealand are popular among the trainees because of the better work-life integration and higher pay scale. Interested candidates can refer to the references for more information.[8]

KEY POINTS

- Patient safety during the perioperative phase is the responsibility of anesthesiologists so much so that they are known as the 'Perioperative guardians of the patients.'
- Anesthesiologists were the front-line warriors in the fight against the COVID-19 campaign because of their skills and leadership talents.
- In teaching institutes, generally, there is a team that divides the work to maintain a better work-life balance.
- Many career options are available abroad.

REFERENCES

1. Davies JI, Vreede E, Onajin-Obembe B, Morriss WW. What is the minimum number of specialist anaesthetists needed in low-income and middle-income countries? BMJ Global Health, 2018;3:001005.
2. Kempthorne P, Morriss WW, Mellin-Olsen J, Gore-Booth J. The WFSA Global Anesthesia Workforce Survey. Anesth Analg. 2017;125:981-90.
3. Law TJ, Lipnick M, Joshi M, Rath GP, Gelb AW. The path to safe and accessible anesthesia care. Indian J Anaesth. 2019;63:965-71.
4. Van Klei WA, Hollmann MW, Sneyd JR. The value of anesthesiologists in the COVID-19 pandemic: a model for our future practice? Br J Anaesth. 2020; 125:652-5.

Chapter 3: Career Opportunities in Anesthesia

5. Garg R, Bajwa SK, Yalagachin G, Jadhav R. Anesthesiology as a career: Surgeons' perspectives. Indian J Anaesth. 2021;65:79-81.
6. Harrington B, Jamie JL. Work-Life Integration. Organizational Dynamics. 2009:38:148-57.
7. Verma R, Mohan B, Attri JP, Chatrath V, Bala A, Singh M. Anesthesiologist: The silent force behind the scene. Anesth Essays Res. 2015;9:293-7.
8. Sood J, Bhatia P, Johnson JE, Lalwani J, Sethi N. Career as a general specialty anesthesiologist. Indian J Anaesth. 2021;65:6-11.

MARK THE STATEMENTS TRUE/FALSE

1. About the complications an anesthesiologist face during the perioperative period?
   a. Circulatory collapse because of surgical bleeding/hemorrhage (T/F)
   b. Bronchospasm or aspiration of stomach content (T/F)
   c. Allergic reaction to drugs (T/F)
   d. An anesthesiologist must recognize the problem and manage it. (T/F)

2. About the number of anesthesiologists per unit population:
   a. WFSA recommends 4–5 anesthesia providers per 100,000 population is a necessary aim for safe anesthesia delivery at a population level (T/F)
   b. India has 4 anesthesiologists for every 100,000 of the population (T/F)
   c. Developed countries have 20 anesthesiologists per 1,00,000 of the population (T/F)
   d. India is short of nearly 40,000 anesthesiologists (T/F)

3. About the courses and entrance examinations available for anesthesia training:
   a. Only 3 year courses are available. (T/F)
   b. NEET-PG offers more than 4000 seats for postgraduate training in anesthesia. (T/F)
   c. INI-CET is organised twice a year. (T/F)
   d. NEET-PG and INI- CET are computer-based format (CBT) tests. (T/F)

4. Following are the area of work for an anesthesiologist:
   a. Intensive care unit (T/F)
   b. Radiology suite for an interventional radiological procedure in a child (T/F)
   c. End-of-life care (T/F)
   d. Operation theater (T/F)

ANSWERS

1. a (T), b (T), c (T), d (T)   2. a (T), b (F), c (T), d (T)   3. a (F), b (T), c (T), d (T)   4. a (T), b (T), c (T), d (T)

CHAPTER 4

Respiratory Physiology

Sandeep Sahu

INTRODUCTION

For proper anesthetic management a basic knowledge of respiratory function is must. This chapter reviews the basic concepts of airway anatomy and respiratory physiology in reference to anesthesia practice.

ANATOMY

There are two openings to the human airway: (1) the nose, which leads to the nasopharynx and (2) the mouth, which continues to the oropharynx. These passages are separated anteriorly by the palate, but they join posteriorly in the pharynx **(Fig. 4.1)**.

Nose

The nose warms, filters, and humidifies incoming air and is the organ of smell. Under normal breathing, nose accounts for two-thirds of total airway resistance.[1]

Glottis is the narrowest portion of upper airway in both adults and pediatrics. However, the relative distensibilty of the glottic tissues and the relatively nondistensible cricoid cartilage gives the feeling

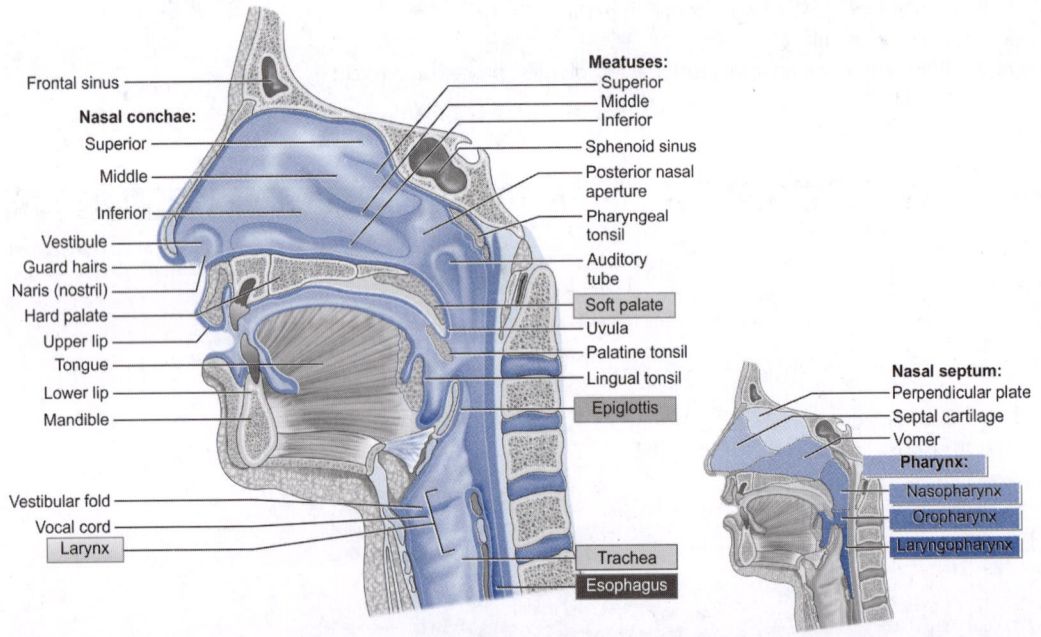

Fig. 4.1: Anatomy of the pharynx and larynx.[1]

that cricoid being functionally the narrowest part of the airway.[2]

Pharynx

The pharynx is a U-shaped fibromuscular structure that extends from the base of the skull to the cricoid cartilage. It opens anteriorly into the nasal cavity and the mouth. At the base of the tongue, the epiglottis functionally separates the oropharynx from the laryngopharynx (or hypopharynx). The epiglottis prevents aspiration by covering the glottis (the opening of the larynx) during swallowing **(Fig. 4.1)**.

Larynx

The larynx is situated at the upper end of the respiratory tract, where it extends from the epiglottis to the lower end of the cricoid cartilage corresponds to vertebral level C_3 to C_6. The larynx is a cartilaginous skeleton held together by ligaments and muscle. The larynx is composed of nine cartilages— three unpaired (thyroid, cricoid and epiglottis) and three paired (arytenoid, corniculate, and cuneiform). Out of these cricoid[Q] is a complete ring **(Fig. 4.2)**.

> **M**nemonic
> All paired cartilages have 'n' in their name.

The cricothyroid membrane joins the thyroid cartilage with the adjacent cricoid cartilage. It is close to the skin, relatively avascular, and is the site of widest gap between the cartilage of the larynx and trachea, so it is the optimal site for invasive airway access during emergency.

Glottis is the narrowest portion of upper airway in both adults and pediatrics. However the relative distensibilty of the glottic tissues and the relatively nondistensible cricoid cartilage gives the feeling that cricoid being functionally the narrowest part of the airway.[2]

Nerve Supply of Upper Respiratory Tract

Anterior aspect of the nasal mucosa is innervated by the ophthalmic division of the trigeminal nerve while maxillary division (sphenopalatine nerve) supplies posterior aspect. Tongue is innervated by lingual nerve (anterior two-thirds) and the glossopharyngeal nerve (posterior one-third). Pharynx, tonsil and under surface of palate are also innervated by glossopharyngeal nerve.

Larynx has both sensory and motor innervation though both motor and sensory supply comes from vagus nerve. Vagus nerve while descending down to the neck gives a branch just above the carotid bifurcation, this branch known as superior laryngeal nerve further divides into external laryngeal nerve and internal laryngeal nerve.

The external branch contains motor fibers that innervate the cricothyroid muscle. While the internal branch pierces through the thyrohyoid membrane and carries sensory fibers that innervate the laryngeal mucosa superior to the vocal cords.[Q]

Vagus nerve gives one more branch in proximity to subclavian artery the recurrent laryngeal nerve (RLN). RLN travel superiorly along the lateral surface of the esophagus and trachea, coursing posterior to the thyroid lobes; cricothyroid joint, to enter the larynx. Once in the larynx, the recurrent laryngeal nerve is referred to as the inferior laryngeal nerve. RLN innervates all the intrinsic musculature of the larynx except for the cricothyroid muscle. RLN is the principal motor supply to vocal production. RLN also provides sensory innervation to the laryngeal portion inferior to the vocal cords **(Fig. 4.2)**.

> **M**nemonic
> **RASCEL Hoarse**
> **R**ecurrent nerve supplies **A**ll muscles and its palsy causes **S**tridor.[Q] **C**ricothyroid is supplied by **E**xternal **L**aryngeal nerve, whose palsy results in **H**oarseness.[Q]

Long tortuous course of RLN makes it vulnerable to injuries during thyroid surgery. Pressure from the endotracheal tube cuff (if cuff lies just below the vocal cords) can also compress RLN **(Table 4.1)**.[3]

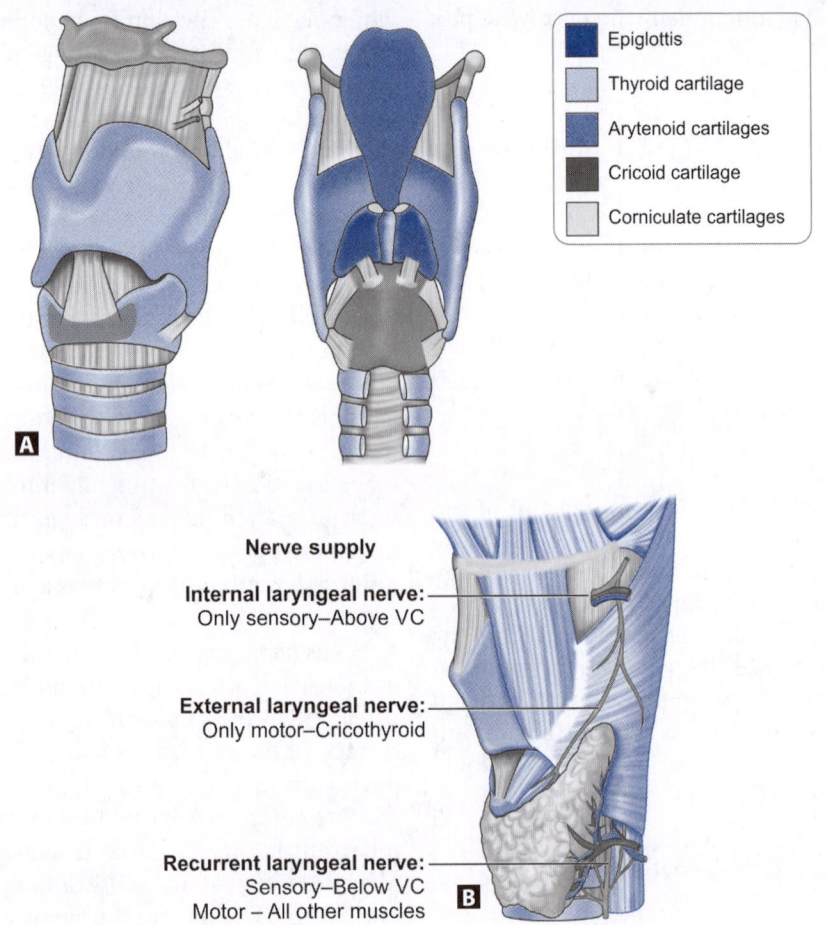

Figs. 4.2A and B: (A) Larynx anterior and posterior view; (B) Nerve supply of larynx.

Table 4.1: Effects of laryngeal nerve paralysis.

Superior laryngeal nerve	
Unilateral	Minimal effects
Bilateral	Hoarseness and tiring of voice
Recurrent laryngeal nerve	
Unilateral	Hoarseness
Bilateral	
• Acute	Stridor and respiratory distress
• Chronic	Aphonia
Vagus nerve	
Unilateral	Hoarseness
Bilateral	Aphonia

Trachea

The trachea extends from the lower edge of the cricoid cartilage to the carina, which corresponds to C_6 and T_5 vertebrae respectively. Anteriorly carina corresponds to angle of Louis. Length of trachea ranges from 10 cm to 12 cm. It consists of U-shaped cartilage joined by fibroelastic tissue and is closed posteriorly by the longitudinal trachealis muscle. The tracheal rings and trachealis muscle are responsible for the characteristic ring-like appearance of the trachea on endoscope.

Bronchial Tree (Fig. 4.3)

Trachea divides into right and left main bronchus. Right bronchus divides at narrow angle, is shorter,

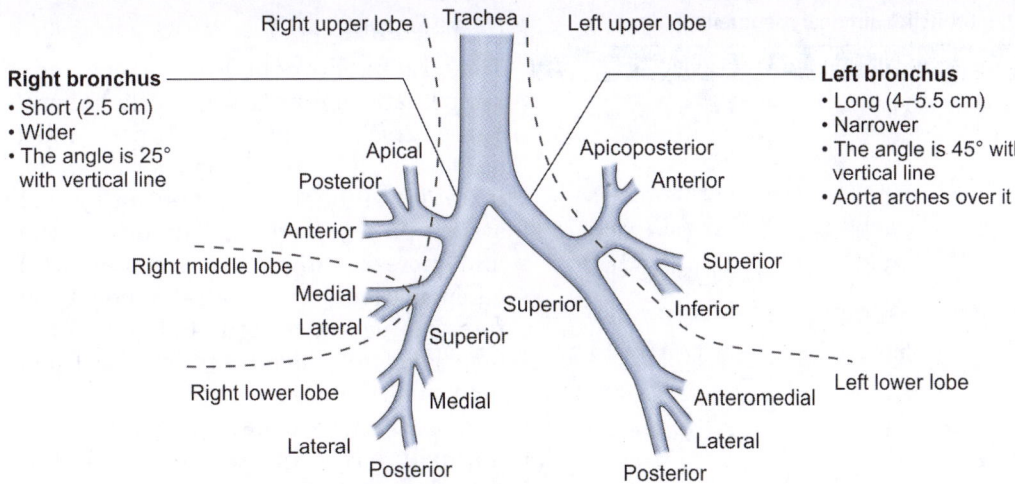

Fig. 4.3: Tracheobronchial tree.

wider in comparison to left bronchus (**Fig. 4.3**). So a blindly passed endotracheal tube is more likely to enter right bronchus.

Right main bronchus divides into upper, middle and lower lobe bronchus, whereas left main bronchus divides into left upper and lower lobe bronchus.

Tracheobronchial tree conducts gas flow from larynx to alveoli. This pathway involves 23 divisions, or generations and results in approximately 300 million alveoli in the adult to provide an area[Q] of 70 m² for gas exchange.

The pulmonary epithelium contains two cell types: (1) type I pneumocytes are flat and form tight (1 nm) junctions with one another thereby preventing the passage of large oncotically active molecules such as albumin into the alveolus and (2) type II pneumocytes, (more in number) have prominent cytoplasmic inclusions containing surfactant, that prevent lung collapse during expiration.

✪ KEY POINTS

In pediatric patients (up to 3 years) the angle of division of both principal bronchus is the same.

Bronchopulmonary Segments (Fig. 4.4)

Each of the principal bronchi divides into lobar (main stem bronchus) bronchi. Primary branches of the right and left lobar bronchi are termed segmental bronchi. Segmental bronchi is a structurally separate, functionally independent

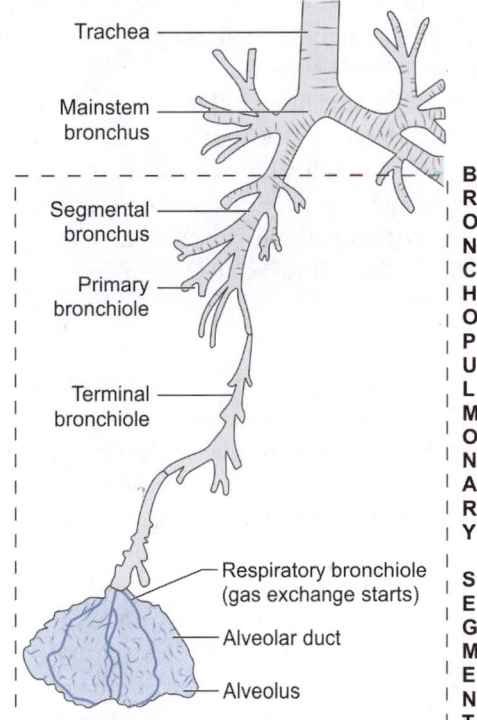

Fig. 4.4: Respiratory tract divisions.

Table 4.2: Bronchopulmonary segments.

	Right lung	Left lung
Superior lobe	Apical	Apical
	Posterior	Posterior
	Anterior	Anterior
Middle lobe	Lateral	Superior lingular
	Medial	Inferior lingular
Inferior lobe	Superior	Superior
	Medial basal	Anterior basal
	Anterior basal	Lateral basal
	Lateral basal	Posterior basal
	Posterior basal	

unit of lung tissue and along with lung parenchyma it constitutes a bronchopulmonary segment.^{Q} Bronchopulmonary segment of right and left lungs are given in **Table 4.2**.

Each segmental bronchus divides into primary bronchiole, which gives rise to terminal bronchiole which further ramifies into respiratory bronchiole. Gas exchange starts from respiratory bronchiole.^{Q} Respiratory bronchiole with alveolar duct and alveolar sac forms the respiratory unit.

Pulmonary Circulation

The lungs are supplied by both pulmonary and bronchial circulation. The bronchial circulation arising from the left heart supplies the tracheobronchial tree up to the level of the bronchioles. Peripheral lung tissue is supplied by pulmonary circulation.

There are two pulmonary arteries which carry deoxygenated blood from heart. Deoxygenated blood passes through the pulmonary capillaries, where O_2 is taken up and CO_2 is eliminated. The oxygenated blood is then returned to the left heart by four main pulmonary veins (two from each lung). Due to the lower pulmonary vascular resistance, pulmonary vascular pressure is only one-sixth of systemic pressure.

Nerve Supply

The tracheobronchial tree receives both sympathetic and parasympathetic innervation. Vagus nerve^Q is responsible for parasympathetic activity which mediates bronchoconstriction and increases bronchial secretion. In sympathetic system β2 receptors mediate bronchodilation and increase bronchial secretion, while α1 adrenergic receptors inhibit secretion. Vasoactive intestinal peptide mediated nonadrenergic, noncholinergic system also exists, which produces bronchodilation.

Regarding perfusion, sympathetic system normally has minimal effect on pulmonary vascular tone. Parasympathetic system has vasodilatory effect on pulmonary vasculature.

The diaphragm is innervated by the phrenic nerves,^{Q} which arise from the C_3–C_5^{Q} nerve roots. Intercostal muscles are innervated by their respective thoracic nerve roots. Spinal cord injuries above C_5 are incompatible with spontaneous ventilation because both phrenic and intercostal nerves are affected.

BREATHING MECHANICS

During normal breathing, the diaphragm and to a lesser extent, external intercostal muscles are responsible for inspiration; expiration is generally passive. Diaphragm is the principal muscle of respiration which normally accounts for 75% of the change in chest volume. Accessory respiratory muscles also increase chest volume (and lung expansion) by their action on the ribs. Accessory muscles of inspiration^Q are sternocleidomastoid, scalene, pectoralis muscles, and latissimus dorsi.

Mechanics of Respiration

The lungs and the chest wall are elastic structures. Lung is similar to an elastic rubber balloon which has an inherent tendency to collapse. The lungs get stretched when they expand at birth and they remain stretched for whole life. At the end of quiet expiration their tendency to collapse from the chest wall is just balanced by the tendency of the chest wall to recoil in the opposite direction. The elastic behavior of the lung is often analyzed in terms of compliance. Compliance is defined as and is expressed as dV/dP (where dV is change in volume and dP is change in pressure). Normal lung compliance is around 0.2–0.3 L/cm of H_2O (2–3 L/kPa). Compliance is increased[Q] in emphysema while reduced in fibrosis.

Inspiration is an active process. The contraction of the diaphragm increases intrathoracic volume. The intrapleural pressure at the base of the lungs, which is normally about –2.5 mm Hg (relative to atmospheric) at the start of inspiration decreases to about –6 mm Hg. The expiration is passive under normal circumstances. However in patients with chronic obstructive respiratory disease (COPD), expiration may be active. COPD patients use accessory expiratory muscles (**external oblique, internal oblique, and transversus abdominis**) to exhale the air through their narrowed airways.[4]

LUNG VOLUMES (TABLE 4.3 AND FIG. 4.5)

Tidal Volume

The amount of air that moves in and out of the lungs during normal breathing.

Inspiratory Reserve Volume

The air inspired with a maximal inspiratory effort in excess of the tidal volume.

Expiratory Reserve Volume

The volume expelled by an active expiratory effort after normal expiration.

Residual Volume

Air left in the lungs after a maximal expiratory effort.

Forced Vital Capacity

The largest amount of air that can be expired after a maximal inspiratory effort, this is the frequently measured clinically index for assessment of pulmonary function. Forced vital capacity (FVC)

Table 4.3: Respiratory volumes and capacities for an average young adult male.

Measurement	Mean value	Definition
Respiratory volumes		
Tidal volume (TV)	500 mL	Amount of air inhaled or exhaled in one breath during relaxed, quiet breathing
Inspiratory reserve volume (IRV)	3,000 mL	Amount of air in excess of tidal inspiration that can be inhaled with maximum effort
Expiratory reserve volume (ERV)	1,200 mL	Amount of air in excess of tidal expiration that can be exhaled with maximum effort
Residual volume (RV)	1,200 mL	• Amount of air remaining in the lungs after maximum expiration • Residual volume keeps alveoli inflated in between breaths
Respiratory capacities		
Vital capacity (VC)	4,700 mL	Amount of air that can be exhaled with maximum effort after maximum inspiration (ERV + TV + IRV); used to assess strength of thoracic muscles as well as pulmonary function
Inspiratory capacity (IC)	3,500 mL	Maximum amount of air that can be inhaled after a normal tidal expiration (TV + IRV)
Functional residual capacity (FRC)	2,400 mL	Amount of air remaining in the lungs after a normal tidal expiration (RV + ERV)
Total lung capacity (TLC)	5,900 mL	Maximum amount of air the lungs can contain (RV + VC)

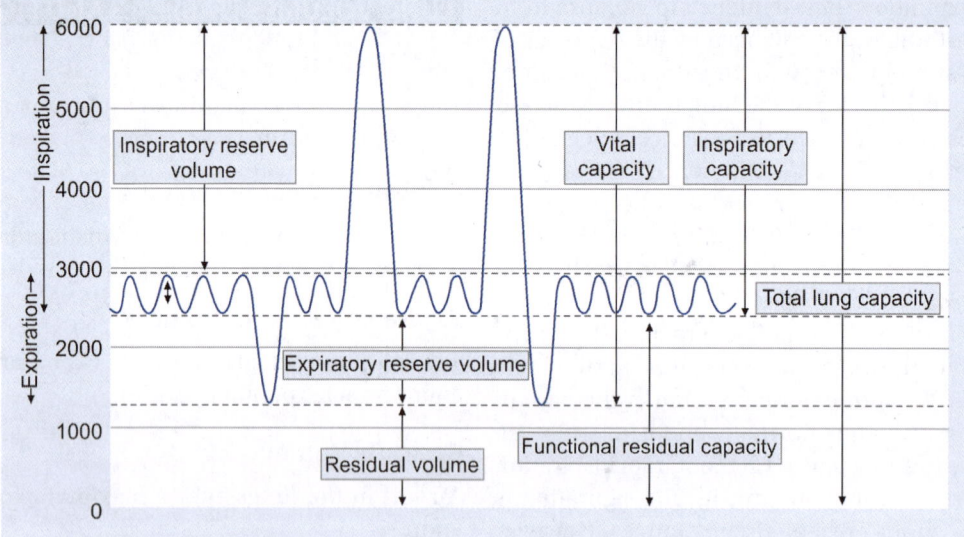

Fig. 4.5: Lung volumes and their relation to breathing.

provides useful information about the strength of the respiratory muscles and other aspects of pulmonary function. The fraction of the vital capacity (VC) expired during the first-second of a forced expiration is referred to as forced expiratory volume (FEV_1)[Q] (formerly the timed VC). The FEV_1 to FVC ratio (FEV_1/FVC)[Q] is a useful tool in the diagnosis of obstructive airway disease.

Minute Volume

The amount of air inspired per minute,[Q] i.e., tidal volume × respiratory rate. It is about 6 L (500 mL/breath × 12 breaths/minutes).

Functional Residual Capacity

There is the amount of air left in the lungs after normal expiration. It is determined by the balance of the inward force of the lung and the outward force of the chest wall. In anesthesia functional residual capacity (FRC) is a very important parameter because it is this air which participates in diffusion when patient is in apnea. Factors affecting FRC includes:

- **Physique**: FRC is directly proportional to height, while obesity markedly decreases FRC (due to reduced chest compliance)
- **Sex**: Males have higher FRC.
- **Position**: FRC is more in upright position in comparison to supine or prone position.
- **Lung disease**: Decreased compliance of the lung, chest, as in restrictive lung disease, reduces FRC.

Closing Capacity

Small airways lack cartilaginous support, if expiration is deep enough, these small airways particularly in dependent regions will eventually close. Once closed the CO_2 from the alveoli of these airways doesn't wash out and oxygen would not come in or these alveoli doesn't contribute much to ventilation. The volume above RV at which airways begin to close during expiration is called closing volume (CV), and the sum of RV and CV is called closing capacity (CC).[Q] In young individuals closing capacity is well below FRC, so after normal expiration lower airways remain open. CC increases with age and in diseases like chronic obstructive pulmonary disease (COPD). At 66 years of age, CC equals FRC in the upright position. When CC encroaches FRC, ventilation-perfusion ratio (V/Q) mismatch begins to occur.

DEAD SPACE AND UNEVEN VENTILATION

Because gaseous exchange in the respiratory system occurs only in the terminal portions of the airways, the gas that occupies the conducting part **(Fig. 4.2)** does not participate in gas exchange. Normally, the volume (100-150 mL) of this anatomic dead space is approximately 30% of tidal volume (500 mL).

Total (physiologic)^Q dead space **(Flowchart 4.1)** includes both anatomical dead space and additional volume of gas that does not equilibrate (alveolar dead space) with blood. In healthy individuals, alveolar dead space is negligible so usually physiological dead space approximates anatomical dead space. However, in disease states, some alveoli may be over ventilated while some remain unperfused, so physiological dead space exceeds anatomical dead space.^{Q} Intermittent positive pressure ventilation (IPPV) also increases alveolar dead space.

Effect of Anesthetics on Dead Space

Anesthesia mask and circuits (by increasing the length of airway) increase the anatomical dead space. Whereas endotracheal intubation and tracheostomy reduces anatomical dead space bypassing upper airways.

Inhalational agents increase both anatomical (because of bronchodilation) and alveolar dead space^Q (by increasing V/Q mismatch).

Positive pressure ventilation and positive end expiratory pressure (PEEP) application also increase both anatomical and alveolar dead space. *Effect of positioning*: When anesthetized patient is placed in lateral position, alveolar dead space is increased (due to increased V/Q mismatch). Trendelenburg position and lithotomy position also increases V/Q mismatch.

VENTILATION-PERFUSION RELATIONSHIP

Ventilation

The air that is inspired gets distributed unevenly in the lung. During quiet breathing in the upright or sitting position, most gas goes to the lower, dependent regions^Q—the basal, diaphragmatic areas. In the left lateral position left lung will receive most of the air and vice versa **(Fig. 4.6)**.

This is due to gravitationally induced gradient in intrapleural pressure. The major factor for which is weight of the lung itself. Alveoli in upper lung areas remain near maximally inflated even after expiration (as lower lung tissue pulls them) and they undergo little more expansion during

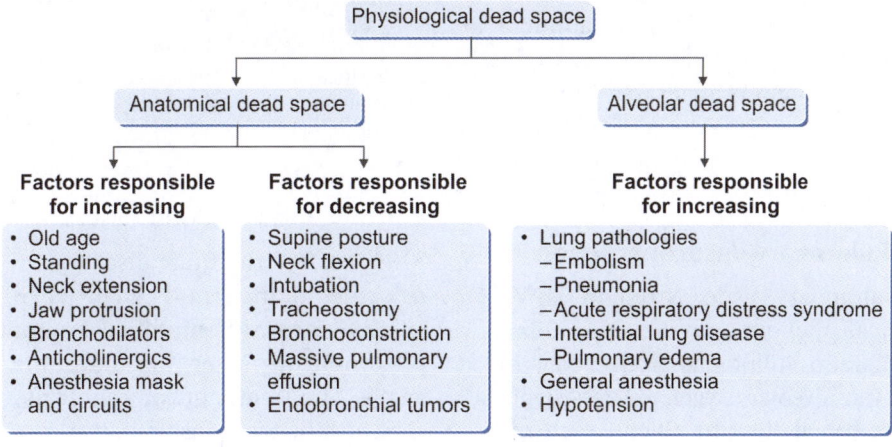

Flowchart 4.1: Factors affecting physiological dead space.

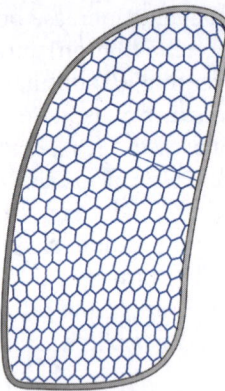

Fig. 4.6: Ventilation and perfusion of the lung in the upright position, expired phase. Note the gradual reduction in alveolar size from top (apex) to bottom. Perfusion increases from apex to base.

inspiration. In contrast, the alveoli in dependent areas are totally deflated after expiration and thus undergo greater expansion during inspiration. However, under anesthesia when individual on IPPV, ventilation is more in nondependent lung and perfusion is more in dependent portion.

Perfusion

Distribution of pulmonary blood flow is also nonuniform. Irrespective of position lower (dependent) portions of the lung receive greater blood flow than upper (nondependent) areas. This is also due to gravitational effect.

Ventilation-Perfusion Ratio

Alveolar ventilation is normally about 4 L/minute and pulmonary perfusion is 5 L/minute, thus overall V/Q ratio is about 0.8. Though both ventilation and perfusion are higher in dependent portion, the V/Q ratio is higher in the upper portions of the lungs.^{Q}

Hypoxic Pulmonary Vasoconstriction

Hypoxic pulmonary vasoconstriction (HPV) is a physiological phenomenon which maintains a normal V/Q ratio. Pulmonary arteries constrict in areas with low alveolar oxygen tension (hypoxia), redirecting blood flow to alveoli with higher oxygen content. All inhalational agents diminish HPV response (maximum with halothane)^Q thereby increase V/Q mismatch.

REGULATION OF RESPIRATION

Spontaneous respiration is produced by rhythmic discharge of motor neurons that innervate the respiratory muscles. Spontaneity of this rhythmic discharge is modulated by alterations in arterial PO_2, PCO_2, and H^+ concentration.

There are two separate neural mechanisms, first one is responsible for voluntary control and is located in the cerebral cortex; this system sends impulses to the respiratory motor neurons via the corticospinal tracts. The second one or automatic system is located in the medulla. Rhythmic respiration is initiated by a small group of synaptically coupled pacemaker cells in the pre-Bötzinger complex. Impulses from these cells activate motor neurons in the cervical (for diaphragm via phrenic nerve) and thoracic (for intercostals) spinal cord. The motor neurons to the expiratory muscles are inhibited when those supplying the inspiratory muscles are active, and vice versa.

KEY POINTS

- In awake patient, ventilation is more in dependent portion
- In anesthetized patient, ventilation is more in non-dependent portion
- In awake patient, perfusion is more in dependent portion
- In anesthetized patient also perfusion is more in dependent portion.

Pontine and Vagal Influences

Although the rhythmic discharge of medullary neurons concerned with respiration is spontaneous, it is modified by impulses from pneumotaxic center (located in the pons) and vagus. The pneumotaxic center plays a role in switching between inspiration and expiration.

Effects of Anesthetics on Respiratory Drive

Spontaneous ventilation is frequently reduced during anesthesia. Both volatile and intravenous anesthetics reduce sensitivity to CO_2. The response is dose dependent. Anesthesia also reduces the response to hypoxia.

MEASURING LUNG FUNCTION

It is essential to estimate lung function in patients with respiratory disease and patients posted for thoracic surgery. Common pulmonary function tests include:

Bedside Pulmonary Function Test

Breath Holding Time of Sabrasez

In this test patient is asked to hold breath after full inspiration. An individual with normal pulmonary function can hold breath for more than 25 seconds. Breath holding time (BHT) less than 15 seconds indicates diminished cardiopulmonary reserve. BHT is not a specific pulmonary function test (PFT) as it is reduced in cardiac dysfunctions too.

Snider Match Blowing Test

Patient is asked to blow off lighted match stick with wide open mouth from a distance of 15 cm.

This test estimates FEV_1 and negative result points towards airway obstructive disease.

Spirometry

With pocket spirometer it is possible to estimate TV, FVC, ERV, IRV, and VC. Lung capacities which have residual volume component [(FRC, RV and total lung capacity (TLC)] cannot be estimated by spirometry.Q

Forced Spirometry

Here measurements of airflow are obtained after maneuvers in which the subject inspires to TLC and then exhales to RV as rapidly as he can and with maximum force. Following measurements are commonly made:
- The volume of gas exhaled during the first second (FEV)
- The total volume exhaled (FVC)
- The average expiratory flow rate during the middle 50% of the VC [forced expiratory flow (FEF) 25–75%, also called as maximal midexpiratory flow rate (MMFR)]
- FEV_1/FVC *ratio*: The ratio of FEV_1 to FVC is proportional to the degree of airway obstruction. Normally, FEV_1/FVC is 80%.

Whereas both FEV_1 and FVC are effort dependent, forced midexpiratory flow (FMFR) (FEF: 25–75%) is effort independent and therefore is a more reliable measurement of obstruction.Q

Helium Dilution and Whole-Body Plethysmography

These are used to measure RV, FRC and TLC. The helium dilution method is easier one but may under estimate the volume of gas in the lungs if there are slowly communicating airspaces, such as bullae. In this situation, lung volumes can be measured more accurately with a whole-body plethysmograph.

> **KEY POINTS**
> - Spirometry cannot measure TLC, RV and FRC.
> - RV, FRC and TLC are measured by helium dilution or whole-body plethysmography.

Diffusing Capacity

This is usually assessed by measuring the diffusing capacity of the lung for carbon monoxide (DLCO). In this test, a small concentration of carbon monoxide (0.3%) is inhaled, usually in a single breath that is held for approximately 10 second. During the breath hold, the carbon monoxide is diluted by the gas already present in the alveoli and is also taken up by blood. The concentration of carbon monoxide is then measured in the gas exhaled after the breath hold, and DLCO is calculated as the quantity of carbon monoxide absorbed per minute per mm Hg pressure gradient from the alveoli to the pulmonary capillaries.

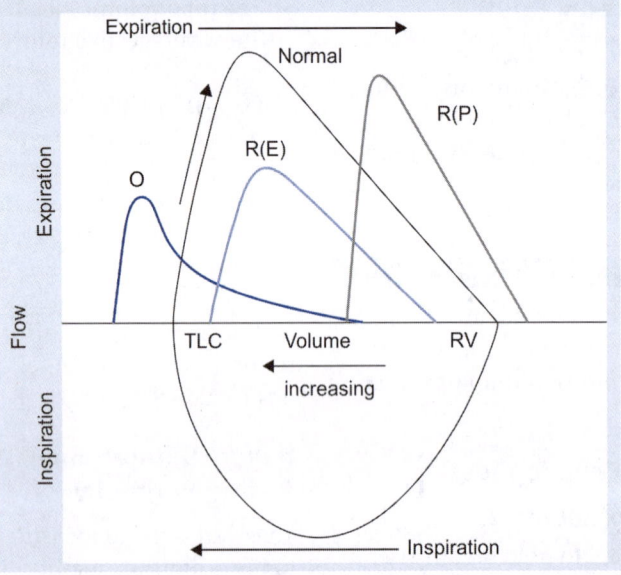

Fig. 4.7: Flow-volume curves in different respiratory diseases—O, obstructive disease; R(P), parenchymal restrictive disease; R(E), extraparenchymal restrictive disease with limitation in inspiration and expiration. By convention, lung volume increases to one moving left.
(TLC: total lung capacity; RV: residual volume)

Flow Volume Curves

Latest microprocessor controlled spirometer automatically generates flow volume loops. These curves are more informative in detecting pulmonary disorders than conventional spirometry (**Fig. 4.7**).

FITNESS FOR ANESTHESIA

Patients with severe respiratory disease should be optimized before anesthesia and surgery. Features suggesting severe respiratory compromise are:

- Dyspnea at rest
- FEV_1 l<15 mL/kg or FVC <20 mL/kg, FEV_1 <50%.[5]
- PaO_2 <60 mm Hg and/or PCO_2 >45 mm Hg. These patients require respiratory exercises, bronchodilator therapy before anesthesia.
- Patients with FEV_1 <10 mL/kg have life-threatening respiratory disease and these patients should be subjected to only life-saving emergency procedures.

LAST-MINUTE REVISION

- Gas exchange starts from respiratory bronchiole.
- Bronchopulmonary segment is the anatomically and functionally separate unit of lung tissue; right lung has ten bronchopulmonary segments, whereas left lung has nine.
- Right bronchus is straighter and wider than left bronchus.
- Normally both ventilation and perfusion are more independent portions of lung.
- Physiological dead space is the sum of anatomical dead space and alveolar dead space.
- Narrowest part of larynx is subglottis in children (up to 5 years) and glottis in adults.
- Inhalational anesthetic agent increases both anatomical and alveolar dead space.
- Breath holding time estimates functional residual volume whereas match blowing test measures forced expiratory volume in 1 second (FEV_1).

REFERENCES

1. Campbell M, Sapra A. Physiology, Airflow Resistance. [Updated 2022 Apr 28]. In: StatPearls [Internet]. Treasure Island (FL): StatPearls Publishing; 2022 Jan-. Available from: https://www.ncbi.nlm.nih.gov/books/NBK554401/
2. Harless J, Ramaiah R, Bhananker SM. Pediatric airway management. Int J Crit Illn Inj Sci. 2014;4(1):65-70. doi: 10.4103/2229-5151.128015. PMID: 24741500; PMCID: PMC3982373.
3. Audu P, Artz G, Scheid S, Harrop J, Albert T, Vaccaro A, et al. Recurrent laryngeal nerve palsy after anterior cervical spine surgery: the impact of endotracheal tube cuff deflation, reinflation, and pressure adjustment. Anesthesiology. 2006; 105(5):898-901. doi: 10.1097/00000542-200611000-00009. PMID: 17065882.
4. Yan S, Sinderby C, Bielen P, Beck J, Comtois N, Sliwinski P. Expiratory muscle pressure and breathing mechanics in chronic obstructive pulmonary disease. Eur Respir J. 2000;16(4):684-90. doi: 10.1034/j.1399-3003.2000.16d20.x. PMID: 11106213.
5. Duggappa DR, Rao GV, Kannan S. Anaesthesia for patient with chronic obstructive pulmonary disease. Indian J Anaesth. 2015 Sep;59(9):574-83. doi: 10.4103/0019-5049.165859. PMID: 26556916; PMCID: PMC4613404.

REVIEW QUESTIONS

1. Dead space is increased by all, *except*:
   a. Anticholinergic drugs
   b. Standing
   c. Hyperextension of neck
   d. Endotracheal intubation
2. Physiological dead space is decreased by:
   a. Upright position
   b. Positive pressure
   c. Neck flexion
   d. Emphysema
3. Which of the statement regarding ventilation-perfusion relationship is not true?
   a. In left lateral position both ventilation and perfusion are more in left lung
   b. In standing position perfusion is more in basal portion of lung
   c. In standing position ventilation is more in apical portion of lung
   d. Ventilation is more in well perfused area in comparison to underperfused area
4. Gas exchange starts from:
   a. Trachea
   b. Bronchi
   b. Terminal bronchiole
   d. Respiratory bronchiole

> **Mnemonic**
> Respiration starts from respiratory bronchiole.

5. True statement regarding closing capacity includes all, *except*:
   a. It is less than residual volume
   b. Reduces with age
   c. If closing capacity encroaches functional residual capacity V/Q mismatch starts
   d. It is not related to residual volume

ANSWERS

1. d   2. c   3. c   4. d   5. a and b

CHAPTER 5

Oxygen and Carbon Dioxide Transport

Shivali Pandey

Under anesthesia the most important goal is to maintain oxygen (O_2) supply to tissues and simultaneously remove carbon dioxide (CO_2).

OXYGEN CASCADE

Oxygen moves along the concentration gradient from a relatively high level in air (PO_2:160 mm of Hg), to the respiratory tract (PO_2:150 mm of Hg) and then alveolar gas (110 mm of Hg), to the arterial blood, capillaries and finally the cell. The partial pressure oxygen (PO_2) reaches the lowest level (4–20 mm Hg) in the mitochondria. This stepwise reduction in PO_2 from air to the mitochondrion is known as the **oxygen cascade** **(Fig. 5.1)**.

OXYGEN TRANSPORT

The O_2 from environment diffuse into the blood through the lungs. O_2 delivery to a particular tissue depends on the amount of O_2 entering the lungs, the adequacy of pulmonary gas exchange, the blood flow to the tissue, and the capacity of the blood to carry O_2. Blood carry O_2 in two forms: (1) dissolved in plasma **(approximately 2%)** and (2) in reversible association with hemoglobin (Hb) **(approximately 98%)**.

Reaction of Hemoglobin and Oxygen

Hemoglobin is a protein made up of four subunits, each of which contains a heme moiety

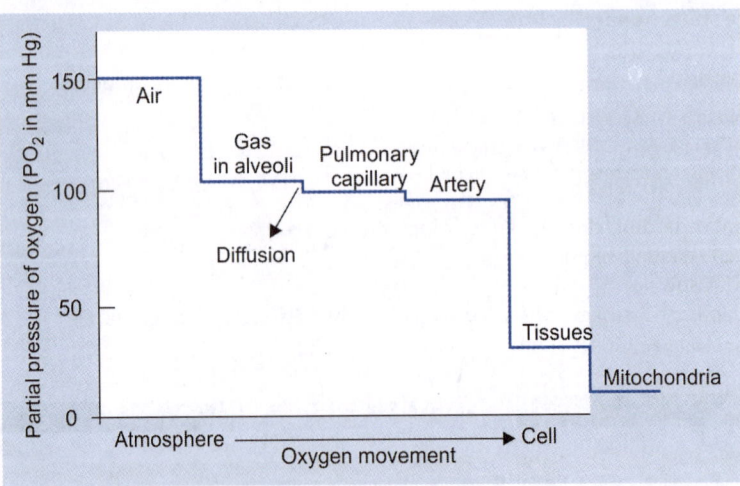

Fig. 5.1: Oxygen cascade.
Note: There is gradual reduction in PO_2 when O_2 moves from air to mitochondria.

(a porphyrin ring complex that includes one atom of ferrous iron) attached to a polypeptide chain. Thus, a Hb molecule contains four iron atoms; each iron atom can reversibly bind one O_2 molecule. The iron stays in the ferrous state, so that the reaction is oxygenation,^{Q} not oxidation.

In deoxyhemoglobin, the globin units are tightly bound in a tense configuration, which reduces the affinity of the molecule for O_2. Combination of the first heme in the Hb molecule with O_2 increases the affinity of the second heme for O_2, and so on.^{Q}

When fully saturated, each gram of normal Hb contains 1.39 mL^Q of O_2. However, in vivo blood normally contains small amounts of inactive Hb, so this figure comes down to 1.34 mL^Q of O_2 **(Hüfner Constant)**. The normal Hb concentration in blood is about 15 g/dL. Therefore, when 100% saturated 1 dL of blood contains 20.1 mL^Q (1.34 mL × 15) of O_2.

Dissolved Oxygen

Oxygen first dissolves in plasma, from there it moves to bind hemoglobin. This dissolved portion determines the PO_2. This portion is readily available to supply tissue. It is also replenished by oxygen that is bound to hemoglobin. The amount of O_2 dissolved in blood is proportional to its partial pressure. Each dL of blood carries 0.003 mL/mm Hg or at arterial partial pressure of oxygen (PaO_2) of 100 mm Hg, the maximum amount of O_2 dissolved in blood is 0.3 mL/dL.

Normally because of slight admixture with venous blood that bypasses the pulmonary capillaries (physiologic shunt), the Hb in systemic arterial blood is only 97% saturated. The arterial blood therefore contains a total of about 19.8 mL of O_2 per dL; 0.29 mL in solution and 19.5 mL bound to Hb.[1]

Oxygen Flux

Amount of oxygen leaving ventricle per minute in the arterial blood is oxygen flux.

In venous blood at rest, Hb is 75% saturated and the total O2 content is about 15.2 mL/dL: 0.12 mL in solution and 15.1 mL bound to Hb. Thus, at rest the tissues remove about 4.6 mL of O2 from each deciliter of blood passing through them (0.17 mL of this is in dissolve form). In this way, approximately 250Q mL [body contains 50 dL (5,000 mL) blood multiplied by 4.6] of O2 per minute is transported from the blood to the tissues at rest.

O_2 flux = CO × SaO_2 × Hb× 1.34 mL/g
= 5,000 mL/min × 98 % × 15.6 g/100 mL × 1.34 mL/g
= 1,000 mL/min (approx)

> ### 🔑 KEY POINTS
> - Presence of Hb increases the O_2 carrying capacity of blood by 70-fold.
> - **Hüfner Constant** is defined as the amount of oxygen that can bind with one gram of hemoglobin when fully saturated. It was found to be (1.34 mL) of oxygen gas as calculated by Gustav von Hüfner.

OXYGEN-HEMOGLOBIN DISSOCIATION CURVE (FIG. 5.2)

The oxygen-hemoglobin dissociation curve is a graphical representation of the relationship between the amount of oxygen bound to hemoglobin and the partial pressure of oxygen. This curve has a characteristic sigmoid shape.^{Q} Sigmoid shape results from the fact that binding of one molecule of O_2 facilitates binding of subsequent molecule.

Important factors affecting the oxygen-hemoglobin dissociation curve are: the pH, the temperature, and the concentration of 2,3-biphosphoglycerate (BPG; 2,3-BPG).

P50 is the convenient index for comparison of such shifts. P50,^{Q} is the PO_2 at which Hb is half saturated with O_2. As P50 increases (curve shift to right) affinity of Hb for O_2 decreases and vice versa. Normal value of P50 is 26.5 mm Hg for adult Hb and 20 mm Hg for fetal Hb **(Fig. 5.2)**.

The decrease in O_2 affinity of Hb when the pH of blood falls is called Bohr effect^Q and is closely related to the fact that deoxygenated Hb binds hydrogen ion (H^+) more actively than oxygenated Hb. As blood enters capillaries, its CO_2 content raises and pH falls, this shifts the curve to right which favors O_2 release **(Fig. 5.3)**.

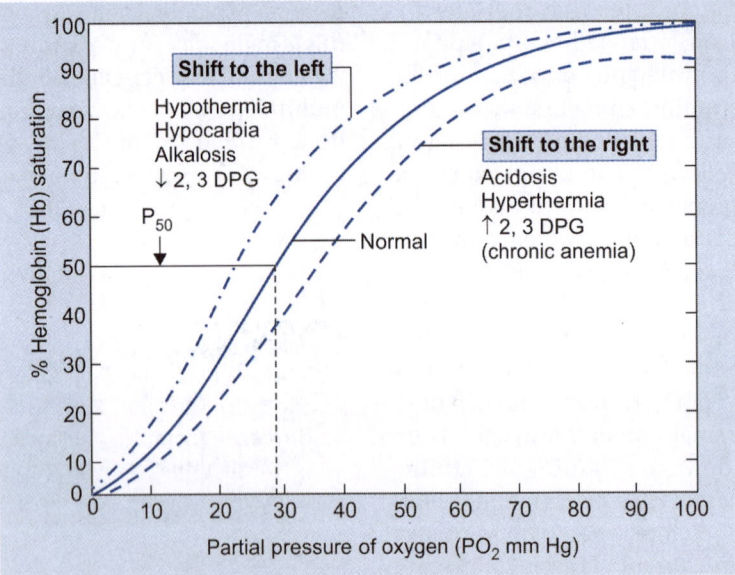

Fig. 5.2: Oxygen-hemoglobin dissociation curve.
(DPG: diphosphoglycerate)

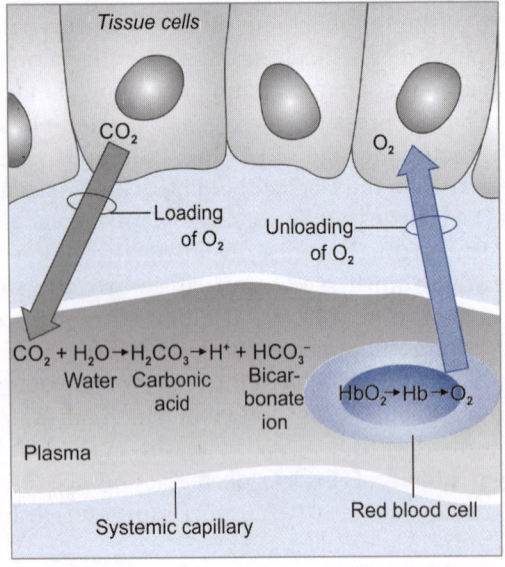

Fig. 5.3: Oxygen and carbon dioxide transport at cellular level.

CARBON DIOXIDE TRANSPORT

Carbon dioxide is transported in blood in three forms:
1. Dissolved in plasma
2. As bicarbonate (maximum)
3. With proteins in the form of carbamino compounds.

The solubility of CO_2 in blood is 20 times that of O_2; therefore, considerably more CO_2 than O_2 is present in simple solution at equal partial pressures. The CO_2 that diffuses into red blood cells (RBCs) is rapidly hydrated to carbonic acid (H_2CO_3) because of the presence of an enzyme carbonic anhydrase. H_2CO_3 then dissociates to H^+ and bicarbonate ion (HCO_3^-), and the H^+ is buffered, primarily by Hb, while the HCO_3^- enters the plasma. Some of the CO_2 in the RBCs reacts with the amino groups of Hb and other proteins (R), forming carbamino compounds **(Fig. 5.3)**.

As deoxyhemoglobin binds more H^+ than oxyhemoglobin and forms carbamino compounds more readily, venous blood carries more CO_2

✦ KEY POINTS
- 100 mL of arterial blood carries 20.1 mL of O_2.
- 100 mL of arterial blood carries 49 mL of CO_2.
- 100 mL of venous blood carries 52.7 mL of CO_2.
- 100 mL of venous blood carries 15.2 mL of O_2.

than arterial blood. Binding of O_2 to Hb in lung reduces its affinity for CO_2 (Haldane effect)^Q and facilitates its release.[2] As HCO_3^- diffuses out from RBC to plasma, Cl^- diffuses in opposite direction to maintain equilibrium. This is called Chloride shift or Hamburger effect.

Summarizing, each dL of arterial blood carries 49 mL of CO_2 out of which 2.6 mL is dissolved, 2.6 mL is in carbamino compounds and 43.8 mL as HCO_3^-. In the tissues, 3.7 mL of CO_2 per dL of blood is added; 0.4 mL stays in solution, 0.8 mL forms carbamino compounds and 2.5 mL forms HCO_3^-. In the lungs, the processes are reversed, and the 3.7 mL of CO_2 is released into the alveoli.

In this manner, (55 × 3.7) 200 mL of CO_2 per minute at rest and much larger amounts during exercise are transported from the tissues to the lungs and exhaled out.

LAST-MINUTE REVISION

- A Hb molecule contains four iron atom and each iron can bind four O_2 molecules.
- When fully saturated, 1 g of Hb contains 1.39 mL of O_2.
- Presence of Hb increase the O_2 carrying capacity of blood by 70-fold.
- P50 for oxygen-hemoglobin dissociation curve at body temperature is 26.7 mm Hg.
- Acidosis, hyperthermia and increased 2, 3-diphosphoglycerate (DPG) shifts hemoglobin-oxygen dissociation curve to right and vice versa.
- Carbon dioxide is transported maximally as bicarbonate.

REFERENCES

1. Collins JA, Rudenski A, Gibson J, Howard L, O'Driscoll R. Relating oxygen partial pressure, saturation and content: the hemoglobin-oxygen dissociation curve. Breathe (Sheff). 2015;11(3):194-201. doi: 10.1183/20734735.001415. PMID: 26632351; PMCID: PMC4666443.

2. Benner A, Patel AK, Singh K, et al. Physiology, Bohr Effect. [Updated 2021 Aug 15]. In: StatPearls [Internet]. Treasure Island (FL): StatPearls Publishing, 2022. Available from: https://www.ncbi.nlm.nih.gov/books/NBK526028/

REVIEW QUESTIONS

1. Oxygen–hemoglobin dissociation curve shifts to right in all of the following conditions, *except*:
    a. Acidosis
    b. Alkalosis
    c. Fever
    d. Anemia

    Mnemonic
    Shift to right is seen in CADET, i.e., CO_2, acid, 2-3DPG, exercise, temperature.

2. Each gram of normal hemoglobin carries:
    a. 1.35 mL of O_2
    b. 1 mL of O_2
    c. 0.35 mL of O_2
    d. 4 mL of O_2

3. Most of the CO_2 is transported as:
    a. Carbamino compound
    b. As bicarbonate
    c. Bound to hemoglobin
    d. Bound to protein

4. 100 mL of blood carries how much O_2:
    a. 10 mL
    b. 20 mL
    c. 30 mL
    d. 40 mL

5. An anesthetized individual is being ventilated with 100%. His 100 mL of arterial blood is supposed to contain:
   a. Approx. 20 mL of O_2
   b. Approx. 50 mL of CO_2
   c. Both a and b
   d. Neither a nor b

   Note: Breathing 100% O_2 affects only dissolves O_2 in blood which forms a very little proportion of total O_2 content in blood.

ANSWERS

1. b   2. a   3. b   4. b   5. c

CHAPTER 6

Operation Theater

Apurva Abhinandan Mittal, Anshul Jain

Operation theater (OT) or operation room (OR) is that specialized portion of the hospital where life-saving or life-improving procedure are carried out on the human body by invasive methods under strict aseptic conditions with maximum safety.

LOCATION

The OT suit of a hospital should be located in an area where flow of nonsurgical patient is minimal. The main points while finalizing the location of the OT complex in a hospital includes accessibilities to surgical wards, Central Sterile Supply Department (CSSD), emergency and blood bank, etc. The grouping of all operating rooms in one central location (in the form of OT complex) provides following advantages:
- Efficient use of staff and facilities
- Improved asepsis
- Better economy
- Better OR discipline
- Better sharing of operative equipment.

NUMBER OF OPERATION THEATERS

Various reports recommended that there should be one OT for each 100 beds, i.e., for 500-bedded hospital five OTs are recommended. However, the exact number can be modified as per need.

DESIGN

Planning of OR complex must ensure the separation of clean restricted area from contaminated area. On the basis of contamination, OR complex is divided into four zones, viz.

Sterile Zones

This includes OR itself. Only aseptic activities are permitted in this zone. Sterile zone also includes sink areas and substerile rooms.

Clean Zone

Around sterile zone lies clean zone. Accessibility of this zone is limited to staff who have changed their outer clothing and footwears. Patient holding and preparation area is provided in this zone. Anesthesia induction rooms (if present) and anesthesia stores are also located here.

Protective Zone

Outside the clean zone lies the protective zone forming a barrier between the clean area of the OT complex and rest of the hospital area. This zone contains the administrative elements, changing rooms. People can enter this area in their streets clothes but no entry is permitted to inner zones without changing clothes and shoes.

Disposal Zone

Disposal zone is the corridor from where the used instrument, linens and operating room debris are removed and taken out. This zone has an independent one way communication to outside. No traffic is allowed from outside to inside via disposal zone.

LAYOUT

Size

A multipurpose OR should be at least 400^Q sq feet in area (20 × 20 feet). For a specialized cardiac or trauma OR, an area of 20 × 30 feet (600 sq feet) is recommended, if area exceeds 600 sq feet efficiency of OR declines. Height should be around 10 feet.

Doors

Sliding doors are preferred as they do not produce the aircurrent. Aircurrent produced by swinging door can dislodge the microorganism on the floor and increases microbial count in air.

Ventilation

In OT with recirculated air, 20–30 air exchanges per hour are recommended. Air change and circulation provide fresh air and prevent accumulation of anesthetic gases in the room. Gas scavenger system is mandatory for OR relying on recirculated air. Ultra-clean laminar airflow is preferred in OR. Blower of airflow is located in the ceiling preferably over OT table, so that patient and surgical team receive maximum fresh air, air leaves through the outlets located at walls just above the floor.

Humidity and Temperature

Relative humidity must be maintained above 45% as moisture provides a conductive medium thereby reducing sparks and fire chances. OT temperature is maintained within a range of 20–24°C. Higher temperature is required during pediatric surgery.

Floors

Floor should be nonporous, suitably hard to permit cleaning by flooding. Tiles should not be used as there are airspaces between their junctions in which microbes may grow.

Walls and Ceiling

Similar to flooring, walls should be hard nonporous, fire resistant and waterproof. The colors used on the walls, floor and ceiling of OR should be light enough to ensure satisfactory reflection and at the same time soothing to eyes.

Lighting

Theater light must be of such quality that the pathologic conditions are recognizable. An anesthesiologist must have sufficient light (at least 200 footcandles) to adequately evaluate the patients. Normally, theater light should produce the white color of daylight. Most surgeons prefer a color temperature of 5,000 K which approximates the white light of cloudless sky at noon.

OPERATION ROOM ASEPSIS

Cleaning, disinfection and sterilization are the cornerstones in ensuring operation asepsis.

Cleaning and Disinfection

Cleaning removes organic matter, visible soils and reduces the bacterial count. Frequency and procedure of cleaning and disinfection have been mentioned in **Table 6.1**.

Table 6.1: Cleaning of operating rooms.

At the beginning of day	Clean floors and all horizontal surfaces (operation table, chairs and cabinets) with a wet cloth
Between patients	Clean operation table, examination couches, trolley tops and any other potentially contaminated surface with a cloth dampened with a disinfectant solution
At the end of day	Dispose all waste. Clean all surface including door handles and anesthesia trolley. Wash floor[Q] with disinfectant such as phenol
Once a week	Clean all the areas inside OT complex with warm water and detergent. Empty the storage shelves wipe them, dry them and then rearrange

Sterilization

Following methods are used for sterilization of:
- **Formaldehyde fumigation**: Each OR should be fumigated weekly.
- **Ultraviolet radiation**:^Q After completion of OT list, ultraviolet (UV) radiation should be started and continued till next day morning. This is to be switched off 2 hours before surgery.

Microbial Monitoring

To check the efficacy of asepsis microbial monitoring is performed with following frequency:
- **Swabbing and culture**: This should be performed once a month. Areas from where sample has to be taken are:
  – OT table at the head end
  – Overhead lamp
  – All walls
  – Floor below the head end of the table
  – Instrument trolley
  – AC duct
  – Microscope handles
- **Air sampling**:^Q This is also performed monthly by settle plate method in which a plate of blood agar and Sabouraud dextrose agar (SDA) is placed in the center of the OR (close to operation table) and the lid is kept open for 30 minutes, the plate is then allow to incubate for 7 days. Bacterial colony count of more than 10 per plate and fungal colony of more than one per plate are considered unacceptable.[1]

LAST-MINUTE REVISION
- Area of operating room should be at least 400 sq feet.
- Operation theater is sterilized by fumigation and UV radiation.

REFERENCE
1. Landrin A, Bissery A, Kac G. Monitoring air sampling in operating theatres: can particle counting replace microbiological sampling? J Hosp Infect. 2005;61(1):27-9. doi: 10.1016/j.jhin.2005.03.002. PMID: 16009457.

REVIEW QUESTIONS

1. As per routine monitoring of operation theater, asepsis by air sampling is performed:
   a. Daily
   b. Weekly
   c. Hourly
   d. Monthly

2. What should be the ideal OT temperature?
   a. 30–35°C
   b. 20–25°C
   c. 15–20°C
   d. 10–15°C

3. Surgeries are carried out in which zone of operation theater complex:
   a. Clean zone
   b. Sterile zone
   c. Protective zone
   d. Any of the above

4. A 100-bedded hospital is constructing neurosurgery OT. What should be the sufficient dimensions for a good neurosurgery OT?
   a. 10 × 15 feet
   b. 30 × 30 feet
   c. 20 × 20 feet
   d. 15 × 15 feet

ANSWERS

1. c   2. b   3. b   4. c

CHAPTER 7

Anesthesia Machine and Vaporizers

Anshul Jain

INTRODUCTION

Anesthesia machine is the device to control the patient's respiratory gas exchange and administer inhalation anesthetics. Over the years, the anesthesia machine has evolved from a simple pneumatic device to a complex multisystem workstation. Anesthesia machine along with vaporizers, the anesthesia breathing circuit, the ventilator, the scavenging system, and respiratory and physiologic monitoring systems form complete anesthesia workstation.

STANDARDS FOR AN ANESTHESIA MACHINE

Due to multiple manufacturers, various guidelines and standards have been imposed for manufacturers regarding their minimum performance and safety requirements. American Society[Q] for Testing and Materials (ASTM) F1850-00 is the latest standard which manufacturers have to follow. To comply with the 2000 ASTM F1850-00 standard, newly manufactured workstations must have monitors, alarm system **(Fig. 7.1)**.

ANATOMY OF AN ANESTHESIA MACHINE

Generic anesthesia machine is a continuous flow[Q] type machine in which fresh gases are delivered via gas cylinder or pipeline source. High pressure gases pass through pressure reducing valve to rotameter. Downstream to rotameter different gases gets mixed and are directed towards the vaporizers, from vaporizers fresh gases gets

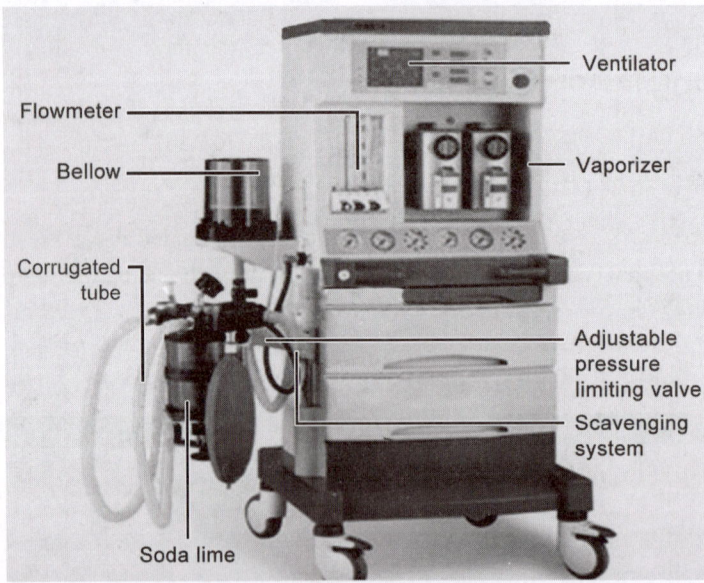

Fig. 7.1: Anesthesia workstation.

volatile anesthetic vapors and whole mixture exits from machine outlet. At outlet lies breathing circuit which conducts the anesthetic mixture from machine outlet to patient. Breathing circuit converts unidirectional continuous flow to bi-direction intermittent flow (normal respiratory pattern). A simplified flow diagram of a basic anesthesia machine is shown in **Figure 7.2**.

On the basis of pressure within the anesthesia machine, it can be divided into three circuits:
1. **High-pressure circuit**: It is confined to the cylinders and the cylinder primary pressure regulators. For oxygen (O_2), the pressure of this circuit range from 2,200 psig to 45 psig and for nitrous oxide (N_2O) it ranges from 750 psig to 45 psig.
2. **Intermediate-pressure circuit** begins from regulated cylinder supply sources at 45 psig, (*it includes the pipeline sources at 50–55 psig*) and extends up to the flow control valves.
3. **Low-pressure circuit** extends from the flow control valves to the common gas outlet. This circuit includes the flow tubes, vaporizers and common gas outlet (**Fig. 7.2**).

High-pressure Circuit

Anesthesia machine atleast contains assembly for two O_2 cylinder and two N_2O cylinders. Additional assembly for carbon dioxide (CO_2) and helium (He) cylinder may be there.

Cylinders are made up of molybdenum steel.[Q] Special need aluminum cylinders are also there, which can be used in magnetic resonance imaging (MRI). As cylinders have to withstand rough handling and high pressure, they are subjected to vigorous test prior to filling. Bend test, tensile test, flattening test and impact test determine the quality of cylinder wall. Hydraulic test[Q] is performed to rule out leak.

O_2, nitrogen (N_2), air and He are kept in cylinders as compressed gases as their critical temperature is very low. N_2O and CO_2 are stored in liquid form.[Q]

Oxygen Cylinder

Internationally white colored cylinder, but black body/white shoulder[Q] is common in many countries including India. According to size there

> **KEY POINTS**
>
> On the basis of gas flow anesthesia machine can be:
> - **Intermittent flow type**: Gas flows only during inspiration, e.g., entonox apparatus.
> - **Continuous flow type**: Gas flows both during inspiration expiration. Most modern anesthesia machines are continuous flow type.

> **KEY POINTS**

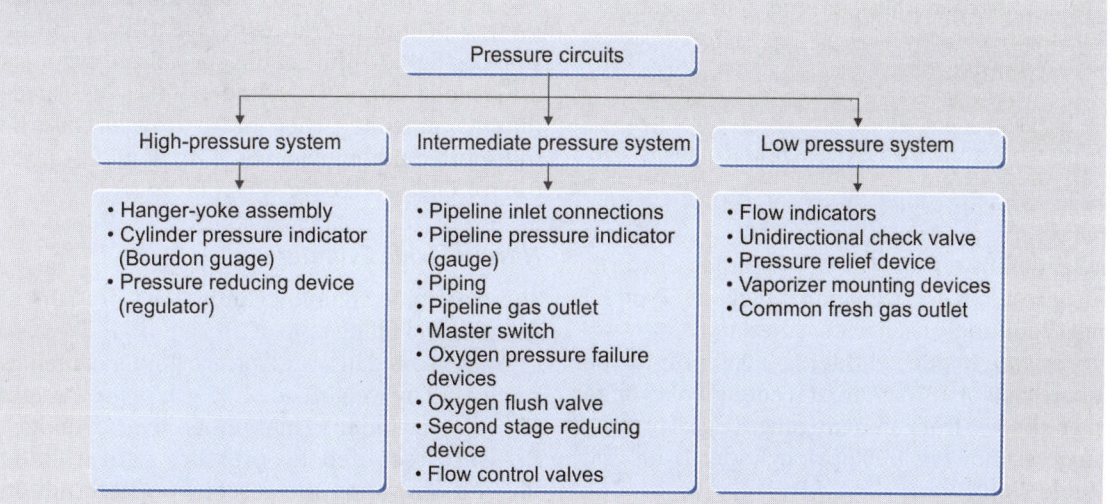

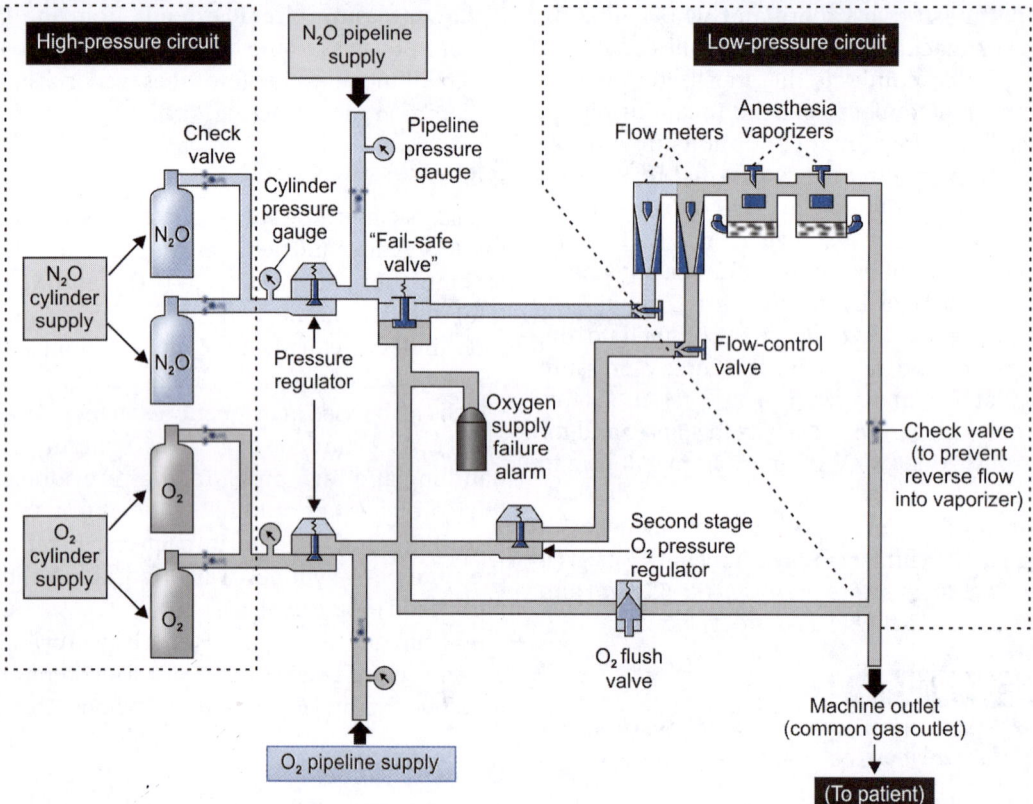

Fig. 7.2: A flow diagram of generic anesthesia machine.

🔑 KEY POINTS

The anesthesia machine performs four essential functions:
1. Provides oxygen
2. Accurately mixes anesthetic gases and vapors
3. Enables patient ventilation
4. Minimizes anesthesia related risks to patients and staff.

Liquid Oxygen

At a pressure of 1,200 kpa and temperature lower then critical temperature^Q (–119°C), O_2 can be stored in liquid form. For this specialized cylinders are needed, liquid O_2 cylinders takes less space thus they are suited when massive oxygen has to be transported in remote areas. 1 mL liquid O_2 gives 840 mL of gaseous oxygen O_2 **(Table 7.1)**.

are different types, viz. AA^Q (smallest for army purpose), A, B, C, D, E, and H (biggest). Type E is most commonly used in anesthesia.

Pressure inside cylinder is 2,000 pounds per square inch or 137 kg/cm². O_2 content of cylinder can be known from pressure gauge (e.g., if pressure gauge is showing 1,000 psi, cylinder is half fill) **(Table 7.1)**.

Nitrous Oxide Cylinder

These are blue colored cylinder with pressure of 760 psi^Q and filling ratio of 0.75.

N_2O is stored in liquid form, cylinder content is calculated by weight, i.e., 1.87 g/L of gas (weight of empty cylinder is mentioned over cylinder). Pressure recorded by pressure gauze would depend only upon the gaseous portion (not on

Table 7.1: Cylinder summary.

Gas	Filled as	Color	Pin index	Pressure (psi)
Oxygen[Q]	Gas	Black with white shoulders	2–5	2,000
Nitrous oxide	Liquid	Blue	3–5	760
Air	Gas	Gray body with black and white shoulder	1–5	760
Carbon dioxide[Q]	Liquid	Gray	2–6	750
Cyclopropane	Liquid	Orange[Q]	3–6	75
Entonox® [50% (O_2) + 50% (N_2O)]	Liquid	Blue body with blue and white shoulder	7	2,000

the actual content of cylinder). Therefore in N_2O cylinders, pressure gauge does not tell about the actual content of gas **(Table 7.1)**.

Cylinder Valves

At the top of cylinder lies valve. Flush-type valve are more common than diaphragm valve. When the valve is opened, content of cylinder exits.

Yoke Assembly (Fig. 7.3)

Especially designed portion of machine where cylinder gets fitted. Assembly consist of pin index system, Bodok seal, and check valve.

Pin index system[Q]: Each hanger yoke has the pin index safety system (PISS), which is a safeguard to eliminate cylinder interchanging. Each gas or combination of gases has a specific pin and holes arrangement. The position of holes over cylinder valve and pins over yoke of machine are fixed and specific for each gas. Cylinder can be fit only when they get align, e.g. yoke for O_2 connection have pins at 2–5 position, so only a cylinder that possess hole at 2–5 position (oxygen cylinder) can be fitted

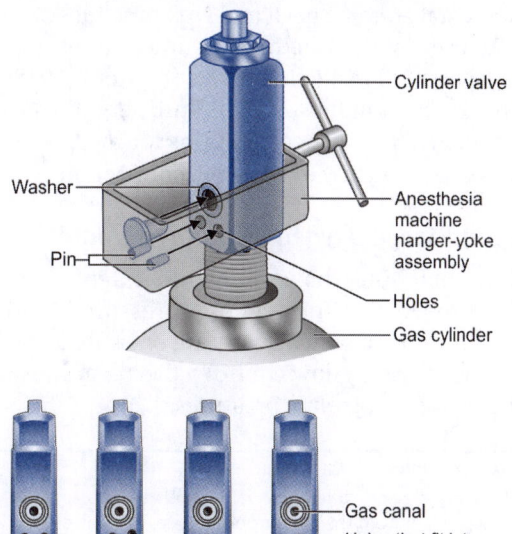

Fig. 7.3: Pin index system and hanger-yoke assembly.

or N_2O cylinder (holes at 3–5 position) cannot be fitted over there **(Fig. 7.3)**.

Pressure Reducing Valves

Gases exits cylinder at a very high pressure so a pressure reducing valve is always needed, otherwise sudden high pressure flow can damage anesthesia apparatus and above all respiratory mucosa of patient. Out of various types of regulators available, Adams[Q] valve is most popular and reliable. Most modern anesthetic machines have two preset pressure regulator. First one reduces pressure to 60 psi while second reduces to 15–20 psi.

> **KEY POINTS**
>
> **Filling ratio:** It is a guide to the maximum amount of gas that can be filled in the cylinder. Technically filling ratio (FR) is the percent ratio of weight of gas in a cylinder to the weight of water the cylinder can hold at 60°F.
> Cylinders in which gases are stored in liquid form must be kept vertical, as liquid content can damage their valves.

Intermediate-pressure Circuit

Pipeline Supply Source

Under normal conditions, the pipeline supply serves as the primary gas source for the anesthesia machine. Most hospitals have a central piping system to deliver medical gases such as O_2, N_2O, and air to the operating room. The most common problems with pipeline system are inadequate O_2 pressure, followed by excessive pipeline pressure whereas most devastating reported hazard is accidental crossing of O_2 and N_2O pipelines.

To prevent this, the pipeline inlet fittings have gas-specific diameter index safety system[Q] (DISS) threaded body fittings. The DISS provides threaded noninterchangeable connections for medical gas lines to minimize the risk of misconnection.

Second-Stage Oxygen Pressure Regulator

Many machines have a second-stage oxygen regulator in the intermediate-pressure circuit. This regulator supplies a constant pressure usually 14 psig to the O_2 flow control valve regardless of fluctuating O_2 pipeline pressures.

> **Fail-safe Valve**
> A safety device called the fail-safe[Q] valve is located downstream from the N_2O supply source. This valve shuts off or proportionally decreases the supply of N_2O (and other gases), if the oxygen supply pressure declines. An alarm device is also there to monitor the O_2 supply pressure. Alarm gets activated when O_2 supply pressure reaches below 30 psig.

Low-pressure Circuit

Flowmeter Assembly (Rotameter) (Figs. 7.4A to C)

Rotameter[Q] precisely controls and measures gas flowing toward low pressure circuit. Flowmeter assembly consists of flow-control valve, flow tube, indicator float (bobbin), and the indicator scale.

In traditional glass flowmeter assemblies, the flow control valve regulates the amount of flow that enters a tapered, transparent flow tube known as a Thorpe tube. A mobile indicator float inside the flow tube indicates the amount of flow passing through the associated flow control valve. The quantity of flow is indicated by a scale imprinted over the flow tube. Due to tapering the gap between tube wall and bobbin (annular space)[Q] is variable, i.e., annular space is more at upper end, and less at lower end. Valve directs flow at the bottom of flowmeter tube; gas flow lifts the bobbin (made of aluminum[Q]), and exits through annular space. The height of bobbin is the balance between upward pressure exerted by gas and weight of bobbin. The higher the bobbin raise greater is the gas flowing around it. At lower flow rates, the gas flow is laminar but at higher flow rates, flow becomes turbulent. Due to difference in viscosity and density of different gases flowmeter assembly are different for different gases.

Proportionating System

This system links flow control valves of O_2 and N_2O mechanically or pneumatically or both, so that minimum O_2 concentration at common gas outlet is at least 25% that of N_2O.

After leaving the flow tubes, both N_2O and O_2 get mixed and the mixture of gases travels through a common manifold and directed to a calibrated vaporizer. Through vaporizers precise amounts of inhaled anesthetic can be added. The total gas flow plus the anesthetic vapor then travel toward the common gas outlet.

Many anesthesia machines have a one-way check valve located between the vaporizer and the common gas outlet. Its purpose is to prevent backflow into the vaporizer during positive-pressure ventilation.

Oxygen Flush Valve

The O_2 flush valve allows direct communication between the O_2 intermediate-pressure circuit and the low-pressure circuit. Flow from the O_2 flush valve enters the low-pressure circuit after the vaporizers. This spring-loaded O_2 flush valve stays closed, until the operator opens it. On opening, valve delivers 100% O_2 at 35–75 L/minute to the breathing circuit. The O_2 flush valve can provide

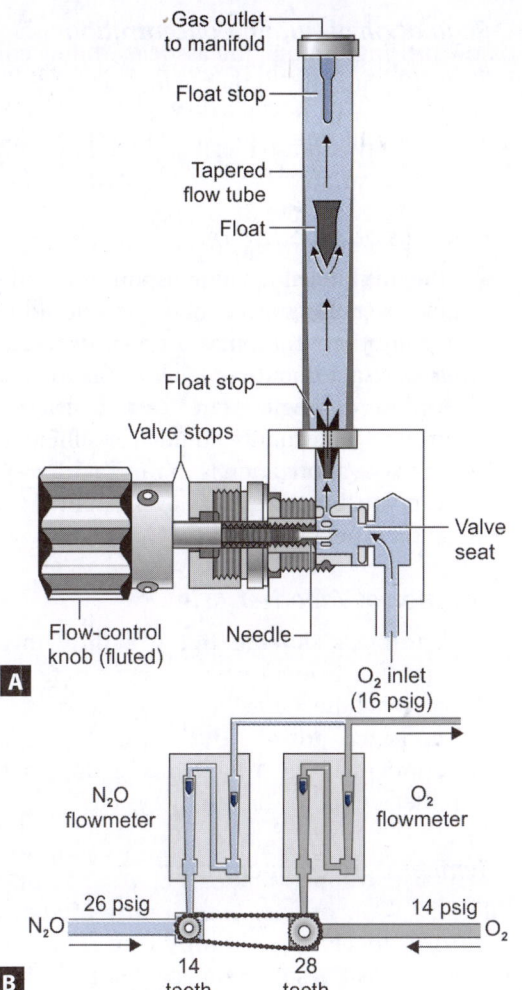
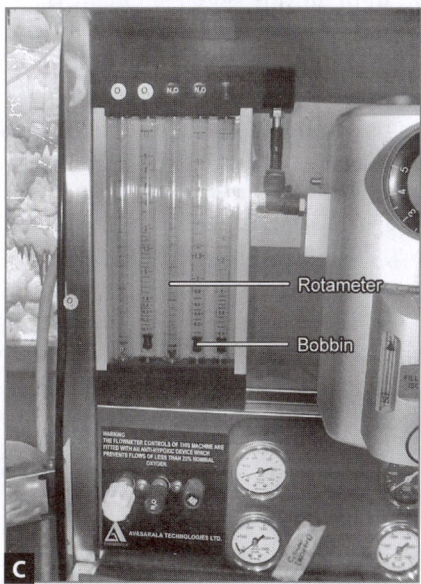

Figs. 7.4A to C: Flowmeter assembly (A) schematic representation; (B) Proportionating system; (C) Rotameter in anesthesia machine (Photograph).

🔑 KEY POINTS

Problems with flowmeters
Leaks, inaccuracy (if float sticks to wall), ambiguous scaling, etc., are the common problems with flowmeters. To overcome this most modern machines have electronic flow and digital displayer rather than conventional glass tubes.

a high-pressure oxygen source suitable for jet ventilation. However, a defective valve can stick in the fully open position and result in barotrauma, whereas sticking in a partially open position can dilute the inhaled anesthetic.

TESTING ANESTHESIA MACHINE

Most of the latest workstation possesses automatic self-check to rule out leak and sensor faults. In generic machines a comprehensive testing must be accomplished atleast daily. The goal of testing is to rule out leak and to ensure the proper functioning of proportionating system and hypoxic guard.

Testing should start from high-pressure system then to low-pressure system.

High-pressure System and Intermediate System

- Oxygen cylinder should be at least half-filled.
- There should be no hissing sound at hanger yoke assembly.
- For central supply pressure should be around 50–60 psi.

Low-pressure System

- Leaks from low-pressure system are difficult to find and some specialized tests are intended for this:
  - *Positive-pressure test*: Start O_2 flow at the rate of 4–5 liters per minute, then occlude the machine outlet. As the result of back pressure height of bobbin drops, provided there is no back pressure valve.
  - *Negative pressure test (universal leak test)*: Close all gas flow and connect the machine outlet to a suction bulb. Keep on squeezing till it collapses completely. This will generate negative pressure in machine and if there is leak in circuit, air will get sucked in leading to inflation of bag. Otherwise it will remain collapse. Do the same test by opening each vaporizes, to rule out leak from vaporizers.

VAPORIZERS

Vaporizer is a device through which volatile liquid anesthetic is converted into vapor, so that it can be delivered to patient in a controlled manner.

Rate of vaporization of a volatile anesthetic agent depend upon:
- Volatility of the agents
- Temperature of the liquid and its surrounding
- Flow rate of gases
- Surface area of contact between the gas and the liquid.

Classification of Vaporizers

Out of many classification, Dorsch and Dorsch classification of vaporizer is most popular. Dorsch and Dorsch classified vaporizers on the basis of:

Regulation of Output Concentration

- **Variable bypass type**: In these vaporizers entire carrier gas flow through the vaporizers.
- **Measured flow type**: Here measured amount of carrier gas pass through vaporizer.

Methods of Vaporization

- **Flow over type**: In these vaporizers carrier gas flow over the surface of anesthetic liquid for vaporization. They may be incorporated with wicks, so as to increase the surface area of contact.
- **Bubble through**: Here carrier gas bubble through anesthetic liquid, its efficiency in terms of vaporization is more than that of flow over type, but the control over extent of vaporization is poor.

Location of Vaporizer

- **Vaporizers outside the breathing system**: Vaporizer is incorporated between flowmeter and machine outlet.
- **Vaporizer inside the breathing system**: Vaporizer is incorporated after the machine outlet within the breathing system.

Temperature Compensation

During vaporization, temperature of anesthetic liquid decreases thereby reducing vapor pressure, as a result there is a gradual reduction in vaporization also. In order to obtain accurate control over vaporization, vapor pressure of anesthetic liquid must be kept constant. This can be achieved either by supplying heat directly or indirectly or by altering the flow of carrier gases.

On this basis vaporizer can be:
- **Noncompensated**: No means for temperature compensated.
- **Temperature compensation by supplying heat**: As by incorporating vaporizers in hot water bath or introducing an electric heater inside vaporizers. However, these techniques increase the risk of explosion hazards.
- **Temperature compensation by regulating flow**: In these vaporizers low temperature

induced decreased vapor pressure is compensated by increasing the flow of carrier gas into vaporizing chamber. This flow can be controlled either manually or via thermo-compensated valve.

Agent Specification

- **Agent specific**: These vaporizers are specific for a particular agent, e.g., sevoflurane vaporizers can be used for sevoflurane only.
- **Multiple agents**: A single vaporizer can be used for multiple agents.

Currently used vaporizers are agent specific, flow over, variable bypass type, temperature compensated, and are located outside the breathing system **(Fig. 7.5)**.

Principle of Vaporization

Most inhalational anesthetics in current use are volatile liquids. They are stored in liquid state and must be vaporized first for administration. Their vapors mixed with O_2 and other gases (if any) are then administered to patient.

Vapor Pressure

When a volatile liquid is kept in a closed container, molecules escape from liquid phase to vapor phase until equilibrium achieve. These molecules in vapor phase exert certain pressure against the wall of closed chamber, this pressure is called saturated vapor pressure. Saturated vapor pressure depends on the temperature and physical properties of liquid and is independent of atmospheric pressure.

Boiling Point

The boiling point of a liquid can be defined as the temperature at which saturated vapor pressure becomes equal to atmospheric pressure.

Latent Heat of Vaporization[Q]

When a molecule is converted from liquid to gaseous phase, energy is consumed. The amount of energy that is consumed is called latent heat of vaporization. The energy for vaporization comes either from the liquid itself or by outside source. In the absence of outside source, temperature of liquid decrease during vaporization. This reduction, if not compensated can markedly diminish subsequent vaporization.

Specific Heat

Specific heat of a substance is the number of calories required to increase the temperature

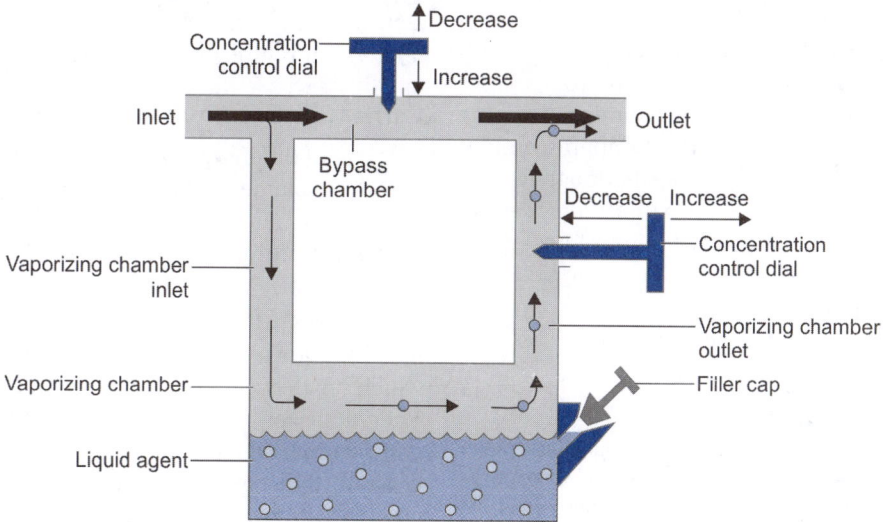

Fig. 7.5: Generic variable-bypass vaporizer.

of 1 g of substance (solid, liquid, or gas) by 1°C. The knowledge of specific heat is important for proper functioning of vaporizers. As this much heat must be supplied to liquid from outsides so as to maintain a constant temperature. Moreover material^Q of vaporizer should be of high specific heat to minimize the temperature changes associated with vaporization.

Thermal Conductivity

It is the measure of the speed at which heat flows through a substance. Vaporizer material should be of high thermal conductivity, so as to maintain uniform internal temperature.

Basic Operating Principle of a Variable Bypass Vaporizer

Most modern vaporizers are variable bypass vaporizers. Modern anesthesia machine use Tec vaporizers for halothane, isoflurane and sevoflurane. Component of Tec type vaporizers include concentration control dial, vaporizing chamber, the filter port, and filter cap **(Fig. 7.5)**.

Liquid anesthetic is poured into vaporizing chamber; through filler port, up to a maximum safe level. Fresh gas from the flowmeter enters the inlet of vaporizers. More than 80% of the flow passes through the bypass chamber to the vaporizer outlet, less than 20% of the flow passes through vaporizing chamber. The concentration control dial is a variable restrictor which controls relative flow of gases through bypass and vaporizing chambers. Depending on the temperature and vapor pressure of the liquid anesthetic agent gases passing through vaporizing chamber carry certain amount of volatiles agents with them. These gases get mixed with bypass chamber gases at outlet.

Most modern vaporizers (Tec 4, 5, 7) have bimetallic strip for temperature compensation, when temperature of liquid falls this strip leans to one side and flow through vaporizing chamber increase. Under hot conditions, reveres happen and flow through bypass chamber increases.

As boiling point of desflurane is below room temperature it require specialized vaporizer viz. Datex-Ohmeda Tec 6 vaporizer, Aladin cassette vaporizer, etc.

Factors Influencing a Vaporizer's Output Concentration

Flow Rate

Under both extremely low and extremely high flow rates, the output concentration is less than that of dial setting.

Temperature

Modern vaporizers possess mechanism for temperature compensation, which minimize the effect of cooling during vaporization.

Intermittent Back Pressure

Intermittent back pressure resulting from positive pressure ventilation can lead to higher than expected vaporizer output. This phenomenon known as pumping effect^Q is more pronounced at low flow rates, low dial setting, and high peak inspired pressure. Newer Tec 4, Tec 5 and Tec 7 are relatively immune from pumping effect.

Carrier Gas Composition

Because of difference in relative solubility of N_2O and O_2 in volatile anesthetic, output concentration changes when carrier gas concentration is changed rapidly.

Aladin Cassette Vaporizer

It is a unique electronically controlled vaporizers which can deliver five different inhalational agents. The vaporizer consists of a permanent internal control unit and an interchangeable agent specific cassette that contains anesthetic liquid. These cassettes are both color coded (for each anesthetic agent) and magnetically coded, so that integrated

> **KEY POINTS**
>
> Vaporizers are and made of copper. Copper has a high specific heat and thermal conductivity. Using copper in vaporizers material provides a physical means of rapid heat transfer.

circuit (IC) can identify which cassette has been inserted. Rest functioning is automatic.[1]

Sequence of Vaporizers

More than one vaporizer can be incorporated in workstation. Vaporizer of the agent with higher boiling point should be placed last otherwise vapors of this agent will condense in vaporizers of other agent with lower boiling point, e.g., sevoflurane will condense into desflurane vaporizer while desflurane will not condense in sevoflurane vaporizers.[2]

SAFETY FEATURES IN AN ANESTHESIA MACHINE

- To reduce fire
  - Antistatic rubber tyres
  - Rotating bobbin (so as to prevent friction charges over bobbin)
- To prevent cylinder swiping
  - Pin index system
- To ensure delivery of O_2
  - O_2 failure alarms
  - O_2 nitrous lock
  - Proportionating system
  - Fail-safe valve
  - O_2 flush
  - Color coding and bigger size of flow controlling knob of O_2
- Miscellaneous
  - Pressure reducing valve
  - Fluorescent back panel of rotameter, so that can be visualized even in the dark.

Safety Features of a Vaporizer

- **Color coding**: All new vaporizers are color coded **(Table 7.2)** and the anesthetic liquid is also packed in the same colored bottle.
- One way check valve at the outlet to minimize the back pressure effect of positive pressure ventilation (pumping effect).

- Permanent fitting in anesthesia workstation to prevent tilting effect.

Table 7.2: Some agent specific vaporizers.

Vaporizers name	Agent
EMO^Q vaporizer	Ether
Goldman^Q	Halothane
Boyle's ether vaporizer	Ether
Tec (red colored)	Halothane
Tec (purple)	Isoflurane
Tec (yellow)^Q	Sevoflurane
Tec 6^Q blue	Desflurane

(EMO: Epstein-Macintosh-Oxford)

LAST-MINUTE REVISION

- ASTM F1850-00 is the latest standard which anesthesia machine manufactures have to follow
- Oxygen cylinder: Black with white shoulder; pressure 2,000 psi and pin index 2–5.
- Nitrous oxide cylinder: Blue, pressure 760 psi and pin index 3–5.
- Moderns vaporizers are agent specific, flow over, variable bypass type and temperature compensated.
- Vaporizer of the agent with higher boiling point should be placed last.
- Color coding: Red: halothane; purple: isoflurane; yellow, sevoflurane; blue: desflurane.

REFERENCES

1. Kundra P, Goswami S, Parameswari A. Advances in vaporisation: A narrative review. Indian J Anaesth. 2020;64(3):171-180. doi: 10.4103/ija.IJA_850_19. Epub 2020 Mar 11. PMID: 32346162; PMCID: PMC7179779.
2. Chakravarti S, Basu S. Modern anaesthesia vapourisers. Indian J Anaesth. 2013;57(5):464-71. doi: 10.4103/0019-5049.120142. PMID: 24249879; PMCID: PMC3821263.

Section 1: Anesthesia

46 Unit I: Basics of Anesthesia

REVIEW QUESTIONS

1. All of the following are safety measures to prevent the delivery of hypoxic gas mixture to the patient, *except*:
   a. Location of O_2 valve after the N_2O valve
   b. Presence of pin index system to prevent wrong attachment of the N_2O and O_2 cylinders
   c. Location of fail-safe valve downstream from the N_2O supply source
   d. Proportionating system

2. Which gas is filled as liquid in cylinder?
   a. O_2
   b. Air
   c. N_2O
   d. Halothane

3. Regarding critical temperature which of the following statement is true:
   a. Critical temperature of O_2 is –119°C
   b. Critical temperature of N_2 is –119°C
   c. Critical temperature of N_2 is –16.5°C
   d. Critical temperature of N_2O is –136.5°C

4. All of the following cylinder colors are correctly matched, *except*:
   a. O_2: Black
   b. N_2O: Blue
   c. CO_2: Black
   d. Cyclopropane: Orange

5. As per hanger yoke assembly, oxygen cylinders of anesthesia machine possess:
   a. Pins at 2 and 5
   b. Holes at 2 and 5
   c. Pins at 3 and 5
   d. Hole at 3 whereas pin at 5

6. Fail-safe valve of anesthesia machine is located in:
   a. High-pressure circuit
   b. Low-pressure circuit
   c. Intermediate-pressure circuit
   d. Any of the above

7. Gas cylinders for anesthesia machine are made up of:
   a. Copper
   b. Bronze
   c. Molybdenum
   d. Iron

8. Epstein-Macintosh-Oxford (EMO) vaporizer had been used for:
   a. Ether
   b. Halothane
   c. Cyclopropane
   d. Trielene

9. Gas stored in liquid form is:
   a. CO_2
   b. N_2O
   c. Cyclopropane
   d. O_2

10. Pin index of nitrous oxide is:
    a. 1–5
    b. 2–5
    c. 3–5
    d. 1–6

ANSWERS

1. b	2. c	3. a	4. c	5. b	6. c
7. c	8. a	9. a and b	10. c		

CHAPTER 8

Anesthesia Breathing System

Anshul Jain

A breathing system can be defined as an assembly of components which connects the patient's airway to the anesthetic machine creating an artificial atmosphere, through and into which the patient breathes. Breathing system is vital as it maintains the oxygen (O_2) supply during anesthesia and simultaneously ensures the removal of carbon dioxide (CO_2).

PROPERTIES OF AN IDEAL BREATHING SYSTEM

- Simple and safe to use
- Provide adequate inspired O_2 concentration and efficient elimination of CO_2
- Easy to sterilize
- Permits spontaneous, manual and controlled ventilation in all age groups
- Should have minimal dead space and low resistance to gas flow
- Should be efficient, and require low fresh gas flow rate
- Protects the patient from barotrauma
- Sturdy, compact and lightweight in design
- Permits easy removal of waste exhaled gases
- Easy to maintain with minimal running cost.

CLASSIFICATION OF BREATHING SYSTEM

On the basis of notational boundaries, breathing system are classified into (Table 8.1):

Open System

It is a breathing system with infinite boundaries and no restriction on the entry of fresh gases or exit of exhaled gases. In this system, patient has access to atmosphere both during inspiration and expiration. Volatile agent is administered to patient with atmospheric air as vehicle. This system has no reservoir or rebreathing bag and hence, there is no rebreathing, e.g., open drop ether anesthesia via. Schimmelbusch mask. This system is least economic and produces maximum theater pollution. Hence, the system and equipment are not used now.

Semiopen System

It is a partially bounded breathing system with some restriction on fresh gas entry. In this system also, respiratory tract of the patient is

Table 8.1: Classification of breathing system.

System	Reservoir bag	Rebreathing	Types
Open	No	No	Bag and bottle
Semiopen	No	Partial (CO_2 build-up)	Bag and bottle with occlusive packing
Semiclosed without absorption	Yes	No/partial	Bains, modified Jackson Rees, Ayre's T-piece, Lack and Magill
Semiclosed with absorption	Yes	Partial	CO_2 absorbers with leak (circle and to and fro)
Closed	Yes	Complete	CO_2 absorbers with no leaks

open to atmosphere both during inspiration and expiration. However, some reservoir is made over the patient mouth/mask, e.g., in open drop anesthesia, if a towel is placed over Schimmelbusch mask to prevent early escape of anesthetic gases, then circuit become semiopen.

Closed System

Closed system is a fully bounded breathing system with no provision for fresh gas flow (FGF). There is total rebreathing in this system. Safety of closed system depends upon replacement of O_2 consumed by patient and removal of CO_2 produced by body. Thus, this system essentially requires CO_2 absorbent.

Semiclosed System

A fully bounded breathing system with some provision for elimination of expired gas. This is further subdivided into:

A. Semiclosed Nonrebreathing System

Here all the expired gases escape to atmosphere through nonrebreathing valve. This type ensures no rebreathing and essentially requires non-rebreathing valve, e.g., Ruben valve and Ambu bag are the examples of this breathing system.

B. Semiclosed Rebreathing System

Here part of expired gas escapes to the atmosphere through expiratory valve and this part passes to rebreathing bag, e.g., Mapleson D circuit.

MAPLESON SYSTEMS

Mapleson analyzed and described five different semiclosed systems according to the position of expiratory valve, fresh gas inlet, presence/position of reservoir bag and reservoir tubing (corrugated tube). They are referred to as Mapleson systems and are designated by letters A–E. Mapleson F system was introduced later as a modification of Mapleson E system **(Table 8.2)**.

Mapleson A (Magill Circuit and Lack Circuit)

It is one of the most widely used breathing system. In this type, reservoir bag is present at machine end while expiratory valve is located at patient end.

Functional Analysis (Figs. 8.1A to D)

- **Spontaneous ventilation**: Breathing system should be filled with fresh gas (FG) before connecting to the patient. During inspiration, patient takes FG breath from reservoir bag and corrugated tube. Expiratory valve remains closed in inspiration. At the start of expiration, gas from airway dead space enters the breathing system, hence, reservoir bag begins to fill with the expired dead space gas and FG from machine. This continues until reservoir bag is filled sufficiently and the pressure in the whole system becomes equal to opening pressure of expiratory valve. When the valve opening pressure is reached, expiratory valve opens and further expiratory gases are vented out through that valve. For a given setting if FGF is increased, pressure of breathing system reaches valve pressure early, and valve opens. Thus FGF can determine the opening of valve. In spontaneous ventilation, expiratory valve is usually kept open and a flow equal to alveolar minute ventilation (or 0.7 times minute volume) is sufficient to void the expiratory gases and prevent rebreathing.
- **Controlled ventilation**: Inspiratory tidal volume is delivered by squeezing reservoir bag, hence, expiratory valve must be partially closed otherwise gas will leak through expiratory valve. Further during controlled ventilation, pressure in breathing system is more in inspiratory phase (due to squeezing of bag) than expiratory phase, thus expiratory valve opens during inspiration and remains closed or open very late in expiration. As a result, the expired gas always returns to circuit and there is marked rebreathing. The extent of rebreathing can be reduced by increasing FGF, however, it is

Table 8.2: Mapleson breathing system.

Circuit	Design	Flow	
		Controlled ventilation	Spontaneous ventilation
Mapleson A	Breathing tube, APL valve, FGI, Breathing bag, Mask	Very high and difficult to predict	≈MV
Mapleson B	FGI, APL valve	2–2.5 MV	2 × MV
Mapleson C	FGI, APL valve	2–2.5 × MV	2 × MV
Mapleson D	APL valve, FGI	1–1.5 × MV	2–3 × MV
Mapleson E	FGI	3 × MV	2–3 × MV
Mapleson F	FGI	2 × MV	2–3 × MV

(FGI: fresh gas inlet; APL: ajustable pressure limiting; MV: minute ventilation)

never totally preventable. These properties make Mapleson A system, a most suited circuit for spontaneous ventilation[Q] and least suited circuit for controlled ventilation (**Figs. 8.1A to D**).

Mnemonic

Mapleson **A** is for an **a**wake patient[Q] (spontaneous ventilation).

Lack Circuit

This is the coaxial modification of Mapleson A. In lack circuit, there is an outer tube which receives FG from anesthesia machine, inside this tube a narrow tube is incorporated which has got expiratory valve at machine end. Patient inspires FG through outer tube and expires in inner tube.

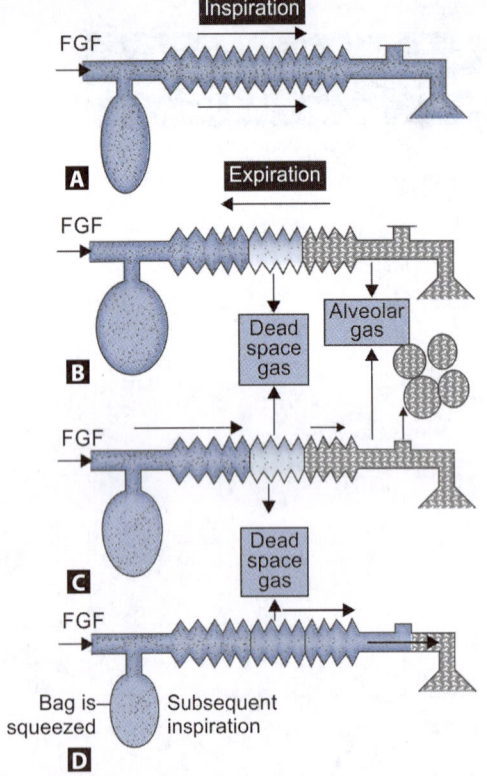

Figs. 8.1A to D: Functional analysis of Mapleson A system (controlled ventilation).
(FGF: fresh gas flow)

Mapleson B and C Systems

In Mapleson B system, both the FG inlet and expiratory valve are toward the patient end. The reservoir bag is present at other end of corrugated tube. Mapleson C system is essentially similar to Mapleson B system except that in C system corrugated tube is omitted and reservoir bag is directly attached to FG inlet. These circuits are less efficient than Mapleson A for spontaneous ventilation. Also for controlled ventilation, their efficiency is below Mapleson D system.

Mapleson D System

In this FG inlet is toward the patient end, expiratory valve and reservoir bag are present at the other end between two ends lies corrugated tube.

Functional Analysis

- **Spontaneous respiration (Figs. 8.2A to D):** The breathing system should be filled with FG before connecting to the patient. When the patient takes an inspiration, the FG from the machine, the reservoir bag and the corrugated tube flow to the patient.
  - During expiration, there is a continuous FGF into the system at the patient end. The expired air initially contains dead space gas which gets mixed with fresh gas and moves back into the corrugated tube and the reservoir bag. Once the pressure of system raises above opening pressure of valve, expiratory valve opens and afterwards expired alveolar excess gas is vented to the atmosphere. During the expiratory pause the fresh gas continues to flow and fill the proximal portion of the corrugated tube.
  - In subsequent inspiration patients breath fresh gas as well as mixed gas from corrugated tube. Thus there is rebreathing. The extent of rebreathing depends upon the volume of corrugated tube, length of expiratory pause, tidal volume of patient and FGF. Among all variables FGF can be controlled very easily. FGF^Q should be at least 1.5–2 times the patient's minute ventilation (MV) in order to minimize rebreathing to acceptable levels (Figs. 8.2A to D).
- **Controlled ventilation (Figs. 8.3A to C):** To facilitate intermittent positive pressure ventilation, the expiratory valve has to be partly closed, so that it opens only after sufficient pressure has developed in the system. Breathing system has to be filled with FG before connecting to the patient. When reservoir bag is squeezed, inspiration is delivered to patient by FG filled in corrugated tube. During expiration, the expired gas continuously gets mixed with the FG that is flowing into the system at the patient end. During the expiratory pause, the FG continues to enter the system and gets accumulated in corrugated tube. When bag is squeezed to deliver next inspiration, this accumulated FG forms

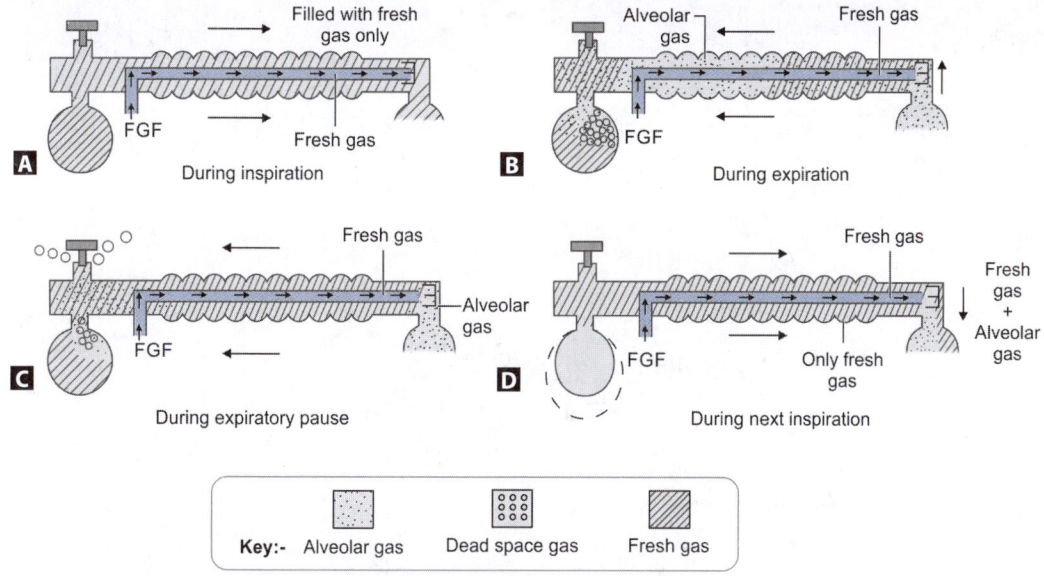

Figs. 8.2A to D: Spontaneous respiration with Mapleson D system (Bain circuit).
(FGF: fresh gas flow)

alveolar part of tidal volume, thus minimizing rebreathing. In inspiratory phase the pressure in the system increases, and expiratory valve opens and reservoir bag gases are discharged into the atmosphere. Thus, Mapleson D system is an ideal system for controlled breathing (Figs. 8.3A to C).

Note: From the above-mentioned functional analysis it should be clear that expiratory valve is not meant to be opened during expiratory phase only. Its opening is determined by the pressure in the system.

Modification of Mapleson D System

Bain Circuit (Fig. 8.4)

This circuit consists of two coaxial tubes, outer one is corrugated plastic tube, which carry expired gases and a second narrow tube of 7 mm diameter is incorporated inside the outer tube, which delivers the FG from anesthetic machine to patient end of circuit. At the other end of outer tube lies expiratory valve followed by reservoir bag.

In this system, the fresh gas flows through the inner tube whereas patient breathes the air collected in the annular space[Q] between the outer and inner tubes along with fresh gas. For spontaneous ventilation a FGF of 2.5 times of minute volume is required to prevent rebreathing. In controlled ventilation, a FGF of 70–100 mL per kg body weight is sufficient.

- **Advantages:** The circuit is light weight, can be used both in children and adults, resistance is very low. Moreover, it is the most economic circuit for controlled ventilation, thus this is the most widely used or universal circuit.[Q]
- **Limitations:** Mainly due to its inner tube which may get kinked, obstructed or disconnected. To overcome this, outer tube should be transparent enough so that inner tube can be visualized.

Penlon Circuit

Modified version of Bain circuit, which can be easily connected to scavenging system. Through scavenging system expired gases are vented outside operation theater (OT) thereby reducing

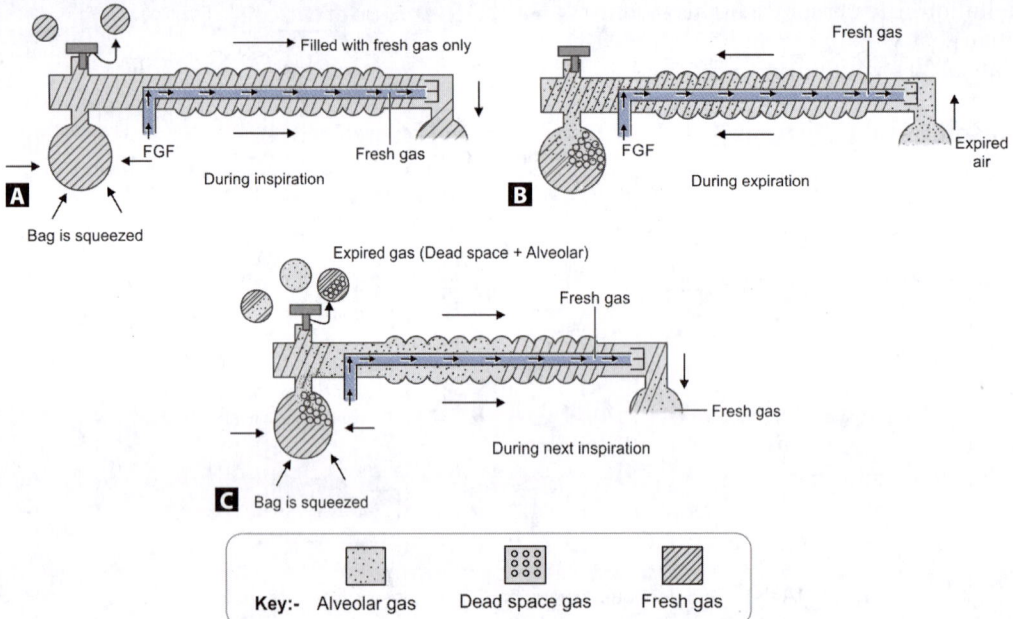

Figs. 8.3A to C: Controlled ventilation with Mapleson D system.
(FGF: fresh gas flow)

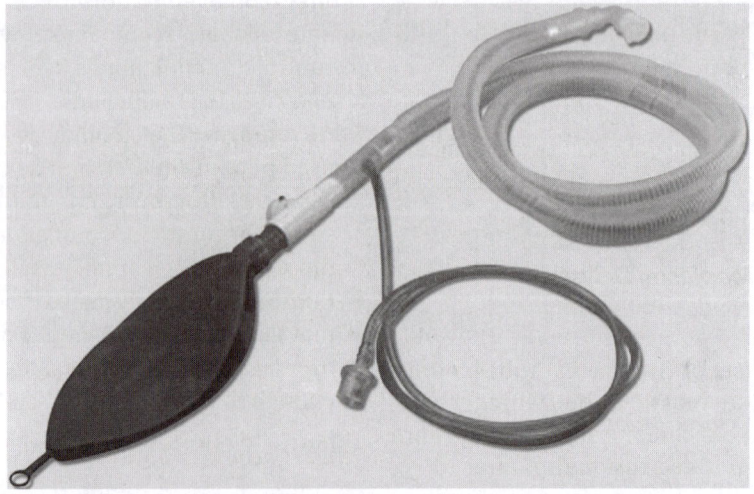

Fig. 8.4: Bain circuit as whole.

OT pollution. The resistance of this system is also less than that of Bain circuit (0.5 cm of H_2O at a flow rate of 30 L/minute).

Mapleson E and F Systems

In this system, Ayre's T-piece is connected to corrugated tube. FG inlet is at patient end. Mapleson type E lacks reservoir bag and expiratory valve. Here corrugated tube acts as reservoir. Due to absence of valve and reservoir bag, this circuit is virtually free of resistance. This absence of reservoir bag also restricts its use only for spontaneous ventilation. Controlled ventilation for brief period can be administered by occluding free end of corrugated tube.[Q] However, due to absence of reservoir bag, it is not possible to predict the tidal volume.

Mapleson type F (In 1950 Jackson Rees modified the original Ayre's T piece by adding an open-ended 500 mL bag to expiratory limb). Through this bag controlled ventilation becomes easy and tidal volume can also be predicted. Mapleson F[Q] requires FGF of 1.6 × minute volume for controlled ventilation and 2.5 × minute volume for spontaneous ventilation.

As both of them are free of resistance, they are mainly used in pediatric patients, where resistance matters a lot. In pediatric patients Mapleson F[Q] (Jackson Rees modification) is the most commonly used breathing circuit.

⚡ KEY POINTS

Efficiency of different mapleson system
- Spontaneous ventilation: A > DFE > CB
- Controlled ventilation: DFE > BC > A

Mnemonic

Mapleson **A**:	**A**wake patient
Mapleson **D**:	**D**octor is ventilating (i. e., controlled ventilation)
Mapleson **E**:	**I**nfant

Other Modifications

Hafnia System

In this system expiratory valve of Mapleson A, B, C and D are replaced by suction port through which expired gases are sucked and vented out of OT to reduce OT pollution.

ABSORBER BREATHING SYSTEM (CLOSED SYSTEM)

The circuits described till now require a minimum flow equal to alveolar ventilation (i.e., at least 5 L/minute in an adult) for proper functioning. If we consider the fact that body consumes only 250 mL O_2 per minute, one must realize that more than 4,500 mL gas is wasted per minute. Along with this fact that beside CO_2 all other exhaled gases (O_2, N_2, etc.) can be inspired again, leads to the development of absorber breathing systems. In these systems, expired gases are reused after absorption of CO_2. Absorber breathing system not only provide advantage in terms of better conservation of anesthetic gases but also humidify gases (through exhaled water vapors), limits OT pollution and conserves heat (FG are usually dry and cold while exhaled gases are warm and humid).

Essential component of absorber system is CO_2 absorbent which absorbs CO_2 from exhaled gases. There are two types of absorber breathing system:

To-and-Fro System (Water's System) (Fig. 8.5)

This system has the basic configuration of Mapleson C. There lies a canister of CO_2 absorber, between expiratory valve and breathing bag. During expiration, expired gases mixed with FG passes into reservoir bag via canister. In canister CO_2 is absorbed, so gases reaching reservoir bag are free of CO_2. Inspiration is provided by the reservoir bag, as CO_2 absorption is there, a flow less than alveolar ventilation can maintain oxygenation. To-and-fro system is a low resistance handy circuit but it is not used nowadays because of following limitations:

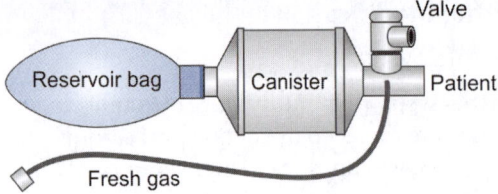

Fig. 8.5: To-and-fro system (water's system).

- **Dead space**: Soda lime consumption begins from patient end and thus there is a progressive increase in dead space of system.
- **Channeling**: When circuit is placed horizontally, soda lime granules settle down creating channels between upper wall of canister and soda lime granules. Through these channels expired gases can flow without being purged of CO_2.
- **Soda lime dust inhalation**: As canister is very near to patient inspired gases may contain soda lime dust.
- **Weight and bulk of apparatus**: Because of heavy canister, there is continuous traction on endotracheal tube.

Circle System

The components of circle system are shown in **Figure 8.6**. System consists of two-unidirectional valves (inspiratory and expiratory valves) that maintain unidirectional flow, CO_2 absorber canister, reservoir bag, an inlet port for FGF and a common outlet connected to patient via Y-piece. Circle system is the breathing system used for:

- **Low flow anesthesia**: FGF is less than half the MV
- **Closed circuit anesthesia**: Delivery of gases in amounts sufficient to replace only the gases consumed by patient.

CARBON DIOXIDE ABSORBENT

Carbon dioxide absorbents are the prime requirement for low flow anesthesia. CO_2 absorbents are soda lime, baralyme, calcium hydroxide lime, etc. Out of these, baralyme is not used nowadays.

Soda Lime

Soda lime is the most widely used CO_2 absorbent. It is a mixture of:
- Calcium hydroxide $[Ca(OH)_2]$—95%
- Sodium hydroxide (NaOH)—4%
- Potassium hydroxide (KOH)—1%
- Silica (to prevent powdering and dust formation)
- Indicators.

Potassium hydroxide is an activator while NaOH acts as catalyst. Soda lime is used in granular form;

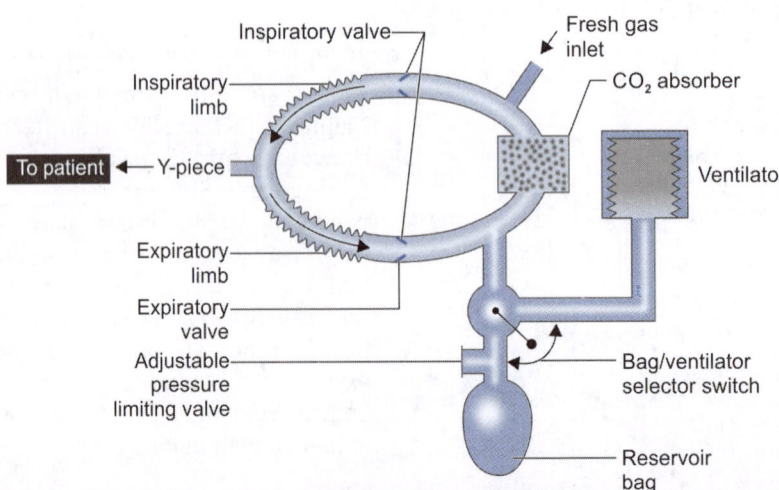

Fig. 8.6: Generic circle system.

Chapter 8: Anesthesia Breathing System

> **KEY POINTS**
>
> **Closed system versus semiclosed system**
> **Advantages:**
> - Economical
> - Less operation theater pollution
> - Conserves heat and humidity
> - Low resistance
> - Same flow is required for both spontaneous and controlled ventilation
> - In conditions where CO_2 production is high only closed system with CO_2 absorber can eliminate expired CO_2.
>
> **Disadvantages:**
> - Bulky, so chance of accidental extubation is always there due to continuous drag on endotracheal tube.
> - If CO_2 absorber gets exhausted, there can be dangerous hypercapnia. So, closed circuit should be used in congestion with inspiratory and expiratory CO_2 concentration monitoring only.
> - Produce carbon monoxide and compound A.
> - Malfunctions of unidirectional valve can lead to sudden increase in resistance.

size of granules should be such that it provides effective surface area without much increase in resistance to airflow. Smaller the granule size, the greater is the absorptive surface area. However, as particle size decreases, airflow resistance increases. Particle size used clinically represents a compromise between resistance to airflow and absorptive efficiency. Clinically, a size of 4–8 mesh[Q] solves the purpose. Hardness number of the granules should be above 75.

Chemical Reactions

Carbon dioxide absorption by soda lime is not a physical process like water (H_2O) absorption by sponge. Rather it occurs via series of chemical reactions. Presence of moisture is essential for these reactions, the equations are as follows:
1. $CO_2 + H_2O \rightleftharpoons H_2CO_3$
2. $H_2CO_3 + 2NaOH\ [KOH] \rightleftharpoons Na_2CO_3\ (K_2CO_3) + 2H_2O + Heat$
3. $Na_2CO_3\ (K_2CO_3) + Ca(OH)_2 \rightleftharpoons CaCO_3 + 2NaOH\ (KOH)$

As the reaction is exothermic, the expired gases automatically get warmed.

Note: 100 g soda lime absorb 24–26 L of CO_2.[Q]

Signs of Soda Lime Exhaustion

- **Indicators**: Indicators are added to soda lime, so that exhaustion of soda lime can be identified easily. Commonly used indicators are:

Indicator	Color	
	Fresh	Exhausted
Ethyl violet	White	Violet
Phenolphthalein	White	Pink
Mimosa Z	Pink	White

- **Physical changes**: After exhaustion, granules become soft and heavy. Temperature of soda lime canister decreases.
- **Clinical signs**: After exhaustion, there is improper absorption of CO_2 or CO_2 is being rebreathed, which can result in hypercapnia. Suggested clinically by tachycardia, hypertension and increased oozing from wound. If capnography is being performed end-tidal carbon dioxide ($EtCO_2$) would increase and graph never reaches baseline.

Baralyme

It is a mixture of 20% barium hydroxide [$Ba(OH)_2$] and 80% $Ca(OH)_2$. Baralyme does not contain silica and NaOH and is less efficient than soda lime. Baralyme may produce fire in breathing system when used with sevoflurane because of these reasons, it is not used nowadays.

Calcium Hydroxide Lime (Amsorb)

It is the newest member of CO_2 absorbents consists primarily of $Ca(OH)_2$ and calcium chloride ($CaCl_2$) and contains two setting agents—calcium sulfate ($CaSO_4$) and polyvinyl pyrrolidone (PVP). Most significant advantage of $Ca(OH)_2$ lime over other agents is its stability with volatile agents. Chances of carbon monoxide (CO) and compound A production are not there, and possibility of fire is also least. Disadvantages include less absorptive capacity and higher cost.

Complications of Carbon Dioxide Absorbents

Interaction with Inhalational Anesthetics

In the presence of alkali and heat, trichloroethylene degrades into the cerebral neurotoxin dichloroacetylene and phosgene, a potent pulmonary irritant. Sevoflurane interacts with soda lime and baralyme to form compound A. Production is more when:
- Low-flow or closed-circuit anesthetic techniques
- Baralyme is being used
- Higher concentrations of sevoflurane is being used
- Higher temperature
- Fresh absorbent.

Carbon Monoxide Production

Strong-base absorbents degrade inhalational anesthetics to produce clinically significant concentrations of CO, as well as trifluoromethane. Higher levels of CO are more likely after prolonged contact between absorbent and anesthetics, as well as after disuse of an absorber for at least 2 days, especially over a weekend. Thus, CO poisoning, if seen is more common in patients anesthetized on Monday morning.

OTHER OXYGEN DELIVERY DEVICES

Circuits and systems described so far requires at least an assistant who applies them to patient. Moreover, they are bulky and prohibit the patient to talk, a situation which is totally unliked by patients in regional anesthesia. In intensive care unit (ICU) setup also, there is requirement for O_2 supplementation. So, O_2 delivery devices were invented, these devices are light, small and can be used in a conscious patient to provide variable degree of inspiratory O_2 concentration.

LAST-MINUTE REVISION

- In current practice, semiclosed and closed systems are the most commonly used.
- Mapleson system is the type of semiclosed system. Mapleson A is ideal for spontaneous whereas Mapleson D is ideal for controlled ventilation. Mapleson E is best for infants.
- Bain circuit and Penlon circuit are the modification of Mapleson D system. Lack circuit is the modification of Mapleson A circuit.
- Soda lime, baralyme and calcium hydroxide lime are the carbon dioxide absorbent. Chances of carbon monoxide and compound A production are least with calcium hydroxide lime.

REVIEW QUESTIONS

1. All reduce carbon dioxide absorption in a closed circuit, *except*:
    a. High flow
    b. Small granule size
    c. Large granule size
    d. Channeling
2. Which of the following devices provides fixed performance oxygen therapy?
    a. Nasal cannula
    b. Venturi mask
    c. Oxygen by T-piece
    d. Edinburg mask
3. Bain circuit is a modification of:
    a. Mapleson A circuit
    b. Mapleson B circuit
    c. Mapleson C circuit
    d. Mapleson D circuit

Chapter 8: Anesthesia Breathing System

4. **Pediatric patients are anesthetized with which circuit:**
   a. Mapleson A circuit
   b. Mapleson E circuit
   c. Mapleson C circuit
   d. Mapleson D circuit

5. **Mapleson breathing circuit represents:**
   a. Open system
   b. Closed system
   c. Semiclosed system
   d. Semiopen system

ANSWERS

1. b   2. b   3. d   4. b   5. c

CHAPTER 9

Airway Management

Anshul Jain, Brijendra Verma

INTRODUCTION

No act can better define an anesthesiologist than the ability to manage patient's breathing and airway.

Airway management is not only limited to anesthetize patients. It is required in any individual in whom normal ventilation is hampered, cause of which ranges from minor facial trauma to septic shock.

AIRWAY ASSESSMENT

The purpose of airway assessment is to identify possible difficulty in direct laryngoscopy (and hence tracheal intubation), mask ventilation and creation of a surgical (percutaneous) airway if required. Airway assessment is made through clinical history, physical examination and a specific airway assessment test. Imaging is valuable in cases with known airway problem but is not indicated for routine assessment.

History

It includes review of previous anesthesia records and direct questioning of the patient. A history of previous airway difficulty is highly suggestive of difficult airway. Similarly snoring usually suggest potentially difficult airway.

Physical Examination

The combined assessment of mouth opening, jaw protrusion and head extension is the core of airway assessment. Physical examination should include:
- **Patency of nares**: Look for masses inside nasal cavity (polyps), deviated nasal septum, etc.
- **Mouth opening**: Mouth opening of at least two finger breadths between upper and lower incisors in adults is desirable. Reduced mouth opening makes both intubation and laryngeal mask airway (LMA) insertion difficult.
- **Teeth**: Prominent upper incisors make alignment of oral and pharyngeal axis difficult. On the other hand in edentulous patients tongue can obstruct hypopharyngeal structures.
- **Temporomandibular (TM) movement**: Restricted TM joint movement reduces mouth opening.
- **Physiological conditions**: Pregnancy and obesity are associated with difficult airway.

Assessing Airway Risk

L.E.M.O.N. the generic mnemonic, the components of LEMON should be assessed before airway management.

L: Look externally: Facial trauma, beard, loose teeth, dentures, large incisors indicates difficult airway.

E: Evaluate the 3-3-2 rule
- Can 3 fingers fit between the incisors?
- Can 3 fingers fit between the tip of the chin and the hyoid bone?
- Can 2 fingers fit from the top of the thyroid notch to the hyoid bone?

A decrease in these distances indicates difficult airway.

M: Mallampati score (see below): Mallampati score >2 indicates difficult airway.

O: Obstruction or obesity: Obesity (body mass index >30) can be a predictor of a difficult airway. Obstruction of the airway, including head and neck cancer, epiglottitis, also point towards a difficult airway.

Chapter 9: Airway Management

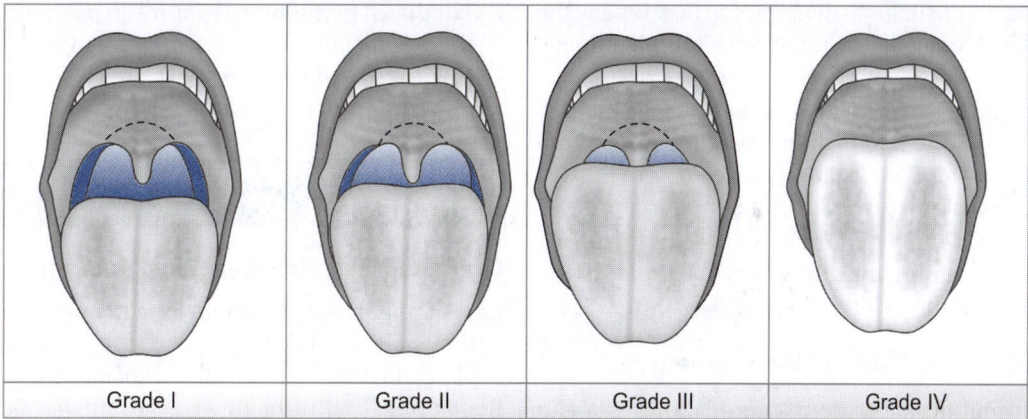

Fig. 9.1: Mallampati grading.

N: Neck mobility: Immobile neck due to trauma, c-collar, or rigidity can lead to difficult airway.[1]

Specific Airway Assessment Tests

Mallampati Classification (Fig. 9.1)

Mallampati score or classification correlates tongue size to pharyngeal size. Test is performed with the patient in the sitting position, head in neutral position, the mouth wide open and the tongue protruding to its maximum. Patient should not be actively encouraged to phonate as phonation can provide false positive results. Classification is assigned according to the visibility of pharyngeal structures. Originally three grades were proposed:
- **Grade I**: Visualization of the soft palate, fauces; uvula, anterior and the **p**osterior **p**illars.
- **Grade II**: Visualization of the soft palate, fauces and tip of **u**vula.
- **Grade III**: Visualization of **s**oft palate and base of uvula.
  In 1987 Samsoon and Young added Grade IV.
- **Grade IV**: Only **h**ard palate is visible. Soft palate is not visible at all.

Mnemonic

> **PUSH**
> **P**osterior Pillar, **U**vula, **S**oft palate, **H**ard palate

Mandibular Protrusion

The protruding ability of the mandible depends on proper functioning of TM joint function. Inability to protrude mandible (the mandibular incisors cannot be brought in line with the maxillary incisors) is associated with difficult intubation.

> **KEY POINTS**
>
> Normal neck mobility:
> - **Extension**: 80°
> - **Flexion**: 30–40°
> - Rotation (occurs at atlanto-axial joint)
>
> Classically, it was taught that flexion and extension occurs at atlanto-occiput joint but latest studies revealed atleast equal or more contribution of atlanto-axial joint.

Neck Movements

Atlanto-occipital extension assesses feasibility to make sniffing position for intubation. Limited head (more accurately described as occipito-atlanto-axial) extension impairs direct laryngoscopy and hence intubation.

Thyromental Distance (Patil's Test)

It is defined as the distance from the mentum to the thyroid notch while the patient's neck is fully extended. Thyromental (T-M) distance measurement helps in determining how readily the laryngeal axis will fall in line with the pharyngeal axis when the atlanto-occipital joint is extended.

Alignment of these two axes is difficult if the T-M distance is <6 cm (less than three finger breadths) in adults. The T-M distance, however, is of limited value as a predictor of difficult laryngoscopy.

Some dental patterns, such as protruding, single or missing maxillary incisors, increase the difficulty of direct laryngoscopy.

Who Require Airway Management?

In normal awake patient, there is always a gap between tongue and soft palate. In an unconscious or semiconscious individual there is hypotonia of genioglossus and geniohyoideus muscle because of which tongue falls back and tends to obstruct the upper airway. Thus patient requires some sort of maneuvers or equipment to maintain the patency of airway.

Manual Airway Maneuvers (Figs. 9.2A to C)

- **Head tilt chin lift maneuver**: Preferred technique for opening the airway of a patient who has sustained trauma.
- **Jaw thrust maneuver**: Preferred in patient when there is suspicion of cervical spine injury.
- **Jaw thrust maneuver with head tilt**: Most efficient, used in operating room.

EQUIPMENT FOR AIRWAY MANAGEMENT

Oral and Nasal Airways (Figs. 9.3A and B)

Loss of upper airway muscle tone in anesthetized patients allows the tongue and epiglottis to fall back against the posterior wall of the pharynx. Repositioning the head or a jaw thrust is the preferred technique for opening the airway.

Oral and nasal airways are the devices which keeps upper airway patent. Awake or lightly anesthetized patients may cough or even develop laryngospasm during airway insertion if laryngeal reflexes are intact. Placement of an oral airway is sometimes facilitated by suppressing airway reflexes and, in addition, sometimes by depressing the tongue with a tongue blade.

Guedel airway (made up of plastic) and Water's airway (metallic) are commonly used airway.

Nasal airways, though well tolerated have got the risk of epistaxis and should not be used in bleeding disorders, children with prominent adenoids and patient with basilar fracture.

Face Mask (Fig. 9.4)

Face mask facilitates delivery of oxygen or anesthetic gas from a breathing system to patient by creating an airtight seal with the patient's face. Transparent masks allow observation of exhaled humidified gas and immediate recognition of vomiting.

Several mask designs are available. They are available in sizes 0–5. Application of appropriate size is must, large size mask would significantly increase dead space, whereas small size produces significant air leak.

Positive pressure ventilation by compressing the bag attached to breathing circuit produces remarkable air entry in esophagus and stomach too. When excessive amount of air enters stomach

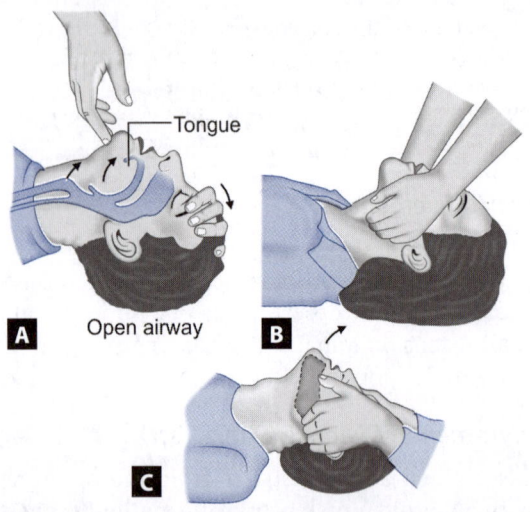

Figs. 9.2A to C: Manual airway maneuvers. (A) Head tilt chin lift; (B) Jaw thrust; (C) Jaw thrust with head tilt.

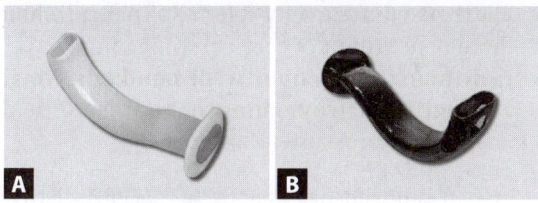

Figs. 9.3A and B: Oropharyngeal airway: (A) Guedel airway; (B) Water's airway

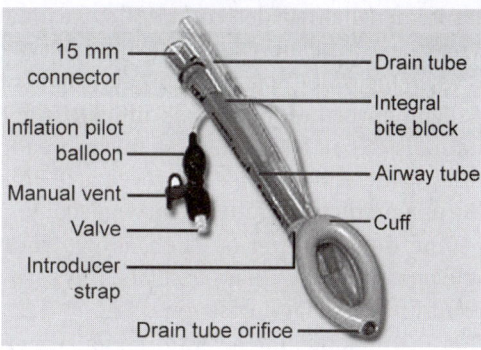

Fig. 9.5: Laryngeal mask airway.

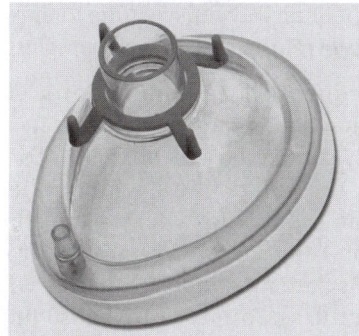

Fig. 9.4: Face mask.

or in condition, where intragastric pressure is already high, patient might vomit and can aspirate the gastric contents. So bag and mask ventilation is contraindicated[Q] in:
- Congenital diaphragmatic hernia
- Tracheoesophageal fistula
- Full stomach patient
- Intestinal obstruction
- Pregnancy
- Hiatus hernia

Supraglottic Airway Devices

These devices are placed above glottis for airway management. The most popular supraglottic airway device is laryngeal mask airway (LMA).

Laryngeal Mask Airway (Fig. 9.5)

Laryngeal mask airway forms a seal in the pharynx between the respiratory and digestive tracts. LMA tends to protect the airway and facilitate gas exchange. So, it has surpassed the combitube as a preferred device to manage a difficult airway.

Three types of LMAs are commonly used:
1. Classic™ LMA
2. ProSeal™
3. Fastrach™/Intubating LMA

Classic™ Laryngeal Mask Airway (Brain Mask)

LMA consists of a wide-bore tube whose proximal end connects to a breathing circuit with a standard 15 mm connector; its distal end is attached to an elliptical cuff which when inflated forms a low-pressure seal around the entrance to the larynx. LMA insertion requires an anesthetic depth slightly greater than required for the insertion of an oral airway. Propofol or sevoflurane provides excellent conditions for LMA insertion. Short-acting narcotics like fentanyl trends to make insertion easy.

The LMA partially protects the larynx from pharyngeal secretions (but not from gastric regurgitation).

Recommended sizes of LMA according to the weight of patient have been mentioned in **Table 9.1**.

ProSeal™ Laryngeal Mask Airway (Fig. 9.5)

The ProSeal™ laryngeal mask airway (PLMA) provides better seal and possesses a separate orifice for nasogastric tube. ProSeal™ LMA provides better laryngeal protection. Moreover, it allows positive-pressure ventilation with higher airway pressure in comparison to Classic™ LMA.

Table 9.1: Recommended sizes of LMA.

Laryngeal mask airway (LMA) size	Patient category	Weight (kg)
1	Infant	<6.5
2	Child	6.5–20
2½	Child	20–30
3	Small adult	30–50
4	Normal adult	50–70
5	Larger adult	>70

Other features include a reinforced airway tube and an integrated bite block.

A greater depth of anesthesia is required for insertion of a PLMA than Classic LMA. The insertion technique is also difficult. **Table 9.2** shows advantages and disadvantages of LMA.

Intubating/Fastrach™ Laryngeal Mask Airway

Special LMA that allows insertion of endotracheal tube (ETT) through it. It is especially indicated for intubating patients with difficult airways. Endotracheal tube up to size 8 can be passed through intubating LMA. Contraindications of PLMA and intubating LMA are same as that of classic LMA.

Contraindications for the Laryngeal Mask Airway

- Patients with oropharyngeal pathology
- Full stomach

Table 9.2: Advantages and disadvantages of LMA.

Advantages	Disadvantages
Less invasive	Increased risk of gastrointestinal aspiration
Very useful in difficult intubations	Less safe in prone or jack-knife positions
Less trauma to tooth and larynx	Limits maximum PPV
Less laryngospasm and bronchospasm	Less secure airway
Does not require muscle relaxation	Greater risk of gas leak and OT pollution
Does not require neck mobility	Can cause gastric distention
No risk of esophageal or endobronchial intubation	

(PPV: positive pressure ventilation; OT: operation theater)

- Patients who are at risk for aspiration (hiatus hernia, pregnancy)
- Low pulmonary compliance conditions (e.g., restrictive airways disease) requiring peak inspiratory pressures >30 cm H_2O.

Note: In bronchospastic and chronic obstructive pulmonary disease (COPD) patient (traditionally considered as contraindication) LMA is associated with less bronchospasm than a tracheal tube.

Combitube (Fig. 9.6)

Most frequently used supraglottic device in prehospital and emergency setting. It consists of two tubes connected side by side. When inserted blindly, the longer and wider tube usually enters the esophagus whereas the shorter and thin tube remains above glottis. By inflating both cuffs patient can be ventilated. Esophageal cuff simultaneously provides protection against aspiration. If esophageal tube enters trachea, combitube behaves like an infraglottic device.

Infraglottic Airway Devices

At the name suggests, these devices are placed below the glottis. Endotracheal tube is the most frequently used infraglottic airway. Tracheostomy tube, cricothyroidotomy cannula are other infraglottic airways devices.

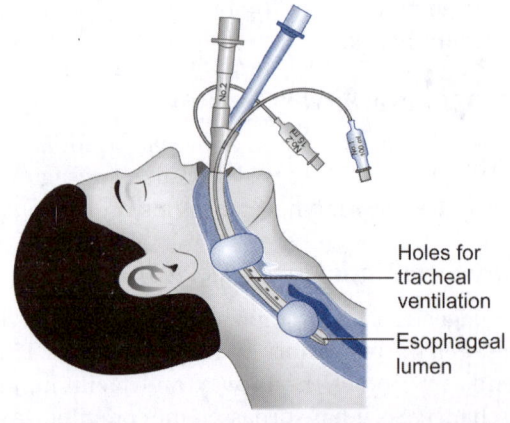

Fig. 9.6: Combitube.

Tracheal Tubes

Tracheal tubes (TT) are the gold standard device[Q] for airway management. They provide a secure channel through the upper airway and ensure maximum airway protection. The tracheal end of tube lies in the mid to lower part of the trachea, whereas the proximal end lies outside the mouth or nose, where it is connected to an anesthesia circuit or other device.

It must be noted though they are the best technique of airway management, they are associated with many adverse effects like sore throat, tracheomalacia, transmission of infection, etc.

Following materials are approved for manufacturing TT—polyvinyl chloride (PVC), red rubber and silicon. Currently, disposable PVC tubes are the most frequent one.

Adult TTs have a cuff near the distal end, which when inflated forms a seal against the tracheal wall to protect the lungs from pulmonary aspiration. Cuff also ensures that the tidal volume delivered ventilates the lungs and do not escape out through the upper airway.

Uncuffed tubes are usually used in children to minimize the risk of pressure injury and postintubation croup.

There are two major types of cuffs:
1. **High pressure low volume**: These are associated with more ischemic damage to the tracheal mucosa and are less suitable.
2. **Low pressure high volume**: They increase the chances of sore throat (larger mucosal contact area), aspiration, spontaneous extubation, and difficult insertion (because of the floppy cuff). But due to the lesser chance of mucosal damage, low-pressure cuffs tubes are preferred **(Fig. 9.7)**.

There are many modifications of TT some important one includes:
- **Armored tubes**: Flexible, spiral-wound, wire-reinforced TTs which resist kinking and are used in head and neck surgeries, surgery in prone position.
- **Microlaryngeal tubes**: For laryngeal surgery.

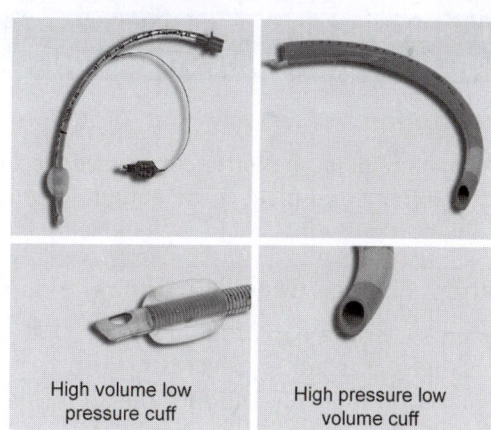

Fig. 9.7: High and low pressure cuffs.

- **Ring-Adair-Elwyn (RAE) preformed tubes for head and neck surgeries**: RAE tube named after (Ring, Adair, and Elwyn) the scientists who invented it. They can be **south facing**, i.e., machine end is toward the foot of patient (used in nasal, neurosurgery); or *north facing*, i.e., machine end is toward the head of patient (used for mandibular surgery and neck surgery).
- **Endotrol tube**: Special tube for nasal intubation, in this tube angle of tip can be changed.
- **Double-lumen TT**: For thoracic surgery.

Estimation of Size of Endotracheal Tubes

As both undersize and oversize tube creates problem, it is must to estimate the appropriate size of the tube before accomplishing intubation:

Patient category	Size of endotracheal tubes
Preterm baby	2.5 mm internal diameter
0–6 months	3–3.5 mm internal diameter
6 months to 1 year	3.5–4 mm internal diameter
1–6 years	Age (in years)/3 + 3.5 mm
6–16 years	Age (in years)/4 + 4.5 mm
Adult male	8.0–9.0 mm internal diameter
Adult female	7.0–8.0 mm internal diameter

TECHNIQUES OF DIRECT LARYNGOSCOPY AND INTUBATION

Preparation

Preparation for intubation encompasses checking of equipment and placing the patient in proper position.

Patient Position (Magill Position)

Patient's airway is curved in three axes: Oral axis, pharyngeal axes and laryngeal axis. When a patient is placed in morning sniffing[Q] position (*Magill position*) in which there is flexion (30–40°) at C_2–C_4 level and extension at (80°) occipito-atlanto-axial complex, these three axes get aligned **(Figs. 9.8A to C)**.

Flexion of lower cervical spine can be achieved by elevating the head by keeping a 8–10 cm thick pillow under occiput.

Preoxygenation[Q]

Before administering any anesthetic agent, the patient is ventilated with 100% O_2, so as to replace nitrogen of lung (denitrogenation)[Q] with oxygen. This increases the apnea tolerability as the excess oxygen in lung will take part in gaseous exchange during the period apnea.

🔑 KEY POINTS

- On room air breathing partial pressure of various gases in lung is: PO_2: 100 mm of Hg, CO_2: 40.0 mm of Hg, H_2O: 47.0 mm of Hg, N_2: 573 mm of Hg.
- After preoxygenation partial pressure of N_2 reduces whereas PO_2 raises.

Direct Laryngoscopy

After inducing general anesthesia with either intravenous or inhalational method, muscle relaxant is administered. Succinylcholine inspite of many adverse effects is still the most commonly used muscle relaxant for intubation.[Q] Amongst nondepolarizers, rocuronium[Q] is the most preferred muscle relaxant. If a nondepolarizer is supposed to be administered anesthetist should check that he would be able to ventilate or not by giving two or three puffs of positive pressure ventilation. As the effect of muscle relaxant comes (which is usually 60 sec for scoline and 120–240 sec for nondepolarizers) tracheal tube is guided

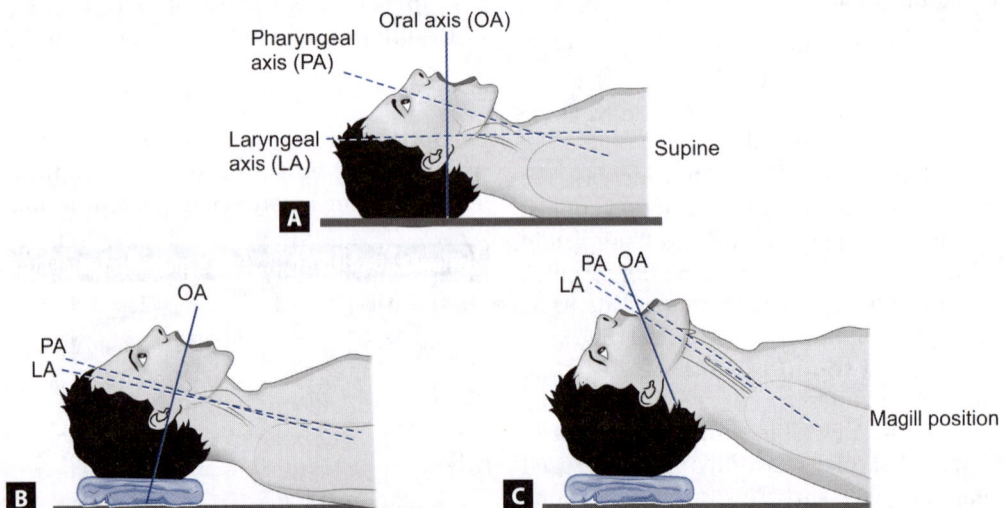

Figs. 9.8A to C: Steps for Magill position. (A) Supine; (B) Supine with flexion at lower cervical vertebrae; (C) Supine with flexion at lower cervical vertebrae and extension at atlanto-occipital joint.

into trachea under direct vision using direct laryngoscopy.

Among the variety of laryngoscopes blades available Macintosh blade[Q] is most preferred.

Technique of Laryngoscopy (Figs. 9. 9A and B)

For a normal right handed person the laryngoscope is held in the left hand. The blade is introduced through the right side of the oropharynx—with care to avoid the trauma to teeth. The tip of a Macintosh blade lies in vallecula, and the straight blade tip covers the epiglottis. Trapping a lip between the teeth and the blade and leverage on the teeth should be avoided. The TT, is passed through the abducted vocal cords under direct vision by the right hand. The laryngoscope is withdrawn, with

KEY POINTS

- **Length of tube to be inserted:** Optimally tracheal end of tube should lie 3–5 cm above carina. To achieve this tube should be inserted 19–21 cm in females and 20–22 cm in males. In children insertion length is calculated by following formula:

$$\frac{Age\ (in\ years)}{2} + 12$$

- **Cuff pressure:** Cuff can be inflated with air or water with pressure which <30 cm H_2O. Pressure >30 cm H_2O can produces tracheal ischemia. When N_2O is being used, it may diffuse in cuff and can increase cuff pressure. So cuff should be deflated intermittently. In children <5 years uncuffed tube should be used.

KEY POINTS

Esophageal intubation
Following features suggest esophageal intubation:
- Absent air entry in chest
- Presence of air entry in epigastrium
- Bulge in epigastrium
- No end-tidal carbon dioxide in the expired air ($ETCO_2$) in capnography or initial presence of $ETCO_2$ (due to swallowed air) which is decreasing.

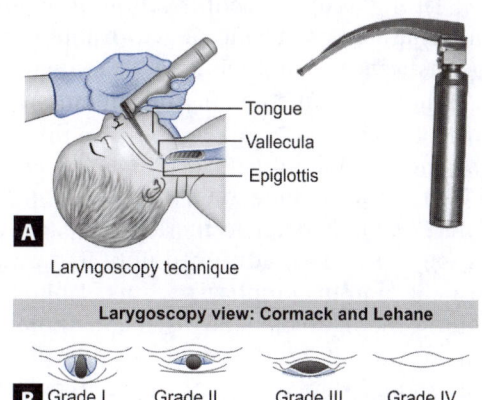

Grades	Extent of visualization
Grade I	Whole glottis is visible
Grade II	Only the posterior extremity of the glottis is visible
Grade III	No part of the glottis and only the epiglottis is visible
Subclass IIIa	Epiglottis can be lifted from the posterior pharyngeal wall
Subclass IIIb	Epiglottis cannot be lifted
Grade IV	Even the epiglottis is not visible

Figs. 9.9A and B: (A) Macintosh laryngoscopy and its technique of use; (B) Cormack and Lehane grades of laryngoscopy.

care. The tube is secured with adhesive tape and tube cuff is inflated with the air or saline.

Confirming the Position of Tube

- **Auscultation:** Immediately after intubation chest is auscultated on both sides for air entry, epigastrium is also auscultated to rule out esophageal intubation. In chest, apex, axilla, inframammary area should be auscultated on both side.
- **Capnography:** The persistent detection of CO_2 by a capnograph is the confirmatory sign of correct placement, though it cannot exclude bronchial intubation.[Q]
- **Fiberoptic bronchoscope:** Tracheal rings and bifurcation of trachea is visible when fiberoptic bronchoscope is introduced through the tube. It is the most accurate method to detect endotracheal intubation.

Difficulty with the Macintosh Technique

The efficacy of direct laryngoscopy is measured in terms of the best view of the larynx achieved **(Fig. 9.9)**. The most widely used scale for this purpose is Cormack and Lehane (CL) scale. Four grades are proposed depending upon the extent of visualization.

Nasotracheal Intubation (Fig. 9.10 and Table 9.3)

Here endotracheal tube is passed through nose in to the trachea.

Indications

- Intraoral surgery like tonsillectomy
- Intraoral space occupying lesion (require fiberoptic guided nasal intubation)
- Inadequate mouth opening (require fiberoptic guided nasal intubation)
- Blind awake intubation (nasal intubation is preferred over oral)
- In intensive care unit (ICU) setting when tube is to be kept for prolong period.

Contraindications

- Basal skull fractures, or in facial trauma where basal skull fracture has not been ruled out. In this condition tube passed through nose may accidentally enter cranium.
- Bleeding disorders
- Nasal polyps abscess
- Adenoids

In nasal intubation TT is advanced through the nose and nasopharynx into the oropharynx before laryngoscopy. Administration of phenylephrine nasal drops or lignocaine with adrenaline vasoconstricts subcutaneous vessels and also shrinks the mucous membrane, thereby minimizes the risk of trauma.

Technique: A TT lubricated with water-soluble jelly is introduced along the floor of the nose, at an angle perpendicular to the face **(Fig. 9.10)**. The tube is gradually advanced until its tip can be visualized in the oropharynx. This is followed by routine laryngoscopy, the distal end of the TT can be advanced into the trachea under direct visualization. If difficulty is encountered, passage of the tip of the tube through the vocal cords may be facilitated by manipulation with Magill forceps.

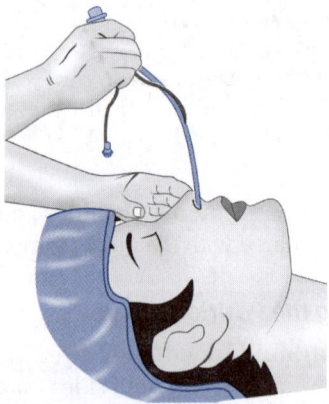

Fig. 9.10: Tube and head positions for nasotracheal intubation.

Complications of Laryngoscopy and Intubation

Laryngoscopy and intubation are associated with many and some potentially serious complications like trauma to airway, bleeding and sympathetic stimulation.

Techniques of Extubation

When to remove a TT is an extremely important part of the practice, as most complications arise during and immediately after extubation.

It is better to extubate patient in deeper plane of anesthesia or in fully awake state. In either

Table 9.3: Advantages and disadvantages of nasotracheal intubation.

Advantages	Disadvantages
Better tolerability	Increased risk of bleeding
Better oral hygiene	More chances of meningitis, sinusitis
Better fixation so less chance of accidental extubation	Chances of nasal deformity
Patient cannot bite the tube	Trauma to nasal structures

case, adequate recovery from neuromuscular blocking agents should be established prior to extubation. Extubation in light plane of anesthesia is associated with increased risk of laryngospasm. Eye opening or purposeful movements imply that the patient is awake.

Extubating an awake patient is usually associated with increase in the heart rate, blood pressure, intracranial pressure, and intraocular pressure. So such extubation is cautious in a cardiac patient, and patient of neurosurgery.

Regardless of timing when the tube is removed, the patient's pharynx should be thoroughly suctioned before extubation to decrease the risk of aspiration or laryngospasm. After extubation, oxygen should be supplemented for at least 5 minutes.

> **KEY POINTS**
>
> **Contraindications for endotracheal intubation**
> As such in emergency condition there is no absolute contraindication. In elective conditions contraindications include:
> - Laryngotracheobronchitis
> - Active upper respiratory tract infection
> - Aneurysm arch of aorta
>
> In first two conditions tracheal intubation can produce laryngospasm and bronchospasm, whereas in a case of aneurysm arch of aorta tracheal intubation can rupture aneurysm.

Tracheostomy

Making an opening on the anterior wall of trachea and converting it into a stoma on the skin surface. Through that stoma a tube (tracheostomy tube) is passed and the other end of which is connected to breathing circuit. For airway management it is indicated very rarely. Few important indications are:
- Major laryngeal surgeries like laryngectomy.
- Space occupying lesion in oropharynx where both oral and nasal intubation seems impossible through conventional means.
- As an elective procedure in ICU when prolonged ventilation is required.

Important Points about Tracheostomy

- Vertical incision is preferred in emergency whereas transverse incision in elective surgery.
- Trachea is opened in the region of third and fourth or third and second ring. First tracheal ring is never divided as it can lead to perichondritis of cricoid cartilage with stenosis.
- Out of various types of tracheostomy tubes available, cuffed (high volume low pressure) plastic tracheostomy tubes are most frequently used. Cuff should be deflated at least once in 5 hours, so as to prevent damage to trachea.
- Common early complications are hemorrhage and malposition. Tracheal stenosis is the most common delayed complication.

Cricothyrotomy

- Almost always done in emergency conditions only.
- In this procedure an opening is created in cricothyroid membrane.
- Most common indication is, cannot intubate, cannot ventilate situation secondary to laryngospasm.
- Cricothyrotomy is accomplished by inserting 12G or 14G needle or cannula in cricothyroid membrane.
- A high flow oxygen source is then connected to cannula with the goal to supply oxygen to patient. Jet ventilation (if available) can accomplish this goal by providing high flow oxygen.

EMERGENCY AIRWAY MANAGEMENT (FIG. 9.11)

Emergency airway management might be required in some patients to ensure adequate oxygenation and ventilation while protecting the patient from the risks of aspiration. Endotracheal intubation is commonly required and is specifically indicated in the following conditions:
- Cardiac or respiratory arrest
- In deep sedation when reflexes get blunt
- Transient hyperventilation of patients with increased intracranial pressure (ICP)

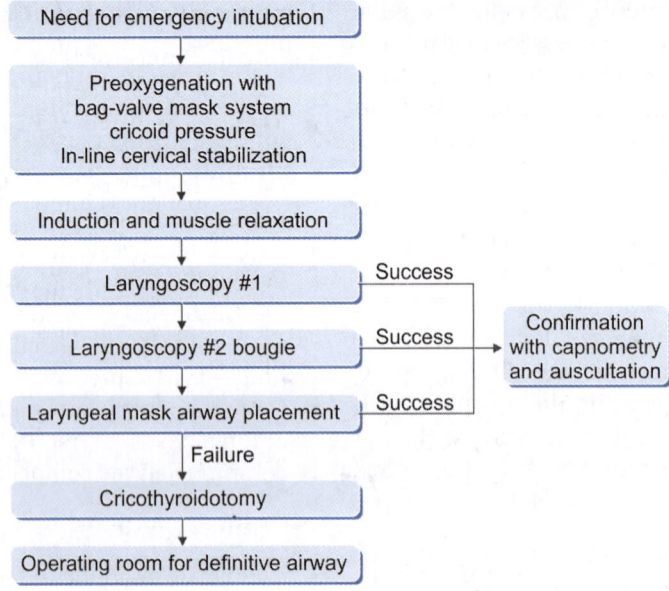

Fig. 9.11: Algorithm for emergency airway management.

- In patients with carbon monoxide poisoning who require 100% oxygen.
- To facilitate diagnostic work-up in uncooperative or intoxicated patients.

Steps for emergency airway management are as per algorithm **(Fig. 9.11)**.[2]

RAPID SEQUENCE INDUCTION AND INTUBATION

Endotracheal intubation using rapid sequence intubation (RSI) is the cornerstone of emergency airway management. RSI is designed to forestall the dangers of vomiting, regurgitation and aspiration of stomach contents. RSI is the preferred method of induction where ever there is risk of gastric aspiration, e.g., in full stomach patients, in pregnancy.

The purpose of RSI is to provide airway protection (by intubation) at the earliest.

Steps

- **Preparation**: This includes patient evaluation, equipment checking, and patient positioning.
- **Preoxygenation**: All patients proposed to be intubated by RSI method should be asked to breathe in 100% oxygen preferably through Mapleson A circuit, purpose is to replace the nitrogen (denitrogenation) of lung by oxygen, which will participate in diffusion when patient is apneic. In direct emergency situation, four vital capacity breath with 100% oxygen are considered as sufficient.

Note: Preoxygenation for 5 minutes permits 3 minutes of apnea after which desaturation starts ($SPO_2 < 90\%$).

KEY POINTS

BURP maneuver: It is slightly different from Selick's maneuver, here pressure is applied over trachea in backward, upward, rightward direction, the goal is to improve the visualization of glottis during laryngoscopy. It does not provide protection against regurgitation.

- **Induction**: Administration of intravenous induction agents provides rapid loss of consciousness. Thiopentone and propofol are the common inducing agent for this purpose.

- **Selick's maneuver**: Firm backward pressure over the cricoid cartilage, so as to compress the proximal esophagus. The goal is to obliterate esophageal lumen by cricoid ring so as to prevent regurgitation of gastric contents. This maneuver should be initiated as the person begins to lose consciousness and pressure must be maintained till the position of tube is verified and cuff is inflated. The force required is variable and is around 25–35 Newton.
- **Paralysis**: Immediately after loss of consciousness muscle relaxant is administered to paralyze the patient. A rapid-acting muscle relaxant is preferred. Succinylcholine is the muscle relaxant of choice for RSI unless contraindicated. Rocuronium is the nondepolarizing muscle relaxant of choice.
- **Intubation**: As the effect of muscle relaxant ensues, patient is intubated with cuffed endotracheal tube. Positive pressure ventilation is contraindicated till the patient is intubated. Cricoid pressure (Selick's maneuver) is only released when the endotracheal cuff is safely inflated.

LAST-MINUTE REVISION

- Mallampati score correlates tongue size to pharyngeal size.
- Guedel airway is the most frequently used airway.
- LMA is contraindicated in full stomach, patients and those risk for aspiration.
- ProSeal™ LMA provides better seal than Classic LMA.
- Currently PVC tube with high volume low pressure cuff are most frequency used endotracheal tubes.
- Magill or Morning Sniffing position (Also called sniffing position): Extension at atlanto-occipital joint and flexion at lower cervical spine (C_2–C_4).
- Capnography is the most sensitive noninvasive technique to know correct placement. Overall fiberoptic bronchoscopy is the most sensitive but invasive technique.
- Macintosh laryngoscope is the most frequently used laryngoscope in anesthesia practice.

Sterilization of airway devices and equipments
- All disposable items like endotracheal tubes, face mask, plastic airways, breathing circuits are best sterilized by ethylene oxide.
- Laryngoscope blades, Magill forceps, metallic airways can be autoclaved.
- Fiberoptic scopes are sterilized by 2% glutaraldehyde.

REFERENCES

1. Schrader M, Urits I. Tracheal Rapid Sequence Intubation. [Updated 2022 May 8]. In: StatPearls [Internet]. Treasure Island (FL): StatPearls Publishing; 2022 Jan-. Available from: https://www.ncbi.nlm.nih.gov/books/NBK560592/
2. Avva U, Lata JM, Kiel J. Airway Management. [Updated 2022 May 1]. In: StatPearls [Internet]. Treasure Island (FL): StatPearls Publishing; 2022 Jan-. Available from: https://www.ncbi.nlm.nih.gov/books/NBK470403/

REVIEW QUESTIONS

1. The laryngeal mask airway can be used for securing the airway of patient in all of the following conditions, *except*:
    a. In a difficult intubation
    b. In cardiopulmonary resuscitation
    c. In a child undergoing an elective/routine eye surgery
    d. In a patient with a large tumor in oral cavity

Unit I: Basics of Anesthesia

2. **True about LMA:**
   a. Available in 8 sizes
   b. Intubation can be done
   c. Size 1 for neonates
   d. Size 3 for weight >70 kg

3. **Which of the following is not an indication for endotracheal intubation?**
   a. Maintenance of a patent airway
   b. To provide positive pressure ventilation
   c. Pulmonary toilet
   d. Pneumothorax

4. **Cormack and Lehane grade is related to:**
   a. Ascitis
   b. Severity of cranial injury
   c. Direct laryngoscopy
   d. LMA insertion

5. **Immediately after epidural anesthesia, a patient lands in respiratory arrest, and emergency endotracheal intubation has been tried after administration of thiopentone and succinylcholine. In the first attempt, intubation was not successful. Which of the following is not a part of management strategy beyond this point?**
   a. Make one more attempt of intubation by using fiberoptic bronchoscope
   b. LMA is the preferred airway device if initial two attempts are unsuccessful
   c. Try to mask ventilate the patient with 100% oxygen
   d. Cricothyroidectomy should be accomplished if other modes of ventilation fail

6. **Merits of nasotracheal intubation is:**
   a. Good oral hygiene
   b. Less infection
   c. Less mucosal damage and bleeding
   d. More movement or displacement of endotracheal tube

ANSWERS

| 1. d | 2. b and c | 3. d | 4. c | 5. a | 6. a |

CHAPTER 10

Preanesthetic Evaluation

Anshul Jain, Shivali Pandey

INTRODUCTION

Preanesthetic assessment is an integral part of safe anesthetic practice. It serves to identify associated medical illness and anesthetic risks with the ultimate aim of reducing morbidity and mortality associated with anesthesia and surgery.

The objectives of the preanesthetic assessment are to:
- Evaluate the patient's medical condition by medical history, physical examination, investigation and when appropriate, past medical records.
- Optimize the patient's medical condition for anesthesia and surgery.
- Identify any associated medical condition that makes anesthesia and surgery risky.
- Plan anesthetic technique and perioperative care.
- Inform and educate the patient about anesthesia, perioperative care and pain management.
- Develop a confident feeling in the patient to reduce anxiety and facilitate conduct of anesthesia.
- Obtain consent for anesthesia.

GENERAL PRINCIPLES

- Preanesthetic assessment should be performed at an appropriate time before the scheduled surgery to allow adequate preparation of the patient. This also applies to day care surgery patient.
- Preanesthetic assessment should preferably be performed by the anesthesiologist who has to conduct anesthesia.
- In cases of emergency surgery where consultation is not always possible, a brief assessment should always be performed.

IMPLEMENTATION OF PREANESTHETIC ASSESSMENT

There are three methods for organizing preanesthetic evaluation efficiently:
1. An anesthetist and/or surgeon who sees the patient before a scheduled procedure can obtain history, perform physical examination and advise investigation accordingly.
2. A clinic can be set up in an outpatient facility; so as to perform these task early enough to ensure that laboratory test can be obtained without delaying schedules. This clinic also ensures the assessment of patient without hospital admission. Hospital admission is indicated in only those patients who require further medical evaluation.
3. Through a questionnaire answered by patient. Among these methods, second method, i.e., a preanesthetic checkup clinic is the most efficient one.

STEPS OF ASSESSMENT

Medical History

History is the first and most important part of any medical examination. This includes:
- Brief medical history—ask specially for respiration system (such as shortness of breath) and those relating to cardiovascular system (CVS) (angina, orthopnea).

- Drugs which patient is consuming (there are some drugs which have to be stopped prior to surgery, e.g., aspirin).
- Any infectious disease like human immunodeficiency virus (HIV), hepatitis B virus (HBV), tuberculosis (TB), etc.

Physical Examination

A rapid general and cardiorespiratory examination/evaluation should be performed. A thorough airway assessment and examination of spine (if central neuraxial block is being planned) should also be performed.

On the basis of physical assessment, patients are categorized into different classes as devised by American Society of Anesthesiologists (ASA) (Table 10.1).

Laboratory Evaluation

The use of laboratory test, electrocardiography (ECG) and X-ray are long been an element of preoperative evaluation of a patient fitness for anesthesia and surgery. However, since few years there is a strong debate regarding the usefulness of routine laboratory testing for healthy asymptomatic patient (ASA class I and II) when history and physical examination fail to detect any abnormality. In 2016, the National Institute for Health and Care Excellence (NICE) issued an updated guideline for preoperation testing considering patient ASA class and nature of surgery. Indian Society of Anaesthesiologists (ISA) also formulated evidence-based practice guidelines for preoperative investigations.[2]

Guidelines for Preoperative Laboratory Testing

Grading of Severity of Surgery

Both NICE guidelines and ISA guidelines suggests preoperative investigations and testing on the basis of extensiveness of surgery. Depending on the invasiveness and stressfulness, operative procedures are classified in three grades (Table 10.2):

Routine Lab Test and Indication

Hemoglobin Concentration and Complete Blood Count

- As per NHS UK guidelines indicated in all patients of ASA class greater than or equal to 3
- All patients over 60 years of age
- All patients posted for grade 3 surgeries. ISA India, on the basis of high prevalence of anemia in India, recommend CBC in all patients irrespective of type of surgery and ASA grading.

Hemostasis Test (Prothrombin Time/Activated Partial Thromboplastin Time)

- Patients of ASA class >3
- Patients on anticoagulants. If clotting status needs to be tested before surgery use point-of-

Table 10.1: American Society of Anesthesiologists classification of a patient's physical status.

Class	Definition
1	A normal healthy patient
2	Patient with mild systemic disease (no functional limitations)
3	Patient with severe systemic disease (some functional limitations)
4	Patient with severe systemic disease that is a constant threat to life (functionality incapacitated)
5	Moribund patient who is not expected to survive without the operation
6	Brain-dead patient whose organs are being removed for donor purposes
E	If the procedure is an emergency, the physical status is followed by "E" (for example, "2E")

Table 10.2: Grading classification of severity of surgery.

Grades	Example
Grade 1 (minor)	Excision of lesion of skin; drainage of breast abscess
Grade 2 (intermediate)	Primary repair of inguinal hernia; tonsillectomy/adenotonsillectomy
Grade 3 (major)	Total abdominal hysterectomy; TURP; thyroidectomy Total joint replacement, lung operations, colonic resection, radical neck dissection, neurosurgery, cardiac surgery

(TURP: transurethral resection of the prostate)

care testing, as direct oral anticoagulants can not be measured by routine testing.
- Patient with coagulopathy or if first degree relatives have coagulopathy.

Renal Function Test (Blood Urea and Creatinine)
- Preoperative serum creatinine estimation is not indicated in patients undergoing minor surgery.
- Preoperative serum creatinine estimation is indicated in patients undergoing intermediate and major surgery.

Random Blood Sugar
Indicated only in diabetic patients. In nondiabetic patients, preoperative blood glucose estimation is not suggested when scheduled to undergo minor, intermediate and major surgery.

12-Lead Electrocardiogram
In noncardiac patients, preoperative 12-lead electrocardiogram testing is suggested at age 45 years and above, when scheduled to undergo minor and intermediate surgery indicated in all patients posted for major surgery.

Chest X-ray
- Patients over 50 years posted for grade intermediate and major surgeries.
- Patient with known cardiorespiratory disease.

Serum Electrolytes
As per both NHS and ISA guidelines, routine measurement of serum electrolytes is not indicated. Serum electrolytes to be measured when there is some condition which can cause electrolyte abnormality or patient is on any medication that may affect serum electrolytes.

Liver Function Test
Preoperative liver function testing is suggested for patients undergoing major surgery or when there is suspicion of liver abnormality, e.g., alcoholism.

Preoperative Ultrasonographic Airway Assessment
Not indicated routinely

Validity of Old Investigations

Many a time controversy arises when patient show the old investigations, he or she should be advised fresh investigation of the old report to be considered, the answer remain controversial. As per ISA guidelines, The acceptable validity time for a previously performed normal complete blood count, renal function tests, liver function tests, coagulation profile, is suggested to be 2 months provided the clinical condition of the patient has not changed in the intervening period.

Instructions after Preanesthetic Assessment

- If patient seems fit for anesthesia following advice is given:
  – Nil orally for a period before surgery
  – Remove artificial dentures, bangles, jewelry, and contact lenses
  – Nail polish and lipstick to be removed (as they can obscure cyanosis)
  – Administer anxiolytic drugs (usually alprazolam) or other premedicant if required.
- If patient require optimization before anesthesia, he/she can be referred to respective speciality [e.g., patients with congestive heart failure (CHF) can be referred to cardiology department for optimization] and repeat preanesthetic assessment is advised after optimization.
- If patient is consuming some drug that can interfere with anesthetic agents, patient can be referred to the specialty doctor who has prescribed the drug with a note "kindly stop 'x' drug 'y' days prior to surgery". By doing so it is ensured that stopping drug would not affect patient disease process. For example,

> **KEY POINTS**
> **The purpose of nil orally is to:**
> Reduce the gastric volume and chances of perianesthetic pulmonary aspiration of gastric contents.

if oral hypoglycemic needs to be stopped, endocrinologist will substitute insulin for oral hypoglycemic.

Fasting Guidelines

Traditionally all patients posted for surgery were advised to remain nil per orally for a period that range from 6–8 hours. The rationale for this was a theoretical risk of aspiration of gastric content that may lead to pneumonia. However now with the availability of better anesthetic agents, recent researches regarding preoperative fasting found that a shorter fasting time is associated with better hemodynamic stability, lowers the risk of dehydration and also lowers the risk of post-operative nausea and vomiting.

So, as per current recommendations for healthy children, the new 6-4-3-1 regimen (6 hours for solids, 4 hours for formula and nonhuman milk, 3 hours for breast milk, 1 hours for clear fluids) is followed. For adults clear liquids (water, fruit juice without pulp, clear tea, clear coffee) can be allowed up to 2 hours prior to surgery, milk and milk tea up to 4 hours, light meal up to 6 hours and for fatty meals 8 or more hours of fasting is recommended.

Any fasting beyond 6 hours should be supplemented with IV fluids.

Various national and international societies recommend that oral intake can be initiated within hours of surgery in most patients.[3,4]

EFFECT OF PRE-EXISTING DRUG THERAPY ON ANESTHETIC MANAGEMENT AND MODIFICATIONS REQUIRED

Antihypertensive Drugs

All antihypertensive drugs[Q] are normally continued till the day of surgery. It should be mentioned clearly in preanesthetic instruction "continue antihypertensive till the day of operation, morning dose to be taken with sip of water". Angiotensin-converting-enzyme (ACE) inhibitors and angiotensin II[Q] antagonist are exception they should be stopped at least 24 hour prior to non-cardiac surgery.[Q] Their continuation increases the chances of intraoperative hypotension.[5]

Antianginal Drugs

All antianginal drugs should be continued including morning dose of day of surgery which should be taken with a sip of water.

Anticoagulants

Vitamin K antagonists (warfarin)[Q] needs to be stopped at least 72 hours[Q] prior to surgery and are substituted by heparin. Heparin is then stopped 12 hours prior to surgery. In case of urgency, effect of warfarin may be reversed by administering vitamin K and in emergency situation transfusion with fresh frozen plasma (FFP) improves coagulability.

Antiplatelet Drugs

In contrary to older recommendations, according to which aspirin[Q] has to be stopped 1 week before surgery. As per latest recommendation, aspirin should be continued unless the bleeding outweighs the risk of thrombus. If removal of platelet inhibition is necessary, then aspirin must be stopped 5–7 days prior to surgery. Further aspirin should never be discontinued in patients with coronary stents. For clopidogrel, recommendations are same as that for aspirin.

Oral Contraceptive Pills

Estrogens containing oral contraceptive pills (OCPs) increase chance of deep venous thrombosis (DVT) and thromboembolism, so they should be stopped 4 weeks before elective surgery. If this is not possible low molecular weight heparin should be considered. Progesterone-only pills need no special precaution.

Oral Hypoglycemics

Oral hypoglycemics can be continued till the day of surgery, in patients with well-controlled diabetes undergoing grade 1 and 2 surgery. But sulfonylureas[Q] and metformin should be stopped for 24–48 hours before surgery because of their long half-lives. Additionally sulfonylureas block myocardial potassium adenosine triphosphate channels, which are responsible for ischemia and anesthetic-induced preconditioning. A meta-analysis however suggested that sulfon for major surgeries,[Q] oral hypoglycemics should be withdrawn 24–48 hours preoperatively and insulin has to be started. Insulin allow more precise control of blood sugar.

Steroids

If patient has taken steroid for more than 1 week in last 1 year, there are chances of suppression of pituitary-adrenal axis, resulting in reduced stress-related steroid secretion. Considering this, it is generally safe to administer hydrocortisone over the period of surgery (as surgery produces stress).

Smoking

Smoking should be stopped. Longer the period of abstinence, greater would be the benefit. Complete recovery of respiratory function takes place only after 8 weeks of abstinence (Also *see* chapter 23).

Antidepressants

Monoamine oxidase (MAO-A) inhibitors[Q] should be stopped 2 weeks before elective surgery as they can precipitate dangerous arrhythmias and hypertensive episodes. Reversible MAO-A inhibitors (moclobemide) and MAO-B inhibitors (selegiline) can be continued up to the day before surgery.

Selective serotonin uptake inhibitors (SSRIs) and tricycle antidepressants can also be continued.

Antiepileptic and Levodopa

To be continued strictly, morning dose to be taken with a sip of water.

Thyroid Supplement

To be continued including morning dose of day of surgery, which has to be taken with a sip of water.

KEY POINTS
Beneficial effects of smoking cessation and time course

Time course	Benefit
12–24 hours	Decreased carbon monoxide and nicotine level
48–72 hours	Carboxy hemoglobin (COHB) levels normalized, improved ciliary function
1–2 weeks	Reduced sputum protection
4–6 weeks	PFT improves
6–8 weeks	Immune function and metabolism normalizes
8–12 weeks	Decreased overall postoperative morbidity and mortality

Lithium

To be stopped 2 days before major as lithium potentiates nondepolarizer muscle relaxants.[Q]

Herbal Medicine

Herbal medicines can affect metabolic and bleeding profile of patient. So, they should to be stopped 1 week prior to surgery.

PREMEDICATION

The main rationale for premeditating patient before anesthesia is to minimize their anxiety, provide good sleep and reduce metabolic rate. Other additional reasons are:
- To provide hemodynamic stability
- To reduce the possibility of aspiration of gastric contents
- To reduce postoperative nausea and vomiting
- To reduce salivary secretion
- To reduce the risk of infection.

Drugs Used for Premedication

To Relieve Anxiety

Benzodiazepines (BZD) are most commonly used for this purpose. Lorazepam[Q] is the BZD of choice. Zopiclone[Q] is a safe nonbenzodiazepine alternative. For proper anxiolytic effect, they should be given 24 hours prior to surgery.

To Reduce Chances of Aspiration

Prokinetic agents (metoclopramide); proton pump blockers (omeprazole); H$_2$ blockers (ranitidine). They should be given prophylactically in patients who are at risk for aspiration.

To Control Secretion

Anticholinergic drugs are used to reduce salivary and tracheobronchial secretions. Following anticholinergic drugs can be used **(Table 10.3)**:
- **Glycopyrrolate**: It is devoid of central nervous system (CNS) effect (does not cross blood brain barrier) and produce minimal cardiac effect. Thus it is the preferred anticholinergic when only antisialagogue effect is required.
- **Atropine**: This is the preferred agent when both vagolytic and antisialagogue effects are required.
- **Scopolamine**: This is used in cases where sedative effects are also required.

Most modern anesthetics do not increase salivary secretions, so routine use of anticholinergics is restricted to oropharyngeal surgery cases only.^{Q}

Table 10.3: Comparison of anticholinergic drugs.

Features	Atropine	Hyoscine	Glycopyrrolate
Duration of action	3 hours	2 hours	6 hours
Effect on heart rate	++++ (maximum)	Moderate	Minimum
Inhibition of salivation	++	++	+++
CNS side effect	+	+	–

(CNS: central nervous system)

Antiemetic

Hyoscine (most potent), ondansetron, metoclopramide are the most widely used antiemetics. Polanosetron^Q is the newer longest acting congener of ondansetron. Antiemetics should be given preoperatively as prophylaxis in patients who are at risk for postoperative nausea and vomiting.

LAST-MINUTE REVISION

- **Medications that should be stopped before surgery**: MAO-A inhibitors (2 weeks), oral anticoagulants, lithium, all herbal medicines.
- **Medications whose morning dose to be omitted**: ACE inhibitors, angiotensin II antagonist, long-acting oral hypoglycemics.
- Glycopyrrolate is the most frequently used anticholinergic to reduce oropharyngeal secretions.
- Metoclopramide is the most frequently used antiemetic for prophylaxis whereas ondansetron in the most effective drug to control postoperative nausea and vomiting.

REFERENCES

1. Umesh G, et aL. Indian J Anaesth. 2022; 66(5):319-43. doi: 10.4103/ija.ija_335_22. Epub 2022 May 19. PMID: 35782661; PMCID: PMC9241185.
2. O'Neill F, et aL. Routine preoperative tests for elective surgery: summary of updated NICE guidance. BMJ. 2016; 354:i3292. doi: 10.1136/ bmj.i3292. PMID: 27418436.
3. Frykholm P, Veyckemans F, Afshari A. Preoperative fasting in children: A guideline from the European Society of Anaesthesiology and Intensive Care. European Journal of Anaesthesiology. 2022; 39(1): 4-25 doi: 10.1097/ EJA.0000000000001599.
4. Practice Guidelines for Preoperative Fasting and the Use of Pharmacological Agents to Reduce the Risk of Pulmonary Aspiration: Application to Healthy Patients Undergoing Elective Procedures: An Updated Report by the American Society of Anesthesiologists Task Force on Preoperative Fasting and the Use of Pharmacologic Agents to Reduce the Risk of Pulmonary Aspiration. Anesthesiology. 2017 ;126(3):376-93. doi: 10.1097/ ALN.0000000000001452. PMID: 28045707.

5. Roshanov PS, et aL. Withholding versus continuing angiotensin-converting enzyme inhibitors or angiotensin II receptor blockers before noncardiac surgery: an analysis of the vascular events in noncardiac surgery patients cohort evaluation prospective cohort. Anesthesiology. 2017;126(1):16-27. doi: 10.1097/ALN.0000000000001404. PMID: 27775997.

REVIEW QUESTIONS

1. In an ASA grade 1 patient posted for anal fissure surgery which of the following investigations should be advised as a part of routine testing:
   a. TLC, hemoglobin (Hb), renal function test
   b. Renal function test and Hb
   c. Liver function test, renal function test, hemogram
   d. CBC
2. All of the following drugs can be continued perioperatively, *except*:
   a. Antihypertensives
   b. Oral hypoglycemics
   c. None
   d. Antiepileptics

ANSWERS

1. d   2. c

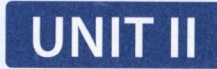

Anesthesia Pharmacology

Unit Outline

11. Inhalational Anesthetics
12. Intravenous Anesthetics
13. Local Anesthetics
14. Muscle Relaxants
15. Additional Drugs in Anesthesia

COMPETENCIES COVERED IN UNIT II

Competency Number	Competency Name	Chapter Number
AS4.1	Describe and discuss the pharmacology of drugs used in induction and maintenance of general anesthesia (including intravenous and inhalation induction agents, opiate and non-opiate analgesics, depolarizing and nondepolarizing muscle relaxants, anticholinesterases).	11-15
PH1.15	Describe mechanism/s of action, types, doses, side effects, indications and contraindications of skeletal muscle relaxants.	14
PH1.17	Describe the mechanism/s of action, types, doses, side effects, indications and contraindications of local anesthetics.	13
PH1.18	Describe the mechanism/s of action, types, doses, side effects, indications and contraindications of general anesthetics, and preanesthetic medications.	15
PY3.5	Discuss the action of neuromuscular blocking agents.	14
PY3.4	Describe the structure of neuromuscular junction and transmission of impulses.	14

CHAPTER 11

Inhalational Anesthetics

Anshul Jain, Pooja Chaubey

INTRODUCTION

Inhalational anesthetics are the agents (either volatile liquid or gases) which when inhaled produce reversible unconsciousness. These agents can be used either for induction or for maintenance of anesthesia or both. This chapter reviews the basic concept of inhalational anesthesia and the pharmacological agents used for the aforementioned purpose.

Classification

As mentioned inhalational anesthetics can be gas or volatile liquids. Chemically inhalational anesthetics could be ether, halogenated hydrocarbons or inert gases **(Fig. 11.1)**.

MECHANISM OF INHALATIONAL ANESTHESIA

Precise mechanism is yet unknown, critical signal proteins (ion channel and receptor) are the most likely target. Other important theories include:

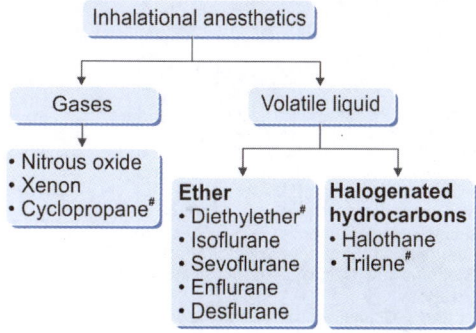

Fig. 11.1: Classification of inhalational anesthetics.
#Not used nowadays.

- **Fluidization theory and lateral phase theory:** Suggest disturbance in membrane form
- **Critical volume hypothesis:** Inhalational anesthetics expand neuronal membrane beyond a critical amount, thereby altering membrane function.

Site of Action

Almost all volatile agents act on central nervous system (CNS) directly to produce unconsciousness; action on dorsal horn[Q] of spinal cord produces analgesia. In high doses, they can block synaptic transmission directly. Two-pore domain potassium channels have recently been suggested as the site of action of volatile anesthetics. These agents augment the effect of the potassium channels, leading to hyperpolarization, and causing anesthesia. Potassium channels have a leaking current which influences the baseline resting membrane potential of cells and neuronal action potentials.[1]

MINIMUM ALVEOLAR CONCENTRATION

Minimum alveolar concentration[Q] (MAC) of an inhaled anesthetic is the alveolar concentration at atmospheric pressure that prevents movement in 50% of subjects in response to a standardized noxious stimulus. It is analogous to the plasma EC50 (concentration which produce unconsciousness in 50% individuals) for intravenous anesthetic.

MAC value also tells about the potency of an agent. Higher the MAC value, higher would be the concentration required to produce anesthesia, or lesser would be the potency.

In general potency of inhalational agents correlates directly with their lipid solubility (Meyer-Overton rule).Q

Similar to standard MAC, each agent has specific MAC intubation (concentration that prevents movement and coughing during endotracheal intubation); MAC awakeQ (alveolar concentration at which patient wakes from anesthesia) MAC awake is usually 0.3–0.4 MAC; MAC-BAR (1.7–2.0 MAC), which is the concentration required to block autonomic reflexes to nociceptive stimuli. MAC is altered by several physiological and pharmacological variables; one of the most consistent factors is age. There is 6% decrease in MAC per decade of age, irrespective of volatile anesthetic **(Fig. 11.2)**.

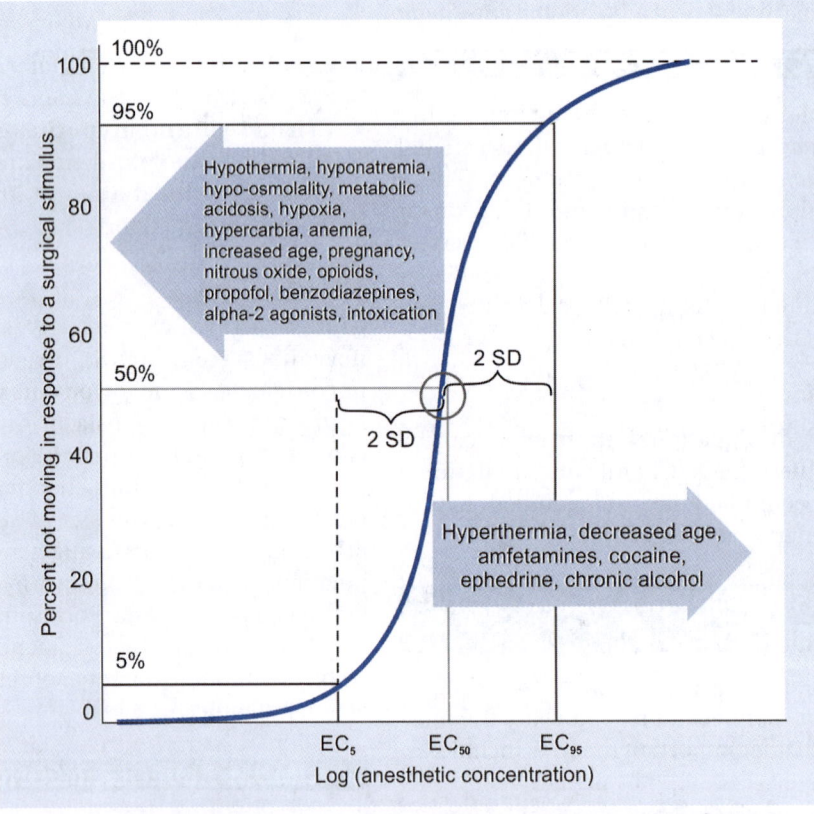

Fig. 11.2: Minimum alveolar concentration and the factors affecting (MAC).

GENERAL PRINCIPLES OF INHALATIONAL ANESTHESIA

Anesthetic gases are taken up in the body through lung. The uptake is determined by physical property of agent. It can be separated into uptake in the lung, diffusion into pulmonary blood, and then distribution into the brain and other organ. Alveolar partial pressure of inhalational anesthetic governs its partial pressure in all other body tissue.

After equilibrium is achieved between brain and blood, alveolar concentration reflect the concentration in brain. Usually, it takes 5–10 minutes to achieve this equilibrium.

$$\text{Uptake} = \frac{\lambda \times Q(P_A - P_V)}{P}$$

λ = Blood gas partition coefficient
Q = Cardiac output
$P_A - P_V$ = Difference between alveolar and venous partial pressure
P = Barometric pressure

Any factor which tends to increase uptake[Q] would result in delayed equilibrium and hence delayed induction. Principally two factors determine how quickly the alveolar concentration of any inhalational agent rise toward MAC during induction:

A. Inspired Concentration

If inspired concentration (F_I) is high, rate of rise of F_A would also be high and it would tend to approaches MAC value rapidly (**Fig. 11.3**). When body gets fully saturated, anesthetic uptake from alveoli ceases and F_A becomes equal to F_I.

However, clinically because of continuous metabolism, F_A usually remains below F_I.

B. Alveolar Ventilation

Alveolar concentration rises rapidly, if alveolar ventilation is increased and rise is slow if there is respiratory depression or obstruction.

However, the physics of volatile induction in not so simple, as from lung volatile anesthetic is taken up and distributed to whole body and for anesthesia it is essential that partial pressure of agent reaches a specific value (different for each agent) in brain. Thus anesthesia is achieved only when alveolar, blood and brain concentration are in equilibrium.

The rapidity of this equilibrium depends on factors that determines anesthetic uptake from lung.

Anesthetic Uptake Factors

- **Blood gas partition coefficient**: This denotes the solubility of gas in blood. Blood gas partition coefficient is specific for each agent; a value of 0.42 (desflurane) means that at equilibrium the concentration of desflurane in blood is 0.42 times (42%) of its alveolar concentration. Agents with high blood gas partition coefficient (highly soluble) diffuse rapidly from alveoli to blood and their F_A raise slowly. As it is the alveolar concentration which determines the speed of induction and recovery, agents with low B/G coefficient show faster induction and recovery. So, induction is fastest with desflurane and slowest with methoxyflurane.
- **Cardiac output**: As cardiac output increases uptake increases or alveolar concentration decreases, hence induction is delayed in states with increased cardiac output.[Q] Learn this thing very clearly as it looks opposite. In low cardiac output states [shock, congestive heart failure (CHF)] alveolar concentration rises rapidly particularly for agents with high B/G coefficient

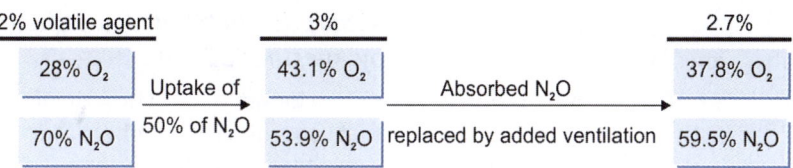

Fig. 11.3: Uptake of an inhalational anesthesia.

> **KEY POINTS**
> In low cardiac output state agent with low blood gas partition coefficient is preferred and vice versa.

and they can achieve dangerously high alveolar concentration. So in low cardiac output state agents with low B/G coefficient are preferred and inspired concentration (F_I) is kept low.

- **Alveolar to venous anesthetic gradient:** Through the lung, volatile agent is transferred to pulmonary vein from where it is distributed to systemic arterial circulation via aorta. In systemic circulation an amount is taken up by various tissues, e.g., muscles, brain, fat. Remaining amount is transferred back to lung through venous circulation via pulmonary artery. Tissue uptake is high initially, so the partial pressure of volatile anesthetic agent in veins is low. In due course of time, tissues get saturated (equilibrium achieved) and partial pressure in veins increases and alveolar to venous pressure difference decreases which results in reduced uptake.

From above discussion, it is not difficult to make you understand that as initially uptake is high, the usual practice is to start volatile agent at high concentration (usually 2–3 MAC), and gradually the concentration is reduced.

Other Factors Affecting F_A/F_I Ratio

Concentration Effect

The inspired anesthetic concentration influences both rate and height of F_A/F_I. Increasing the inspired concentration accelerates rate of raise.

This effect results from two factors:
1. A concentrating effect.
2. Augmentation of inspired ventilation.

To understand these effect *see* **Figure 11.3**.
- **Step I**: If we consider a perfused lung, and fill it with 70% nitrous oxide (N_2O) (70 volumes per 100 volumes), 28% O_2, 2% volatile agent
- **Step II**: In a cardiac cycle, if half (35 volumes) of N_2O is taken up, 35 volumes remain left in a total of 65 volumes (28 + 2 + 35), resulting in concentration of 53.9%. Thus, uptake of half of N_2O does not half the concentration as the remaining gases are concentrated in a smaller volume. Further this enhanced the concentration of N_2O.
- **Step III**: Further, the void created by uptake of 35 volumes is filled by drawing an equal volume (35 volumes) of same gas mixture (70% N_2O; 28% O_2; 2% volatile agent) into lung. The volumes would be 35 × 70/100 N_2O (= 24.5 volumes); 28 × 35/100 O_2 (= 9.8 volumes) and 2 × 35/100 volatile agent = 0.7 volume.

The resulting 100 volumes would be the mixture of:
- N_2O: 35 + 24.5 = 59.5%
- O_2: 28 + 9.8 = 37.8%
- **Volatile agent**: 2 + 0.7 = 2.7%

So, it can be seen that concentration of N_2O is not reducing in the proportion of its uptake. This phenomenon is called augmenting inflow effect[Q] (N_2O augmenting its inflow).

Second Gas Effect

Factors that govern concentration effect also influence the concentration of volatile anesthetic agent given concurrently. As seen above inspired concentration of volatile agent is 2% but uptake of N_2O results in final concentration of 2.7%. This phenomenon by which a gas affects the concentration of other is called second gas effect.[Q]

Clinical implication of second gas effect:

Addition of N_2O[Q] to volatile agent hasten (by increasing its concentration) the onset of anesthesia.

Absorption of Inhaled Anesthetic by Anesthetic Circuit

This delays induction by reducing actual F_I.
- **Absorption by rubber**: Maximum for methoxyflurane and halothane

- **Absorption by plastic**: Maximum for halothane[Q]
- **Absorption by PVC (endotracheal tube)**: Maximum for halothane.

RECOVERY FROM INHALATIONAL ANESTHESIA

All factors that govern the rate of rise of alveolar anesthetic concentration at the time of induction apply to recovery also. Therefore, recovery is earliest with desflurane[Q] and slowest with methoxyflurane.[Q] It must be noted that metabolism of volatile agent play very little role (if any) in recovery and it is mainly elimination through lung that determines recovery.

Diffusion Hypoxia (Fink Effect)[Q]

It is just reverse to concentration effect and is seen at the time of recovery. At the time of recovery, as N_2O is stopped, diffusion gradient reverses and there is outpouring of large volume of N_2O from blood into the lung. This out pouring has two effects:
1. As lung volume is constant out pouring would displace O_2 and tends to decrease O_2 concentration in alveoli (P_AO_2).
2. By diluting alveolar CO_2, Fink effect may decrease respiratory drive and hence ventilation.

    Both factors increase the chances of hypoxia. As large volume of N_2O is released only during the first 4–8 minutes of recovery, this is the period of greatest risk. To avoid diffusion hypoxia, 100% O_2 should be supplemented for 5 minutes after discontinuing N_2O.

METABOLISM OF INHALED ANESTHETICS

Only few inhalational anesthetics are metabolized by human tissue. CYP2E1[Q] is the main enzyme series responsible for oxidative metabolism of halogenated inhalational agent (phase I). Glucuronidation is the most important phase II conjugation reaction. Among currently used inhalational agents halothane[Q] is maximally metabolized, desflurane[Q] and isoflurane are metabolized minimally (<1%) where as N_2O is not metabolized by human tissue.

ORGAN SYSTEM EFFECTS AND TOXICITIES

Liver

All volatile agents reduce portal blood flow to some extent. Halothane[Q] by producing hepatic artery vasospasm reduces arterial flow too. Halothane (more) and enflurane reduce total hepatic blood flow. Halothane also reduces O_2 delivery and hepatic venous O_2 saturation. Sevoflurane, desflurane, isoflurane preserve hepatic blood flow and function.

> **KEY POINTS**
> - Halothane is the most hepatotoxic inhalational agent.
> - Desflurone is the most hepatofriendly inhalational agent.

Hepatocellular Damage

Incidence of liver injury follows following order: halothane[Q]>enflurane>isoflurane>desflurane. Chloroform, methoxyflurane, carbon tetrachloride were other older hepatotoxic agents.

Hepatitis

Halothane produces two types of hepatitis: First one (common) is mild and is due to direct hepatocellular damage. Second one is rare immunologically mediated fulminant form. In second form, halothane metabolites bind irreversibly with tissue proteins to form haptens that can induce immune response. For unknown reason, this severe hepatitis is usually seen in adults, particularly with repeated exposure. Very rarely other halogenated hydrocarbons (isoflurane, enflurane and desflurane) can also produce idiosyncratic hepatitis.

Kidney

All current inhalational agents reduce renal blood flow and glomerular filtration rate (GFR). Metabolism of certain inhaled halogenated anesthetics produces inorganic fluoride, which is directly nephrotoxic. Fluoride production is maximum with methoxyflurane[Q] (so it is most nephrotoxic). It is not only the peak (fluoride level >50 mol/L is required for nephrotoxicity) fluoride concentration that determines injury but the duration of systemic increase in fluoride concentration is equally important. Fluoride production with sevoflurane is also high, but due to its low blood solubility and rapid elimination fluoride concentration falls very quickly, thus reducing its risk of nephrotoxicity. Desflurane[Q] does not produce fluoride at all.

In addition to fluoride, nephrotoxicity has been attributed to compound A [fluoromethyl 2-2-difluoro-1 (trifluoromethyl) vinyl ether] also. The dehydrofluorination of sevoflurane to form compound A is initiated by soda lime and baralyme (more). So, sevoflurane[Q] is contraindicated in patients with pre-existing renal disease. Production of compound A is higher when fresh gas flow is kept low (< 2 L/minute), at high temperatures, and if high concentration of sevoflurane is being used.

> **KEY POINTS**
> Among currently used volatile agents, sevoflurane is most nephrotoxic.

Hematopoietic System

Except N_2O, inhalational agent does not affect hematopoietic system.

Nitrous oxide oxidize vitamin B_{12} and inactivate methionine synthase.[Q] Inhibition of methionine synthase reduce synthesis of thymidine and hence DNA. The clinical outcome includes megaloblastic anemia[Q] and subacute combined degeneration of spinal cord,[Q] secondary to reduced myelin synthesis.

> **KEY POINTS**
> - Hematopoietic effects of N_2O are seen only after prolong exposures (days) so are more common in anesthetics working in operation theater not equipped with scavenging system.
> - In patients as exposure is for limited period only, these side effects are extremely rare in them.

Neurotoxicity

Until now, inhalational anesthetics are supposed to be devoid of neurotoxicity, recent studies however suggest inhalational anesthetics can be neurotoxic to developing and senescent brain through accelerated apoptosis. Halothane and isoflurane increase the generation of amyloid, a protein strongly implicated in the pathogenesis of Alzheimer's diseases. Combined degeneration of spinal cord is the known neurotoxicity of N_2O.

Pregnancy

- **Teratogenicity**: N_2O[Q] is the only teratogenic inhalational anesthetic, that too only under experimental conditions which are very extreme.
- **Abortion**: N_2O increase the incidence of spontaneous abortions.
- **Tocolysis**: All current inhalational agents relax uterus. Halothane, isoflurane, desflurane[Q] possess equal tocolytic potential.

Note: Many older books had mentioned that halothane has got maximum tocolytic potential, because of which it is the agent of choice for internal and external versions, and manual removal of placenta. Recent studies have proved that other agents (isoflurane, desflurane) are equally tocolytic. Currently desflurane[Q] due to its extreme short duration has emerged as agent of choice for above mentioned procedure. Desflurane maintain uteroplacental blood flow (crucial during versions) and carries lower risk of postpartum hemorrhage (PPH)[Q] (known complication of halothane after manual removal of placenta).

METABOLIC EFFECT

Currently used inhalational anesthetics are devoid of metabolic effect. Among older agents ether, cyclopropane, chloroform (maximum) produce hyperglycemia.

OTHER EFFECTS

Analgesia

Except N_2O, none of the present day inhalational agent possesses analgesic activity. Among older agents, trielene[Q] (maximum analgesic activity) and ether[Q] have analgesic activity.

Reaction with CO_2 Absorbents

- Sevoflurane reacts with soda lime and baralyme to produce compound A.
- All volatile agents interact with strongly basic soda lime to produce some carbon monoxide (CO). CO production is maximum with desflurane[Q] followed by enflurane>isoflurane >>sevoflurane, halothane.
- Newer, calcium hydroxide based CO_2 absorbents are chemically inert and do not produce CO neither they degrade sevoflurane to compound A.
- Trielene (obsolete now) produce dichloro-acetylene[Q] (neurotoxic) and phosgene[Q] gas in closed circuit. So it was contraindicated in closed circuit.

> **KEY POINTS**
>
> **MAC value of important agents**
> N_2O (105); Halothane (0.75); Isoflurane (1.2); Desflurane (6.0); Sevoflurane (2.0)

Inflammability

Ether, cyclopropane, ethylene, ethyl chloride (all obsolete now) are inflammable inhalational agents.

INDIVIDUAL ANESTHETIC AGENTS

Nitrous Oxide (Laughing Gas)

N_2O is the only inorganic anesthetic gas in clinical use. First prepared by Joseph Priestley, its anesthetic properties and name laughing gas were suggested by Humphrey Davy.[Q]

Manufacturing

N_2O is manufactured by heating ammonium nitrate to 240°C. At higher temperature, the percentage of impurities [nitric oxide (NO), nitrogen dioxide (NO_2) and carbon monoxide (CO) increases. Starch iodide test[Q] is performed to exclude impurities of NO_2.

Physical Properties

- It is colorless, odorless[Q] and nonirritant[Q] with molecular weight 44 (*Note: some books have mentioned it as sweet smelling, which is wrong*).
- 1.5 times heavier than air.
- Solubility in blood is 35 times more than nitrogen.
- Critical temperature is –36.5°C (critical temperature of a gas is **the temperature at or above which vapor of the gas cannot be liquefied, no matter how much pressure is applied**).
- Neither flammable nor explosive but supports the combustion of other agents, if high temperature is supplied. At temperature greater than 450°C N_2O decompose into N_2 and O_2, perhaps which aids combustion.
- In fully filled cylinder, 4/5 of N_2O is in liquid state and only 1/5 is gas. Cylinders are filled to a filling ratio (ratio of weight of N_2O to weight of water the cylinder could hold) of 0.75. The resulting pressure in cylinder is 760 psi.[Q]

> **KEY POINTS**
>
> Among all agents (currently used and historic) ether is the only complete anesthetic agent, i.e., it produces the triad of amnesia, analgesia and muscle relaxation.

Metabolism

N_2O is not metabolized by human tissue. It is eliminated unchanged from the body, mostly via lungs, partly through the skin.[Q] It is not degraded by soda lime.

Anesthetic Properties

- N_2O is a weak anesthetic agent with a MAC value between 100 and 105. However, it is a potent analgesic. Analgesic effect is seen at concentration above 50%.
- Maximum concentration that can be given is 70% (as minimum 30% O_2 has to be given). Because of easier calculation, usually 66% N_2O and 33% O_2 is administered (flow of O_2 is half of N_2O, e.g., in a total flow of 6 L/minute, 2 L/minute O_2 and 4 L/minute N_2O are delivered).
- Blood gas coefficient is 0.47[Q] (solubility in blood is very low) which relates to its property of faster induction and recovery.
- Not a good muscles relaxant.[Q]
- Associated with second gas effect[Q] and concentration effect[Q] at the time of induction, and diffusion hypoxia[Q] at the time of recovery.

Systemic Effects

Cardiovascular System

Depresses myocardial activity *in vitro*. *In vivo* this effect is masked by its property of mild sympathetic stimulation. Thereby, arterial blood pressure, cardiac output and heart rate (HR) remain unchanged or increase slightly, so it can be used in cardiac patients and patients in shock.

Respiratory System

- Nitrous oxide increases respiratory rate and decrease tidal volume (minute ventilation change only minimally) through its effect on CNS.
- Hypoxic drive is markedly depressed.
- Impurities of N_2O can lead to laryngospasm and pulmonary edema.

Central Nervous System

Increases cerebral blood flow,[Q] increases cerebral blood volume,[Q] and produces a small rise in intracranial pressure (ICP). N_2O increases cerebral metabolic rate too.

Neuromuscular

In contrast to other inhalational agents, N_2O does not relax muscle, rather high concentration can produce muscles rigidity.

Liver and Kidney

No significant effect.

Immune System

Reduce chemotaxis and motility of polymorphonuclear leukocytes.

Other Effects

Effect on Delivery of Other Volatile Agents

Decreasing N_2O concentration (i.e., increasing O_2 concentration) mildly increases the delivered concentration of volatile agents, despite a constant vaporizer setting. This is due to difference in relative solubility of volatile anesthetics in N_2O and O_2.

Effect on Closed Gas Space

During anesthesia, appreciable volume of N_2O can move into closed gas spaces and expand them resulting in grievous sequelae.

There are two types of closed gas space:

1. **Those enclosed by compliant walls**: Bowel, pneumothorax, pneumoperitoneum, air emboli and blood vessel.

> **KEY POINTS**
>
> **Why N_2O diffuses?**
> Normally air cavities contain N_2, a gas whose low solubility limits its absorption by blood (O_2 and CO_2 are absorbed readily by blood). When N_2O is administered, say 60% its ratio in blood is also 60%, but in closed space it is zero. So, just following principle of equilibrium N_2O diffuses in closed space to achieve 60% ratio. N_2O is 35 times more soluble than N_2 in blood or 1 mole of N_2 is removed per 35 moles of N_2O entered. Thus equilibrium is achieved mainly by addition of N_2O; not by removal of N_2. Subsequently, there is expansion of compliant air space and increase in the intercavity pressure in noncompliant air spaces.

2. **Those enclosed by poorly compliant walls**: Middle air cavity, cranial cavity (may cause pneumocephalus so should be stopped at the time of closure in craniotomy).

When N_2O diffuses into complaint air spaces they expand and compress nearby structures. However, there is no effect on intracavitary pressure. In contrary when N_2O diffuses into a noncompliant air space, they do not expand but intracavitary pressure increase markedly.

Contraindications

- **Pneumothorax**: N_2O doubles the pneumothorax volume in 10 minutes and triples in 30 minutes.
- Pneumoperitoneum
- Postpneumoencephalogram
- **Middle ear surgery and tympanoplasty**: Pressure in middle ear cavity may exceed 50 mm Hg, which can displace the tympanic membrane graft.
- **Posterior fossa surgeries**: There is high risk of air embolism, and N_2O can increase the size of air embolism.
- **Acute intestinal obstruction**: Distends the obstructed bowel and may result in its perforation.
- **Ophthalmic surgeries**: When sulfur hexafluoride has to be used.
- **In laparoscopic surgeries**: N_2O is relative contraindicated, as chances of air embolism are there. Beside this N_2O-induced bowel distension reduces space for work through laparoscope.

Note: N_2O diffuses into the cuff of endotracheal tube (when air is used for inflation) and may increase cuff volume. This is of particular concern in surgeries of long duration. In laryngeal surgery also, increased cuff volume can aggravate laryngeal edema.

Side Effects

- By inactivating vitamin B_{12}, N_2O produces megaloblastic anemia and subacute degeneration of spinal cord. Inactivation is seen if N_2O is used for more than 8 hours.
- By activating chemoreceptor trigger zone N_2O increases the chances of postoperative nausea and vomiting.
- Teratogenic effects have been observed in animals, so N_2O should be avoided in first trimester of pregnancy.

- N_2O contributes to global warming and ozone depletion and some countries have started focusing on other alternatives.

Uses of Nitrous Oxide

- As a carrier gas for volatile agents.
- As a supplement, 65% N_2O decreases the MAC of volatile anesthetics by approximately 50%.
- As an analgesic for labor analgesia, dental pain, burn dressing, acute trauma.

Entonox®

Premixed 50:50 mixture of O_2 and N_2O. Cylinders of Entonox® needs to be stored horizontally (other cylinders are stored vertically) and above 10°C. At low temperature (<7°C), some N_2O settles down as liquid. This may lead to delivery of uneven mixture, i.e., too much O_2 at the beginning and too much N_2O at the end of cylinder life. This can be avoided by immersing the cylinder in hot water at 52°C and inverting it four times before using.

Uses

Painful dressings, removal of chest drains, dental surgeries.

Poynting Effect

In 50:50 mixture of nitrous oxide/oxygen. (entonox), gaseous oxygen bubbled through liquid nitrous oxide increases the vapour pressure of the mixture to form a gas at pressures where nitrous oxide normally remains in liquid form (called as Poynting effect). Because of this effect, Entonox has a pseudocritical temperature of -6°C at a cylinder pressure of 137 bar (13700 kPa) and is therefore a compressed gas at room temperature. However below its pseudocritical temperature (<6°C) it will separate under a process called 'lamination'. Where nitrous oxide will remain as liquid and oxygen as gas.[2]

Xenon

Only inert gas that possesses anesthetic properties under normobaric conditions (krypton and argon show anesthetic properties in hyperbaric condition). Xenon was first identified as an anesthetic agent in 1951 but was largely forgotten, and then was rediscovered in 1990. The gas cannot be manufactured but is recovered from air by the process of fractional distillation. Its cost of production is 100 times that of N_2O, which makes xenon a costly affair.

Physical Properties

- Inert gas with high density (heavier than air) and high viscosity (increase work of breathing).
- Noninflammable and nonexplosive.

Anesthetic Properties

- Possess analgesic effect, MAC—70%
- Blood gas coefficient is lowest (0.14), therefore induction and recovery is very rapid, (three times faster than desflurane).

Metabolism

Not metabolized by human tissue and is excreted as such through lungs.

Organ System Effects

- Xenon exhibit better cardiovascular and hemodynamic stability in both cardiac and noncardiac patients. Xenon possesses both neuroprotective and cardioprotective effects. It has no effect on liver, kidney and is not teratogenic.
- Because of high density and viscosity, xenon increase pulmonary resistance and work of breathing, so should better be avoided in patient with severe chronic obstructive pulmonary disease (COPD), asthma, and morbid obesity.
- During xenon anesthesia, N_2 released from patient body accumulates in anesthesia circuit and reduce the concentration (fraction) of O_2, thereby increase risk of hypoxia. So, preoxygenation (denitrogenation) is mandatory before administration of xenon.
- By depressing both sympathetic and parasympathetic nervous system xenon blunts the laryngoscopic reflexes. Beside this it does not contributes to greenhouse effect nor depletes ozone.
- Thus except one main disadvantage that is cost there is no limitation. So it is now widely accepted as future anesthetic gas.

KEY POINTS

Why is xenon a future anesthetic gas?
- Noninflammable, nonexplosive
- Very rapid induction and recovery
- No adverse side effect on any organ system
- No metabolism
- Provides hemodynamic stability

Halothane

Halothane is a noninflammable, nonexplosive halogenated alkane. It is the first member of modern volatile agents and also cheapest of all.

Physical Properties

- Colorless, pleasant smelling, nonirritating[Q] liquid. Thus, excellent for induction in pediatric patients.
- To prevent spontaneous decomposition, it is stored in amber[Q] colored bottle with thymol 0.01% as preservative. It has highest blood gas and fat/blood partition[Q] coefficient among currently used volatile agents, consequently both induction and recovery are delayed. This also contributes to its accumulation in adipose tissue after prolong exposure.

Anesthetic Properties

Potent anesthetic with MAC value of 0.74.[Q] Produces good muscle relaxation, but not a good analgesic.

Metabolism[Q]

Approximately 25–30% of halothane, administered undergoes oxidative metabolism into trifluoroacetic acid, chloride and bromide. Less than 1% is metabolized via reductive pathway. 70–75% is eliminated unchanged via lung.

Systemic Effect

Cardiovascular System[Q]

- Decreases HR,[Q] decreases cardiac output,[Q] decreases BP, decreases coronary blood flow.
- Sensitizes[Q] the heart to arrhythmogenic effect of epinephrine.
- Blunts the baroreceptor reflex to hypotension.
- Most of the cardiac effects are mediated by reduced activity of slow calcium channel.[Q]

Respiratory System

- Increases respiratory rate, decreases TV, decreases minute ventilation (produce rapid shallow breathing).
- Both hypoxic and hypercapnic respiratory derive are reduced.
- Among all volatile agents, halothane is the most potent bronchodilator;[Q] halothane attenuates airway reflexes and relaxes bronchial smooth muscles by inhibiting intracellular calcium mobilization (volatile agent of choice in asthmatics).[Q]
- Halothane depresses mucociliary function, thereby increases chance of postoperative atelectasis.

Nervous System[Q]

- Increases cerebral blood flow, increases intracranial pressure,[Q] decreases cerebral O_2 demand. Hyperventilation before halothane administration can prevent or at least attenuate the raise in ICP.
- Halothane relaxes skeletal muscles and potentiates nondepolarizing neuromuscular blocking drugs.
- It is a triggering agent for malignant hyperthermia.[Q]

Uterus

Produce uterine relaxation and increase chances of postpartum hemorrhage,[Q] so should better be avoided in cesarean section. Surprisingly due to its tocolytic property, it is *the agent of choice*[Q] for external version and manual removal of placenta in centers where desflurane is not available.

Temperature

There is drop in core temperature, after halothane induction. Among all inhalational anesthetics chances of postoperative shivering (halothane shakes)[Q] is maximum with halothane.

Liver

Halothane produce two types of hepatotoxicity[Q] (*see* above). Halothane hepatitis is extremely rare but severe form seen after repeated exposure in patients (particularly middle aged obese women) with familial pre-disposition. Histology in halothane hepatitis reveals **centrilobular necrosis**.[Q] Hypoxia and preexisting liver disease increases the severity. Evidence suggests autoimmune mechanism, trifluoroacetic acid combines with hepatic microsomal portions forming a haptene which can induce immune response in susceptible individual.[3]

Note: If the patient with halothane hepatitis has to undergo surgery, than sevoflurane is the volatile agent of choice (as it does not produce trifluoroacetic acid).

Uses

- To maintain the depth of anesthesia
- **As an inducing agent**: Halothane is the second volatile agent of choice for inhalational induction in pediatric patients.
- **Agent of choice for**:
  - Asthmatic patients
  - External cephalic version.

Contraindications

- History of halothane hepatitis
- Intracranial mass lesion (increases ICT)
- Fixed cardiac output disease (aortic stenosis)
- Patient with angina
- When exogenous epinephrine administration is planned (as lignocaine with adrenaline) or endogenous catecholamines are increased (as in pheochromocytoma)
- Patient susceptible to malignant hyperthermia.

Drug Interactions

- β blockers, calcium channel blockers potentiates myocardial depression of halothane
- Tricyclic antidepressants and MAO inhibitors increase risk of halothane related arrhythmias. Similarly combination of aminophylline and halothane may result in serious ventricular dysrhythmias.

Isoflurane

Chemically fluorinated methyl-ethyl ether. It is an isomer of enflurane.

Physical Properties

- Noninflammable,^{Q} colorless volatile liquid with saturated vapor pressure similar to that of halothane. So (though not recommended), it can be administered with halothane vaporizer.
- Pungent smell,^{Q} induction may be accompanied by breath holding, laryngospasm.^{Q} This is of particular importance in children.
- Isoflurane is a stable compound, therefore no preservative is added neither it react with rubber or metal of breathing system.

Anesthetic Properties

- MAC value of 1.15^Q makes isoflurane a moderately potent volatile agent. B/G coefficient is 1.38 which explain its delayed (but faster than halothane) induction and recovery.
- Produce good muscle relaxation but not a good analgesic.

Systemic Effects

Cardiovascular System

- Isoflurane in contrast to halothane produce lesser myocardial depression. Heart rate^Q tends to increase as a result of which cardiac output usually remain unchanged. Simultaneously, it does not sensitize the myocardium to arrhythmogenic effect of adrenaline.
- The most prominent effect is hypotension, secondary to reduced systemic vascular resistance.
- Isoflurane dilates coronary artery. This dilation is prominent in normal coronary artery, as coronary arteries of ischemic areas are already dilated *(ischemia is the most potent stimulus for coronary dilatation)*. Dilation of normal coronary artery shifts the blood away from ischemic area to nonischemic area. The phenomenon called as *coronary steal syndrome*^{Q} theoretically increases the risk of infarction. However, it is not so significant *in vivo* and isoflurane is second agent of choice^Q (first being sevoflurane) for cardiac patients.

Respiratory System

- Effect are same (but less marked) as that of halothane.
- Due to its irritating property, incidence of laryngospasm is high. Isoflurane also produce bronchodilation but of lesser degree than that of halothane.

Cerebral

For concentrations up to 1 MAC cerebral blood flow is not increased, hence ICP is maintained. At a higher concentration both cerebral blood flow (CBF) and intracranial pressure (ICP) increases, but this increase can be reversed by hyperventilation. Isoflurane reduces cerebral O_2 demand, and provide some degree of brain protection. Due to all these properties, isoflurane^Q is the most commonly used volatile agent in neurosurgery.

Hepatorenal System

Not much affected.

Metabolism

Only 0.2% of isoflurane administered is metabolized. Trifluoroacetic acid is the principal metabolic product.

Contraindications

Except in patient susceptible to malignant hyperthermia, there is no other absolute contraindication. However, it should be avoided in hypovolemic patients as they might not tolerate its vasodilating effect. In asthmatic patients also isoflurane should be avoided.

Enflurane

It is a sweet smelling isomer of isoflurane with similar anesthetic effects. Noninflammable at clinical concentration, but inflammable[Q] at concentration above 4.25%.

Systemic Effect

Cardiovascular System

- Depresses myocardium, decrease BP, decrease cardiac output, increase HR
- Sensitizes heart to arrhythmogenic[Q] effect of adrenaline, but potential is less than that of halothane.

Respiratory System

Effects (including bronchodilation)[Q] are same as that of halothane.

Cerebral

Increases CBF, increase ICP, increase CSF production. In high doses, enflurane can produce tonic clonic type of seizures.[Q] This epileptiform activity is exacerbated by high anesthetic concentration and hypocapnia. Therefore, hyperventilation is not recommended to attenuate enflurane induced intracranial hypertension. Due to these effects, it is contraindicated[Q] in epileptic patient and avoided in neurosurgery.

Hepatorenal System

Reduce hepatorenal blood flow.

🔑 KEY POINTS

Anesthetic agents with epileptic potential
- Enflurane
- Etomidate
- Ketamine
- Meperidine

Metabolism

About 5% of enflurane administered is metabolized. Fluoride is an end product; however, fluoride concentration usually remains below nephrotoxic concentration. Even then, it should be avoided in patient with pre-existing renal disease.

Sevoflurane

- Sevoflurane is fluorinated ether. Sweet smelling,[Q] nonirritant, so induction is smooth, rapid and is well-tolerated by both pediatric and adult patients.
- Blood gas coefficient[Q] of 0.63 makes sevoflurane a rapid acting volatile agent. Recovery is also rapid, and all these properties have made sevoflurane a volatile agent of choice[Q] in pediatric patients and patients posted for day care surgery.
- Metal and environmental impurities, glass bottles packing and anesthesia equipment, degrade sevoflurane into hexafluoride which can produce acid burn to respiratory mucosa. To prevent this degradation, water is added to sevoflurane during manufacturing and it is packed in a special plastic container.

Systemic Effect

Cardiovascular System

Effects are similar (but in lesser degree) to isoflurane. Absence of coronary steal syndrome makes sevoflurane the volatile agent of choice[Q] in cardiac patients.

Respiratory

Depresses respiration and reverses bronchospasm to an extent same as that of isoflurane.

🔑 KEY POINTS

Agent	Important side effect
N_2O	Megaloblastic anemia
Halothane	Bradycardia
Isoflurane	Coronary steal phenomenon
Enflurane	Epilepsy
Sevoflurane	Compound A production
Methoxyflurane	Most nephrotoxic

Liver

Sevoflurane reduce portal vein blood flow but simultaneously increase hepatic artery blood flow so usually total hepatic blood flow remains relatively unchanged.

Kidney

Sevoflurane minimally reduce renal blood flow. Under low flow and hypoxic conditions baralyme and soda lime degrade sevoflurane to form potentially nephrotoxic compound A.

Cerebral

Increases cerebral blood flow, increase ICP, decrease cerebral metabolic rate of oxygen ($CMRO_2$), there is no seizure potential. These properties make sevoflurane an excellent choice in neurosurgery.

Metabolism

About 5% of total sevoflurane administered is metabolized mainly by liver to from inorganic fluoride. Fluoride concentration may exceed renal threshold (50 mol/L) but due to its rapid washout, nephrotoxicity is very rare. Compound A[Q] is another nephrotoxic product produced by soda lime, baralyme induced degradation of sevoflurane.

Factors increasing compound A production are:
- Hypoxic conditions
- Low gas flow (< 2 L/minute)
- High temperature
- Fresh CO_2 absorbent.

Contraindications

Susceptibility to malignant hyperthermia and hypovolemia.

Desflurane

Fluorinated ether; structurally similar to isoflurane. In desflurane chlorine atom of isoflurane is substituted by fluorine.

Physical Properties

- Desflurane is a unique volatile agent with boiling point of 23°C (i.e., below room temperature).
- Blood gas solubility is lowest, perhaps making desflurane a volatile agent with most rapid onset.[Q] Desflurane is least[Q] (MAC = 6) potent among volatile anesthetics, this is also related to its low fat solubility. Requires no preservative and is stable in soda lime.
- Due to its low boiling point, special vaporizer is required for desflurane. Tec 6[Q] is a specialized vaporizer for desflurane, though Aladin™ cassette vaporizer can also be used *(See chapter 7)*.
- Desflurane has got pungent smell, due to which induction is often accompanied by coughing laryngospasm, this makes desflurane slightly less suitable for pediatric patients.

Systemic Effects

Cardiovascular

- Increase HR, decrease systemic vascular resistance, cardiac output remains unchanged or decrease only slightly. Rapid increases in desflurane concentration can sometime lead to transient but worrisome elevations in HR, BP and catecholamine levels. This is more pronounced in patients with cardiovascular disease and are due to sympathetic stimulation.
- Unlike isoflurane, desflurane does not increase coronary artery blood flow.

Respiratory

Decrease TV, increases minute ventilation.

Cerebral

Increases CBF, increases ICP, there is marked reduction in cerebral O_2 consumption rate,[Q] thus even during hypotension, aerobic metabolism is maintained.

Hepatorenal Function

Not much affected.

Metabolism

Among all volatile agents, desflurane is least[Q] metabolized. However, CO_2 absorbents (baralyme>soda lime) degrade desflurane to produce CO.

Indications and Contraindications

Rapid inset and recovery, makes desflurane an ideal agent for day care surgery.[Q] Due to its sympathetic stimulating properties, it can be used in shock patients.[Q]

Contraindications

Beside susceptibility to malignant hyperthermia, desflurane should be avoided in cardiac patients (tachycardia increase myocardial O_2 demand) and asthmatics (more chances of bronchospasm).

AGENTS NO LONGER USED

As details of these agents are not much useful, go through only main points and reason of their withdrawal.

Ether

- First anesthetic agent used in modern anesthesia.
- Diethyl ether (commonly called as ether) is a pungent smelling,[Q] highly inflammable[Q] and explosive.[Q]
- It is a very good muscles relaxant[Q] and provides intense analgesia.[Q] It is a potent bronchodilator[Q] and the only agent that preserves mucociliary activity of respiratory mucosa. Thus it is the only complete anesthetic agent.[Q] So one must be thinking despite all advantage why ether had been withdrawn, well here are the reasons:
  - Highly inflammable and explosive, may catch fire when cautery is being used.
  - Tracheobronchial secretions are markedly increased.
  - Among all inhalational agents, ether has got maximum[Q] chances of nausea and vomiting.
  - Induction is very irritating and unpleasant and is often accompanied by sympathetic stimulation (tachycardia, hypertension).
  - Due to high blood/gas coefficient, both induction and recovery are delayed.[Q]

Methoxyflurane

First fluorinated ether used as anesthetic agent. Blood/gas coefficient is highest (15). So, both induction and recovery are delayed. Most potent[Q] (MAC: 0.16) and toxic[Q] among all fluorinated ethers. Fluoride[Q] production is highest with methoxyflurane. Exhibit both hepatotoxicity and nephrotoxicity (high output renal failure secondary to high fluoride levels).

Cyclopropane

A highly inflammable and explosive[Q] anesthetic gas which was stored in orange[Q] colored cylinders. As such induction with cyclopropane is pleasant and is accompanied by sympathetic stimulation, which increases HR and blood pressure, so it was the agent of choice[Q] for shock patients. At emergence when cyclopropane is discontinued, there is abrupt withdrawal of sympathetic support and patient may land in shock, called as cyclopropane shock.[Q] Therefore cyclopropane should be stopped slowly. Beside this cyclopropane increase chances of nausea and vomiting, sensitizes myocardium to arrhythmogenic effect of adrenaline, can produce bronchospasm, increases surgical bleeding (due to raised BP). So, its withdrawal was not unusual.

Trielene

Colorless sweet smelling liquid, noninflammable, nonexplosive. Second most potent inhalational agent (first being methoxyflurane) and the most potent[Q] analgesic among all inhalational agents. Induction is slow and irritating. Trielene stimulates respiration, produces tachypnea, sensitizes myocardium to adrenaline. Biggest disadvantage of trielene was its reaction with soda lime. Trielene reacts with soda lime of closed circuit to produce:

- **Dichloroacetylene**:[Q] A neurotoxic compound which can affect V, VII (most commonly), and rarely III, IV, X, XI, XII cranial nerves.

- **Phosgene:**[Q] A gas which has got direct toxic effects on lung.

  In older days, it was used for labor analgesia. To prevent this, older anesthesia machine had trielene lock, which assures that closed circuit cannot be used when trielene is being used.

Chloroform

It is the most toxic[Q] inhalational anesthetic ever used. Chloroform is cardiotoxic, hepatotoxic,[Q] produces[Q] respiratory arrest. Surprisingly, chloroform was the first agent used for labor analgesia that too in Royal family of Great Britain.

NONANESTHETIC GASES IN ANESTHESIA

Beside inhalational anesthetics, an anesthetized individual requires other gases also, in which O_2 is mandatory, whereas other gases like CO_2, helium have definitive indication.

Oxygen

Physical Properties

- Colorless, odorless gas with boiling point –183°C, critical temperature –118.4°C.
- Not flammable by self but encourages fire production.
- Medical O_2 is manufactured by fractional distillation of air.
- Oxygen concentrators are the cheaper device, which concentrate O_2 from ambient air by preferential absorption of nitrogen on zeolites. This can generate the concentration up to 95% of O_2. However, the resultant mixture contains 4–6% of harmless impurities (mostly argon).
- Oxygen concentrators are suitable for use in hospitals, remote areas and in military.

Storage

- Medical O_2 is stored in cylinders with white shoulders and black body at a pressure of 2,000 psi, as a gas.

🔧 KEY POINTS

Agent	Why it is no longer used
Ether	Explosive, inflammable, nauseating
Methoxyflurane	Nephrotoxicity
Cyclopropane	Explosive, may produce shock
Trielene	Produce phosgene and dichloroacetylene

- In specialized cylinders, O_2 can be stored as liquid, at a temperature below the critical temperature (–119°C).

Medical Air

- Medical air contains gases in same concentration as atmosphere; however, it lacks infective spores, dust particles and H_2O.
- Medical air is used as a respiratory gas and to drive ventilators.
- It is supplied in gray cylinders with black and white shoulder quadrants compressed to 137 bar.

Helium

- Inert, colorless, odorless gas with boiling point –269°C, critical temperature –268°C.
- Specific gravity is one-sixth of that of air. So it is less dense than air.
- Its low density enables the mixture of 21% O_2 and 79% helium to flow through an orifice three times as fast as air. This is beneficial in patients with upper airway obstruction.
- Its low solubility has led to its use in the measurement of lung volumes by gas dilution.

Hyperbaric Oxygen

Delivering the O_2 above atmospheric pressure (>760 mm Hg). It is delivered in special hyperbaric chamber.

Indications

- **Decompression sickness:** Most common use
- In severe cases of carbon monoxide poisoning

- Gas gangrenes
- Gas embolism.

Therapeutic Principles

Hyperbaric O_2 increases dissolve O_2 in blood this competes with other gases and tends to shift equilibrium in favor of O_2 (principal behind CO poisoning treatment). Moreover this enhanced PaO_2 is directly toxic to anaerobic organism like *Clostridia*.

Contraindications

The only absolute contraindication is tension pneumothorax. Hyperbaric O_2 therapy should be avoided in patients consuming cisplatin, doxorubicin, disulfiram.

Limitations

Main limitations are its availability and cost.

Oxygen toxicity

Oxygen, though essential for life, when inhaled in higher concentration for prolonged period, is associated with many complications affecting multiple organ systems:
- Respiratory system
  - First system to get affected
  - Toxic radical of O_2 damage capillary membrane affecting diffusion
  - Clinically manifest as tracheobronchitis, atelectasis, acute respiratory distress syndrome (ARDS)
  - In neonates prolong oxygen therapy can lead to bronchopulmonary dysplasia.
- Nervous system: Acute O_2 toxicity can produce convulsions, this is called as Paul Bert effect.[4]
- Eyes: Retinolental fibroplasia seen in neonates particularly premature one, can produce blindness.

LAST-MINUTE REVISION

- Cyclopropane, N_2O, xenon are the anesthetic gases, rest all are liquids.
- Halothane is the most hepatotoxic volatile agent.
- Methoxyflurane is the most nephrotoxic volatile agent.
- N_2O is the only anesthetic agent with teratogenic potential.
- N_2O: MAC—0.5%; blue cylinder, associated with second gas effect and diffusion hypoxia.
- Fastest induction and recovery: xenon.
- Fastest induction and recovery with volatile agent: desflurane.

REFERENCES

1. Gruss M, et al. Two-pore-domain K+ channels are a novel target for the anesthetic gases xenon, nitrous oxide, and cyclopropane. Mol Pharmacol. 2004; 65(2):443-52. doi: 10.1124/mol.65.2.443. PMID: 14742687.
2. Litwin PD. The effects of temperature on nitrous oxide and oxygen mixture homogeneity and stability. BMC Anesthesiol. 2010;10:19. doi: 10.1186/1471-2253-10-19. PMID: 20950473; PMCID: PMC2967548.
3. LiverTox: Clinical and Research Information on Drug-Induced Liver Injury [Internet]. Bethesda (MD): National Institute of Diabetes and Digestive and Kidney Diseases; 2012-. Halothane. [Updated 2018 Jan 1]. Available from: https://www.ncbi.nlm.nih.gov/books/NBK548151/
4. Chawla A, Lavania AK. Oxygen toxicity. Med J Armed Forces India. 2001;57(2):131-3. doi: 10.1016/S0377-1237(01)80133-7. Epub 2011 Jul 21. PMID: 27407317; PMCID: PMC4925834.

Unit II: Anesthesia Pharmacology

REVIEW QUESTIONS

1. True about N_2O:
   a. Pin index 3, 5
   b. Cylinder blue in color
   c. Stored as liquid
   d. MAC 105
2. Which of the following is not true about xenon anesthesia?
   a. Nonexplosive
   b. Minimal cardiovascular side effects
   c. Slow induction and slow recovery
   d. Minimal renal side effects
3. Which of the following fluorinated anesthetics corrodes metal in vaporizers and breathing system?
   a. Sevoflurane
   b. Enflurane
   c. Isoflurane
   d. Halothane
4. Which of the following inhalational agents has the minimum blood gas solubility coefficient?
   a. Isoflurane
   b. Sevoflurane
   c. Desflurane
   d. Nitrous oxide
5. All the following are the disadvantages of anesthetic ether, *except*:
   a. Induction is slow
   b. Irritant nature of ether increases salivary and bronchial secretions
   c. Cautery cannot be used
   d. Affects blood pressure and is liable to produce arrhythmias
6. Use of N_2O is contraindicated in all the following surgeries, *except*:
   a. Cochlear implant
   b. Microlaryngeal surgery
   c. Vitreoretinal surgery
   d. Exenteration operation
7. True about halothane, all *except* that it:
   a. Is nonirritant
   b. Is antiarrhythmic
   c. Antagonizes bronchospasm
   d. Is a vasodilator

ANSWERS

| 1. a, b, c, d | 2. c | 3. d | 4. c | 5. d | 6. c |
| 7. b | | | | | |

CHAPTER 12

Intravenous Anesthetics

Anshul Jain, Pooja Chaubey

The drugs which on intravenous (IV) administration can produce reversible loss of consciousness at a dose which is relatively nontoxic to other organ system.

Intravenous anesthetics are used in anesthesia for:
- **Induction, i.e., loss of consciousness**: Propofol and thiopentone are the common inducing agent.
- **Analgesia**: Opioids, ketamine
- **Anxiolysis and amnesia**: Benzodiazepines (BZD)
- **Sedation**: Opioids, benzodiazepines
- **To blunt the sympathetic response of intubation and surgery**: Opioids.

The classification of intravenous anesthetics is shown in **Table 12.1**.

BARBITURATES

History
- Barbituric acid, a combination of urea and malonic acid was first synthesized in 1864 by JFW Adolph von Baeyer. Barbital (diethylbarbituric acid) was the first barbiturate with sedative properties.
- In anesthesia practice, thiopental became the most widely used barbiturate. It was initially used during the attack on Pearl Harbor as "the ideal form of euthanasia in war surgery".
- Today thiopental is one of the most commonly used inducing agents.

The two major divisions of barbiturates are:
1. Oxybarbiturates with oxygen at position two
2. Thiobarbiturates with a sulfur at position two. Sulfur increases the lipid solubility.

The classification of hypnotically active barbiturates is given in **Table 12.2**.

THIOPENTONE THIOPENTAL (PENTOTHAL)

Thiopentone is an ultrashort acting thiobarbiturates and is one of the most commonly used IV induction agents.

Metabolism
- All barbiturates (except phenobarbital) are metabolized in liver. The metabolites are inactive, water soluble, and excreted in urine. Renal excretion is important in the elimination of phenobarbital[Q] which is further enhanced by alkalinization of urine.
- Oxidation is the most important pathway, for metabolism. Drugs that induce oxidative microsomes enhance the metabolism of barbiturates. Chronic administration of barbiturates itself induce the enzymes. This enzymes induction property of thiopentone is

Table 12.1: Classification of intravenous anesthetics.

Barbiturates	Benzodiazepines	Opioids	Others
Thiopentone, methohexitone	Midazolam, diazepam	Morphine, pethidine, fentanyl, sufentanil, remifentanil, alfentanil	Propofol, ketamine, etomidate, phenothiazines, adrenergic agonist

Table 12.2: Classification of hypnotically active barbiturates.

Ultrashort-acting	Short-acting	Long-acting
Thiopental	Pentobarbital	Phenobarbital
Methohexital	Secobarbital	Mephobarbital
Thiamylal	Butalbital	Barbital
	Hexobarbital	Metharbital
		Primidone
	Mnemonic	
TMT	BSP Hathi	

responsible for its contraindication in patient with acute intermittent porphyria. Barbiturates may precipitate an attack by stimulating α-aminolevulinic acid synthetase,[Q] the enzyme responsible for the production of porphyrins.

Physicochemical Properties

- Sulfur analog of phenobarbiturate, (sulfur enhances the lipid solubility). It is prepared as sodium salts (mixed with 6% anhydrous sodium carbonate by weight to prevent its reaction with atmospheric CO_2) and then mixed with either water or normal saline to produce a 2.5% solution of thiopental.
- Thiopentone is administered in 2.5% solution[Q] as it is nearly isotonic[Q] (2.8% solution is isotonic which is difficult to form). pH of 2.5% solution is 10.4.[Q]
- It is highly alkaline (pH 10.4).
- Any decrease in alkalinity (or acidic solutions) can lead to precipitation of thiopentone, as free salts. This is why thiopentone should not be prepared in Ringer lactate.[Q]

> **KEY POINTS**
> - Drugs that are not to be coadministered or mixed in solution with barbiturates (thiopentone) are succinylcholine,[Q] pancuronium,[Q] vecuronium, atracurium, alfentanil, sufentanil, and midazolam.
> - In blood 80–90% of thiopentone is bound to plasma protein.

Pharmacokinetics

Thiopental and methohexital are most lipid soluble barbiturates, which account for their rapid onset of action. Unconsciousness is produced with in one arm brain circulation time (15 sec).[Q]

The two most important factors governing the onset of duration are:
1. Dose administered
2. Rate (speed) of administration.

However, if the initial dose is high, patient wakes up at high plasma concentration and requires subsequent dose more frequently, this phenomenon is known as *acute tolerance*.[Q]

The most important factor for the termination of thiopentone anesthesia is *redistribution*[Q] of the drug to other less perfused tissues (first muscle and then fat).

In addition, there is constant (first order) metabolism in liver. Clinically, patients wake after 5–10 minutes[Q] of thiopentone administration. Elimination half-life is 9 hours.

In the case of infusion or repeated injection, tissue sites get saturated and patients wake after a long period because first-order hepatic metabolism begins to play a larger role.

Pediatric patients (younger than 13 years) metabolize thiopentone with a higher rate which may result in earlier awakening.

Mechanism of Action[Q]

- Barbiturates mediate their action through gamma-aminobutyric acid (GABA).[Q] At low concentrations, barbiturates enhance the effects of GABA thus increasing the duration of GABA-activated chloride ion channel opening.
- At higher concentrations, barbiturates directly activate chloride channels thus, acting as the agonist themselves. The GABA-mimetic effect at slightly higher concentrations is responsible for "barbiturate anesthesia".[Q] Barbiturates also inhibits the synaptic transmission of excitatory neurotransmitter, such as glutamate and acetylcholine **(Fig. 12.1)**.[1]

Systemic Effects

Central Nervous System

- Thiopentone produces a dose-related depression[Q] in cerebral metabolic rate of oxygen

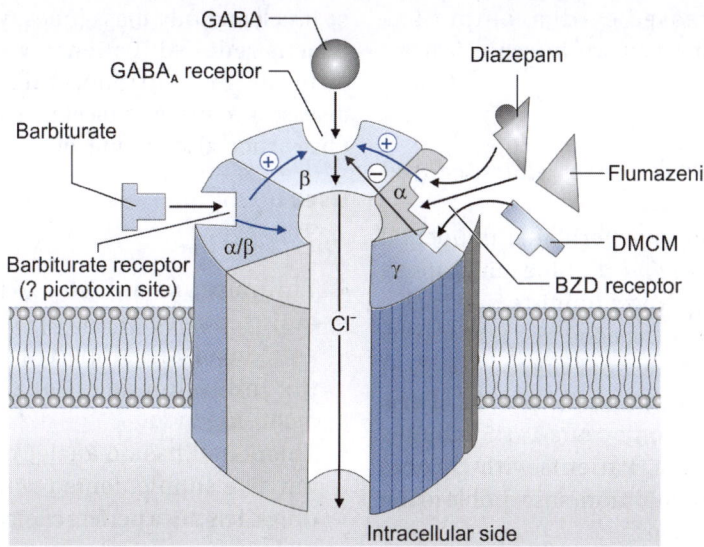

Fig. 12.1: Schematic depiction of GABAA-benzodiazepine receptor-chloride channel complex. The chloride channel is gated by the primary ligand GABA acting on GABAA receptor located on the ß subunit. The benzodiazepine (BZD) receptor located on the interface of α and Γ subunit modulates GABAA receptor in either direction: agonists like diazepam facilitate, while inverse agonists like DMCM hinder GABA mediated Cl- channel opening, and BZD antagonist flumazenil blocks the action of both. The barbiturate receptor, located either on α and ß subunit also facilitates GABA and is capable of opening Cl- channel directly as well. Bicuculline blocks GABAA receptor, while picrotoxine blocks the Cl- channel directly, DMCM (methyl 6,7-dimethoxy-4-ethyl-β-carboline-3-carboxylate).

($CMRO_2$). There is concomitant reduction in cerebral blood flow with reduction in $CMRO_2$. The ratio of cerebral blood flow (CBF) to $CMRO_2$ is unchanged, thus reducing the rate of adenosine triphosphate (ATP) consumption, and protection from cerebral ischemia.

- Even though mean arterial pressure (MAP) decreases, barbiturates do not compromise overall cerebral perfusion pressure [mean blood pressure minus intracranial pressure (ICP)]. Thiopentone decreases ICP to a greater extent relative to the decrease in MAP, thus preserving cerebral perfusion pressure.
- Thiopentone does not reduce basal metabolic rate.Q The only way to suppress the baseline metabolic cellular activity is through hypothermia.
- Due to the presence of phenyl group thiopentone is a potent anticonvulsant.Q
- Thiopentone does not provide analgesia, rather barbiturates actually decrease the pain threshold (*antianalgesic action*).Q

Cardiovascular System

- Barbiturates are cardiovascular depressant. The primary cardiovascular effect of thiopentone induction is peripheral vasodilation thus decreasing blood pressure secondary to pooling of blood.
- A decrease in contractility (*myocardial relaxant*)Q is another effect related to reduced availability of calcium to myofibrils leading to direct *negative inotropic action*.

KEY POINTS

Anesthetic agents with antiepileptic property
- Thiopentone
- Propofol
- Isoflurane, sevoflurone desflurome
- Benzodiazepines

- In few cases there is increase in heart rate secondary to baroreceptor-mediated sympathetic response to hypotension. This tachycardia along with decreased cardiac output has deleterious effect particularly in ischemic heart disease patients.

Respiratory System
- Barbiturates produce dose-related central respiratory depression.
- The usual ventilatory pattern after thiopental induction is "*double apnea*".[Q] The initial apnea that occurs during drug administration lasts a few seconds and is succeeded by a few breaths of reasonably adequate tidal volume, followed by a more lengthier apneic period. Peak respiratory depression occurs 1–1.5 minutes after administration. Patients with chronic lung disease are slightly more susceptible to the respiratory depression.
- If laryngoscopy or any other painful stimuli is given at lighter planes, severe laryngospasm[Q] and bronchospasm may occur. Bronchospasm may be seen in chronic obstructive pulmonary disease (COPD), asthmatic patients even at adequate depth. Thiopentone laryngospasm can be treated with positive pressure ventilation. Small dose of succinylcholine may be required in some cases.[Q] Rarely cricothyroid membrane puncture may be required for emergency airway management.

Eyes
Pupils first dilate then contract. It reduces intraocular pressure. *Loss of eye lash reflex*[Q] is an excellent sign of adequate induction of anesthesia.

Other Effects
Thiopentone stimulates antidiuretic hormone (ADH) action. Thiopentone due to presence of sulfur was thought to possess antithyroid property but recent studies have failed to demonstrate any such effect. Even though it is induction agent of choice in hyperthyroid patients[Q] because of its excellent hypnotic property.

Dosing
The usual dose of thiopental is 3–4 mg/kg.[Q] In patient with less blood volume (shock, dehydration) or less lean body mass (obesity, elderly females) dose is reduced. Patients with severe anemia or burns, malnutrition, widespread malignant disease, uremia, and ulcerative colitis or intestinal obstruction also require lower induction dose.

Uses

Anesthetic Uses
- Thiopentone is used for induction and maintenance (rarely) of anesthesia. Its anticonvulsant property makes thiopentone the induction agent of choice in *elective neurosurgery*.[Q]
- Thiopental has no analgesic[Q] properties and must be supplemented with other analgesic drugs. It is not a perfect choice, during balanced anesthesia as analgesic supplementation is required more often.
- Basal narcosis: Not used nowadays.

Other Uses
- As lie detector (*narcoanalysis*)[Q]
- As anticonvulsant[Q] when other drug fails
- As an *execution agent*[Q] where it is used along with pancuronium and potassium chloride
- To facilitate verbal communication with psychiatric patients.

Side Effects

Systemic
- Cardiorespiratory depression
- Laryngospasm and bronchospasm
- Garlic or onion taste (40% of patients)
- An urticarial rash[Q] that lasts a few minutes may develop on the head, neck, and trunk. More severe reactions and anaphylaxis are extremely rare.
- Postoperative delirium, euphoria.

Local
Most of the local complications are due to high alkalinity. These include:
- Pain on injection[Q] (seen in 10%)

- Thrombophlebitis.
- **Perivenous or intramuscular (IM) injection**: This can lead to tissue necrosis and ulceration. This can be prevented by assuring that IV cannula is properly placed, use 2.5% solution, inject drug slowly and in incremental doses.
  - *Treatment*: Inject 10 mL of 1% lignocaine with 100 units of hyaluronidase.
- **Intra-arterial injection**:Q This is one of most severe complication which can lead to gangrene and subsequent loss of limb. Usually intra-arterial injection occurs when cannula is misplaced in brachial artery instead of antecubital vein. So special precaution should be taken while injecting thiopentone in antecubital vein.
  - *Mechanism*: In artery, thiopentone gets precipitated which irritates the small vessels and stimulates noradrenalineQ secretion which causes arteriolar spasm severe enough to cease blood flow and thus cause ischemia.
  - *Symptoms*: Sudden severe burning pain in the limb, which is accompanied by pallor, cyanosis and gangrene of limb.
  - *Treatment*: Stop further injection, leave cannula or needle at site, through same cannula or needle inject:
    i. 10–20 mL of saline, so as to dilute the drug.
    ii. 500 unit of heparin to prevent thrombus formation.
    iii. Papaverine 40–80 mg to produce vasodilation.
    iv. Other vasodilators like tolazoline, phenoxibenzamine, if nothing is available inject lignocaine.
  - Brachial plexus block or stellate ganglion block for pain relief and vasodilation.
  - Defer elective surgery
  - Give oral anticoagulant.
- **Intraneural injection**:Q Mostly median nerve is injured. Treatment: 10–15 mL of 1% lignocaine.

Contraindications

Absolute

- Acute intermittent porphyriaQ and variegate porphyria (can be used in porphyria cutanea tarda)
- Known hypersensitivity to thiopentone
- Nonavailability of airway equipment.

Relative

- Patients with respiratory obstruction or anticipated difficult airway
- Severe cardiovascular instability or shockQ
- Asthma and COPD patients
- **Dystrophia myotonica**: Prolong apnea can be seen
- **Familial hypokalemic periodic paralysis**: It can cause severe hypokalemia.

In severe liver and kidney disease, dose is reduced but it is not contraindicated.

METHOHEXITONE

- The only other IV barbiturate used for induction. 2–3 times more potent than thiopentone.
- Similar to thiopentone in regard to distribution, which may explain the similar wake-up time. However, the total-body clearance of methohexital is faster, so it is superior to thiopental for maintenance of anesthesia and for brief infusion (<60 minutes).Q This is why methohexital is preferred barbiturate for Day care surgery.Q
  - Dose is 1–1.5 mg/kg (half that of thiopental).
  Incidence of cough, hiccough, tremors, and twitching is higher in comparison to thiopentone but chances of bronchospasm are less. So it is preferred barbiturate in asthma patients.

PROPOFOL

Propofol (chemically 2,6-diisopropylphenolQ) is most frequently used IV hypnotic today. It is used for induction and maintenance of anesthesia, as well as for sedation in and outside the operating room.

Physicochemical Characteristics

- Propofol belongs to the group of alkylphenols that have hypnotic properties. The alkyl-phenols are oils at room temperature and insoluble

in aqueous solution, but they are highly lipid soluble. So it is marketed as lipid base emulsion.
- The mostly widely used formula consist of 1 or 2% (weight/volume) propofol, 10% soybean oil, 2.25% glycerol, and 1.2% purified egg phosphatide.^{Q} The presence of oil makes the injection painful and presence of egg and glycerol make this formulation a perfect medium for microbial growth. Because of this disodium edetate^Q (0.005%) or sodium metabisulfite is added as antimicrobial.
- If a dilute solution of propofol is required, it is compatible with 5% dextrose in water. Propofol has a pH of 7 and appears as a slightly viscous milky white substance **(Fig. 12.2)**.
- Due to high susceptibility of microbial growth, once open ampoule should not be stored and the remaining drug must be discarded.

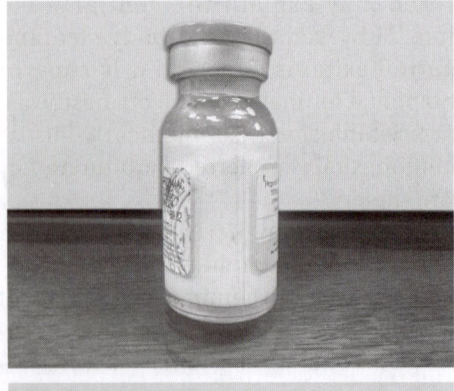

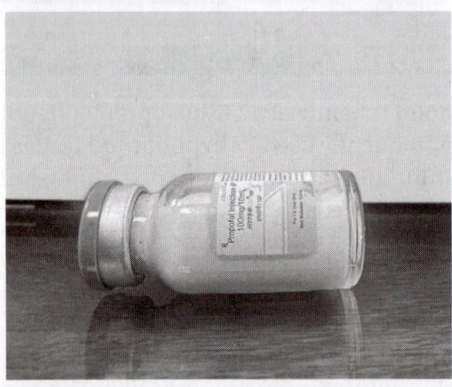

Fig. 12.2: Propofol vial (Note the white milky emulsion).

Mechanism of Action

Propofol is primarily a hypnotic. The exact mechanism is unknown, however, evidence suggest following mechanism:
- Potentiation of GABA^Q induced chloride current through binding to the α-subunit of the GABA receptor (hypnotic action).
- Through its action on GABA receptors, propofol inhibits acetylcholine release in the hippocampus and prefrontal cortex (sedative effects).
- Inhibition of N-methyl-D-aspartate (NMDA) receptor which contribute to the CNS effects.
- Decrease in serotonin levels in the area postrema (antiemetic effect).

Pharmacokinetics

Propofol onset is immediate and induction is achieved in one arm-brain circulation time (15 sec), peak effect seen at 90–100 seconds. Redistribution is responsible for termination of its effect and consciousness is regained in 4–8 minutes.

The *context sensitive half-time* (the time for the plasma level of the drug to drop 50% after cessation of infusion) of propofol for infusions lasting up to 8 hours is less than 40 minutes. So the recovery from propofol remains rapid even after prolonged infusions.

Doses^Q

- **Induction**: 1–2.5 mg/kg IV
- **Maintenance**: 50–150 µg/kg/min IV combined with N$_2$O or an opiate
- **Sedation**: 25–75 µg/kg/min IV
- **Antiemetic**: 10–20 mg IV

✎ KEY POINTS

Condition	Intravenous anesthetic agent of choice
Neurosurgery	Thiopentone
Day care surgery	Propofol
Cyanotic heart disease	Katamine
Asthmatic patient	Ketamine
Ischemic heart disease	Opioid ± Benzodiazepines (BZD)

For propofol infusion[Q] the scheme is:
- 1 mg/kg over a period of 20 seconds followed by
- 170 µg/kg/min (10 mg/kg/hr) for 10 minutes then
- 130 µg/kg/min (8 mg/kg/hr) for 10 minutes and then.
- 100 µg/kg/min or 6 mg/kg/hr.

Children younger than 3 years show greater systemic clearance values than adults or older children. So dose requirements are higher in them.

Metabolism

- Mainly metabolized in the liver[Q] by glucuronide conjugation to produce inactive compounds, which are excreted by the kidneys. Less than 3% of propofol is excreted unchanged in urine, and feces.
- Propofol also exhibits extrahepatic metabolism through *lungs*[Q] which contributes for 30% of its uptake and first-pass elimination.
- Propofol inhibit cP450 in a concentration-dependent manner and alter the metabolism of other P450 dependent drugs (e.g., opiates). Propofol impair its own clearance by decreasing hepatic blood flow owing of its effects on cardiac output.

Pharmacology

Central Nervous System

- Propofol decreases ICP[Q] in patients with either normal or increased ICP. It reduces the $CMRO_2$ by 36%.
- Cerebral protective effects are of same degree[Q] as of thiopentone.
- Unlike barbiturates, propofol is not anti-analgesic. In subhypnotic doses, propofol provides sedation and amnesia and helps in the diagnosis and treatment of central, but not neuropathic pain.
- Propofol lacks anticonvulsant property, rather associated with grand mal seizures. This feature makes it useful for cortical mapping of epileptogenic foci. Sometimes propofol induction can be accompanied by muscle twitching or myoclonic activity.

Effects on the Cardiovascular System

- The most prominent effect of propofol is a decrease in blood pressure[Q] by 25–40%, which is due to vasodilation (secondary to a reduction in sympathetic activity) and possibly myocardial depression.
- Propofol either resets or inhibits the baroreflex as a result heart rate does not change even after reduction in blood pressure (BP). It also attenuates the heart rate response to atropine in a dose-dependent manner.[2]

Effects on the Respiratory System

- Apnea occurs after an induction dose of propofol, in 25–30% cases. The incidence of prolong apnea (>30 seconds) is more than thiopentone and is further increased by the addition of an opiate. It abolishes the upper airway reflexes to a level that laryngoscopy and endotracheal intubation can be performed without muscle relaxant.
- Propofol induces bronchodilation[Q] but less than halothane.

Ocular Effects[Q]

Propofol reduces intraocular pressure more than thiopentone, it is more effective in preventing a rise in intraocular pressure secondary to succinylcholine and endotracheal intubation.

Other Effects

- Propofol, like thiopental, does not potentiate the neuromuscular blockade and has no effect on the evoked electromyogram or twitch tension. It does not trigger malignant hyperpyrexia and is the *anesthetic agent* of *choice*[Q] in patients with this condition.
- At subhypnotic doses, it exhibits antipruritic property, and can relieve cholestatic pruritus or pruritus induced by spinal opiates.
- Propofol decreases neutrophil chemotaxis, but not adherence, phagocytosis, and killing. However, propofol inhibits phagocytosis and killing of *Staphylococcus aureus* and *Escherichia coli*.

Uses

- Quick onset, early and smooth recovery, and antiemetic property has made propofol a commonly used IV anesthetic agent. It is *inducing agent of choice for*: Day care surgery,[Q] total IV anesthesia,[Q] patient susceptible for malignant hyperthermia.[Q]
- It has been approved for use in neurologic and cardiac anesthesia. As a precaution to prevent hypotension in sick patients or those undergoing cardiac surgery intravascular volume has to be restored before its injection and it should be administered in small incremental doses.
- It is also agent of choice for sedation in intensive care unit (ICU) patient.[Q] A potential advantage of propofol for sedation of ICU patients is its antioxidant properties.
- Recently, propofol has been shown to be valuable in the treatment of chronic refractory headache in doses of 20–30 mg every 3–4 minutes (400 mg maximum).

Side Effects and Contraindications

- Induction of anesthesia with propofol is associated with several side effects, including pain on injection,[Q] myoclonus[Q] (but less than that after etomidate), apnea, decrease in arterial blood pressure, and rarely, thrombophlebitis of the vein into which propofol is injected.
- **Pain on injection:** Can be reduced by using a large vein, avoiding veins in the dorsum of the hand, and adding lidocaine to the propofol solution or using cold solution.
- The most significant side effect of propofol induction is the decrease in BP; slow administration and smaller doses in adequately prehydrated patients may attenuate the decrease.

Propofol Infusion Syndrome[Q]

Propofol infusion syndrome[Q] is a rare, but lethal syndrome associated with infusion of propofol in a dose of 4 mg/kg/hr or greater for 48 hours or longer in an infant, younger child or critically ill adult. Clinical features include acute refractory bradycardia leading to asystole, in the presence of one or more of the following: metabolic acidosis, rhabdomyolysis, hyperlipidemia, and enlarged or fatty liver. Other features are cardiomyopathy with acute cardiac failure, metabolic acidosis, skeletal myopathy, hyperkalemia, hepatomegaly, and lipemia. This syndrome occurs as a result of failure of free fatty acid metabolism[Q] and failure of the mitochondrial respiratory chain.

Note: Propofol can be safely administered to individuals with history of egg white allergy. However, it should be avoided in persons with allergy to egg lecithin.

Mnemonic

- **P** : Painful
- **R** : Reflex suppressant
- **O** : Oil containing
- **P** : Pressure reducing (BP, intraocular pressure, decreasing ICP)
- **O** : Onset is rapid
- **F** : Fast action
- **O** : Open injection not to be used again
- **L** : Liver and lung metabolism

KEY POINTS

Propofol versus Thiopentone	
Advantages	**Disadvantages**
Rapid and smooth induction	Costly
Early wake-up, even after infusion	More chances of prolong apnea
Antiemetic and antipruritic	Injection is painful
Bronchodilator	Associated with myoclonic activity
Effective suppression of upper airway reflexes	Chances of microbial growth is high
Can be used in porphyria	Hypotension may be severe

KETAMINE

Ketamine (Ketalar) is a phencyclidine derivative.[Q] It is different from most other induction agents in following:

- It has significant analgesic effect[Q]
- Does not depress the cardiovascular system[Q]

- Does not depress respiratory systems^Q
- Can be given IM, IV, orally.^Q

But it is associated with some embarrassing psychological side effects and this is the reason because of which it is not used routinely.

Physicochemical Characteristics

Ketamine consists of two stereoisomers: S-(+) and R-(-). The S(+) isomer^Q is more potent and is associated with fewer side effects.

Ketamine is highly lipid soluble (5–10 times that of thiopental). It is prepared in a slightly acidic (pH 3.5–5.5) solution with benzethonium chloride as preservative.

Pharmacokinetics and Metabolism

Onset is rapid and patient gets induced within 30 seconds of IV injection. Maximal effect occurs in about 1 minute. The duration of ketamine anesthesia is 5–10 minutes.

Termination of effect after a single bolus is a result of drug redistribution. Elimination half-life is 2–3 hours. Clearance is also relatively high and is approximately equal to liver blood flow. Thus drugs which reduces hepatic blood flow (e.g., halothane), decreases ketamine clearance.

Ketamine is metabolized in liver. The major pathway involves N-demethylation to form norketamine (metabolite I), which has less activity (20–30%) than the parent compound. Norketamine is then hydroxylated and conjugated and is excreted in urine.

Ketamine can be administered intravenously, intramuscularly, orally, nasally, rectally, and as a preservative free solution epidurally. The dose depends on the desired therapeutic effect and the route of administration.

Ketamine shows additive interaction with propofol and tends to counteract the propofol induced hypotension. The dose of each would be reduced by about half when used together for induction.

Mechanism of Action (Fig. 12.3)

- The primary site of CNS action of ketamine is thalamoneocortical projection system.^Q
- The drug selectively depresses cortex (especially association areas) and thalamus (analgesia) while stimulates parts of the limbic system (emergence reaction), including the hippocampus creating functional disorganization in the midbrain and thalamic area. Ketamine also depresses the transmission of nociception from the spinal cord to higher brain centers.
- Ketamine acts by blocking NMDA receptor^Q (NMDA antagonist) and HCN1 receptors. It also blocks opiate receptors in the brain and spinal cord.

Pharmacology

Central Nervous System

- Ketamine produces dose-related unconsciousness and analgesia. The anesthetized state has been termed dissociative anesthesia^Q because patients who receive ketamine appear to be in a cataleptic state; they have profound analgesia but keep their eyes open and maintain many reflexes. Corneal, cough, and swallow reflexes may all be present but should not be assumed to be protective. But among all inducing agent chances of aspiration are minimum^Q with ketamine.

Note: Though cough reflex is preserved it should not be used in full stomach patient as ketamine increases chance of vomiting and also increases muscle tone, thus chances of aspiration are high in full stomach.

- Ketamine increases cerebral metabolism,^Q $CMRO_2$ CBF, and ICP because of its excitatory CNS effects. But ICP response to CO_2^Q is preserved, so hyperventilation can attenuate the increase in ICP. The increase in $CMRO_2$ and CBF can be blocked by use of diazepam or thiopental. It can cause petit-mal seizure-like activity and was supposed to deteriorate outcome in CNS ischemia. However recently in animal models ketamine has shown to improve neurologic outcome in cerebral ischemia by reducing necrosis. The neuroprotection observed with ketamine involve antiapoptotic mechanisms.

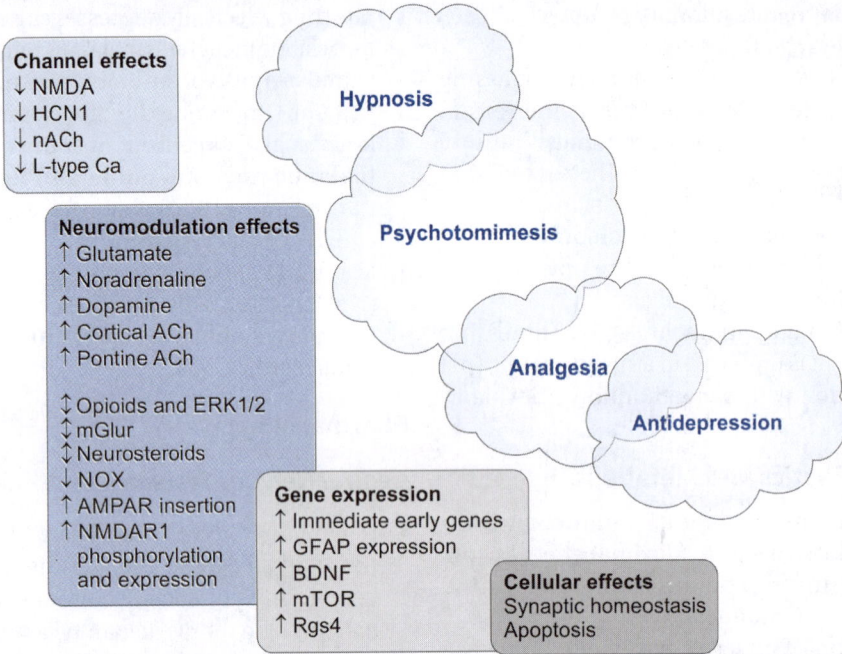

Fig. 12.3: Modes of action of ketamine, and the resultant clinical effects. The rapid effects (the top left), to delayed and prolonged effects (the bottom right). (NMDA: N-methyl-d aspartate; HCN1: hyperpolarization-activated cyclic nucleotide channels; ACh: acetylcholine; nACh: nicotinic acetylcholine receptors; AMPA: α-amino-3-hydroxy-5-methylisoxazole-4-propionic acid; mGluR: metabotropic glutamate receptors; ERK1/2: extracellular signal-regulated kinases; NOX: NADPH oxidase; BDNF: brain-derived neurotrophic factor; mTOR: mammalian target of rapamycin; Rgs4: regulator of G protein signaling 4; L-type Ca^{2-} L-type calcium channels; GFAP: glial fibrillary acidic protein).

- The plasma level for analgesia is lower than that required for anesthesia, so there is considerable postoperative analgesia[Q] after ketamine general anesthesia and its subanesthetic dose can be used to produce analgesia. Ketamine has got a rapid and delayed antidepressant effect too.[3]

Cardiovascular System

- Ketamine stimulates the cardiovascular system and is associated with increase in blood pressure, heart rate, and cardiac output. This increases myocardial work and oxygen consumption.
- Directly ketamine exhibits negative inotropic effects (myocardial depressant[Q]) by inhibiting calcium channel. However, it is least cardiac depressant among all induction drugs.
- There may be transient dysrhythmias[Q] after ketamine administrations which are due to increased noradrenaline.
- Cardiac diseases that can be well managed with ketamine anesthesia are cardiac tamponade[Q] and restrictive pericarditis due to its property of preserving the heart rate and right atrial pressure.
- Ketamine[Q] is the preferred drug in patients with right-to-left shunting [e.g., tetralogy of Fallot (TOF)] as it increase systemic vascular resistance and reduce shunt fraction.

Respiratory System

- Ketamine has minimal effect on the central respiratory drive and only a high dose can produces apnea.
- Ketamine is a profound *bronchodilator*.[Q] When given to patients with reactive airway disease, pulmonary compliance is improved. Bronchodilating effect of ketamine is due to its sympathomimetic action. Ketamine has been

used to treat status asthmaticus[Q] unresponsive to conventional therapy.

Eyes

After ketamine administration, pupils dilate moderately and nystagmus occurs. There is transient increase in intraocular tension.[Q] Nystagmus[Q] can be used as a sign of adequate induction.

Other Effects

- Ketamine increases the chances of nausea[Q] and vomiting. There is increase in salivation too, which can be prevented by prior administration of glycopyrrolate.
- Ketamine increases skeletal muscle tone.[Q] Nonpurposeful movement may be seen in light ketamine anesthesia.

Uses (Table 12.3)

Induction and Maintenance of Anesthesia

Due to the high incidence of unwanted emergence reaction, ketamine is rarely used as an inducing agent in routine surgeries. Poor-risk patients [American Society of Anesthesiologists (ASA), Class IV)] with respiratory and cardiovascular system disorders (excluding ischemic heart disease) represent the majority of candidates for ketamine induction. It is particularly appropriate for patients with:

- Reactive airway disease[Q]
- Patient in shock either due to hypovolemia or cardiomyopathy (not coronary artery disease).
- Healthy trauma victims in whom blood loss is extensive.
- Patients in septic shock.
- In patient susceptible to malignant hyperthermia when spontaneous ventilation is required.
- In remote places where airway equipment are not available.

Sedation

- Ketamine is particularly suited for the sedation in pediatric patients[Q] for minor procedures as they exhibit fewer emergence reactions.
- Ketamine can be used as a supplement or an adjunct to regional anesthesia in the dose of 0.5 mg/kg IV combined with diazepam or midazolam.

Other Uses

- Low-dose ketamine has been used as an analgesic after thoracic surgery and in opioid addict patients.
- Ketamine in doses of 10–20 mg preoperatively decreases postoperative pain (pre-emptive analgesia).[Q]
- Epidural/caudal administration of preservative free ketamine (0.5–1 mg/kg) as an adjuvant is increasingly being reported.

Table 12.3: Uses and doses of ketamine.

Use	Route	Dose	Onset	Peak effect	Duration
Induction	Intravenous Intramuscular	0.5–2 mg/kg[Q] 4–6 mg/kg	30–60 sec 8–10 min	1–2 min 15 min	5–10 min 10–30 min
Maintenance	Incremental bolus IV infusion	0.5–1 mg/kg IV with N$_2$O 50% in O$_2$ 15–45 µg/kg/min with N$_2$O 50–70% in O$_2$ 30–90 µg/kg/min without N$_2$O			
Sedation	IV (slow) IM Oral	0.2–0.8 mg/kg 2–4 mg/kg 3–10 mg/kg	1 min 10 min 20 min	30 min 30 min	10 min 30 min
Pre-emptive analgesia	IV	0.2–0.25 mg/kg			

(IV: intravenous; IM: intramuscular)

Side Effects

- **Emergence reaction:**[Q]
  - Ketamine has got high incidence (10–30%) of undesirable psychological reactions when patient regains consciousness. These are called emergence reactions.[Q] Common manifestations of these reaction are vivid dreaming, extracorporeal experiences (sense of floating out of one's body), and illusions. They usually occur in the first hour of emergence.
  - Factors that affect the incidence of emergence reactions are age, dose, gender, psychological susceptibility, and concurrent drugs. Pediatric patients have lower incidence compared to adults and it is more frequent in females than males.
  - Benzodiazepines[Q] are the most effective drugs to attenuate ketamine emergence reactions and hallucinations.
- **Hallucinations:**[Q] Most common side effect (seen in 30–40%). Both auditory (common) and visual hallucinations are common.
- Ketamine's preservative, chlorobutanol, is neurotoxic, so its intrathecal administration is contraindicated.
- Other side effects include increased muscle tone, salivation (so administered after an antisialagogue), increased intraocular pressure, increased incidence of nausea and vomiting.

Contraindications

- Head injury,[Q] intracranial mass lesion or other conditions in which ICP is increased (as it further increases ICP and can cause seizures).
- Open eye injury, or other ophthalmologic disorder, in which an increase in intraocular pressure is deleterious.
- Ischemic heart disease (as it increases myocardial oxygen demand).
- Hypertensive patients.
- Psychiatric disease such as schizophrenia.
- History of adverse reactions to ketamine or one of its congeners.

Mnemonic
- K : Kataleptic
- E : Epileptic
- T : Tensor (increase intraocular tension, intragastric tension, intracranial tension)
- A : Analgesic
- M : Myotonic (increase muscle tone)
- I : Inotropic, chronotropic
- N : Nystagmus, nauseating
- E : Emergence reactions

BENZODIAZEPINES

- Benzodiazepines commonly used in the anesthesia are diazepam, lorazepam midazolam and tamezepam.
- Diazepam (Valium) was the first benzodiazepine which was used as an anesthetic. Midazolam (Versed), is the first clinically used water-soluble benzodiazepine.

Pharmacokinetics and Metabolism (Table 12.4)

- Biotransformation of the benzodiazepines occurs in the liver. The principal pathways involve either hepatic microsomal oxidation or glucuronide conjugation.[Q]
- The termination of action is primarily a result of redistribution of the drug from the CNS to other tissues.
- Aging decreases and smoking increases the clearance of diazepam, but neither has a significant effect on midazolam biotransformation. Habitual alcohol consumption increases the clearance of midazolam.
- The metabolites of benzodiazepines can be active. Diazepam forms two[Q] active metabolites while midazolam has one.[Q] These metabolites are excreted in urine and can cause profound sedation in patients with renal impairment.

Mechanism of Action (Fig 12.1)

- BZD acts by stimulating GABA receptor. BZD alter the conformation of the GABA receptor

Table 12.4: Benzodiazepines at a glance.

Features	Midazolam	Diazepam	Lorazepam
Physicochemical			
Lipid solubility	++++^{Q}	+++	++
Water solubility	++ (in acidic medium)	--	--
Pharmacokinetics			
Onset (after IV)	30–60 sec	30–60 sec	1–2 min
Duration	Short	Long	Intermediate
Elimination $t_{1/2}$	2–3 hours	20–50 hours	10–20 hours
Context sensitive $t_{1/2}$	70–90 min^Q	Very high (not used for infusion)	Very high (not used for infusion)
Dose			
Induction	0.05–0.15 mg/kg	0.3–0.5 mg/kg	0.1 mg/kg
Maintenance	0.05 mg/kg prn	0.1 mg/kg prn	0.02 mg/kg prn
Sedation	0.5–1.0 mg repeated	2 mg repeated	0.25 mg repeated
Receptor affinity (Potency)	+++	++	+++(max)^Q
Metabolism	Oxidation	Oxidation	Conjugation
Active metabolite	Hydroxymidazolam	Oxazepam,^{Q} Desmethyldiazepam	None
Disadvantages			
Pain on injection	–^{Q}	++	++
Hypotension	+	–/+	–/+
Flumazenil reversal	Effective	Effective	Poor (due to high affinity)

(PRN : As required to keep patient hypnotic)

complex so that binding affinity for GABA is increased (GABA facilitatory action).^{Q}
- The benzodiazepine binding site is located on the γ-2 subunit.
- BZD antagonists (e.g., flumazenil) occupy the benzodiazepine receptor, but they have no activity and therefore block the actions of both agonists and inverse agonists.
- Long-term administration of benzodiazepines produces tolerance (decrease in efficacy of the drug) due to decreased receptor binding and function.

Pharmacology

Central Nervous System
- All BZDs have hypnotic, sedative, anxiolytic, amnesic and anticonvulsant property.
- Increase stage 2 sleep, decrease stage 3, 4 and REM sleep.
- The benzodiazepines reduce $CMRO_2$ and CBF in a dose-related manner maintaining a relatively normal ratio of CBF to $CMRO_2$.
- Midazolam and to a lesser extent diazepam induce a dose-related protective effect against cerebral hypoxia.
- The best method of monitoring depth with midazolam is use of the bispectral index (BIS).^{Q}
- They possess no analgesic property, so must be used with other analgesics.

KEY POINTS
- Both barbiturates and benzodiazepines reduces REM sleep. Reduction is more with barbiturates.
- Nitrazepam is the only benzodiazepine which increases REM sleep.

Cardiovascular System
- BZDs itself have no significant cardiovascular effect except slight reduction in arterial BP

(maximum with midazolam[Q]) which results from reduced systemic vascular resistance.
- Heart rate, ventricular filling pressure, and cardiac output remains unchanged after midazolam induction.
- In patients with elevated left ventricular filling pressure, diazepam and midazolam produce a "nitroglycerin-like effect"[Q] by lowering the filling pressure and increasing cardiac output. These properties make BZD a suitable agent for cardiac anesthesia and in cardiac patients.

Respiratory System

- Produce dose-related central respiratory system depression which is greater with midazolam than with diazepam and lorazepam. It is more pronounced and of longer duration in patients with chronic obstructive pulmonary disease. BZD and opioids produce additive or supra-additive (synergistic) respiratory depression.
- The peak of depression is rapid (approx. after 3 min), and significant depression remains for about 60 to 120 minutes. The rate of midazolam administration affects the time of onset of peak ventilatory depression; the faster the drug is given, the more quickly this peak depression occurs.

Muscular System

BZD itself produce muscle relaxation through central action (at medulla and spinal cord). BZD potentiates nondepolarizers.

Uses

Sedation and Anxiolysis

- Benzodiazepines are used for sedation as preoperative premedication, intraoperatively during regional or local anesthesia, and postoperatively.
- Assessment of adequacy of sedation is by Verill sign,[Q] when the upper eyelid droops to halfway across the pupil.
- Midazolam[Q] is the most commonly used agent. It has got lowest context sensitive half-time among BZD, so is the most suitable agent for infusion.
- Despite the wide safety margin with benzodiazepines, respiratory function must be monitored when used for sedation.

Oral Sedation[Q]

Recently, an oral formulation of midazolam has been used for oral premedication in pediatric patients. The dose is 0.5 mg/kg. It provides reliable amnesia within 10 minutes and effectively sedates children for induction of anesthesia.

Induction and Maintenance of Anesthesia

Though induction with BZD is hemodynamically stable, it takes time because of which they are not used routinely for induction purpose. Midazolam due to its rapid onset is BZD of choice for induction of anesthesia.[Q]

Other Uses in Anesthesia

- As anticonvulsant, to control convulsions after local anesthetic toxicity.
- As adjuvant to regional blockade.
- To control emergence reaction of ketamine.

Side Effects and Contraindications

- Benzodiazepines have a relatively high margin of safety, especially when compared with barbiturates.

> **KEY POINTS**
> - Cimetidine reduces the metabolism of diazepam.
> - Erythromycin inhibits the metabolism of midazolam and prolongs its duration by 2–3 folds.
> - Heparin displaces diazepam from protein binding sites and increases the free drug fractions, so does respiratory depression.

- They are free of allergic effects, do not suppress adrenal gland and are hemodynamically stable.
- The most significant problem with midazolam is respiratory depression.[Q] Diazepam and lorazepam cause venous irritation and thrombophlebitis due to presence of propylene glycol as solvent.

- It is also important to mention that respiratory depression and sedation of BZD can be readily reversed with flumazenil.

FLUMAZENIL

- Flumazenil (Anexate) is the first benzodiazepine competitive antagonist approved for clinical use. It binds to GABA at BZD binding site and has minimal intrinsic activity.
- Used for diagnostic and therapeutic reversal of the benzodiazepine effects.
- Antagonizes respiratory depression, sedation, hypnosis but amnesia is minimally reversed.
- *Dose*: Incremental IV doses of 0.2–0.5 mg up to 3 mg.
- *Onset*: 1–3 min.

Side Effects and Contraindications

- Due to its shorter half-life (1–2 hours) an important caution is resedation^Q particularly when given after longer agents like diazepam. It does not antagonize lorazepam optimally because of high receptor affinity of lorazepam.
- It is free of local or tissue irritant properties, and it has no known organotoxicities.

ETOMIDATE

Etomidate was introduced in 1972. Its unique properties include hemodynamic stability, minimal respiratory depression, cerebral protection, and pharmacokinetics enabling rapid recovery after either a single dose or a continuous infusion.

This enthusiasm for etomidate, was tempered by reports that it can cause temporary inhibition of steroid synthesis after both single doses and infusions. This effect, combined with other minor disadvantages (e.g., pain on injection, superficial thrombophlebitis myoclonus, nausea and vomiting) waned the use. Recently because of rediscovery of beneficial physiologic profile combined with a lack of any new reports gives etomidate a new birth as an inducing agent.

Physicochemical Characteristics

Etomidate is an imidazole^Q derivative which is water insoluble and is unstable in a neutral solution. To increase its solubility, it is formulated as a 0.2% solution either in 35% propylene glycol or in a lipid emulsion.

Pharmacokinetics and Metabolism

- Etomidate is a rapid and short-acting^Q inducing agent. The onset of anesthesia is rapid (one arm-brain circulation) and effect usually last about 100 seconds.
- It is 75% protein bound, thus in patients with low serum proteins etomidate exhibits an exaggerated effect.
- Etomidate is metabolized in the liver primarily by ester hydrolysis. The metabolites are excreted through kidney (85%), bile (13%). The drugs affecting hepatic blood flow alter its elimination.

Dose

- **Induction**: 0.2–0.6 mg/kg IV
- **Maintenance**: 10 µg/kg/min IV with N_2O and an opiate
- **Sedation**: 5–10 µg/kg/min IV.
- Limited to periods of brief sedation because of inhibition of corticosteroid synthesis.

Mechanism of Action

Etomidate depresses reticular activating system and mimics the inhibitory effects of GABA. It binds to GABA type A receptors and increases the affinity of the inhibitory neurotransmitter (GABA) for the receptors.

Pharmacology

Central Nervous System

- Etomidate reduces ICP and $CMRO_2$ without altering mean arterial pressure. Thus, cerebral perfusion pressure (MAP-ICP) is maintained or increased.
- It is associated with grand mal seizures and produce increased EEG activity in epileptogenic foci. This feature is useful for intraoperative mapping of seizure foci before surgical ablation. It is also associated with a high incidence of myoclonic movement.
- Etomidate exhibits no analgesic activity.

> **KEY POINTS**
>
> **Anesthetic agents and enzymes**
> - **Thiopentone**: Stimulates D-aminolevulinic acid (ALA) synthetase.
> - **Etomidate**: Inhibits 11-β-hydroxylase.

Cardiovascular System[Q]

- Etomidate in regular doses has no effect on heart rate, cardiac output, and other cardiovascular parameters in both normal and cardiac patients.
- The hemodynamic stability seen with etomidate is due its lack of effect on the sympathetic nervous system and baroreceptor function.
- Etomidate is thus useful in patient with valvular heart disease and ischemic heart disease undergoing noncardiac surgery and in patient with poor cardiac function.

Respiratory System

Etomidate has minimal effect on respiratory system. However, hiccups or coughing may sometime accompany etomidate induction.

Endocrine Effects

- Etomidate results in adrenocortical suppression by producing a dose-dependent reversible inhibition of the enzyme 11 β-hydroxylase,[Q] which converts 11-deoxycortisol to cortisol. This reduces cortisol level. The temporary adrenocortical suppression, last up to 6 hours after the dose of etomidate.
- Vitamin C supplementation restores cortisol levels to normal after the use of etomidate.

Other Effects

- Reduces intraocular pressure which lasts 5 minutes.
- In a very few cases, etomidate resulted in inhibition of platelet function with increased blood loss.

Uses

- Etomidate is most appropriate in hemodynamically unstable patients, e.g., cardiovascular disease.
- It is inducing agent of choice for aneurysm surgery,[Q] cardiothoracic procedures, especially cardiac and lung transplantation.
- For cardioversion too, quick recovery, and maintenance of blood pressure makes it an acceptable choice.
- Sedation with etomidate is useful in hemodynamically unstable patients, such as those with acute myocardial infarction or unstable angina who require sedation for a minor operative procedure, or those who require intubation in the emergency room or the ICU.

Side Effects and Contraindications

- Etomidate induction is associated with nausea and vomiting. It has got highest incidence[Q] of nausea and vomiting among all currently available inducing agents.
- Pain on injection,[Q] superficial thrombophlebitis, myoclonic movement, and hiccups are other side effects.
- Pain on injection maybe reduced by injecting lidocaine 20–40 mg immediately before induction with etomidate.
- Myoclonus is reduced by premedicaion with midazolam.
- Prolonged sedation for patients in the ICU, is contraindicated because of the inhibition of corticosteroid and mineralocorticoid activity.

NEUROLEPTANALGESIA (FLOWCHART 12.1)

- In 1950s a concept was proposed to use drugs that would produce neurovegetative blockade (artificial hibernation) of the cellular, autonomic, and endocrine mechanisms normally activated in response to stress.
- The first combination was the lytic cocktail, of an analgesic (meperidine), two tranquilizers (chlorpromazine and promethazine), and atropine. But this combination produced respiratory depression and was abandoned.
- Later a combination of fentanyl and droperidol was used and found to be superior. This fixed combination of droperidol and fentanyl,

Chapter 12: Intravenous Anesthetics

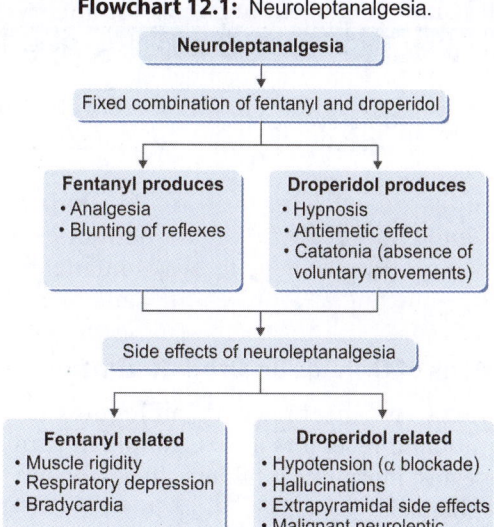

Flowchart 12.1: Neuroleptanalgesia.

marketed as Innovar[Q] was primarily used for neuroleptanalgesia (NLAN).

Innovar contains droperidol and fentanyl in the ratio of 50:1[Q] (Droperidol 2.5 mg + Fentanyl 0.05 mg).

With the invention of better agents, the use of NLAN has largely disappeared in modern anesthetic practice.

Neuroleptanesthesia

When an inhalational agent (nitrous oxide or halothane) is added to innovar, it constitutes neuroleptanesthesia.[Q]

DROPERIDOL

- Droperidol, a phenothiazines derivative which produces CNS depression characterized by marked tranquility and cataleptic immobility along with potent antiemetic effect. In present scenario the primary use of droperidol in anesthesia is limited only as an antiemetic, sedative and antipruritic.
- It has got little effect on the respiratory system. However, it prolongs the QT interval and may precipitate torsades de pointes.[Q]

Uses

- As an antiemetic,[Q] the dose for which varies between 10 µg/kg and 20 µg/kg. In pediatric patients it can be given orally.
- For the treatment and prevention of pruritus secondary to opioids.

OPIOID ANESTHETICS

Opiates include the natural products **(Table 12.5)** like morphine, codeine, and thebaine which are derived from the juice of the *Papaver somniferum* and many other semisynthetic or synthetic congeners derived from them.

In anesthesia, they are used for:
- Analgesia (both intraoperative and postoperative)
- Premedication

Table 12.5: Classification of opioids.

Class	Natural	Semisynthetic	Synthetic		
Agonist			Benzomorphans	Phenylpiperidine	Morphinan derivative
	Codeine	Heroin		Pethidine	Levorphanol
	Papaverine	Dihydromorphone		(meperidine)	
	Morphine			Fentanyl	
	Thebaine			Alfentanil	
	(Mnemonic: CPMT)			Sufentanil	
				Remifentanil	
				Tramadol	

Contd...

Contd...

Class	Natural	Semisynthetic	Synthetic		
Agonist-antagonist		Buprenorphine	Pentazocine		Butorphanol
			Other synthetic agonist-antagonist		
			Nalbuphine		
			Nalorphine		
Antagonist (all synthetic)			Nalmefene	Naloxone	Naltrexone

- Sedation in ICU
- To blunt intubation reflex
- As an adjuvant to local anesthetic in intrathecal or epidural space
- To prevent and control shivering.

Physicochemical Properties

Opioids are weak bases that are to some extent bound to plasma proteins, either albumin or α-acid glycoprotein.

Opioid Receptors (Table 12.6)

- The opioid receptors belong to the G protein-coupled receptor family. They all inhibit adenylate cyclase[Q] and reduce cellular cyclic adenosine monophosphate (cAMP) content.
- Opioid receptors[Q] are expressed in amygdala, the mesencephalic reticular formation,[Q] the periaqueductal gray matter (PAG), and the rostral ventral medulla.[Q]

Table 12.6: Physiological effects of opioid receptor.

μ (mu)	κ (kappa)	δ (delta)
Analgesia	Analgesia	Analgesia
Constipation	Miosis	Nausea
Euphoria	Dysphoria	
Sedation	Sedation	
Miosis	Diuresis	
Respiratory Depression		
Increase growth hormone and prolactin		

Actions of Opioids on Other Receptors

Opioids can interact with molecules other than opioid receptors also. Example in cardiac myocytes, morphine inhibits voltage-dependent Na^+ channels.

Mechanism of Analgesia and Other Effects

- Opioids produce analgesia through spinal, supraspinal and peripheral mechanism.
    - *Supraspinal*:[Q] They activate pain control circuits that descend from the midbrain, via rostral ventromedial medulla (RVM), to the spinal cord.
    - *Spinal*: Opioid receptors are present in substantia gelatinosa[Q] where they inhibit substance P release and directly inhibit the ascending transmission of nociceptive information from the spinal cord dorsal horn.
    - *Peripheral mechanism*: Through opioid receptors located on primary sensory neuron.
- Opioid produce euphoria, tranquility, and other alterations of mood through dopaminergic pathways in the nucleus accumbens.[Q]

Systemic Effects of Opioids

Central Nervous System

- **Analgesic action**: Opioids produce analgesia, drowsiness, changes in mood, and mental clouding. Nociceptive pain responds much better than neuropathic pain.
    - Intrathecal or epidural administration of opioids can produce profound segmental analgesia without significantly altering motor function.

- Opioids generally decrease cerebral metabolic rate (CMR) and ICP.
- Animal studies of neurologic injury suggest that anesthesia with opioids improves neurologic outcome.
- They do not alter sensory evoked potentials (SEPs). Therefore, SEP monitoring can be used for spinal cord function monitoring during anesthesia using opioids.
- **Muscle rigidity:**[Q] Opioids can increase muscle tone and may cause muscle rigidity. It is due to activation of central μ-receptors. Opioid-induced rigidity usually begins just as, or after, a patient loses consciousness. However it may be delayed too.
- **Neuroexcitatory phenomena**: Morphine can produce tonic-clonic activity after epidural and intrathecal administration. Meperidine[Q] can also cause convulsions which are due to its metabolite normeperidine. Fentanyl can cause neuroexcitation ranging from delirium to grand mal seizure-like activity.

Respiratory System

- Opioids are respiratory-depressant which is their most serious adverse effect.
- Some respiratory effects of opioids are therapeutic while some are deleterious.

Therapeutic Effects

- Opioids, by decreasing both pain and central ventilatory drive, are effective agents in preventing hyperventilation induced by pain or anxiety.
- They possess effective antitussive actions and are excellent agents for depressing upper airway, tracheal, and lower respiratory tract reflexes. However, fentanyl, sufentanil, and alfentanil may cause a brief cough in up to 50% of patients.
- Opioids blunt sympathetic response responses to tracheal intubation, allowing patients to tolerate endotracheal tubes without coughing or "bucking".
- Opioids can reduce the bronchomotor tone in asthma. Fentanyl has antimuscarinic, antihistaminergic, and antiserotonergic actions and is more effective than morphine in asthma or other bronchospastic diseases.

Nontherapeutic/Deleterious Effects

Opioids depress respiration through a direct action on brainstem respiratory centers. There is decrease in both hypercapnic and hypoxic ventilatory drives.

Factors increasing opioid induced respiratory depression:
- High dose
- Sleep
- Old age
- Other CNS depressant
- Renal insufficiency
- Hyperventilation
- Respiratory acidosis
- Chronic obstructive pulmonary disease (COPD)
- Inhaled anesthetics, alcohol, barbiturates and benzodiazepines.

Note: Droperidol, scopolamine, and clonidine, though CNS depressant do not enhance the respiratory depressant effects of opioids.

Cardiovascular System (Table 12.7)

- Opioids provide hemodynamic stability throughout the operative period. They maintain myocardial perfusion and the O_2 supply/demand ratio. They decrease heart rate through vagal stimulation. Opioids do not effect preload and afterload.
- Opioids may depress cardiac conduction. Fentanyl slows atrioventricular node conduction, and prolongs the PR interval.
- **B**utorphanol, **p**entazocine, **p**ethidine (*Mnemonic:* BP **p**otentiates BP) in contrast to other opioids, cause tachycardia[Q] and increase myocardial oxygen requirement. So they should be avoided in cardiac patients.

KEY POINTS

Nucleus accumben is located in the region of basal forebrain. It has an important role in pleasure including laughter, reward as well as fear of aggression, impulsivity.

Table 12.7: Hemodynamic effects of agonist-antagonist compounds compared with morphine.

Drug	HR	Cardiac workload	BP	PAP
Morphine	↓	↓	↓	↓
Buprenorphine	↓	↓	↓	–
Butorphanol	–	↑	↑	↑
Nalbuphine	↓	↓	–	–
Pentazocine	↑	↑	↑	↑

(HR: heart rate; BP: blood pressure; PAP: pulmonary artery pressure)

Endocrinologic Effects

- Opioids reduce the stress response by reducing pain and modulating centrally mediated neuroendocrine responses. Sufentanil^Q is the most effective opioid in diminishing stress responses.
- Opioids are potent inhibitors of the pituitary-adrenal axis.

Renal and Urodynamic Effects

μ-receptor activation causes antidiuresis while κ-receptor stimulation predominantly produces diuresis.

Gastrointestinal Effects

- Opioids decrease gastrointestinal motility. Patients receiving parenteral opioid therapy preoperatively should be considered "full stomach" regardless of their "nil per orally (NPO)" status. Among all opioids, tramadol^Q has got least inhibitory effect on gastric emptying.
- Opioid agonists increase biliary duct pressure and sphincter of Oddi tone in a dose dependent manner.

Other Effects

- **Nausea and vomiting**: Opioids stimulate the chemoreceptor trigger zone (CTZ)^Q in the area postrema through δ receptors, leading to nausea and vomiting which is a serious problem with opioid induction. Ondansetron, is effective in preventing and treating opioid-induced nausea and vomiting. Alfentanil, has lowest incidence of postoperative nausea and vomiting among opioids.
- **Pupil size**: Most μ- and κ-receptor agonists cause constriction of the pupil by an excitatory action on the parasympathetic nerve innervating the pupil.
- **Thermoregulation and shivering**: Pethidine and tramadol^Q are very effective in controlling and preventing shivering by reducing the shivering threshold. They are very effective in treating postoperative shivering too.
- **Pruritus**: Opioids cause pruritus mediated by the μ-receptor. Naloxone reverses opioid-induced itching. Nalbuphine and butorphanol, have least pruritic potential. Ondansetron (an antiemetic) can treat spinal or epidural morphine-induced pruritus.
- **Immune effects**: Opioids have immunosuppressive effects mediated by decreased activation of NF-κB (nuclear factor kappa-light-chain-enhancer of activated B cells).

Factors Affecting Pharmacokinetics of Opioids

Age

- Neonates eliminate opioids at a lower rate, due to immature cytochrome P450 system.
- In elder age group also dose has to be reduced due to decreased central volume of distribution and increased sensitivity of brain to opioids.

Renal Failure

- Kinetics and dynamics of fentanyl congeners is not affected.
- Morphine toxicity is increased and patient can develop very high levels of M6G and life-threatening respiratory depression.

- Pethidine metabolism is also significantly altered and its chief metabolite normeperidine, gets accumulated which can cause seizures.

Hepatic Failure
- Remifentanil is the only opioid whose metabolism is not affected in liver disease.
- Morphine pharmacokinetics also remains relatively unchanged because of the significant extrahepatic metabolism.

Anesthetic Uses

Sedation and Analgesia
- The most common use of opioid in anesthesia is as an analgesic. At the time of induction, the short-acting potent agent (commonly fentanyl) are used.
- Long-acting agents such as morphine, pethidine are used for maintaining intraoperative and postoperative analgesia.
- For doses *see* **Table 12.8.**
- **Choice of opioid**: The ideal agent permit rapid titration, should not depress cardiovascular function, permit the return of adequate spontaneous ventilation in a timely manner. Alfentanil[Q] and remifentanil are nearest to ideal due to immediate onset, and rapid recovery. Compared with alfentanil, sufentanil provides greater hemodynamic stability and requires less supplementation.
  Remifentanil also reliably suppress somatic and autonomic responses to noxious stimulation and allows rapid emergence from anesthesia.

Table 12.8: Opioids dose for intraoperative analgesia.

Drug	Dose
Morphine	0.2–0.5 mg/kg/IV
Pethidine	2.5–5 mg/kg/IV
Fentanyl[Q]	2 µg/kg/IV
Sufentanil	0.20 µg/kg/IV
Alfentanil	20 µg/kg/IV(loading)(least potent)[Q]
Remifentanil	1 µg/kg/IV

(IV: intravenous)

> **Mnemonic**
> Learn the dose of fentanyl-**s**ufentanil is required in **s**mall dose (1/10 of fentanyl); **a**lfentanil is required in large dose (10 times as that of fentanyl).

Inducing Agent
- Opioids are not preferred inducing agent due to their slower onset, high incidence of nausea and vomiting.
- As an inducing agent, they are used mainly in cardiac patients undergoing cardiac surgery. In cardiac surgery morphine is inducing agent of choice.
- ASA III and IV are other subset of patient in which opioids can be used as an inducing agent.

As Adjuvant to Local Anesthetic
Morphine, fentanyl can be administered in intrathecal, epidural, peripheral nerve blocks along with local anesthetics. They increase the duration of block.

CLINICAL PHARMACOLOGY OF IMPORTANT AGONISTS

Morphine
- **Protein binding**: 20–40% (mostly albumin)
- **Metabolism**:
  - Mainly by conjugation in the liver, but the kidney also plays a role in the extrahepatic metabolism.
  - Morphine 3-glucuronide (M3G) is the major metabolite of morphine, which is inactive. Morphine 6-glucuronide[Q] (M6G) accounts for nearly 10% of morphine metabolite. It is a more potent µ-receptor agonist than morphine. Both of these metabolites are excreted in urine.
  - In patients with renal dysfunction, M6G accumulation can increase incidence of adverse effects, including respiratory depression.

KEY POINTS
Potency of opioid: Sufentanil > Remifentanil ≥ Fentanyl > Alfentanil > Morphine > Pethidine.

Pethidine (Meperidine)

- **Protein binding**: 70% (α1-acid glycoprotein)
- First pass metabolism occur in lung after IV injection.
- **Metabolism**:
  - Mainly in liver.^{Q} Metabolite is excreted through urine.
  - The major metabolite norpethidine^Q (normeperidine) has analgesic activity and has got convulsive activity too.
  - The $t_{1/2}$ of normeperidine is considerably longer than that of meperidine, and thus repeated doses can produce accumulation of this toxic metabolite in patients with renal disease.

Fentanyl, Alfentanil and Sufentanil

- **Protein binding**: 80–85%
- The lungs exert a significant first-pass effect and take up 75% of an injected dose of fentanyl. Significant amount is also taken up by red blood cells.
- **Metabolism**: In liver by N-dealkylation and hydroxylation.
- Fentanyl can produce significant muscle rigidity (called as wooden chest syndrome).

Remifentanil

- Remifentanil is structurally unique because of its ester linkages which make it susceptible to hydrolysis by blood and tissue nonspecific esterases,^{Q} resulting in rapid metabolism. Remifentanil thus constitutes the first "ultrashort-acting"^{Q} opioid.
- Its context-sensitive half-time is independent of duration of infusion and is about 4 min.
- The remifentanil is formulated as a solution with glycine. Glycine is an inhibitory neurotransmitter that causes a reversible motor weakness when injected intrathecally, so remifentanil is not approved for spinal or epidural use.

AGONIST-ANTAGONIST OPIOIDS

Nalorphine, was the first agonist-antagonist opioid, synthesized and was found to be strong antagonist to almost all the properties of morphine except analgesia. Despite of this it was unsuitable for clinical uses because of its psychotomimetic effects.

Agonist-antagonist opioids are less prone (but not immune) to abuse. They also depress respiration however with *ceiling effects*^{Q} (After a certain dose there is no further increase in respiratory depression).

Pentazocine

- κ^Q (mainly) and δ-receptor stimulant and antagonist at μ receptor. Its potency is one-third of that of morphine.
- Abuse potential is less than with morphine, but prolonged use of pentazocine can lead to physical dependence.

Systemic Effects (Table 12.7)

- Pentazocine produces tachycardia and hypertension by stimulating sympathetic system. Thus, it should not be used in cardiac patients.
- Both analgesia and respiratory depression shows *ceiling effect*.
- It is associated with a high incidence of postoperative nausea and vomiting. Though biliary spasm and constipation are less severe.

Dose

0.5–1 mg/kg can be given IM or IV

Use

Mainly for intraoperative analgesia, sequential analgesia (where it is administered after fentanyl).

It has limited application due to high incidence of PONV, limited analgesia, undesirable cardiovascular and psychomimetic effect.

Butorphanol

- Kappa^Q receptors agonist, 5–8 times^Q as potent as morphine. It has got less abuse and has less addictive potential than morphine.
- Its activity at μ-receptors is either antagonistic or partially agonistic.
- Systemic effects are similar to pentazocine though tachycardia is less. Respiratory depression of butorphanol shows ceiling effect after 1.2 mg.

Dose

- 1–2 mg IV in an adult patient
- Side effects after butorphanol include drowsiness, sweating, nausea and CNS stimulation.

Buprenorphine

- Buprenorphine is a thebaine derivative, μ-receptor partial agonist (agonist at low dose and antagonist at higher dose)[Q] and is 33 times more potent than morphine.
- Systemic effects are similar to morphine except respiratory effects which shows ceiling effect. Infact there is an increase in ventilation on increasing dose due to μ-receptor antagonism.
- Its onset of action is slow, its peak effect may not occur until 3 hours, and its duration is more than 10 hours.

Dose

0.3 mg slow IM or IV.

Nalbuphine

Nalbuphine is an agonist-antagonist opioid related to naloxone. It is kappa-receptor agonist[Q] and μ-receptor antagonist.[Q] The onset of effect is rapid (5–10 minutes), and its duration is long (3–6 hours).

> **KEY POINTS**
> - Opioids showing ceiling effect on respiratory depression
> - Buprenorphine and pentazocine.

OPIOID ANTAGONISTS

Naloxone

Pure opioid receptor antagonist, active against μ, δ, and κ-receptors, has the greatest affinity for μ-receptors:

- Clinically, used to restore spontaneous ventilation in patients who have respiratory depression after opioid overdoses or opioid anesthesia. In addition, opioid antagonists can reduce or reverse opioid-induced nausea and vomiting, pruritus, urinary retention, rigidity, and biliary spasm.
- Naloxone has short half-life and this accounts for recurrence of respiratory depression (renarcotization) when it is used to reverse long acting opioid.

Naltrexone

Naltrexone is a longer acting μ, δ and κ-receptor antagonist which can be taken orally.

α_2 ADRENERGIC AGONISTS

α_2 adrenergic agonists provide sedation, anxiolysis, hypnosis, analgesia and sympatholysis. Dexmedetomidine and clonidine are the α_2 adrenergic agonists which are being used in anesthesia. They are mainly used as an adjuvant to reduce the dose requirements of other agents.

Dexmedetomidine

Dexmedetomidine is a selective α_2-agonist,[Q] (1600-fold selectivity) with the properties of:

- Sedation
- Anxiolysis
- Analgesia
- Sympatholysis
- Hypnosis (at high doses).

Dexmedetomidine is rapidly distributed and extensively metabolized in the liver and excreted in both urine and feces. These parameters remain unaltered in renal failure and elderly.

Pharmacology

Central Nervous System

α_2-agonists produce their sedative-hypnotic effect and analgesic effect by stimulating α_2-receptors in the locus ceruleus and the spinal cord.[Q]

Respiratory System

Dexmedetomidine reduces minute ventilation but maintains the ventilatory response to CO_2. Respiratory rate remains unchanged.

Cardiovascular System

Dexmedetomidine decrease heart rate, systemic vascular resistance, myocardial contractility, cardiac output, and systemic BP.

Other Effects

Dexmedetomidine decreases saliva production resulting in dry mouth, which is due to α blockade.

Uses and Doses

Dexmedetomidine is not indicated for induction as dose required exceeds toxic dose. Presently it is used for:
- Sedation in the dose of 0.4–0.7 µg/kg given 15 minutes before surgery. This dose effectively reduces the hemodynamic response to intubation.
- Intraoperatively, it is used as an adjuvant because its maintenance can reduce volatile anesthetic requirement by more than half.
- For sedation of patient in ICU.

Clonidine

Imidazoline derivative with predominantly α_2 adrenergic agonist activity. *Site of action* is rostral ventrolateral medulla where it activates inhibitory neurons.

It is less selective on α_2 receptors than dexmedetomidine, so chances of hypotension and bradycardia are more.

Currently, it is used as an adjuvant for epidural infusions in pain management particularly in neuropathic pain.

LAST-MINUTE REVISION

- **Thiopentone** (a sulfur containing barbiturate) is one of the most commonly used inducing agents. It is used in 2.5% solution, as it is nearly isotonic.
  - Contraindicated in acute intermittent porphyria (as thiopentone stimulate α-aminolevulinic acid synthetase)
  - Inducing agent of choice in hyperthyroid patient, elective neurosurgery
- **Propofol:**
  - 2,6 diisopropylphenol, contains egg phosphatide and disodium acetate.
  - Agent of choice in day care surgery. Patient with suspicion of malignant hyperpyrexia; ICU sedation.
  - Complications include hypotension; propofol infusion syndrome.
- **Ketamine:**
  - Unique inducing agent, because of its intense analgesia, multiple routes of administration (IV, IM, oral, per rectal).
  - Increase cerebral blood flow, intracranial pressure, depress myocardium, induces bronchodilation. Reflexes remain intact.
  - Contraindication includes epileptic patients, elective neurosurgery, ischemic heart disease, psychiatric patients.
  - Induction agent of choice for asthmatic patients, cyanotic heart disease.
- **Benzodiazepines:**
  - Midazolam is the most frequently used BZD in anesthesia practice. It is most lipid soluble, and has shortest context sensitive half time, however it is maximally bound to plasma protein.
- **Etomidate:**
  - Rapid, short-acting, highly cardiostable inducing agent, which inhibits 11α hydroxylase. Thus reduces cortisol synthesis.
  - Induction agent of choice for aneurysm repair surgery, major cardiothoracic surgery, cardioversion.
- **Opioids:**
  - Morphine, fentanyl, sufentanil, remifentanil are cardiofriendly opioids, whereas pethidine, pentazocine, butorphenol increase BP causes tachycardia and should be avoided in cardiac patients.
  - Remifentanil is the shortest acting opioid and is opioid of choice in pediatric patients, renal patients and cardiac patients.
  - Sufentanil is most potent opioid, and is the most effective opioid in depressing stress response.

Summary of systemic effects of commonly used intravenous anesthetic.

Agent	HR	MAP	Vent	B'dil	CBF	CMRO$_2$	ICP
Barbiturates	↑↑	↓↓	↓↓↓	↓	↓↓↓	↓↓↓	↓↓↓
Benzodiazepines	0/↑	↓	↓↓	0	↓↓	↓↓	↓↓
Ketamine	↑↑	↑↑	↓/↑	↑↑↑	↑↑↑	↑	↑↑↑
Etomidate	0	↓↑	↓	0	↓↓	↓↓	↓↓
Propofol	0	↓↓↓	↓↓↓	0	↓↓↓	↓↓↓	↓↓↓
Droperidol	↑	↓↓	0	0	↓	0	↓
Opioids							
Meperidine*	↑	*	↓↓↓	*	↓	↓	↓
Morphine*	↓	*	↓↓↓	*	↓	↓	↓
Fentanyl	↓↓	↓	↓↓↓	0	↓	↓	↓
Sufentanil	↓↓	↓	↓↓↓	0	↓	↓	↓
Alfentanil	↓↓	↓↓	↓↓↓	0	↓	↓	↓
Remifentanil	↓↓	↓↓	↓↓↓	0	↓	↓	↓

(HR: heart rate; MAP: mean arterial pressure; Vent: ventilatory drive; B'dil: bronchodilation; CBF: cerebral blood flow, CMRO$_2$: cerebral metabolic rate of oxygen; ICP: intracranial pressure)
* Effect of meperidine and morphine on MAP and bronchodilator depends upon a extent of histamine release.

REFERENCES

1. Hao X, et al. The effects of general anesthetics on synaptic transmission. Curr Neuropharmacol. 2020;18(10):936-65. doi: 10.2174/1570159X18666200227125854. PMID: 32106800; PMCID: PMC7709148.
2. Kanaya N, et al. Differential effects of propofol and sevoflurane on heart rate variability. Anesthesiology. 2003; 98:34-40.
3. Zorumski CF, et al. Ketamine: NMDA receptors and beyond. J Neurosci. 2016;36(44):11158-64. doi: 10.1523/JNEUROSCI.1547-16.2016. PMID: 27807158; PMCID: PMC5148235

REVIEW QUESTIONS

1. Induction agent that may cause adrenal cortex suppression is:
    a. Ketamine
    b. Etomidate
    c. Propofol
    d. Thiopentone
2. Which anesthetic induction agent produces cardiac stability? In other words cardiostable anesthesia agent is:
    a. Ketamine
    b. Propofol
    c. Thiopentone
    d. Etomidate
3. An intravenous anesthetic agent that is associated with hemodynamic stability, maintenance of cerebral perfusion pressure CPP with postoperative nausea, vomiting and myoclonus:
    a. Ketamine
    b. Etomidate
    c. Propofol
    d. Opioids
4. Characteristics of Remifentanil:
    a. Metabolized by plasma esterase
    b. Short half-life
    c. More potent than Alfentanil
    d. Dose reduced in hepatic and renal disease
    e. Duration of action more than Alfentanil

Unit II: Anesthesia Pharmacology

5. Cerebral metabolism and O_2 consumption are increased by:
   a. Propofol
   b. Ketamine
   c. Atracurium
   d. Fentanyl

6. All are true about thiopentone except:
   a. $NaHCO_3$ is a preservative
   b. Contraindicated in Porphyria
   c. Agent of choice in shock
   d. Has cerebroprotective action

7. Which of the following anesthetic agent lacks analgesic effect?
   a. N_2O
   b. Thiopentone
   c. Methohexitone
   d. Ketamine
   e. Fentanyl

8. Which of the following intravenous anesthetic agents has/have good analgesic property?
   a. Ketamine
   b. Nitrous oxide
   c. Thiopentone
   d. Propofol
   e. Midazolam

9. With regard to ketamine, all of the following are true, *except*:
   a. It is a direct myocardial depressant
   b. Emergence phenomena are more likely if anticholinergic premedication is used
   c. It may induce cardiac dysrhythmias in patients receiving tricyclic antidepressants
   d. Has no effect on intracranial pressure

10. A 20-year-old patient presented with early pregnancy for medical termination of pregnancy MTP in day care facility. What will be the anesthetic induction agent of choice?
    a. Thiopentone
    b. Ketamine
    c. Propofol
    d. Diazepam

11. The following anesthetic drug causes pain on intravenous administration:
    a. Midazolam
    b. Propofol
    c. Ketamine
    d. Thiopentone sodium

12. Regarding features of propofol, which of the following statement is correct?
    a. It suppresses adrenocortical hormone secretion
    b. IM injection is painful
    c. Undergoes hepatic metabolism
    d. Chemically it is derivative of D-isopropylphenol
    e. Cerebral protector action

13. Anesthetic agent causing bradycardia:
    a. Halothane
    b. Isoflurane
    c. Thiopentone
    d. Ketamine

14. Thiopentone is administered in conc. of:
    a. 2.5%
    b. 5%
    c. 2%
    d. 3%

15. Anesthetic of choice for status asthmatics is:
    a. Ketamine
    b. Thiopentone
    c. Ether
    d. N_2O

ANSWERS

1. b	2. d	3. b	4. a, b and c	5. b	6. c
7. b, c	8. a	9. d	10. c	11. b	12. c, d, e
13. a		14. a	15. a		

CHAPTER 13

Local Anesthetics

Anshul Jain

INTRODUCTION

Local anesthetics (LAs) block propagation of both afferent and efferent nerve impulses that carry pain and other sensation.

To abolish sensation, LAs must be placed in closed vicinity of nerve so they can be absorbed, viz:
- **Topical application**: LAs are readily absorbed by mucosal surface, and results in desensitization of mucosa.
- Injection in the vicinity of peripheral nerve endings and major nerve trunks, or
- **Injection within the epidural or subarachnoid spaces**: This is called epidural anesthesia or spinal anesthesia respectively. Term central neuraxial blockade includes both spinal and epidural anesthesia.

It should not be presumed that LAs have no systemic effects. When LA agents are given systemically, they can alter the function of cardiac, skeletal and smooth muscle, as well as transmission of impulses in the central and peripheral nervous systems.

Toxicity may be local or systemic. The central nervous and cardiovascular systems are most commonly involved organ systems.[Q]

BASIC PHARMACOLOGY

Chemistry

The typical LA molecule contains a tertiary amine attached to a substituted aromatic ring by an intermediate chain that contains either an ester or an amide linkage.

Based on this intermediate chain LAs can be classified as aminoester[Q] or aminoamide compounds. The aromatic[Q] ring system imparts lipophilic character, whereas the tertiary amine end is relatively hydrophilic.

On the basis of their site of application, they are broadly divided into injectable and topical anesthetic **(Table 13.1)**.

Structure-Activity Relationships and Physicochemical Properties

Potency and duration of action depends on certain structural and chemical features:

Lipophilic-Hydrophilic Balance

Compounds with "lipophilicity" or hydrophobic nature are more potent and produce longer-lasting blocks.

Hydrogen Ion Concentration

Local anesthetics exist in an equilibrium state between the basic uncharged form (B) and the charged cationic form (BH^+). At a pH specific for each drug, the concentration of uncharged base in solution is equal to the concentration of charged cation. This pH called pKa, is specific for each drug. There are dual effects of pH on clinical effectiveness (described later).

MECHANISM OF ACTION (FIG. 13.1)

Local anesthetics block nerve conduction by decreasing the entry of Na^+ ions during upstroke of action potential (AP). As the concentration of LA increase, the rate of rise of AP and maximum depolarization decreases, thereby slowing and finally blocking conduction.

In solutions, the LA molecule is partly ionized. The equilibrium between the unionized base form

Table 13.1: Classification of local anesthetics.

Class	Injectable			Surface	
	Low potency (short duration)	Intermediate potency and duration	High potency long duration	Soluble	Insoluble
Amide		Lignocaine (lidocaine)	Tetracaine	Lignocaine	Oxethazaine
		Prilocaine	Bupivacaine	Tetracaine	Butylaminobenzoate
			Ropivacaine	Benoxinate (oxybuprocaine)	Benzocaine
			Dibucaine		
Ester	Procaine Chloroprocaine			Cocaine	

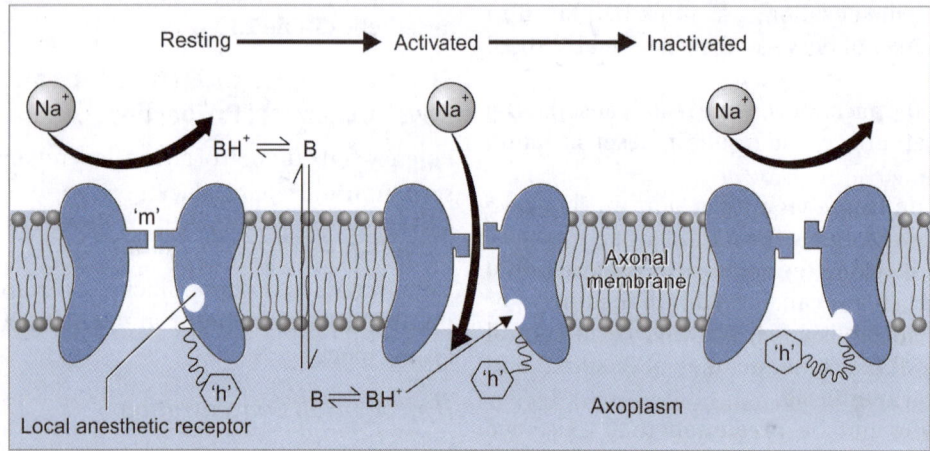

Fig. 13.1: Mechanism of action of local anesthetics. The Na+ channel has an activation gate ('m' gate) near its extracellular mouth and an inactivation gate ('h' gate) at the intracellular mouth. In the resting state, the activation gate is closed. Threshold depolarization of the membrane opens the activation gate allowing Na+ ions to flow in along the concentration gradient. Within a few milliseconds, the inactivation gate closes and ion flow ceases. The channel recovers to the resting state in a time-dependent manner.

(B) and the ionized cationic form (BH+) depends on the pKa of the LA. Most LAs are weak bases with pKa between 7 and 9.

So, at pH greater than 7, concentration of basic form is more, while at pH less than 7 concentration of ionized form is high. The unionized form is lipid soluble and can spread through tissue and penetrates membrane; however, the active is the ionized cationic form.Q

The receptor for LAs are located on the intracellular aspect of sodium channel, which means LA has to traverses the membrane to reach the receptor site (**Fig. 13.1**). Only unionized lipophilic form (B) can traverse the membrane. In the axoplasm, some of the unionized form of LA again dissociate into active cationic form. It is, this cationic form, which binds to the receptor. The receptor has higher affinity or is more accessible to the LA in the activated state compared to resting state. Due to this fact, repeated stimulation of nerve (which is supposed to be blocked) accelerates the onset of block.

Few Interesting Facts

Though the ionized cationic form is active, its intracellular concentration is directly proportional to extracellular concentration of unionized form or inversely proportional to extracellular concentration of cationic form. Addition of weak base (sodium bicarbonate) increases the concentration of unionized base form, and in turn intracellular cationic form, thereby accelerating the onset of block and simultaneously increasing the depth too.

In myelinated nerve fibers the site of action of LA is node of Ranvier. Two or three adjacent nodes must be blocked to prevent conduction. For this at least 6 mm or perhaps 10 mm of nerve fiber must be exposed to the LA solution.[1]

Minimum concentration of LA necessary to block a nerve fiber of a given diameter is called "Cm". Cm depends on myelination and diameter. Myelinated fibers are more sensitive to LA.

Aα fibers are the thickest one, so have the highest Cm. Cm of Aδ fiber[Q] is half as that of Aα fiber. It is, therefore, possible that the concentration at which Aδ fibers are blocked might be ineffective for Aα fibers (carries vibration and pressure sensation) or they get spared. It is evident clinically, when patient fells no pain but says something is happening over surgical site, due to intact proprioception (carried by Aα fibers).

🔑 KEY POINTS

Sequence of blockade
- Type B fibers are most sensitive
- Aα fibers are most resistant
- Among sensory fibers, sequence of blockade is temperature (cold before and hot) → pain → touch → deep pressure.

CLINICAL PHARMACOLOGY

Anesthetic Potency

Directly proportional to the hydrophobicity of the drug.

Onset of Action

Time of onset of blockade mainly depends upon the physicochemical properties of the individual agents and type of nerve fibers. *In vivo* on increasing the concentration of LA, onset is accelerated.

Types of Nerve Fibers

Thinner fibers are more susceptible than thicker ones, however myelinated fibers (*thicker than unmyelinated*) are more susceptible to blockade than the unmyelinated ones. It is because local anesthetic acts at nodes of Ranvier.

Duration of Action

The duration of action of the various LAs differs markedly. Procaine and chloroprocaine have a short duration of action. Lidocaine, mepivacaine and prilocaine produce a moderate duration of anesthesia, whereas tetracaine, bupivacaine,[Q] ropivacaine,[Q] and etidocaine produce block which last up to 6 hours (longer duration).

Differential Sensory/Motor Blockade

Ropivacaine (more) and bupivacaine when used in dilute solutions, block sensory fibers while motor fibers are minimally affected. This differential blockade produces sufficient analgesia with mild muscle paralysis.

FACTORS INFLUENCING ANESTHETIC ACTIVITY IN HUMANS

Dose

As the dose of LA increases, duration of anesthesia increases and the onset of block is accelerated. The dose of LA can be increased either by increasing concentration or by increasing volume. Increased concentration also increases the intensity of block.

Addition of Vasoconstrictors

Addition of vasoconstrictors, usually epinephrine (5 µg/mL or 1:200,000), to local anesthetic solutions increase the duration of anesthesia. They do so by reducing the rate of vascular absorption, thereby allowing more anesthetic molecules to reach the nerve membrane. They also act as a marker for inadvertent intravascular injection, e.g., when there is an inadvertent intravascular injection of lignocaine with adrenaline, heart rate would increase due to presence of adrenaline. However, this can generate false negatives and false positives particularly in parturients in labor, and patients receiving β-blockers. Other vasoconstrictor agents, such as norepinephrine and phenylephrine, have also been used to increase duration of anesthesia, but they do not appear to be superior to epinephrine.

The extent to which epinephrine prolongs the duration of anesthesia also depends on the local anesthetic being used and the site of injection. Epinephrine significantly prolongs the duration of both infiltration anesthesia and peripheral nerve blockade of shorter-duration agents (e.g., lidocaine); effect is mild when it is used with bupivacaine.

> **KEY POINTS**
>
> Adrenaline should not be used in ring block, penile block, pinna, toes (as they get supply from end arteries which gets constricted by adrenaline).

Carbonation and pH Adjustment of Local Anesthetics

The addition of sodium bicarbonate to LA solution accelerates the onset and decreases the minimum dose required for blockade.

Mixtures of Local Anesthetics

Mixtures of LAs for regional anesthesia are sometimes used as an effort to accelerate onset. Mixing rapidly acting agents such as chloroprocaine and lidocaine with long-acting agents like bupivacaine results in early blockade which last for a longer period.

Pregnancy

The spread and depth of both epidural and spinal anesthesia are more in pregnant than in nonpregnant women. This is due to combined effect of mechanical factors associated with pregnancy[Q] (i.e., dilated epidural veins decrease the volume of the epidural and subarachnoid spaces) and direct effects of hormones[Q] (more important), especially progesterone. Progesterone increases the susceptibility of nerves to conduction blockade by LAs.

CHOICE OF LOCAL ANESTHETICS

Due to wide difference in pharmacological properties, LAs choice for a regional procedure depends on many variables. The most important one is the type of regional procedure being used. On the basis of anatomic considerations, regional anesthesia can be divided into:

Infiltration Anesthesia

In this LA, solution is injected intradermally or subcutaneously into the proposed incision site. Epinephrine will prolong the duration of infiltration anesthesia of all LA drugs, although this effect is most pronounced when epinephrine is added to lignocaine. The choice of a specific drug for infiltration anesthesia largely depends on the desired duration of action. In general, lidocaine with adrenaline is drug of choice.

Intravenous Regional Anesthesia (Bier's Block)

Intravenous regional anesthesia (IVRA) involves the intravenous administration of a LA into a vein of tourniquet-occluded limb. The local anesthetic diffuses from the vascular bed to nonvascular tissue such as axons and nerve endings. Both success and safety of IVRA depend upon proper application of tourniquet.

As accidental rapid systemic transfer may occur, least cardiotoxic drug is most suitable. So, lidocaine is the local anesthetic of choice for IVRA.[Q] Bupivacaine is the most cardiotoxic and can cause cardiovascular collapse, thus bupivacaine is contraindicated[Q] in IVRA.

Dose

3 mg/kg (40 mL of a 0.5% solution) of preservative-free lidocaine without epinephrine is used

for upper extremity procedures. For surgical procedures on the lower limbs, 50-100 mL of a 0.25% lidocaine solution has been used.

Peripheral Nerve Blocks

These include procedures that inhibit conduction in fibers of the peripheral nervous system.

Brachial plexus blockade for upper limb surgery is the most commonly performed major peripheral nerve block.Q Lignocaine has most rapid onset (10-20 minutes) while bupivacaine provides maximum duration.

Central Neural Blockade

Central neural blockade (CNB) includes epidural and spinal (intrathecal) anesthesia.

Any of the LA drugs may be used for epidural anesthesia but bupivacaine, lidocaine, and ropivacaine remain the most commonly used. Lidocaine has fast onset while bupivacaine has delayed onset.

Bupivacaine and ropivacaine exhibit differential blockade in different concentrations. In a concentration of 0.0625-0.125%Q, bupivacaine blocks sensory fibers only, i.e., adequate analgesia with only mild motor blockade. Differential blockade is much more with ropivacaine, this combined with its less cardiotoxic nature makes ropivacaine a most suited LA for labor analgesia.Q

For spinal anesthesia, bupivacaineQ is the most common LA used. The usual dose is 2-4 mL of 0.5%Q hyperbaric solution which provides intense blockade for 2-4 hours.Q

Topical Anesthesia

Topical application of LA can desensitize mucous membranes. Lignocaine,Q tetracaine and benzocaine are the most commonly used drugs. Lidocaine and tetracaine sprays are commonly used for endotracheal anesthesia before intubation or for mucosal analgesia during bronchoscopy or esophagoscopy.

Eutectic mixture of local anesthetics (EMLA)—a eutecticQ mixture of 2.5% lidocaineQ base and 2.5% prilocaineQ base can penetrate intact skin. It is widely used for intravenous cannulation, skin grafting, and other minor procedures like circumcision. In order to obtain effective anesthesia, EMLA must be applied with occlusive dressing, 45-60 minutes prior to surgery. Methemoglobinemia is very rare with EMLA and it is quite safe in neonates too.

SyneraQ is a formulation of lidocaine and tetracaine, this formulation has a rapid onset and evokes vasodilatation which may facilitate IV cannulation.

Tumescent Anesthesia

This technique is used by plastic surgeons during liposuction. Here large volumes of diluted LA in combination with epinephrine and other agents are injected in the subcutaneous fat tissue. As fat tissue is relatively avascular, systemic absorption is slow and thus chances of toxicity are rare. Additional LAs by infiltration or other routes must be avoided for at least 12-18 hours of the use of this technique.

PHARMACOKINETICS

The concentration of LAs in blood depends upon the amount injected, rate of absorption, rate of tissue distribution, rate of biotransformation and excretion. Patient-related factors such as age, cardiovascular status, also influence the resultant blood concentration of LAs.

Absorption

Absorption of LA depends upon the site of injection; dose and volume injected, addition of a vasoconstrictor agent, and drug itself. On giving same dose in different site, blood concentration is highest after intercostal nerve blockade.Q Addition of vasoconstrictor such as epinephrine decreases the rate of vascular absorption and thus lowers the potential of their systemic toxicity.

However, adrenaline does not influence the peak blood levels of bupivacaine and etidocaine.

Distribution

Initially, there is a rapid disappearance phase related to uptake by rapidly equilibrating tissues (i.e., tissues that have high vascular perfusion). This is followed by slower phase which is mainly a function of the metabolism.

Biotransformation and Excretion

All ester drugs except cocaine are metabolized by pseudocholinesterase[Q] enzyme, while amide drugs undergo enzymatic degradation primarily in the liver. Cocaine is the only ester drug which is metabolized in liver.

Amide type local anesthetics are metabolized in liver and the metabolites are excreted through kidney.

> **KEY POINTS**
> - Most cardiotoxic: Bupivacaine
> - Most neurotoxic: Chloroprocaine
> - Protoplasmic poison: Cocaine

> **KEY POINTS**
> CNS is more susceptible to local anesthetic toxicity than CVS. However, CVS toxicity is more serious than CNS toxicity.

Pharmacokinetic Alterations by Patient Status

In elder patient, the half-lives of almost all LAs are increased.

Newborn infants have immature hepatic enzyme systems and hence elimination of lidocaine, bupivacaine, and ropivacaine is delayed. The toxic potential of lidocaine (particularly infusions) is high in neonates. This is due to the accumulation of its principal metabolite, monoethylglycinexylidide (MEGX), which can precipitate seizures.

Chloroprocaine is rapidly cleared from plasma, even in preterm neonates. So it is drug of choice for epidural anesthesia in neonates.[Q]

TOXICITY

Local anesthetic drugs are relatively safe, if used in right manner. However, systemic and localized toxic reactions can occur, which usually follows accidental intravascular or intrathecal injection or administration of an excessive dose. In addition, specific adverse effects such as allergic reactions to the aminoester drugs and methemoglobinemia after the use of prilocaine can be seen.

Systemic Toxicity

Local anesthetics exhibit central nervous system (CNS) and cardiovascular system (CVS) toxicity. Central nervous system is more susceptible than the CVS and hence toxicity can be seen, at a dose lower than that can produce circulatory collapse.

Central Nervous System Toxicity

When large quantity of LAs is injected in systemic circulation, they block neuronal function in brain. Inhibitory pathways are blocked first, due to their susceptible nature.

Central nervous system excitation is the result of an initial blockade of inhibitory pathways[Q] and stimulation of release of glutamate[Q] (an excitatory amino acid neurotransmitter). A further increase in the dose of LA leads to inhibition of both the inhibitory and excitatory circuits, resulting a generalized state of CNS depression. Earliest symptoms are light headedness, circumoral numbness[Q] and dizziness followed frequently by visual and auditory disturbances such as difficulty in focusing and tinnitus.

Early signs include shivering, muscular twitching, and tremors (initially involving muscles of the face and distal parts of the extremities). Ultimately, generalized convulsions of a tonic-clonic nature may occur. Excitation is usually followed by a state of generalized CNS depression characterized by cessation of seizure activity, respiratory depression and ultimately respiratory arrest. In some patients, CNS depression can be seen without a preceding excitatory phase, particularly, if other CNS depressant drugs have been administered.

Respiratory or metabolic acidosis increases the risks for CNS toxicity from LAs. It must be noted that seizures further aggravate acidosis and thus CNS toxicity.

Convulsions of LA respond well to IV midazolam, and small IV doses of thiopental.

Transient neurological symptoms, which consist of dysesthesia, burning pain and aching in the lower extremities and buttocks, may follow spinal anesthesia. These symptoms are due to LA related radicular irritation which usually resolves spontaneously. Risk is higher after lidocaine (versus mepivacaine, bupivacaine or tetracaine), lithotomy position and obesity. Chloroprocaine is the most neurotoxic LA.

KEY POINTS

Bupivacaine is the most cardiotoxic LA currently used. The ratio of the dosage required for cardiovascular collapse (CC) to the dose that produce CNS toxicity (convulsions), known as CC/CNS ratio is lowest for bupivacaine. Lidocaine is most cardiostable.

Cardiovascular System Toxicity

Local anesthetics effect CVS via direct actions on heart and peripheral blood vessels and through indirect actions secondary to autonomic blockade.

Direct cardiac effects: LA decreases the rate of depolarization in the fast conducting tissues of Purkinje fibers and ventricular muscle. In extreme high concentrations, they depress sinoatrial (SA) node, thereby resulting in sinus bradycardia and sinus arrest.

The effect is more with bupivacaine than lidocaine does. In addition, the rate of recovery is also slower with bupivacaine. These differential effects of lidocaine and bupivacaine on heart can explain the antiarrhythmic properties of former and the arrhythmogenic potential of bupivacaine.

In addition, LAs depress myocardial contractility by inhibiting cardiac sarcolemmal Ca^{2+} currents and Na^+ currents. This myocardial depressant effect of each drug is roughly proportional to conduction blocking potency of that drug. Thus, bupivacaine is more cardiodepressant than lidocaine.

Direct Peripheral Vascular Effects

Local anesthetics exert biphasic effects on peripheral vascular smooth muscle. Low concentrations of lidocaine and bupivacaine produce mild vasoconstriction, whereas high concentrations produce vasodilation in both isolated tissue models and *in vivo*.

Cocaine inhibits the uptake of norepinephrine by premotor neurons and potentiates neurogenic vasoconstriction. Cocaine is the only LA that produce vasoconstriction at all concentrations.[Q]

Autonomic Effects

Local anesthetics block autonomic fibers. Thus, high levels (above T6) of spinal anesthesia can produce severe hypotension with or without bradycardia.

Contributing Factors

As with CNS toxicity, hypercapnia, acidosis and hypoxia potentiate cardiotoxicity too. Pregnancy increases the cardiotoxic potential of all LAs.

Guidelines for Preventing and Managing Bupivacaine Cardiotoxicity

- Negative aspiration of the syringe does not always exclude intravascular placement. Incremental, fractionated dosing is the rule for all procedures requiring high dosage of bupivacaine. Continuous attention to the electrocardiography (ECG) (including changes in QRS complex, rate, rhythm or ectopy) may be lifesaving as injection can be terminated before a lethal dose is administered. Treatment of bupivacaine induced cardiac arrhythmias is very difficult. It must be mentioned that lidocaine should not be used to treat these arrhythmia. Bretylium[Q] is the only antiarrhythmic which is consistently effective in bupivacaine cardiac toxicity.
- If arrest or arrhythmia occur, first follow basic principles of cardiopulmonary resuscitation

including attention to securing the airway, providing oxygen and ventilation, and performing chest compressions, if needed.
- There are sufficient reports that intralipid^Q 20%, if administered early can terminate or at least decrease the cardiovascular toxicity of bupivacaine, ropivacaine and other LAs.

Methemoglobinemia

It is seen mainly with prilocaine.[Q] O-toluidine, a metabolite of prilocaine oxidizes hemoglobin to methemoglobin. In general, a dose above 600 mg is required to produce significant methemoglobinemia in adults. Methemoglobinemia, if severe, requires treatment with intravenous methylene blue. Risk of methemoglobinemia is high in newborns, patients with metabolic disorders or after the concomitant administration of other drugs.

Allergies

Mainly seen with ester local anesthetics as they are derivatives of para-aminobenzoic acid (PABA), which is a known allergen. Some aminoamide solutions may contain a preservative, methylparaben, which is similar to that of PABA, and may lead to allergic reactions. For most aminoamides, preservative-free solutions are available.

Local Tissue Toxicity

Local anesthetics can produce direct toxicity to nerves, if they are injected intraneurally. So, direct intraneural injection should be avoided.

LOCAL ANESTHETIC FAILURE

Many times it is seen that even after correct technique LAs fails to produce effective anesthesia. Failure of LA can be due to technical failure of delivery, insufficient volume or concentration of drug. In addition, there are clinical situations in which biologic processes contribute to fail LA, even with proper technique:

Inflammation at Site of Application

Local anesthetics are often ineffective in inflammatory areas like cellulitis, tooth abscess. It is due to:
- Increased local blood flow in inflamed areas, which leads to accelerated removal of drug.
- **Acidic environment**: Local tissue acidosis reduce the proportion of basic form.
- **Local tissue edema**: This increases diffusion distances of drug from injection site to nerves.
- **Sensitization**: Inflammation sensitizes both peripheral nerves and central neurons, and facilitates pain impulses, thereby increase the LA requirement.

Genetic Variability

Occasional patients report that LA do not work for me. Though this claim may reflect previous technical failures or a variety of other processes, but rarely these failures may involve genetic variation in LA responsiveness. Ehlers-Danlos syndrome[Q] is a connective tissue disorder in which responses to topical LA are reduced.

INDIVIDUAL AGENTS (TABLE 13.2)

Ester Group

Cocaine
- Cocaine was the first LA used clinically. In the year 1884, it was used in ocular surgery.
- Cocaine is a natural alkaloid derived from leaves of *Erythroxylum coca*. Cocaine is a good surface anesthetic and is rapidly absorbed from mucous membranes.
- It is the only ester LA which is metabolized in liver. One of its metabolite (ecognine) is CNS stimulant.
- Cocaine should never be injected, as it is a protoplasmic poison and can cause tissue necrosis.
- Cocaine stimulates CNS, sympathetic nervous system (raise in BP), vagal center (bradycardia), vomiting center (nausea and vomiting). It is

Table 13.2: Clinical use of local anesthetic agents.

Agent	Applications	Concentrations available	Maximum dose (mg/kg)	Typical duration of neural blockade (hour)
Esters				
Chloroprocaine	Epidural, infiltration, peripheral nerve block	1%, 2%, 3%	12	0.5–1
Cocaine	Topical	4%, 10%	3	0.5–1
Amides				
Bupivacaine	Epidural, spinal, infiltration, peripheral nerve block	0.25%, 0.5%, 0.75%	3	1.5–8
Lidocaine (Lignocaine)	Epidural, spinal infiltration, peripheral nerve block, intravenous regional, topical	0.5%, 1%, 1.5% 2%, 4%, 5%	4.5* or 7 (with epinephrine)	0.75–2
Prilocaine	Peripheral nerve block (dental)	4%	8	0.5–1
Ropivacaine	Epidural, spinal, infiltration, peripheral nerve block	0.2%, 0.5%, 0.75%, 1%	3	1.5–8

*without epinephrine

the only LA that produces vasoconstriction that is due to its ability to inhibit the uptake of norepinephrine[Q] by premotor neurons which subsequently produce vasoconstriction. In the eyes, cocaine produces mydriasis, blanching of conjunctiva, corneal clouding and rarely sloughing of cornea.
- Recurrent use leads to strong psychological but little physical dependence.
- Due to above-mentioned effects, it is almost out from anesthesia practice.

Procaine Hydrochloride

- First synthetic LA introduced.
- Procaine has been recommended as the agent of choice for patient with a history of malignant hyperthermia.[Q] Procaine intravenously in very high doses has also been used for the treatment of malignant hyperpyrexia.
- Procaine forms poorly soluble salt with benzyl penicillin. Procaine penicillin, injected intramuscularly reduces the pain of injection. Elsewhere, it is not used nowadays.

Chloroprocaine

- Short-acting

- Most acidic of all LAs (pH 3.3) produce prompt blockade which last for short duration.
- Most neurotoxic
- So, contraindicated in spinal anesthesia.

Amethocaine Hydrochloride

- A potent and toxic PABA ester which is highly lipid soluble. Like cocaine, it can produce ventricular fibrillation and cardiac asystole.
- Can be used as both surface and conduction block anesthetic, but clinically use is restricted to topical application to the eye, nose, throat, tracheobronchial tree. It is present in most sore mouth formulation.

Oxybuprocaine

- Surface anesthetic used for corneal analgesia.
- Less irritant than amethocaine.

Amide Group

Lignocaine Hydrochloride

Tertiary amide introduced in 1943, it is currently the most widely used LA and perhaps most versatile too. Lignocaine is a very stable compound

and is not decomposed by boiling, acids, alkalis. The pKa is 7.86. Many formulations^Q are available which differ in concentration and perhaps uses:
- 1–2% with adrenaline for infiltration
- 4% for topical analgesia
- 1.5–2% for epidural block
- 5% (heavy) for spinal anesthesia
- 2% jelly for urethral analgesia
- 5% ointment for tracheal tubes

It is metabolized in the liver^Q by oxidases and amidases. Clearance is reduced and toxicity is increased in patients taking propanolol.^{Q}

Lignocaine facilitates release of calcium from sarcoplasmic reticulum and therefore it should not be used in patients susceptible to malignant hyperthermia.^{Q}

- Lignocaine decreases coagulation, enhances fibrinolysis and reduces chances of thromboembolization. In contrary to other LAs, it has no effect on blood vessels^Q (vasoineffective)
- Addition of adrenaline enhances its duration of action by reducing its systemic absorption. As systemic absorption is delayed, its toxicity is also reduced or one can say that safe dose is increased. Maximum safe dose is 7 mg/kg^Q with adrenaline and 4.5 mg/kg^Q without adrenaline.

Prilocaine

- Similar to lignocaine both structurally and pharmacologically, due to large volume of distribution, it is less neurotoxic than lignocaine.
- One of its metabolite has potential to cause methemoglobinemia. Its eutectic mixture with lignocaine is commonly used for surface analgesia.
- Exhibits both hepatic and extrahepatic metabolisms, so is considered as safest LA.

Bupivacaine

- A potent and long-acting LA used for infiltration, nerve block, epidural and spinal anesthesias of long duration. It is four times more potent than lignocaine.
- Among current LAs bupivacaine is most cardiotoxic.^{Q} Moreover, its high lipid solubility and high degree of protein binding, makes resuscitation difficult and prolonged. Hypoxia, acidosis and pregnancy tend to increase its cardiotoxicity. Addition of epinephrine does not greatly prolong the duration but reduces its toxicity.
- Commercial bupivacaine is a racemic mixture of (R) and (S) stereoisomers. S-bupivacaine, called as levobupivacaine (chirocaine), is less cardiotoxic than racemic mixture.
- Metabolized in liver, $t_{1/2}$ is 3.5 hours; a small amount is excreted in urine also.

Levobupivacaine

Levobupivacaine is an enantiomer of the bupivacaine, which is less cardiotoxic than bupivacaine. Equivalent dose of levobupivacaine was less arrhythmogenic than the same dose range of bupivacaine in healthy volunteers. Its effects on the corrected QT interval were significantly less than that of bupivacaine. Levobupivacaine was less cardiotoxic than bupivacaine.

The CNS depressant effect of 40 mg intravenous levobupivacaine was less than that of bupivacaine 40 mg in healthy volunteers both in terms of the magnitude of the effect and the regions of the cortex affected. The level of sensory and motor block were clinically similar to that of bupivacaine in patients requiring anesthesia during surgery.[2]

KEY POINTS

- Safest local anesthetic: Prilocaine
- Maximum differential blockade: Ropivacaine
- Maximum methemoglobinemia: Prilocaine

Ropivacaine

- An equipotent congener of bupivacaine with similar duration. Single S-enantiomer drug rather than a racemic mixture (as in bupivacaine).

- For same concentration, ropivacaine produce differential blockade of greater degree than bupivacaine. Motor block is slower in onset, less intense and shorter in duration.
- Ropivacaine is less cardiotoxic,^Q less arrhythmogenic, less toxic to CNS^Q than bupivacaine. Maximum safe dose is 250 mg (approximately 3–4 mg/kg).

OTHER LOCAL ANESTHETICS NOT IN ANESTHESIA PRACTICE

Dibucaine

Most potent,^Q most stable and longest^Q acting LA. Dibucaine inhibits pseudocholinesterase, so is used to estimate pseudocholinesterase activity (dibucaine number). Clinically, it is used as surface anesthetic for anal canal.

Oxethazaine

A potent LA, unique in ionizing to a very small extent even at low pH values. It is therefore effective in anesthetizing areas with low pH, e.g., gastric mucosa. Swallowed along with antacids it affords symptomatic relief in gastritis, gastroesophageal reflux disease and heartburn.

NOVEL LOCAL ANESTHETICS

Lecithin^Q coated microdroplets of methoxyflurane produces long-lasting local analgesia which is stable and localized.

STERILIZATION OF LOCAL ANESTHESIA

Commonly used local agents are stable and all can be autoclaved. They can also be sterilized by γ-radiation.

KEY POINTS

Levobupivacaine (chirocaine):
- S isomer of bupivacaine. Less potent and expensive than bupivacaine
- Less cardiotoxic than bupivacaine
- Less neurotoxic than bupivacaine
- Vasoconstrictor (bupivacaine is vasodilator)
- Produce blockade of lesser duration than bupivacaine
- Maximum safe dose is 3 mg/kg

LAST-MINUTE REVISION

- **Esters:** Cocaine, procaine, chloroprocaine, amethocaine, oxybuprocaine. All are metabolized in plasma except cocaine, which is metabolized in liver. Allergy is common with ester LA.
- **Amides:** Lignocaine, bupivacaine, prilocaine, ropivacaine.
- Preganglionic sympathetic fibers are most sensitive to LA; whereas A α-fibers are most resistant.
- Cocaine is the only LA which is natural, produces vasoconstriction, possess addictive potential.
- Bupivacaine, most cardiotoxic LA which is contraindicated in Bier's block, it is the most commonly used LA in spinal anesthesia.
- Ropivacaine is the LA of choice in labor epidural, due to its propensity to produce differential blockade.
- Prilocaine is the safest LA, but it produces methemoglobinemia.
- Chloroprocaine is the most neurotoxic LA, and is short-acting too.
- Dibucaine is the longest acting LA.
- **Procaine:** Anesthetic agent of choice in malignant hyperthermia.

REFERENCES

1. Vadhanan P, Tripaty DK, Adinarayanan S. Physiological and pharmacologic aspects of peripheral nerve blocks. J Anaesthesiol Clin Pharmacol. 2015;31(3):384-93.

2. Foster RH, Markham A. Levobupivacaine: a review of its pharmacology and use as a local anaesthetic. Drugs. 2000;59(3):551-79.

REVIEW QUESTIONS

1. All the following are long-acting local anesthetics (> 2 hours), *except*:
   a. Bupivacaine
   b. Prilocaine
   c. Tetracaine
   d. Dibucaine

2. Correct statement regarding bupivacaine includes all, *except*:
   a. Less cardiotoxic than prilocaine
   b. It is an amide
   c. The maximum tolerable dose is 3 mg/kg body weight
   d. Duration more than 2 hours

3. From which of the following routes absorption of local anesthetic is maximum?
   a. Intercostal
   b. Epidural
   c. Brachial plexus block
   d. Caudal

4. Sodium bicarbonate when given with local anesthetics has which of the following effect?
   a. Increases speed and quality of anesthesia
   b. Decreases diffusion of the anesthetic drug
   c. Causes rapid elimination of the local anesthetic
   d. Decreases speed and quality of anesthesia

5. True about EMLA:
   a. Can be used for intubation
   b. Mixture of local anesthesia
   c. Faster acting
   d. Used in children

6. Bupivacaine toxicity treated with:
   a. Esmolol
   b. Epinephrine
   c. Lignocaine
   d. 5% dextrose
   e. Benzodiazepines

7. Following drugs are advocated after accidental IV injection of bupivacaine, *except*:
   a. Lignocaine
   b. Bretylium
   c. Epinephrine
   d. Intralipid

8. Advantages of ropivacaine over bupivacaine include all, *except*:
   a. Less cardiotoxicity
   b. Less hypotension
   c. More intense blockade
   d. Less neurotoxic

9. All of the following drugs enhances the duration of action of local anesthetic, *except*:
   a. Adrenaline
   b. Clonidine
   c. Opioids
   d. Ondansetron

10. Effectivity of local anesthetic is reduced in:
    a. Acidic environment
    b. Edematous tissue
    c. Neither a nor b
    d. Both a and b

11. Local anesthetic that is not used topically is:
    a. Lignocaine
    b. Cocaine
    c. Tetracaine
    d. Bupivacaine

12. Dose of lignocaine for spinal anesthesia is:
    a. 0.5%
    b. 2.5%
    c. 4%
    d. 5%

13. Most cardiotoxic local anesthetic is:
    a. Lignocaine
    b. Bupivacaine
    c. Prilocaine
    d. Procaine
14. Concentration of adrenaline used with lidocaine is:
    a. 1:200
    b. 1:2,000
    c. 1:20,000
    d. 1:200,000
15. All are amides, *except*:
    a. Lignocaine
    b. Procaine
    c. Prilocaine
    d. Etidocaine

> **Mnemonic**
> All amide local anesthetic have two "i" in their spelling

ANSWERS

| 1. b | 2. a | 3. a | 4. a | 5. b, d | 6. b |
| 7. a | 8. c | 9. d | 10. d | 11. d | 12. d |

CHAPTER 14

Muscle Relaxants

Anshul Jain, Manish Kumar Singh

INTRODUCTION

Neuromuscular blockers are routinely used to facilitate endotracheal intubation, mechanical ventilation and to provide muscle relaxation during surgery in conjunction with general anesthetics.

Neuromuscular blockers have no analgesic or amnesic properties. So they should be administered only to anesthetized individuals to provide relaxation of skeletal muscles. Administering muscle relaxant in an unanesthetized individual means patient will feel pain, can hear all sounds, but cannot breath of his own, cannot speak neither can move any of his body part. A state that is wholly unacceptable for the patient.

Most neuromuscular blockers function by blocking transmission at the end plate of the neuromuscular junction.

δ-tubocurarine (dTc) was the first relaxant used by Griffith and Johnson in 1942. Succinylcholine, introduced by Thesleff and Foldes and colleagues in 1952, changed anesthetic practice drastically. Its rapid onset of effect and ultrashort duration of action permit early endotracheal intubation and thus control of airway. Commonly used neuromuscular blockers are mentioned in **Table 14.1**.

MECHANISM OF ACTION OF NEUROMUSCULAR BLOCKERS AT THE NEUROMUSCULAR JUNCTION

Normal Physiology

In mammalian skeletal muscle, the nicotinic acetylcholine receptor (nAChR) is a pentameric complex of two α-subunits and single β-, δ-, and ε-subunits **(Figs. 14.1A and B)**. These subunits are organized to form a transmembrane channel. α-subunit possesses extracellular binding pockets, for acetylcholine and other agonists or antagonists. Functionally, this ion channel is closed in the resting state. Normally, a nerve impulse arriving at the motor nerve terminal, initiates an influx of calcium ions which triggers

Table 14.1: Classification of neuromuscular blockers.[a]

Class of blocker	Long-acting (>50 min)	Intermediate-acting (20–50 min)	Short-acting (15–20 min)	Ultrashort-acting (10–12 min)
Depolarizers			Decamethonium	Succinylcholine
Nondepolarizers				
Steroidal compounds[a]	Pancuronium	Vecuronium[a]		
	Pipecuronium	Rocuronium		
Benzylisoquinolinium compound	Tubocurarine Metocurine Doxacurium	Atracurium[a] Cisatracurium	Mivacurium	Gantacurium[a]
Others		Alcuronium	Gallamine	

the exocytosis of acetylcholine containing synaptic vesicles. Acetylcholine then diffuses across the synaptic cleft. Simultaneous binding of two acetylcholine molecules to the α-subunits initiates conformational changes that open the sodium-potassium channel of the nicotinic receptor. This allows Na^+ and Ca^{2+} ions to enter the cell and K^+ ions to leave the cell, thereby depolarizing the end plate, which is subsequently followed by muscle contraction **(Fig. 14.1 and Flowchart 14.1)**.

The acetylcholine molecules are then rapidly hydrolyzed by acetylcholinesterase into acetic acid and choline. It should be noted that although acetylcholine produces depolarization, it results in muscle contraction only under physiological conditions because it has a very short duration of action (a few milliseconds). Administration of large doses of acetylcholine in experimental animals, produces neuromuscular blockade.

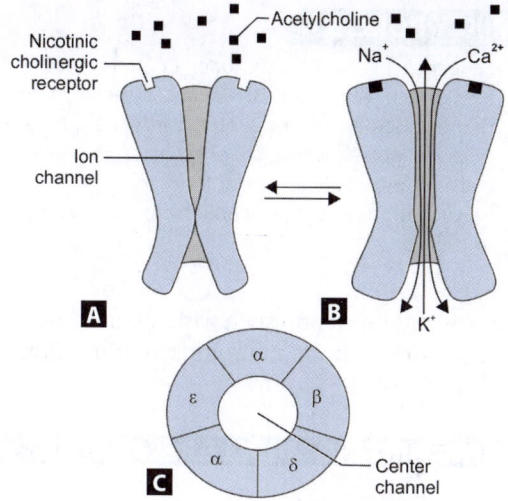

Figs. 14.1A to C: (A) Structure of acetylcholine receptor; (B) Binding of acetylcholine to nicotinic cholinergic receptors which then leads to ion flux (C) As seen from above.

Flowchart 14.1: Steps in neuromuscular transmission.

Discharge of motor neuron
↓
Release of transmitter (acetylcholine) at motor end-plate
↓
Binding of acetylcholine to nicotinic acetylcholine receptors
↓
Increased Na^+ and K^+ conductance in end-plate membrane
↓
Generation of end-plate potential
↓
Generation of action potential in muscle fibers
↓
Inward spread of depolarization along T tubules
↓
Release of Ca^{2+} from terminal cisterns of sarcoplasmic reticulum and diffusion to thick and thin filaments
↓
Binding of Ca^{2+} to troponin C, uncovering myosin-binding sites on actin
↓
Formation of cross-linkages between actin and myosin and sliding of thin on thick filaments, producing muscle contraction

Depolarizing Muscle Relaxants (Leptocurare)

Depolarizing neuromuscular blockers (succinylcholine) physically resemble acetylcholine and therefore bind to ACh receptor, generating a muscle action potential and muscle contraction. Unlike ACh they are not metabolized by acetylcholinesterase. Thus they produce prolonged depolarization of the end-plate region, which leads to:

- Sensitization of the nAChR[Q]
- Inactivation of voltage-gated sodium channels[Q] at the neuromuscular junction, and
- Increase in the potassium permeability in the surrounding membrane.

The end result is failure of action potential generation, and blockade ensues. Initial muscle contractions appear clinically as fasciculation,[Q] a feature characteristic of depolarizing muscle relaxants.

Nondepolarizing Muscle Relaxants (Pachycurare)

Nondepolarizing agents occupy the nicotinic receptor and prevent[Q] the binding of ACh. They themselves are incapable of producing conformational changes necessary for depolarization. Therefore there is no end plate potential and block ensues.

Summarizing depolarizing muscle relaxants acts as ACh receptor agonist,[Q] while nondepolarizing muscle relaxant acts as competitive antagonist.[Q]

Prejunctional Effects

Acetylcholine release by nerve ending not only stimulates motor end plate, but also produces prejunctional effects. ACh activates prejunctional nicotinic receptors which facilitate further release of ACh, this positive feedback system maintains the availability of ACh when demand is high (e.g., during tetany).

Blockade of these receptors by nondepolarizing neuromuscular blockers (NDMB) explain the fade phenomenon seen with tetanic and train of four stimulation in neuromuscular monitoring (*see* Chapter 16).

> **KEY POINTS**
> - *Sequence of muscle blockade*: Central muscles (neck, face, jaw, eyelids) are most sensitive to neuromuscular blockers afterwards peripheral muscles get blocked. Diaphragm is the most resistant muscle to muscular blockade.
> - Fasciculations of succinylcholine are seen earliest in eyelids.

DEPOLARIZING MUSCLE RELAXANTS

Succinylcholine

Succinylcholine (SCh) is composed of two molecules of acetylcholine linked back to back through the acetate methyl groups making a long, thin, and flexible molecule. Like ACh, SCh stimulates cholinergic receptors at the neuromuscular junction. However, it also stimulates nicotinic (ganglionic) and muscarinic autonomic sites, which contributes to its side effects.

Pharmacokinetics and Pharmacodynamics

Succinylcholine is the only neuromuscular blocker which exhibit rapid onset with ultrashort duration of action.

Administration of 1 mg/kg of SCh produces complete paralysis in 60 seconds which normally last only for 3–5 minutes.

The short duration of action of SCh is due to its rapid hydrolysis by butyrylcholinesterase[Q] (pseudocholinesterase) into succinylmonocholine and choline.[Q] Succinylmonocholine, is then metabolized into succinic acid and choline. Infact due to enormous capacity of pseudocholinesterase only 10% of the administered SCh reaches the neuromuscular junction.

There is no butyrylcholinesterase at the neuromuscular junction; the neuromuscular blockade of succinylcholine is terminated by its diffusion away from the neuromuscular junction back into the circulation. However, rapid fall in circulating SCh (due to its continuous metabolism) creates a gradient which dictates the diffusion of SCh away from neuromuscular junction to circulation, this also explains its ultrashort action.[Q]

Butyrylcholinesterase is synthesized by the liver[Q] and found in plasma, intestine, liver,[Q] orbit, white matter (*Mnemonic*: PILOW). Factors that reduce[Q] pseudocholinesterase activity are liver disease, advanced age, malnutrition, pregnancy, burns, anticholinesterase drugs. The β-blocker esmolol also inhibits pseudolocholinesterase but causes only minor prolongation of SCh blockade.

Pseudocholinesterase activity is increased in obesity, toxic goiter, nephrosis, depression, psoriasis and alcoholism.[Q] In these conditions duration of action of SCh is reduced.

Dibucaine Number and Atypical Pseudocholinesterase Activity

SCh-induced neuromuscular blockade can be significantly prolonged if the patient has an abnormal genetic variant of pseudocholinesterase. A local anesthetic dibucaine inhibits normal butyrylcholinesterase to a far greater extent than it inhibits the abnormal enzyme **(Table 14.2)**. This leads to development of a test for detection of atypical pseudocholinesterase called as dibucaine number (cinchocaine number).[Q] The dibucaine number indicates the percentage of enzyme inhibited by 10^{-5} molar concentration of dibucaine. Dibucaine inhibits expression of the normal enzyme by about 80% and the abnormal enzyme by about 20%.[Q]

Homozygous atypical state is extremely rare and therefore, dibucaine number estimation is not performed routinely.

Side Effects

Cardiovascular Effects

- SCh simulates the effects of acetylcholine. At low doses, both negative inotropic and chronotropic responses may occur. These responses can be attenuated by prior administration of atropine.
- SCh can cause cardiac dysrhythmias,[Q] also. Sinus bradycardia, junctional rhythms, and ventricular dysrhythmias might be seen. Bradycardia is due to stimulation of cardiac muscarinic receptors in the sinus node. This is particularly problematic in children as they have high vagal tone. In adults it is seen only after a second dose. The bradycardia may be prevented by the administration of atropine and NDMBs. Incidence of bradycardia is higher after second dose of succinylcholine which suggests that the hydrolysis products of succinylcholine sensitize the heart to a subsequent dose.

> ### KEY POINTS
>
> Fluoride number: Estimates pseudocholinesterase activity and is defined as percentage inhibition of cholinesterase by 5×10^{-5} molar sodium fluoride.

- Suppression of sinoatrial node allows emergence of the atrioventricular node as the pacemaker and this may lead to junctional rhythms.[Q] The incidence of junctional rhythm is also greater after a second dose of succinylcholine.
- Ventricular dysrhythmias though rare can occur due to increase in catecholamine and potassium levels after administration of succinylcholine. Other autonomic stimuli, such as endotracheal intubation, hypoxia, hypercapnia, and surgery, may be additive to the effect of succinylcholine.

Table 14.2: Relationship between dibucaine number and duration of succinylcholine.

Type of butyrylcholinesterase	Dibucaine number	Response to succinylcholine
Homozygous typical	70–80	Normal
Heterozygous atypical	50–60	Lengthened by 50–100%
Homozygous atypical	20–30[Q]	Prolonged to 4–8 hours

- Digitalis, tricyclic antidepressants, monoamine oxidase (MAO) inhibitors, exogenous catecholamines, and halothane increase the arrhythmogenic effect of SCh.

Hyperkalemia

- SCh administration increases plasma potassium levels by 0.5 mEq/dL.[Q] This is due to its depolarizing action. Depolarization produces inward movement of sodium into the cells which is accompanied by outflux of potassium.[Q] This slight increases in potassium is well tolerated by normal individuals. However severe hyperkalemia (to an extent that cardiac arrest ensues) may be seen in patients with:
  - Severe metabolic acidosis
  - Hypovolemia
  - Intra-abdominal infections of more than 1 week
  - Any conditions that result in the proliferation of extrajunctional acetylcholine receptors, such as neuromuscular disease, hemiplegia or paraplegia, muscular dystrophies, and Guillain-Barré syndrome.
- In patients with severe trauma and burns, risk of hyperkalemia begin after 1 week, maximum at 3 week and subside after 3 months.

Increased Intraocular Pressure

- Succinylcholine (Sch) Sh increases[Q] intraocular pressure (IOP) which peaks after 2–4 minutes of injection, and subsides by 6 minutes. The mechanism involves contraction of tonic myofibrils or transient dilatation of choroidal blood vessels.
- Despite this, SCh is not contraindicated in ocular surgeries unless the anterior chamber is open. Moreover prior administration of a small dose of NDMB (precurarization) will prevent SCh induced increase in IOP.[Q]

Increased Intragastric Pressure

- SCh can increase[Q] intragastric pressure (IGP) due to fasciculation's of abdominal skeletal muscle. This increase in IGP is particularly risky in patients prone for gastroesophageal reflux (pregnancy, ascites, bowel obstruction, hiatal hernia, etc.). In these, patient's stomach contents may regurgitate and pulmonary aspiration is a distinct possibility. Precurarization can prevent this increase too.
- In infants and children, due to minimal or absent fasciculation, SCh does not[Q] increase IGP.

Increased Intracranial Pressure

Succinylcholine produces a mild increase[Q] in intracranial pressure (ICP) by unknown mechanisms, but the rise is not seen after pretreatment with NDMBs.

Myalgias

Muscle pain is common after SCh administration. Chances are more after minor surgery, in women and in ambulatory rather than bedridden patients. Pain is due to fasciculation induces damage produced in muscle. Precurarization is not much effective in decreasing myalgia. However, pretreatment with a prostaglandin inhibitor decreases the incidence of muscle pain. This suggests a possible role of prostaglandins and cyclooxygenases in SCh-induced myalgias.

Masseter Spasm

- Masseter spasm is the frequent response to succinylcholine in adults and children and is supposed to be due to exaggerated muscle contraction secondary to SCh induces depolarization.
- Although an increase in tone of the masseter muscle may be an early sign of malignant hyperthermia, but it is not consistently associated with that syndrome.

Clinical Uses

- Despite its many adverse effects, even today SCh is the most commonly used muscle relaxant for intubation. This is due to its rapid onset, the profound neuromuscular blockade that it produces, and its ultrashort duration of action.[Q]

- It is the neuromuscular blocker of choice for rapid-sequence induction of anesthesia. Even in head injury patients it is the drug of choice for emergency airway management.[Q] A small dose of NDMB is commonly given 2 minutes before the intubating dose of succinylcholine. This defasciculating dose of NDMB (called as precurarization)[Q] minimizes the incidence of fasciculation's and will attenuate any increase in IGP and ICP.[Q] However, precurarization renders the muscle relatively resistant to succinylcholine, so the dose of SCh have to be increased by 50%.
- Typically after administration of succinylcholine for intubation, a NDMB is used subsequently for maintaining neuromuscular blockade.
- In high and repeated dose SCh can produce phase[Q] II or nondepolarizing[Q] type of blockade. Train-of-four (TOF) stimulation is a very safe and useful guide for detecting the transition from phase 1 to phase 2 blocks. A phase 2 block is suggested by TOF ratio < 0.4[Q] **(Table 14.3)**.

Interactions with Anticholinesterases

Interaction of SCh with neostigmine or pyridostigmine (drugs used to reverse NDMB paralysis) is very important. For example, pancuronium has been used for intra-abdominal surgery of long duration and the neuromuscular blockade has been reversed by neostigmine, the surgeon announces that another 15 minutes are needed to do something extra.

Sch should never be administered to re-establish neuromuscular blockade because it produces relaxation that will last up to 60 minutes when given soon after the administration of neostigmine. This is due to inhibition of butyrylcholinesterase by neostigmine and pyridostigmine.

Contraindications

Absolute

- **Malignant hyperthermia:**[Q] SCh is one of the most common triggering agents for malignant hyperthermia
- **Hyperkalemia:**[Q] Serum K⁺ more than 5.5 mEq/L
- **Duchenne muscular dystrophy:**[Q] SCh can lead to severe life-threatening hyperkalemia.
- **Dystrophia myotonica:**[Q] SCh exacerbates this condition and produce rigidity severe enough to make ventilation and intubation impossible.
- Diagnosed case of pseudocholinesterase deficiency

Table 14.3: Clinical characteristics of phase 1 and phase 2 neuromuscular blockade during succinylcholine infusion.

Characteristic	Phase 1	Phase 2
Tetanic stimulation	No fade	Fade[Q]
Post-tetanic facilitation	None	Yes
Train-of-four ratio	>0.7	<0.4
Edrophonium	Augments	Antagonizes[Q]
Recovery	Rapid	Prolonged

Mnemonic

Contraindications					Properties
Rhythm abnormalities	R	S	T		Three minute duration
Burns	B	C	D		Depolarizer
Neuromuscular disorders	N	O	P		Pseudocholinesterase metabolism
Ch (K)olinesterase deficiency	K	L	M		Myalgia
Hyperkalemia	H	I	J		Junctional rhythm
Malignant hyperthermia	M	N	O		One minute onset
Dystrophies	D	E	F		Fasciculation

Relative

- **Newborn and infants**: The potential for rhabdomyolysis and hyperkalemia (particularly in children younger than 8 years, who might have unrecognized muscular dystrophy), as well as risk for masseter spasm and malignant hyperthermia suggest SCh should not be used routinely in children.
- Elective neurosurgery
- Shock and acidosis
- Prolong intra-abdominal infection.

NONDEPOLARIZING NEUROMUSCULAR BLOCKERS

Nondepolarizing neuromuscular blocking drugs (NDMB) are bulky molecule, so were originally called as pachycurare. They bind the nicotinic receptor and prevent ACh binding. Origin of NDMB lies in the South American Indians' arrow poisons or curare. Several NDMBs are still purified from naturally occurring sources. Example, dTc from the Amazonian vine *Chondrodendron tomentosum*.

Individual Agents (Table 14.4)

Pancuronium

- Long-acting steroidal muscle relaxant, rarely used nowadays.
- Mainly bound to γ globulin
- Possess vagolytic activity, so may produce tachycardia and hypertension.
- Also releases noradrenaline, so use with halothane is theoretically not advocated (halothane increase the arrhythmogenic potential of adrenaline).
- Metabolized in liver (20%), 80% is excreted through kidney.
- Duration is prolonged in renal failure.

Tubocurarine

- First nondepolarizing skeletal muscle relaxant used in human.
- Possess antifibrillatory property as it gets concentrated in heart muscle.
- Among all (NDMB), dTc is most toxic, it has highest propensity to produce ganglion blockade and results in maximum histamine release.
- Due to these potential side effects it is rarely used nowadays.

Vecuronium

- Intermediate acting steroidal muscle relaxant
- It is the most commonly used muscle relaxant for maintenance of perianesthetic muscle relaxation.
- Highly cardiovascular stable
- It is metabolized mainly in liver[Q] by deacetylation to produce an active metabolite 3-desacetylvecuronium, which is then excreted through kidney. In intensive care unit (ICU) patients with renal failure, 3-desacetylvecuronium can accumulate and produce prolonged neuromuscular blockade. About 30% of vecuronium is excreted unchanged through bile, and 25% undergoes renal excretion.

Rocuronium

- Steroidal muscle relaxant with onset of action, comparable to that of succinylcholine (i.e., 60–90 sec).
- This early onset makes rocuronium, the NDMB of choice for intubation and precurarization.
- Only NDMB which can be given by intramuscular (IM) route too.
- Rocuronium[Q] is eliminated primarily by the liver, and only a small fraction (~10%) is eliminated through urine. It has no active metabolite, so it is preferred over vecuronium for infusion.
- Lacks histamine release, ganglion blockade, but possess some vagolytic activity.

Atracurium

- Intermediate acting muscle relaxant, belonging to benzylisoquinolinium class.
- Main side effect is histamine release, that becomes significant at doses >0.5 mg/kg and

Table 14.4: Summary of neuromuscular drugs.

Drug	Initial dose (mg/kg)	Onset (min)	Duration (min)	Metabolism	Excretion Kidney	Excretion Liver	Histamine release	Ganglion block	Vagal block
Long-acting									
δ-Tubo curarine	0.2–0.4	4–6	60–90	None	80%	20%	+++	++	±
Pancuronium	0.08–0.1	4–6	60–120	Liver	85%	15%	±	±	++
Intermediate duration									
Vecuronium	0.08–0.1	2–4	20–40	Liver (30–40%)	40% (bile)	40%	−	−	±
Atracurium	0.3–0.6	2–4	20–35	Hofmann elimination Ester hydrolysis	20%	−	+	−	−
Cisatracurium	0.15–0.2	4–7	20–40	Hofmann elimination	15%	−	−	−	−
Rocuronium	0.6–0.9	1–2	25–40	None	10–15%	70%	−	−	−
Short duration									
Mivacurium	0.2–0.25	2–4	15–20	Pseudocholinesterase	10%	−	+	−	−
Ultrashort duration									
Succinylcholine	1–1.5	0.5–1.5	3–6	Pseudocholinesterase	<2%	−	++	Stimulates ganglia	Stimulates vagii
Gantacurium*	0.2 mg	2–3	4–10	Cysteine and ester hydrolysis			+		

*Not yet marketed
Cisatracurium is the most potent, but has most delayed onset[a]
Rocuronium is least potent but has most rapid onset[a] among nondepolarizers

can produce bronchospasm particularly in asthmatics.
- Atracurium is an unique NDMB as it is metabolized by two pathways: (1) Hofmann elimination and (2) ester hydrolysis by nonspecific esterases. Hofmann degradation[Q] is a pH[Q] and temperature-dependent spontaneous reaction where higher pH and temperature favor degradation. The resulting compounds monoquaternary acrylate, are devoid of clinical activity. It plays role both *in vivo* and *in vitro*. Because of which, atracurium has to be stored at pH <3.0 and temperature <4°C under cold chain.[Q]
- Laudanosine, a degradation product of Hofmann elimination has central nervous system (CNS) stimulating properties. Laudanosine is dependent on the liver and kidney for its elimination and has a long elimination half-life. Laudanosine concentration is elevated in patients with liver disease who have received atracurium for many hours as in an ICU.

Cisatracurium

- Cis-isomer of atracurium, it is 4 times more potent than atracurium.
- It is also metabolized by Hofmann elimination to produce laudanosine and a monoquaternary acrylate. However, there is no ester hydrolysis. Hofmann elimination accounts for three-fourth of the total clearance. Rest one-fourth is excreted through kidney.
- Cisatracurium is approximately four times as potent as atracurium, because of which dose requirement is less and thus less laudanosine is produced. Moreover, unlike atracurium, it does not induce release of histamine at the clinical doses.
- Cisatracurium is muscle relaxant of choice in:
  - Renal failure
  - Hepatic failure
  - Myasthenia gravis
  - Infants
  - Old age

Mivacurium

- Shortest acting NDMB, metabolized by plasma cholinesterase.
- Effect is prolonged in patients with pseudo-cholinesterase deficiency.
- Side effects include histamine release, hypotension.
- Due to its short duration, it is the muscle relaxant of choice in short procedures. Furthermore reversal is seldom required to reverse its effect. However, whenever required edrophonium is preferred over neostigmine for reversal (as neostigmine inhibits pseudocholinesterase).

KEY POINTS
Muscle relaxants releasing histamine
- dTc
- Mivacurium
- Atracurium

Doxacurium

- Bisquaternary muscle relaxant, having the least rapid onset and longest action.
- It is the most potent muscle relaxant.
- It is primarily eliminated by kidney though hepatic metabolism also occurs.

Pipecuronium

- Another steroidal muscle relaxant with a slow onset and long duration of action.
- Side effects include hypotension and bradycardia.

Gantacurium

- Gantacurium represents a new class of nondepolarizing neuromuscular blockers called asymmetric mixed-onium chlorofumarates. Gantacurium has an ultrashort[Q] duration of action. The time to onset of 90% blockade ranged from 1.5 to 2.0 minutes, with durations ranged from 4.7 to 10.1 minutes.
- Metabolized by cysteine and ester hydrolysis.
- Devoid of side effects like histamine release, ganglion blockade.

Other Agents No Longer Used

Gallamine
- Muscle relaxant with highest vagolytic potential.
- Crosses placenta and can produce muscular blockade in infant.
- Primarily eliminated by kidney.

Repacurium
- Less potent analog of vecuronium.
- In some patients produce severe bronchospasm because of which it was withdrawn.

Alcuronium
Associated with anaphylactic reactions and ganglion blockade. So was withdrawn.

CLINICAL USES

Endotracheal Intubation
- The duration of onset of neuromuscular blockade is most important factor for tracheal intubation. Among all NDMB, rocuronium has most rapid onset and is the nondepolarizer of choice^Q for tracheal intubation.
- Though not suitable for rapid-sequence induction, other NDMB can also be used for routine tracheal intubation. The onset of action of nondepolarizing neuromuscular blocking drugs can be accelerated by following methods:
  - *Priming technique*:^{Q} In priming 10% of the intubating dose of NDMB is given 2–4 minutes prior to intubating dose for tracheal intubation. This accelerates the onset of blockade for most NDMB by 30–60 seconds. However, priming is uncomfortable for the patient and carries the risks of aspiration; moreover the intubating conditions after priming are inferior to those after succinylcholine.
  - *High dose regimen*: Larger doses of NDMB (eight times of ED), can accelerate the onset of intubating conditions. This, however, is associated with prolonged duration and increased cardiovascular side effects.

Maintenance of Relaxation
Vecuronium^Q is the most commonly used muscle relaxant for maintenance of relaxation in routine surgery because of its cardiovascular stability. In liver and kidney patients cisatracurium is the drug of choice. If cisatracurium is not available atracurium can be used as a second choice.

> **KEY POINTS**
>
> Neuromuscular blockade develops faster, lasts a shorter time, and recovers more quickly in neck muscles (that are relevant for endotracheal intubation) than hand muscles which are typically monitored (adductor pollicis). The pattern of blockade in the orbicularis oculi is similar to that in the larynx. By monitoring the onset of blockade at the orbicularis oculi, one can predict the intubating conditions.

Other Uses
- **ICU patients**: Critically ill patients in ICU often need muscle relaxant for endotracheal tube and ventilator tolerance.
- **Electroconvulsive therapy (ECT)**: ECT can produce trauma, joint dislocations in non-paralyzed patient. Muscle relaxants reduce incidence of these complications and are routinely being used for this purpose. SCh due to its ultrashort action is most commonly used drug for this purpose. Mivacurium is suitable nondepolarizing alternate.
- Severe cases of tetanus.
- Status epilepticus refractory to benzodiazepines.

ADVERSE EFFECTS

Autonomic Ganglionic Blockade
As the cholinergic receptors in autonomic ganglia are nicotinic, nondepolarizing neuromuscular blocking agents may interact with these receptors to produce varied degree of ganglion blockade. These autonomic responses are dose related and additive overtime.

Histamine Release

Histamine release is seen with dTc (max), mivacurium, and atracurium. With large doses these muscle relaxants can lead to erythema of the face, neck along with hypotension and tachycardia. The effect is usually of short duration and is clinically insignificant in healthy patients. Tachyphylaxis, is an important characteristic of histamine release and subsequent doses of same relaxant does not release histamine.

Hypotension

It is seen with atracurium, mivacurium (due to histamine release), dTc (histamine release and ganglion blockade) and pipecuronium.

Tachycardia

Pancuronium produces maximum tachycardia,[Q] it is due to its vagolytic[Q] action, and sympathetic stimulation. Pancuronium increases the heart rate, hence, blood pressure and cardiac output raise. Other histamine releasers can also produce tachycardia.

Bradycardia

Bradycardia may be seen after vecuronium, atracurium particularly when they are administered after opioids.

Respiratory Effects

Rapacurium was associated with reports of severe bronchospasm[Q] because of which it was withdrawn. Atracurium and dTc are associated with histamine release, which may result in increased airway resistance and bronchospasm in patients with hyperactive airway disease.

Central Nervous System

Chemically neuromuscular blockers are quaternary compounds and do not cross blood brain barrier, thus are devoid of direct CNS effects. Laudanosine, a metabolite of atracurium and cisatracurium has got CNS stimulating properties.

Complications of Long-term Administration of Nondepolarizing Neuromuscular Blockers (as in Intensive Care Unit)

In addition to specific drug related side effects, long-term administration is associated with:
- **Complications of immobility**: Deep venous thrombosis, pulmonary embolism, decubitus ulcers, etc.
- **Inability to cough**: Retention of secretions and atelectasis, pulmonary infection.
- Dysregulation of nicotinic acetylcholine receptors.
- Prolonged paralysis after stopping relaxants.
- **Critical illness myopathy (CIM)**: Usually seen in patients with asthma and other lung diseases. Affected individuals typically have been treated with corticosteroids and NDMBs. Prolonged immobility is the key risk factor. The major feature of CIM is flaccid weakness that tends to be diffuse and sometimes also includes facial muscles and diaphragm. The clinical features resemble critical illness polyneuropathy (CIP), from which it is differentiated on the basis of increased serum creatine kinase concentration, which remain normal in neuropathy. Avoiding steroids in ICU patients receiving NDMB is the best prevention.

FACTORS AFFECTING RESPONSE TO NEUROMUSCULAR BLOCKERS

Drug Interactions

- **Interactions among NDMBs**: Mixtures of two NDMBs are considered to be either additive or synergistic. Additive interactions are seen after the administration of chemically related agents, such as atracurium and mivacurium, or among various steroidal neuromuscular blockers. Combinations of structurally dissimilar (e.g., atracurium and rocuronium) produce a synergistic response.
- **Interactions between succinylcholine and NDMBs**: The interaction between SCh and

NDMB depends on the order of administration and the dose. NDMB before succinylcholine prevents fasciculation's and have an antagonistic effect on the subsequent block produced by Sch. When NDMB is used for maintenance, after intubation with SCh, there is potentiation of the effects of vecuronium, and atracurium.

- **Interactions with inhaled anesthetics**: Inhaled anesthetics enhance the effects of NDMB, the order of potentiation is desflurane[Q] >sevoflurane >isoflurane >halothane.
- **Interactions with antibiotics**: Aminoglycosides (maximum), tetracycline, polymyxins, lincomycin and clindamycin potentiate muscular blockade.
- **Interactions with antiepileptic drugs**: Patients receiving antiepileptics demonstrated resistance to NDMB[Q] (except mivacurium and atracurium). This is due to increased binding of the neuromuscular blockers to α1-acid glycoproteins[Q] and upregulation of neuromuscular acetylcholine receptors.
- **Interactions with lithium**: Lithium prolongs[Q] blockade of both SCh and NDMB by inhibiting neuromuscular transmission presynaptically.
- **Interactions with other drugs**: Azathioprine and steroids antagonize the effects of NDMB. Tamoxifen potentiate the effects of NDMBs.
- **Interactions with magnesium and calcium**:
  - Magnesium sulfate, given for the treatment of preeclampsia, potentiates NDMBs while antagonizes the blockade of succinylcholine.
  - Increasing calcium concentrations reduce the sensitivity of neuromuscular junction to NDMB, thus more dose is required.

Temperature

Hypothermia prolongs the duration of action of NDMB.

Special Population

- **Pediatric patients**: Neuromuscular junctions are immature at birth. Maturation of neuromuscular transmission occurs after the first 2 months of age. However, neuromuscular blockers can be used safely in term and preterm infants with following precautions:
  - Routine administration of SCh to healthy children is risky as they may have undiagnosed muscular dystrophies. In such case SCh can cause, rhabdomyolysis, hyperkalemia, acidosis which can progress to cardiac arrest. So, US Food and Drug Administration (FDA) restricts the use of SCh in pediatric patient except for emergency control of the airway.
  - Neonates and infants are more sensitive to vecuronium. Vecuronium acts as a long-acting neuromuscular blocker[Q] in neonates. In contrast, pharmacokinetics of atracurium and rocuronium remains unaffected in pediatric patients.
- **Elderly patients**: Due to physiological effects of ageing, the usual doses of relaxant produce more profound block of prolong duration. So, dose must be reduced for all those agents whose clearance depends on liver or kidney. Kinetics and dynamics of atracurium and cisatracurium remain unaltered in elderly.
- **Obese patients**: Neuromuscular blockers should be administered to obese patients on the basis of their lean body mass, so as to avoid overdose.

Coexisting Conditions (Table 14.5)

- **Renal disease**: Renal failure increases the duration of action of all NDMB except atracurium and cisatracurium.
- **Hepatobiliary disease**: Blockade of pancuronium, vecuronium, rocuronium, and mivacurium gets prolonged. Elimination of atracurium and cisatracurium remain unaffected or may rather be increased (or duration of action is reduced) due to increase in Hofmann elimination (as volume of distribution increases).
- **Burns**: Within 48 hours, thermal injury produces upregulation of both fetal and mature acetylcholine receptor. This upregulation is associated with resistance to NDMBs and increased sensitivity to succinylcholine. Therefore, it is better to avoid the use of succinylcholine in

Table 14.5: Muscle relaxant choice and coexisting conditions.

Characteristic	Preferred	Contraindicated	Better avoided
Renal failure	Cisatracurium, Atracurium, Rocuronium	Gallamine, pancuronium, dTC, Doxacurium, Metocurane	Vecuronium
Liver disease	Cis Atracurium, Atracurium	Vecuronium (Relative), Rocuronium	Mivacurium
Biliary obstruction	Cis Atracurium, Atracurium	Rocuronium	
Pregnancy	Cis Atracurium, Atracurium	Gallamine*	Long acting drugs
Myasthenia	Mivacurium, cis-Atracurium	Long acting drugs	Vecuronium, rocuronium

*Because gallamine crosses placenta.
(dTc: d-tubocurarine)

patients 24–48 hours after a thermal injury for at least 1 or 2 years.

RECOVERY FROM NEUROMUSCULAR BLOCKADE

- After the administration of nondepolarizing neuromuscular blocking drugs, adequate return of normal neuromuscular function occurs only when effect of drug weans off. Internationally TOF ratio of 0.60 suggests adequate recovery of neuromuscular strength while a ratio of 0.9 has been considered as an end point for recovery.
- Recovery from muscle relaxation of NDMB results from an increase in the acetylcholine concentration relative to that of the relaxant to overcome the competitive neuromuscular blockade. Though neostigmine will increase the acetylcholine concentration, and antagonize muscle relaxation. Ultimately, recovery depends on elimination of the neuromuscular blocker from the body.

ANTAGONISM OF RESIDUAL NEUROMUSCULAR BLOCKADE

NDMB competes with ACh to produce blockade, thus if ACh concentration is increased at neuromuscular junction equilibrium tends to oppose NDMB or favor transmission across neuromuscular function.

- Anticholinesterases by inhibiting acetylcholinesterase increase the concentration of acetylcholine at neuromuscular junction. Three anticholinesterases are currently being used to antagonize residual neuromuscular blockade: neostigmine[Q] (most commonly used), pyridostigmine, and edrophonium. Speed and adequacy of this antagonism depends on many factors, major ones are:
  - *Depth of the blockade when the antagonist is administered*: Generally, more time is required to antagonize profound levels than lesser levels of blockade.
  - *Anticholinesterase being administered*: The order of rapidity of antagonism is edrophonium[Q] >neostigmine >pyridostigmine. However, edrophonium is not as effective as neostigmine in antagonizing profound blockade.
  - *Dose of anticholinesterase*: Larger doses antagonize neuromuscular blockade more rapidly and more completely, however this relationship is true up to the point of the maximum effective dose only, beyond which increase dose will not produce any further antagonism. For neostigmine, this maximum effective dose is 80 µg/kg and for edrophonium, it is 1.5 mg/kg.
  - *Neuromuscular blocker used*: Reversal is rapid after intermediate duration NDMB in comparison to long acting NDMB.
  - *Acid-base state*: Both metabolic and respiratory acidosis[Q] augment nondepoarizer blockade, but only respiratory acidosis prevents adequate antagonism.

- *Other factors*: Hypothermia, hypokalemia, volatile anesthetics and antibiotics (particularly aminoglycoside or polypeptide classes) makes antagonism difficult.

KEY POINTS

Mixing or combining neostigmine and edrophonium do not potentiate each other. Therefore, when inadequate reversal occurs, one should not be tempted to add a different anticholinesterases but ensure that the maximum dose of the original drug has been administered.[1]

- Increased acetylcholine produce both nicotinic and muscarinic effects. As only nicotinic effects are desired, the muscarinic effects (bradycardia, increased secretions) must be blocked by atropine or glycopyrrolate. Atropine is better suited for administration with the rapid-acting edrophonium, while glycopyrrolate is better suited for administration with the slow-acting neostigmine and pyridostigmine.

OTHER ANTAGONISTS OF NONDEPO-LARIZING NEUROMUSCULAR BLOCKERS

Sugammadex

Sugammadex the molecular antagonist[Q] of rocuronium, is the most exciting drug in clinical neuromuscular pharmacology. It is the first selective relaxant binding agent which binds steroidal neuromuscular blocking agents (rocuronium >vecuronium >pancuronium) to form very tight complexes. During rocuronium induced neuromuscular blockade, intravenous administration of sugammadex results in rapid removal of free rocuronium molecules from plasma. The combination of rocuronium and sugammadex could replace succinylcholine for rapid-sequence induction of anesthesia.

It is also worthy to mention that, sugammadex is ineffective against succinylcholine and nonsteroidal NDMB as it does not form inclusion complexes with these drugs.

LAST-MINUTE REVISION

- Broadly classified as depolarizers (succinylcholine and decamethonium) and nondepolarizers (atracurium, cisatracurium, vecuranium, pancuronium). All NDMBs have 'r' in their spelling.
- Sch produces hyperkalemia, increase intraocular pressure, intracranial pressure, and intragastric pressure.
- C/I in muscular dystrophies, hyperkalemia, elective neurosurgery.
- **Rocuronium**: NDMB of choice for rapid sequence induction, due to its most rapid onset among nondepolarizers.
- **Atracurium and cisatracurium**: Undergoes Hofmann elimination, cisatracurium: Muscle relaxant of choice in liver disease, renal disease.
- **Pancuronium**: Long-acting NDMB produces tachycardia due to its vagolytic property.
- **dTC, mivacurium, atracurium**: Produce histamine release.
- **Gantacurium**: Ultrashort-acting nondepolarizing muscle relaxant.
- **Rapacuronium**: Muscle relaxant associated with bronchospasm.

REFERENCE

1. Nag K, Singh DR, Shetti AN, Kumar H, Sivashanmugam T, Parthasarathy S. Sugammadex: A revolutionary drug in neuromuscular pharmacology. Anesth Essays Res. 2013;7(3):302-6.

REVIEW QUESTIONS

1. Bradycardia may be the problem after injection of:
   a. Midazolam
   b. Succinylcholine
   c. Dopamine
   d. Isoprenaline

2. Which of the following is the neuromuscular blocking agent with the shortest onset of action?
   a. Mivacurium
   b. Vecuronium
   c. Rapacuronium
   d. Succinylcholine

3. Mivacurium when given in high doses, can produce all are true, *except*:
   a. Bronchospasm
   b. Hypertension
   c. Flushing
   d. Increase in dose increase the rapidity of onset

4. Which of the following skeletal muscle relaxants undergo Hofmann's elimination?
   a. Atracurium
   b. Cisatracurium
   c. Mivacurium
   d. Vecuronium

5. An ICU patient on atracurium infusion develops seizures after 2 days. The most probable cause is:
   a. Accumulation of laudanosine
   b. Allergy to drug
   c. Due to prolong infusion
   d. Allergy to atracurium

6. Administration of small dose of succinylcholine 5 minutes prior to full dose of succinylcholine is called:
   a. Precurarization
   b. Self-taming
   c. Reversal
   d. Induction

7. Cisatracurium has following advantages over atracurium, *except*:
   a. More potency
   b. Less chances of laudanosine accumulation
   c. Duration less than 1 hour
   d. Less histamine release

8. Sugammadex is a novel module introduced for:
   a. Reversing succinylcholine paralysis
   b. Reversing atracurium paralysis
   c. Reversing rocuronium paralysis
   d. Less mivacurium induce histamine

9. Which of the following relaxant has got biliary excretion?
   a. Vecuronium
   b. Rocuronium
   c. Atracurium
   d. Mivacurium

10. Muscle relaxant consistently linked with reports of bronchospasm:
    a. Atracurium
    b. Rocuronium
    c. Rapacuronium
    d. Pancuronium

11. Skeletal muscle relaxant of choice in liver and renal disease is:
    a. Mivacurium
    b. Atracurium
    c. Gallium
    d. Vecuronium

12. All statements are true about skeletal muscle relaxants, *except*:
    a. Mivacurium is hydrolyzed by plasma cholinesterase
    b. Rocuronium is largely excreted unchanged in bile
    c. Pancuronium blocks the uptake of norepinephrine
    d. Atracurium degraded by Hofmann's elimination

13. Hofmann degradation is seen in which muscle relaxant?
    a. Atracurium
    b. Succinylcholine
    c. Gallamine
    d. Pancuronium

14. Gallamine is excreted mainly through:
    a. Bile
    b. Liver
    c. Kidney
    d. Pseudocholinesterase

15. **Which muscle is most resistant to neuromuscular blockage?**
    a. Diaphragm
    b. Ocular
    c. Adductor pollicis
    d. Intercostal muscles

ANSWERS

1. b	2. d	3. b	4. a, b and c	5. a	6. b
7. c	8. c	9. a	10. c	11. b	12. c
13. a	14. c	15. a			

CHAPTER 15

Additional Drugs in Anesthesia

Anshul Jain

SYMPATHOMIMETICS

These drugs are used to treat perioperative hypotension, bradycardia and/or to counteract myocardial depressant effects of anesthetic drugs. They include:

- **Direct sympathomimetics**: They act directly as agonist on adrenoceptors. For example, adrenaline, noradrenaline (NA), isoprenaline, phenylephrine.
- **Indirect sympathomimetics**: These drugs act on adrenergic neurons and increase catecholamine secretion, which then acts on the adrenoceptors. For example, tyramine.
- **Mixed action**: They act directly as well as indirectly. Ephedrine, dopamine (DA), and mephentermine are the mixed acting sympathomimetics. Vasopressor effect of all these drugs is accompanied by tachycardia (**Table 15.1**).

Overall mixed acting drugs are used more commonly, while direct acting drugs are reserved for conditions unresponsive to mixed-acting drugs or in specific medical conditions where mixed agents cannot be used.

Adrenaline (Fig. 15.1)

Naturally occurring hormone synthesized in adrenal medulla. Adrenaline increases the stroke volume, heart rate and cardiac output. It increases the systolic blood pressure and has variable effect on diastolic BP. Produce vasoconstriction in skin, mucosa and hepatorenal bed (α_1 mediated). While vasodilation in skeletal muscles is β_2 mediated (**Fig. 15.1**). Overall effect is reduced systemic vascular resistance SVR and preferential distribution of cardiac output to skeletal muscles.[1]

Uses

Primary indication of adrenaline is cardiac arrest where it is administered IV in the dose of 1 mg in

Table 15.1: Comparative evaluation of different sympathomimetics.

Drug	Heart rate	MAP	Cardiac output	PVR	Bronchodilation	RBF
Epinephrine	↑↑	↑	↑↑	↑/↓	↑↑	↓↓
Norepinephrine	↓	↑↑↑	↓/↑	↑↑↑	–	↓↓↓
Isoprenaline	↑↑↑	↓	↑↑↑	↓↓	↑↑↑	↓/↑
Ephedrine	↑↑	↑↑	↑↑	↑	↑↑	↓↓
Phenylephrine	↓	↑↑↑	↓	↑↑↑	–	↓↓↓
Dopamine	↑/↑↑	↑	↑↑↑	↑	–	↑↑↑/↓*
Dobutamine	↑	↑	↑↑↑	↓	–	↑

(MAP: mean arterial pressure; PVR: pulmonary vascular resistance; RBF: renal blood flow)
Note: ↑ increase mild, moderate, marked; ↓ decrease mild, moderate, marked; ↓/↑ variable effect; ↑/↑↑ mild-to-moderate increase; ↓* In high does dopamine also reduces renal blood flow

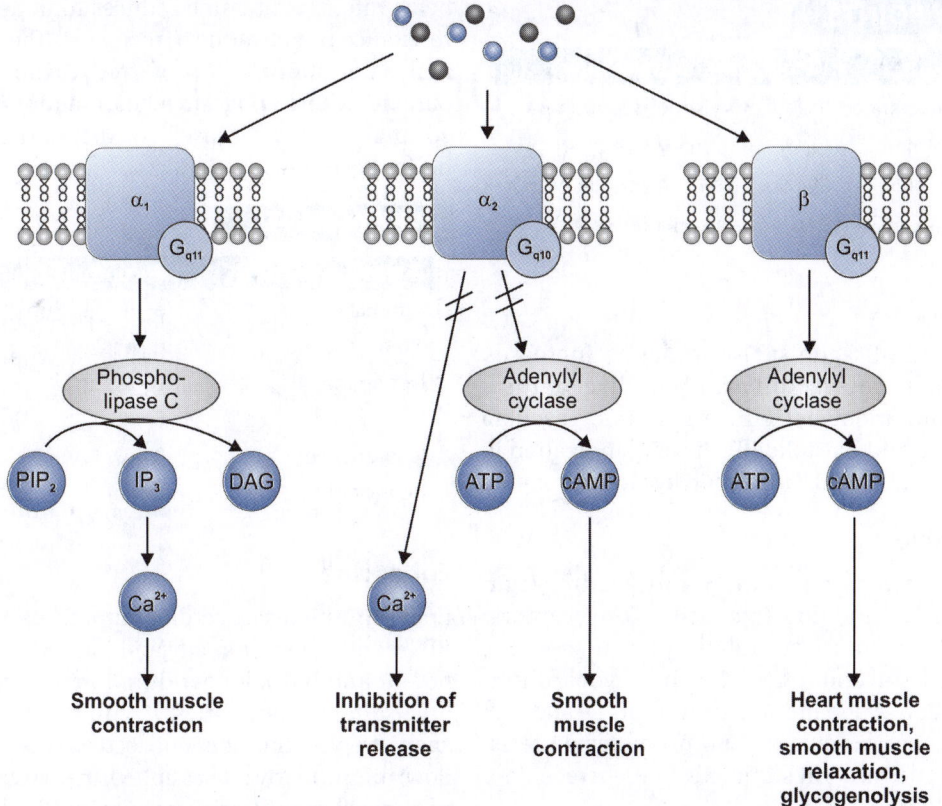

Fig. 15.1: Adrenaline effects; mechanism and receptors mediating the effect.

1 mL (1 in 1,000). Dose may be repeated every 2–5 minutes. Adrenaline can also be administered via endotracheal route or through direct intracardiac injection for this purpose.

Other Uses

- **Along with local anesthetics**: When combined with local anesthetics, adrenaline tends to prolong block by reducing its absorption in systemic circulation and reduce toxicity too.
- **Anaphylaxis**: Adrenaline provides quick relief in urticaria, angioedema, laryngeal edema.
- **Control of local bleeding**: Adrenaline 1 in 10,000 soaked in cotton, can control arteriolar and capillary bleeding during surgery.

Adrenaline (as a vasoconstrictor) should be avoided during anesthesia with halothane, enflurane, chloroform and cyclopropane as these agents sensitize the myocardium to the arrhythmogenic effects of adrenaline and can precipitate cardiac dysrhythmias.

Noradrenaline

Noradrenaline is a potent vasoconstrictor, which increase both systolic and diastolic BP. NA lacks β_2 action so, heart rate usually decreases due to the effect of increased BP on baroreceptors. NA reduces renal, hepatic and cerebral blood flow whereas increase systemic vascular resistance. Primary indications for NA are septic and spinal shock[Q] in which there is abrupt reduction in SVR.

KEY POINTS

Drug	Vasopressor of choice in
Norepinephrine	Vasodilatory shock septic shock
Epinephrine	Cardiopulmonary resuscitation
Dobutamine	Shock with reduced cardiac output
Vasopressin	Resistant vasodilatory shock

Isoprenaline

It is a pure β agonist. Isoprenaline increases heart rate, contractility and cardiac output, and simultaneously reduce systemic vascular resistance and diastolic BP. Primary indication is sudden bradycardia[Q] unresponsive to atropine.

Dopamine

Dopamine acts on both α and β adrenergic receptors in addition to specific DA receptors. α and β receptors stimulation produce direct positive inotropic effect on the myocardium. Stimulation of dopaminergic receptors D_1 and D_2.[Q] dilates renal vasculature and promotes diuresis. Different doses of DA stimulate different receptors **(Table 15.2)**.

Table 15.2: Dopamine: Doses and receptor-stimulated.

Dose	Receptor	Effect
<2 µg/kg/minute	D_1 and D_2 receptor only	Promotes diuresis[Q]
2–10 µg/kg/minute	β stimulation D1 receptor	↑ myocardial contractility ↑ Heart rate ↑ Cardiac output
10–20 µg/kg/minutes	α effect becomes prominent	↑ BP but renal blood flow is reduced

Dopamine is commonly used in the treatment of shock to support BP, improve cardiac output and maintenance of renal function.

Dobutamine

Relatively selective $β_1$ agonist $β_1:β_2 = 3:1$. Dobutamine increases cardiac output by increasing myocardial contractility and has minimal effect on heart rate. Dobutamine reduces total peripheral resistance by activating $β_2$ receptors. These effects make dobutamine a preferred vasopressor in patients where congestive heart failure CHF and coronary artery disease[Q] coexist, particularly if heart rate is already high.

KEY POINTS

Agent	Receptor stimulated
Adrenaline	$α_1, α_2, β_1, β_2$ no $β_3$
Noradrenaline	$α_1, α_2, β_1$, no $β_2$
Dopamine	$D_1, D_2, α_1, β_1$
Dobutamine	$β_1 > β_2$
Isoprenaline	β only
Phenylephrine	α only

Ephedrine

Ephedrine increases cardiac output, heart rate and BP by acting both directly and indirectly. It is less potent and has a longer duration of action than other direct acting drugs. In contrary to other $α_1$ agonist, ephedrine does not decrease uterine blood flow; this property makes ephedrine, a vasopressor of choice[Q] in obstetric patients, particular when patient is under spinal anesthesia.[Q]

Mephentermine

Increase cardiac output and BP, with minimal effect on heart rate, renal blood flow may be increased. It is the most commonly[Q] used drug to treat hypotension secondary to spinal anesthesia.

ANTIHYPERTENSIVES

Perioperative hypertension is a rare but serious problem. Among the variety of antihypertensive available, only few drugs can be used in perioperative period. For which drug should possess following properties:
- Rapid onset, short duration
- Can be administered by IV route
- Should not interact with anesthetic agents
- Effect is titrable.

For commonly used antihypertensives in perioperative period **(Table 15.3)**.

Table 15.3: Commonly used antihypertensives.

Drug	Dose	Comments
Sodium nitroprusside	50–100 μg bolus followed by 0.5–10 μg/kg/minute as infusion	Generates nitric oxide which relaxes both arteriolar and venous smooth muscles. Action begins within 1–2 minutes. Side effects include methemoglobinemia and rarely cyanide toxicity
Nitroglycerin	Same as nitroprusside	Venous dilation is the prominent mode of action. Drug of choice when hypertension and chest pain[Q] coexist. Headache due to dilation of cerebral of vessels is the common side effect
Esmolol	1 mg/kg bolus followed by 50–30 μg/kg/minute	Used when hypertension and tachycardia coexist particularly in condition with increased catecholamines hyperthyroidism. Bradycardia is a prominent side effect
Labetalol	0.1–0.25 mg/kg IV over 2 minutes	Combined α + β blocker which preserves uterine blood flow, so is a drug of choice[Q] for controlling BP in pre-eclampsia and eclampsia
Diltiazem	0.25 mg/kg bolus over 2 minutes. Can be repeated after 15 minutes	Lacks effect on heart rate. So, it is preferred when hypertension occurs in conjunction with normal heart rate as it does not reduce heart rate. Contraindicated in patients with pre-existing AV nodal or myocardial disease, sick sinus syndrome

ANTIEMETICS

Postoperative nausea and vomiting (PONV) is one of the common problems. Though not serious PONV limits oral intake and increase hospital stay. Antiemetics are being used commonly to prevent and/or treat PONV. Commonly used drugs are:

- **Metoclopramide:** Dopamine D_2 antagonist with prokinetic properties. Extrapyramidal side effects are its main limitation. Dose is 10–50 mg/IV.
- **Droperidol:** Highly potent D_2 antagonist with sedative properties. Most effective drug to combat opioid induced vomiting. Effective dose is 0.625–1.25 mg. It is contraindicated in patients with known or suspected QT prolongation.
- **Hyoscine or scopolamine:** Hyoscine an anticholinergic is a well-known antiemetic drug for motion sickness. In addition to injectable preparation, transdermal patches are also available. Blurred vision, dizziness and dry mouth are the main side effects.
- **Ondansetron:** Serotonin antagonist that blocks emetogenic impulses at their peripheral origin and their central relay too. It is the most effective antiemetic for treatment and prevention of PONV. Dose is 4 mg/IV
  - Granisetron and polanosetron are other serotonin antagonist being used for PONV. Polanosetron because of its long life 40 hours can prevent postdischarge nausea and vomiting too.[2]
- **Dexamethasone:** In doses of 4–8 mg dexamethasone effectively prevents nausea and vomiting.

Promethazine, cyclizine, clonidine also possess antiemetic properties. Among anesthetic drugs, propofol has got substantial antiemetic property.

LAST-MINUTE REVISION

- Adrenaline, lacks effect on $β_3$, NA lacks $β_2$ action. Isoprenaline is pure β-agonist.
- All vasopressors reduce renal blood flow except dopamine in doses <2 mg/kg/minute.
- Noradrenaline vasopressor of choice in septic shock.
- Dobutamine vasopressor of choice in cardiogenic shock.
- Ephedrine vasopressor of choice to treat spinal anesthesia induced hypotension in cesarean section.
- Sodium nitroprusside is associated with methemoglobinemia and cyanide toxicity.
- Labetalol is the preferred antihypertensive to control BP in pregnant female.
- Diltiazem is preferred antihypertensive to control BP when heart rate is normal.

REFERENCES

1. Lynch GS, Ryall JG. Role of beta-adrenoceptor signaling in skeletal muscle: implications for muscle wasting and disease. Physiol Rev. 2008; 88(2):729-67. doi: 10.1152/physrev.00028.2007. PMID: 18391178.

2. Shetti AN, et al. Improved prophylaxis of postoperative nausea vomiting: Palonosetron a novel antiemetic. Anesth Essays Res. 2014; 8(1):9-12. doi: 10.4103/0259-1162.128894. PMID: 25886096; PMCID: PMC4173575.

REVIEW QUESTIONS

1. A patient posted for cesarean section, develops hypotension 8 minutes after administration of spinal anesthesia, the most suitable drug to treat hypotension in this patient is:
   a. Adrenaline
   b. Noradrenaline
   c. Ephedrine
   d. Mephentermine
2. Which of the following vasopressor increase renal blood flow?
   a. Noradrenaline
   b. Ephedrine
   c. Dopamine in doses of 20 µg/kg/minute
   d. Dopamine in doses of 5 µg/kg/minute
3. Similarities of nitroglycerine and nitroprusside are all, *except*:
   a. Rapid onset
   b. Rapid recovery
   c. Infusion dose is 0.5–1.0 µg/kg/minute
   d. Both produces methemoglobinemia
4. Longest acting antiemetic:
   a. Dexamethasone
   b. Polanosetron
   c. Scopolamine
   d. Metoclopramide
5. Which of the following drug possess the triple action of antiemetic, sedative, anticholinergic?
   a. Scopolamine
   b. Promethazine
   c. Propofol
   d. Droperidol

ANSWERS

1. c
2. d
3. d
4. b
5. a and b

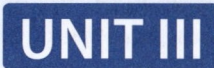

Perioperative Care

Unit Outline

16. Monitoring Under Anesthesia
17. Perioperative Fluid Therapy and Blood Transfusion
18. Blood Salvage Techniques
19. Anesthesiologist as a Perioperative Physician

COMPETENCIES COVERED IN UNIT III

Competency Number	Competency Name	Chapter Number
AS1.2	Describe the roles of anesthesiologist in the medical profession (including as a perioperative physician, in the intensive care and high dependency units, in the management of acute and chronic pain, including labor analgesia, in the resuscitation of acutely ill).	19
AS4.5	Observe and describe the principles and the steps/techniques in monitoring patients during anesthesia.	16
AS9.3	Describe the principles of fluid therapy in the preoperative period.	17
AS9.4	Enumerate blood products and describe the use of blood products in the preoperative period.	17–18

CHAPTER 16

Monitoring Under Anesthesia

Anshul Jain, Sandeep Sahu

INTRODUCTION

Patient monitoring is key aspect of anesthesiology since its beginning as medical specialty. In present scenario of complex surgical procedures, anesthesia monitors are also sophisticated. Anesthesiologist must be able not only to understand and interpret the data from the monitors, but also to anticipate and recognize errors associated with their use. However, it must be very clear that, even in the presence of sophisticated monitors, fundamental monitor is still anesthesiologist sense of sight, hearing and touch.

CLINICAL MONITORING

As mentioned above, clinical monitoring by inspection, palpation and auscultation provides information regarding almost all vital parameters. Simple observations are included in **Table 16.1**.

Now, let you know about the important aspects of systemic monitoring.

CARDIOVASCULAR MONITORING

Arterial Blood Pressure

The rhythmic contractions of the left ventricle eject blood into vascular system in pulsatile manner, this results in pulsatile arterial pressures. The peak pressure generated during systolic contraction is systolic arterial blood pressure (SBP) while the trough pressure during diastolic relaxation is the diastolic arterial blood pressure (ABP). The difference between systolic and diastolic pressure is pulse pressure. The time weighted average of arterial pressure during a pulse cycle is the mean arterial pressure (MAP). MAP is calculated by following formula:

$$MAP = \frac{SBP + 2(DBP)}{3}$$

Mean arterial pressure is important for estimating organ perfusion (e.g., kidney), while diastolic blood pressure (DBP) is useful for estimation of coronary flow.

Arterial blood pressure estimation is a fundamental monitoring, and is indicated in all patients. Methods for measuring arterial pressure can be invasive and noninvasive.

Noninvasive Arterial BP Monitoring

Indication

In all patients.

Table 16.1: Vital parameter and their clinical monitoring.

Cardiac performance, BP	Pulse rate, character and volume
Peripheral volume	Capillary refill time
Circulatory volume	Degree of jugular vein filling
PaO$_2$	Color of skin and blood
Lung function	Movement and compliance of reservoir bag of anesthesia circuit
Renal function	Urine output (also tells about circulatory volume)
Depth of anesthesia	Lacrimation, muscle tone, perspiration, pupil size

Frequency

It should be checked every 5–10 min.

Contraindication

As such, there is no contraindication, but cuff should be avoided in extremities with vascular abnormality.

Techniques

Following noninvasive techniques are used for estimation of blood pressure (BP):

- **Mercury sphygmomanometer**: Most commonly used method for BP estimation in clinical practice. BP can be estimated by palpating (tells about systolic BP only) the pulse while deflating the cuff, or by auscultating Korotkoff sounds. In palpatory method, mercury level at which pulse appears, marks the systolic BP. Size of cuff is very important for accurate measurement. It should cover^Q approximately 2/3rd of length of upper arm, enough to encircle 1/2 of arm and centered over brachial artery. Narrow cuff will overestimate while broad cuff will underestimate BP.
- **Doppler probe**: This technique is same as palpatory method; with the exception, which substitute anesthesiologist finger with Doppler probe for detecting pulse.
- **Oscillometry**: When blood flows in an artery which is compressed by inflated cuff, it produces oscillations, and these oscillations can be detected by automatic oscillometers. This is the principle by which oscillometers determine BP. Oscillometers are much more accurate than conventional mercury sphygmomanometers and are preferred mode of measuring BP, intraoperatively.
  - In these, cuff gets inflated automatically to a pressure level where oscillation ceases (i.e., above systolic pressure). After this cuff deflates automatically, the pressure at which oscillation starts is systolic pressure, oscillations are maximum at MAP and ceases again at diastolic pressure.
  - *Limitations*: Oscillometry is not useful in patient on cardiopulmonary bypass (as there is nonpulsatile flow), when patient has shivering, tremor or when there are frequent movement on the extremity used for measurement.

Note: Most automated BP monitors are based on oscillometry.

- **Arterial tonometry**: Arterial tonometry non-invasively measures beat-to-beat BP by sensing the pressure required to partially flatten a superficial artery that is supported by a bony structure. Continuous recording produces tracing which is similar to an invasive BP waveform. However, the limitations being sensitivity to movement artefact and need for frequent calibrations have restricted its use in routine anesthesia practice.

Invasive Arterial BP Monitoring (Fig. 16.1)

Direct measurement of BP by catheterization of an artery is the gold standard^Q method for BP measurement, and allows continuous beat-to-beat measurement. Further it is the most sensitive^Q technique for early detection of hypovolemia.

As it requires catheterization of artery and costly monitors, it is not used in all patients. Indications for invasive blood pressure (IBP) monitoring include:

- Procedures in which huge blood loss or fluid shifts is expected.
- When wide swings in arterial pressure is expected.
- Nonpulsatile arterial flow (cardiopulmonary bypass).
- Hypotensive anesthesia is being planned.
- Frequent need of arterial blood sampling.

Contraindications

- Catheterization should be avoided in arteries without documented collateral flow.
- Patients with coagulopathy
- **Preferred artery**: Radial artery^Q > dorsalis pedis
- **Complications**: Hematoma, bleeding, thrombosis, infection, accidental intra-arterial injection.

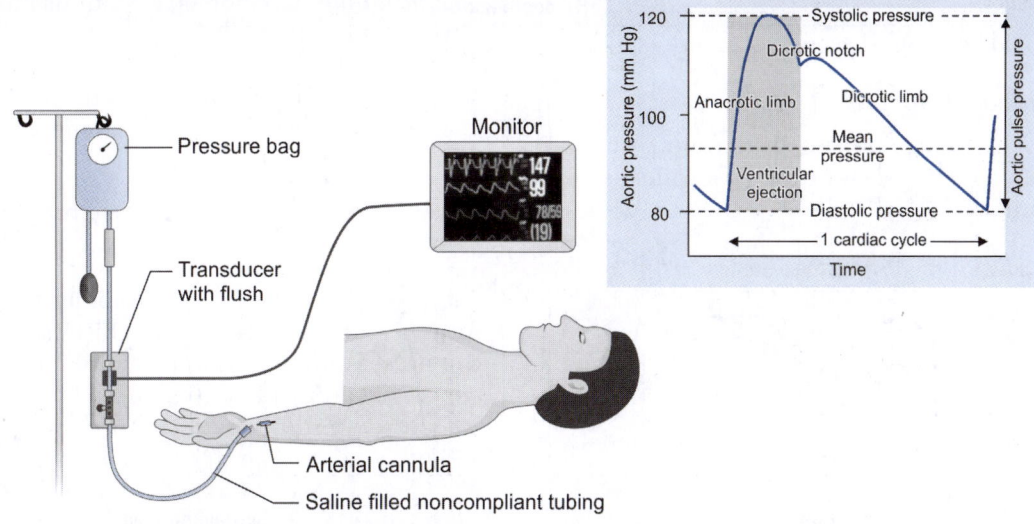

Fig. 16.1: Invasive arterial BP monitoring. Note the technique and the graph.

Technique (Fig. 16.1)

Artery can be catheterized by specialized intra-arterial catheters or usually by 20 G IV cannula, which is then connected to a low volume high pressure extension line. The other end of extension line is connected to IBP module of monitor. Correct measurement requires slightly under damped monitor with frequency more than 20 Hz.[Q] Overdamping underestimates systolic BP while underdamping overestimates systolic BP, though measurement of mean BP remain unaffected.

To prevent thrombus, arterial line must be flushed continuously with pressurized saline at a rate of 2–3 mL/hour.

Electrocardiography (Fig 16.2)

Electrocardiography (ECG) of all patients should be monitored and there is no contraindication. For proper diagnosis, lead selection is important. In most monitors, one can see two leads display simultaneously. Lead (II) parallels the atria, this result in maximum P wave voltages of any surface lead. This lead is best[Q] for detection of dysrhythmias and inferior wall ischemia.[Q] Lead V5 is highly sensitive for anterior and lateral wall ischemia. If only single channel monitor is available than lead (II) is the preferred lead. Perioperative ECG can successfully diagnose arrhythmias, ischemia and also aids in the diagnosis of electrolyte abnormalities (Fig. 16.2).

✦ KEY POINTS

Criteria for diagnosing intraoperative ischemia
Flat or down sloping ST segment depression >0.1 mV 60 or 80 millisecond after the J point (end of QRS complex) exceeding 1 mm.[Q] Predictability is high, if this occurs in conjunction with T-wave inversion.

Central Venous Pressure

Pressure in great veins [inferior vena cava (IVC) and superior vena cava (SVC)] approximately equals to right atrial pressure which in turn is a major determinant of right ventricular end diastolic volume. In normal healthy heart, right ventricular and left ventricular performance are parallel. Thus central venous pressure (CVP) indirectly tells about left ventricular filling.[Q] CVP estimation requires catheterization of either SVC or IVC, an invasive and technically challenging procedure. Due to this CVP monitoring and perhaps central venous catheterization is not a routine. Indications of central venous

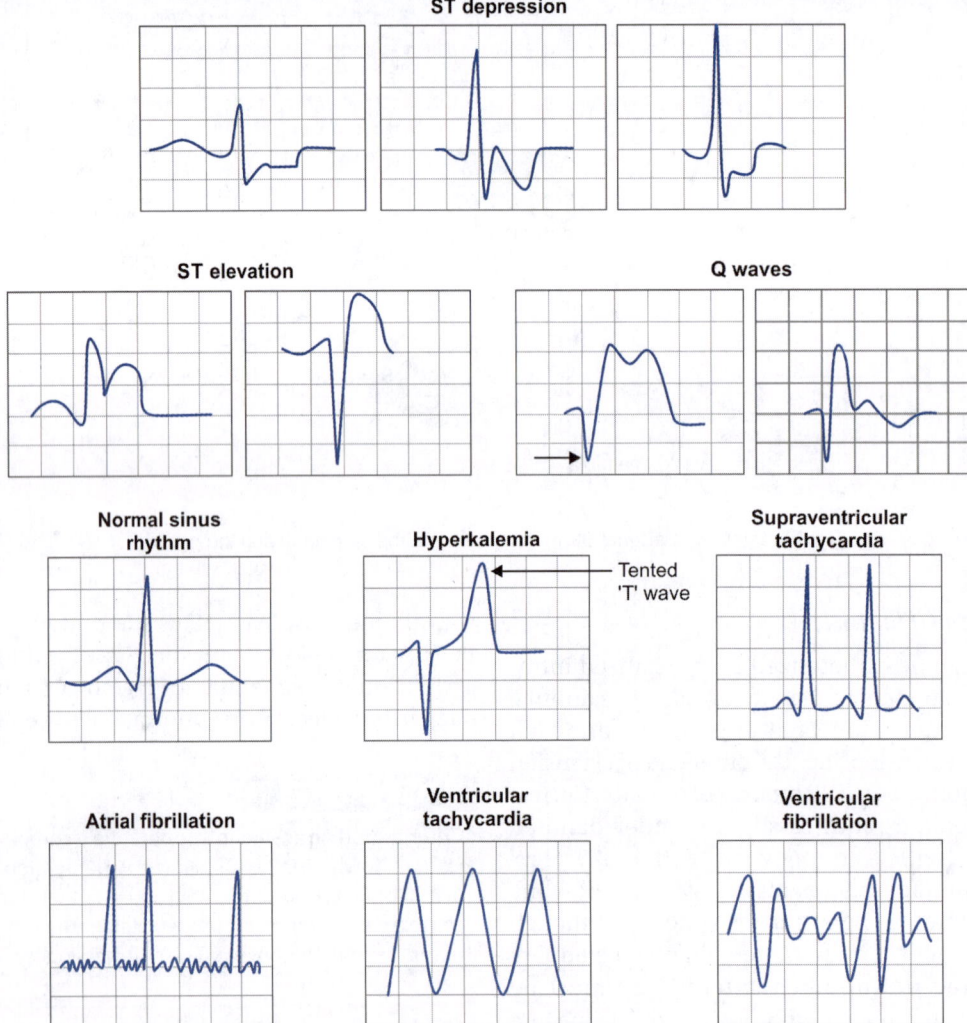

Fig. 16.2: Perioperative ECG abnormalties.

catheterization have been mentioned in **Table 16.2.**

One can see that therapeutic indications are more for central venous catheterization. Nowadays, use of ultrasound for vascular puncture has significantly reduced the associated complications as compared to the landmark guided technique.

Selection of Veins

Selecting the best site for safe and effective central venous cannulation requires consideration of the indication for catheterization (monitoring versus therapeutic), the patient's underlying medical condition, the clinical setting, and the skill and experience of the doctor performing the procedure.

Following veins can be catheterized:
- **Internal jugular vein**: Most frequently used, as catheterization is technically easy. However, *internal jugular catheterization carries maximum risk of infection and arterial puncture (carotid), and moreover it is vulnerable to kinking too.* Right internal jugular vein (IJV)

Table 16.2: Central venous catheterization.

Indications	Contraindications
For monitoring CVP	Renal cell tumor extension in right atrium
For placement of pulmonary artery catheter	Tricuspid valve endocarditis
Infusion of caustic drugs and total parenteral nutrition*	Severe coagulopathy
Aspiration of air embolism*	
Insertion of transcutaneous pacing leads*	
When fluid therapy has to be guided according to CVP*	

*Therapeutic indications
(CVP: central venous pressure)

is preferred over left IJV as cupola of the pleura is higher on the left, thereby theoretically increasing the risk for pneumothorax. Beside this left IJV is often smaller than the right and chances of thoracic duct injury are higher with left-sided catheterization.

- **Subclavian vein**: Technically most challenging, but has least chances of kinking and infection.^Q However, due to its deeper location and technical difficulty chances of pneumothorax are high. Advantages of subclavian venous cannulation include the ease of insertion in trauma patients who may be immobilized in a cervical collar, and increased patient comfort, especially for long-term intravenous therapy as in hyperalimentation and chemotherapy.
- **Basilic**: Peripherally inserted central venous catheters (PICCs) have become a popular alternative to centrally inserted catheters in patients requiring long-term intravenous therapy. Advantages include easier technique, an extremely low risk of vascular and other serious complications. Venous access for a PICC is obtained usually through the basilic vein, because of its more linear course. Most PICCs are placed for long-term therapeutic indications and use very flexible, nonthrombogenic silicone catheters.
- **Femoral vein**: Measures pressure of inferior vena cava technically easy but carries risk of thrombus, kinking and pseudoaneurysm.

KEY POINTS

What is central venous pressure?
Pressure in the intrathoracic portion of great veins (IVC and SVC).
From where should the sample for mixed venous oxygen saturation be taken ideally?
Pulmonary artery.

Waveform

Normal CVP waveform is characterized by three ascents (waves) and two descents (**Fig. 16.3**), viz:
- **'a' wave:** Atrial contraction.
- **'c' wave:** Tricuspid valve elevation due to isovolumic contraction of right ventricle.
- **'x' descent:** Downward displacement of tricuspid valve in ventricular contraction.
- **'v' wave:** Venous return against closed tricuspid valve.
- **'y' descent:** Opening of tricuspid valve during diastole.

Normal central venous pressure
- Normal CVP is 3–10 cm of H_2O.
- For correct measurement, reference level (i.e., zero level) should be at midaxillary line at the manubriosternal angle.
- For proper waveform catheter tip should be at junction of SVC and right atrium.

Pulmonary Artery Catheterization

Through central vein, specialized catheter can be advanced further into pulmonary artery. Swan-Ganz catheter which has balloon on its tip, is the most frequently used catheter for pulmonary artery catheterization (PAC). Pulmonary artery catheterization is not an easier technique and is associated with many

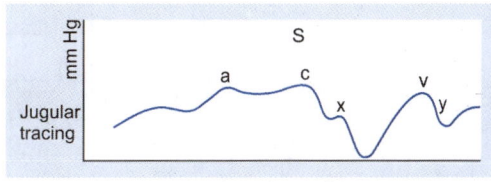

Fig. 16.3: Normal central venous pressure (CVP) waveform.

serious complications, including pulmonary artery rupture which carries a mortality rate of 50–70%. The most recent recommendations of American Society of Anesthesia conclude PAC monitoring to be appropriate in surgical patients undergoing procedures associated with a high-risk of complications from hemodynamic changes (e.g., cardiac surgery) or patients with advanced cardiopulmonary diseases that would place them at increased risk for adverse perioperative events. PAC should be considered only when cardiac index, preload, left atrial pressure or the degree of mixed venous blood oxygenation need to be monitored.

Pulmonary artery catheterization is contra-indicated in conditions where central venous line insertion is contraindicated. Relative contraindications to PAC include complete left bundle branch block (PAC can produce complete heart block), Wolff–Parkinson–White syndrome, and Ebstein's malformation (risk of tachyarrhythmias).

Clinical Uses

Pulmonary artery catheterization allows accurate measurement of left ventricular preload. After attaining a pulmonary artery position, minimal advancement of PAC with inflated balloon extends the catheter tip to right pulmonary artery and results in a pulmonary artery occlusion pressure (PAOP) waveform **(Fig. 16.4)**. This, wedge pressure (PCWP or PAOP) in effect, measure the pressure at the point at which blood flow resumes from the pulmonary artery to the pulmonary vein. Because resistance in the large pulmonary veins is negligible, PAWP provides an accurate, indirect measurement of both pulmonary venous pressure and left atrial pressure.Q Pulmonary edema develops when PAOP is more than 25 mm Hg.

Pulmonary artery catheterization can detect myocardial ischemia in several ways. Ischemia impairs left ventricular relaxation and results in diastolic dysfunction, which in turn leads to increased left atrial and pulmonary capillary wedge pressure (PCWP).Q Morphology of pulmonary artery catheter waveforms also changes. Right ventricular ischemia also increases PCWP, right ventricular ischemia increases CVP too. In fact, right ventricular ischemia is one of the few situations where CVP may be higher than wedge pressure. Pulmonary artery is the site for mixed venous blood sampling (mixture of blood from IVC and SVC). Mixed venous oxygen tension/saturation is the best guide to assess tissue perfusion. Normal MVO_2 saturation is 75%; saturation less than 60% indicates reduced oxygen delivery to tissue.

Cardiac output can also be determined via PAC through thermodilution technique.

Complications

In addition to complications associated with central venous cannulation, PAC can lead to bacteremia, endocarditis, pulmonary infarction, pulmonary artery rupture, arrhythmias, conduction abnormalities, and damage to pulmonary valve. Transient arrhythmias are the most common while pulmonary artery rupture is the most serious complication. The risk of

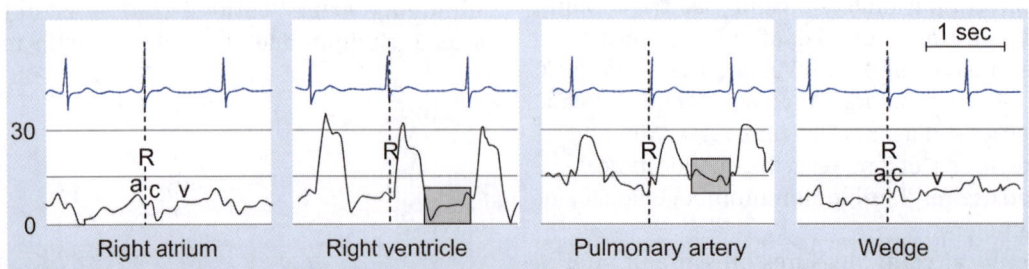

Fig. 16.4: Characteristic waveform recorded during passage of pulmonary artery catheter from right atria to pulmonary capillary wedge.

complications increases with the duration of catheterization, which usually should not exceed 72 hours. As pulmonary artery rupture carries a 50–70% mortality rate and can occur because of balloon overinflation, the frequency of wedge readings should be minimized.

Any degree of hemoptysis should not be ignored, as it may herald pulmonary artery rupture.

> **KEY POINTS**
>
> Mixed venous oxygen saturation
> - **Normal value**: 60–80%
> - **Reduced**: Cardiac disease, hypoxia, anemia
> - **Increased**: Septic shock; cyanide poisoning (Tissues are unable to extract the oxygen).

Cardiac Output

Indications are same as that of PAC. Following techniques are used to determine cardiac output:
- **Thermodilution**: Through pulmonary artery catheter
- **Dye dilution**
- **Thoracic bioimpedance**
- **Ultrasonography**: Transesophageal echocardiography (TEE) is the technique of choice to determine cardiac output. Moreover TEE is the most sensitive technique to detect air embolism[Q] (including paradoxical emboli). Ischemic myocardium does not exhibit normal inward movement or thickening during systole. As TEE requires esophageal probe, it is necessary to sedate the patient before insertion. Beside this, there is variability in interpretation and esophageal probes can compress aorta in infants and small children. Despite these limitations, TEE is routinely being used in complex surgical procedures, perhaps due to its wider range of applications.

RESPIRATORY MONITORING

Stethoscope

Chest auscultation provides information regarding both cardiac and respiratory functions. It is a noninvasive and most economical of all monitors. Precordial stethoscope is perhaps the only monitor which is found in all operation theaters irrespective of specialty and advancement.

Esophageal stethoscope is a specialized variant which has a soft plastic catheter with balloon covered distal openings. Though the quality of breath and heart sounds is much better than with a precordial stethoscope, its placement is an invasive, technique and due to availability of better monitors, esophageal stethoscope is now out of use.

Oxygen Saturation

Measurement of oxygen saturation provides rapid and useful information regarding oxygenation status. Via oxygen-hemoglobin dissociation curve percentage saturation of the O_2 can be corelated to PaO_2. Thus, oxygen saturation indirectly tells about arterial oxygen tension. Techniques used to measure oxygen saturation include:

Co-oximetry

Co-oximetry is accomplished through a traditional blood gas analyzer which is capable of measuring concentration of oxygenated hemoglobin (HbO_2), reduced hemoglobin (HbR), carboxyhemoglobin and methemoglobin.[Q] It is the current gold standard for measuring SaO_2.[1]

Pulse Oximetry

Pulse oximetry combines the principles of oximetry and plethysmography to noninvasively measure oxygen saturation in arterial blood. Oxygenated and deoxygenated hemoglobin absorb light of different wavelength, perhaps the principle on which pulse oximetry works. HbO_2 absorb, more infrared light (wavelength 960 nm) while deoxygenated hemoglobin absorbed more red light (wavelength 660 nm).

Monitor includes a sensor containing light source emitting light of specific wavelength and a photo diode that senses the transmitted light on the opposite side. This sensor is placed across a well perfused tissue that can be transilluminated, e.g., finger, toe, earlobe, nose tip.

Arterial pulsations are identified by plethysmography. Light detector analyzes the wavelength absorbed by pulsatile component arterial blood and nonpulsatile component. The ratio of the absorptions at the red and infrared wavelengths for pulsatile component is analyzed by a microprocessor to provide the oxygen saturation (SpO_2) of arterial blood, expressing it as percentage.

Indication

Indicated in all cases. Preferably in postoperative period also.

Clinical Applications

SpO_2 more than 95% signifies adequate oxygenation while SPO_2 less than 90% indicates PaO_2 less than 65 mm Hg and cyanosis usually corresponds to an SpO_2 less than 80%.[Q]

In addition to arterial saturation, pulse oximetry tells about pulse rate,[Q] perfusion status.

Limitations

Many a times, pulse oximetry is unable to estimate oxygen saturation correctly. Some of these conditions are:
- **Abnormal hemoglobin**
  - *Carboxyhemoglobinemia*: Carboxyhemoglobin absorbs infrared light similar to oxyhemoglobin, thus pulse oximeters display false high saturation.
  - *Methemoglobinemia*: Methemoglobin absorbs both light in equal fraction so pulse oximeters display fix saturation of 85%.[Q]
- **Anemia**: Underestimates saturation
- **Reduced blood flow**: False low reading
- **Henna (mehndi)**: Red henna has no effect where as black henna blocks transillumination and precludes the measurement.
- **Nail polish**: Slight decrease[Q] in SpO_2 reading, maximum effect is with blue nail polish.
- **Movements**: Fast movements like tremors and shivering results in false reading or sometimes totally preclude measurement.
- **SpO_2 <60%**: Below 60% most pulse oximeter gives false low reading. Ear probe gives better reading at low PO_2 than finger probe.

CAPNOGRAPHY

Continuous analysis of end-tidal carbon dioxide ($ETCO_2$) and its waveform is called capnography.[Q] (Fig. 16.5).

Indication and Technique

Due to its noninvasiveness and great clinical importance, it is indicated in all cases of general anesthesia. Capnograph absorbs expired gas via continuous suction, infrared red light is then transmitted through expired gas and CO_2 tensions is derived on the basis of intensity of the transmitted light.

> **Note:** Today's infrared gas analyzers are capable of measuring all currently used inhalational anesthetic agents in addition to CO_2. Oxygen does not absorb infrared light and therefore must be measured by other means, such as electrochemical or paramagnetic analysis.

For correct measurement suction port should be near to patient, so as to prevent mixing of expired gas with fresh gas.

Utilization

- **Shape of expired capnogram**: In most capnograph, PCO_2 is plotted against time. The tracing

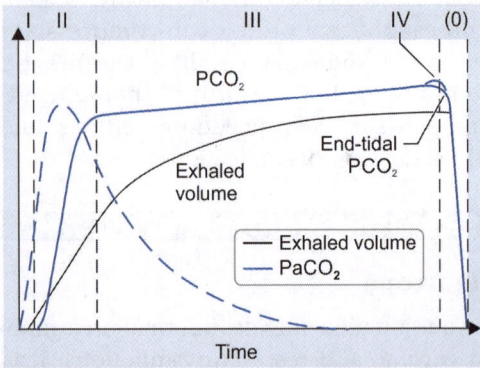

Fig. 16.5: End-tidal carbon dioxide ($ETCO_2$) graph.

can be divided into an inspiratory phase and three expiratory phases **(Fig. 16.6)**:
- *Phase 0*: Inspiratory phase
- *Phase I*: Dead space gases with little or no CO_2
- *Phase II*: Mixture of alveolar and dead space gas
- *Phase III*: Alveolar plateau, with the peak (Phase IV) → representing end-expiratory (*end-tidal*) CO_2 (PETCO$_2$).

Applications

- **Spontaneous inspired effort**: When effect of muscle relaxant weans, there is dip in phase III due to inspiratory effort. This dip acts as guide to administer further dose of muscle relaxant.
- In patients with emphysema slope of phase III is increased.
- Dual plateau (i.e., tails-up pattern) may be seen when there is leak in the sample line.
- If CO_2 absorbent is exhausted,[Q] the inhaled CO_2 concentration is greater than zero, and capnogram never touches baseline.
- **End-tidal CO_2 concentration**: ETCO$_2$ indirectly represent alveolar CO_2. ETCO$_2$ estimation is very important as it not only tells that gas is exchanging in lung but also tells about many perioperative problems where it is altered **(Flowchart 16.1)**.
- **Inspired portion**: Inspired portion, i.e., phase 0 tells about the concentration of CO_2 in inspired air. Normally, inspired air contains very little (zero for practical purpose) CO_2. Raised CO_2 in inspiratory phase suggests rebreathing, exhausted CO_2 or incompetent valves of breathing circuit **(Fig. 16.6)**.

Other Applications

- Most sensitive, noninvasive technique that can predict successful endotracheal intubation. In endotracheal successful[Q] intubation, ETCO$_2$ is almost always more than 20. In esophageal intubation, ETCO$_2$ is less than 10, which then decreases further.
- For detection of air embolus, or pulmonary embolus. In air embolism, ETCO$_2$ suddenly drops to zero.
- Tells about lung compliance.
- Gradient between arterial CO_2 (PaCO$_2$) and ETCO$_2$ (equivalent to alveolar CO_2), which is normally 2–5 mm Hg, represent alveolar dead space. This gradient is increased in conditions of ventilation/perfusion mismatch, decreased cardiac output, decreased BP.

Note: Overall most sensitive method to detect successful intubation is fiberoptic bronchoscope.

ANESTHETIC GAS ANALYSIS

Analysis of anesthetic vapors/gases (N$_2$O, halothane, etc.) concentration in expired gases is very useful. This correctly tells about the alveolar concentration and guides the optimal dose, simultaneously preventing overdose.

Techniques

- Mass spectroscope
- Gas chromatography.

BLOOD GAS ANALYSIS

Analysis of arterial and mixed venous blood to determine partial pressure of dissolved gases in blood.

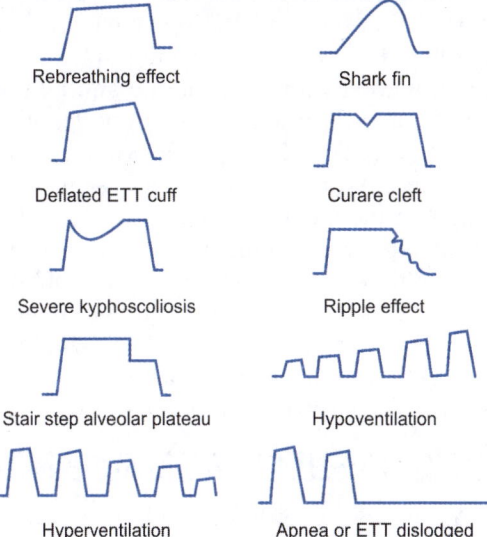

Fig. 16.6: Shapes of few pathological ETCO$_2$ waveforms.

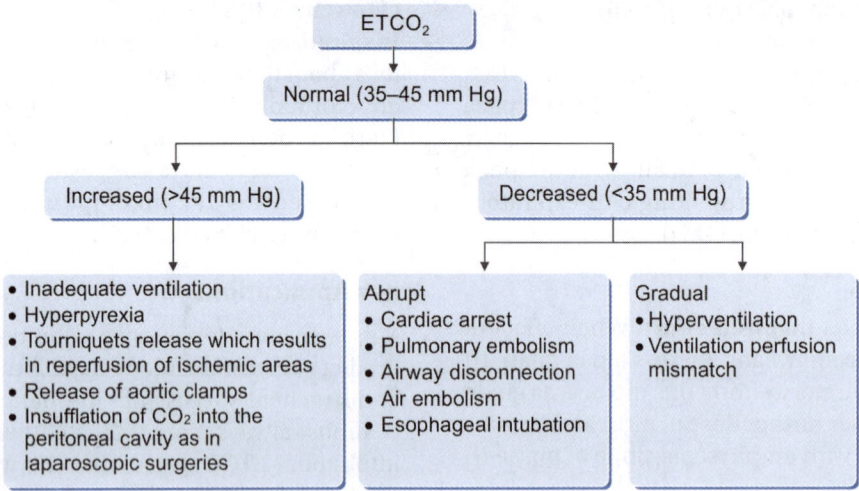

Flowchart 16.1: Conditions where end-tidal carbon dioxide (ETCO$_2$) is altered.

Remember: End-tidal carbon dioxide falls abruptly when there is gross reduction in blood or air supply to lung which results in cessation of diffusion. So the CO$_2$ concentration of exhaled air becomes almost equal to inspired air, i.e., approximately zero

This requires frequent blood sampling from peripheral artery [for arterial BGA (blood gas analysis)] or pulmonary artery (for analysis of mixed venous blood).[Q] Thus, BGA is an invasive procedure and should be done only when benefit outweighs risk. For arterial sampling, radial artery[Q] is preferred site. Femoral artery can be used in pediatric patient, but there is high-risk of pseudoaneurysm formation.

KEY POINTS

Under anesthesia, the dose of inhalational anesthetic is guided by anesthetic gas analyzer. If one wants to administer 1 MAC of halothane then goal is to make end-tidal concentration of halothane around 0.8% (1 MAC of halothane).

KEY POINTS

Normal values of arterial blood gas analysis

pH	7.35–7.45
PaO$_2$	80–100 mm Hg
SaO$_2$	95–100%
PaCO$_2$	35–45 mm Hg
HCO$_3^-$	22–26 mEq/L
Base excess	–2 to +2 mEq/L

For mixed venous blood, pulmonary artery[Q] is the preferred site, however, if pulmonary artery is not catheterized normal venous blood can be also be used.

INTRAOPERATIVE SPIROMETRY AND AIRWAY PRESSURE MONITORING

Latest anesthesia ventilators provide information regarding tidal volume, respiratory rate, airway pressure along with flow volume and pressure volume curves. This aids in better ventilation and prompt diagnosis of any problem in respiratory mechanics. As there is no adverse effect, when available it should be used in every patient.

Peak airway pressure should be kept low, as high inspiratory pressure can produce barotrauma. Very high airway pressure signifies blockade in endotracheal tube or circuit or kinking of endotracheal tube, while sudden drop in airway pressure is suggestive of tube disconnection.

NEUROMUSCULAR MONITORING

In patient where muscle relaxants are being used, neuromuscular monitoring aids in proper dosing and maintenance of relaxation without toxicity.

Principle is very simple; if a nerve is stimulated with sufficient intensity, all muscle fibers supplied by that nerve will contract, and the maximum response will be triggered. After administration of a neuromuscular blocking drug, this contractile response of the muscle ceases in proportion to the number of fibers blocked.

Patterns of Nerve Stimulation (Fig. 16.7)

For evaluation of neuromuscular function, the commonly used stimuli patterns are:

Single Twitch

In this mode of stimulation, single supramaximal electrical stimuli is applied to a peripheral motor nerve at frequencies ranging from 1.0 Hz (once every second) to 0.1 Hz (once every 10 seconds). As intensity of block increases contractile response diminishes. Both depolarizers and non-depolarizers exhibit same type of response to single twitch, thus it cannot be used to differentiate the type of blockade **(Fig. 16.7)**.

Train-of-Four

In train-of-four (TOF), four supramaximal stimuli are given every 0.5 second (2 Hz). Each stimulus in the train causes the muscle to contract, and "fade" in the response provides the basis for evaluation. TOF is a sensitive indicator of intensity of blockade of nondepolarizers. Disappearance of response to 4th twitch represents 75% blockade[Q] while 2nd twitch disappearance signifies 90% blockade.[Q] The

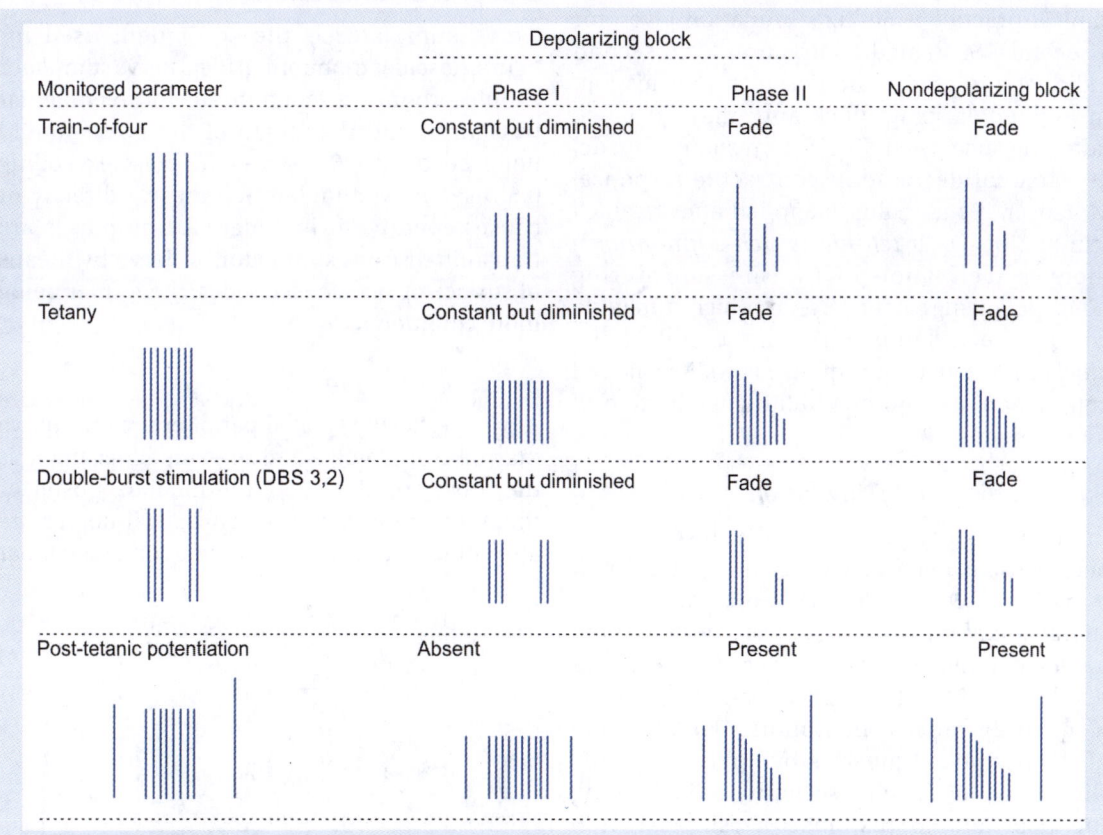

Fig. 16.7: Neuromuscular monitoring—parameter and response in different types of blockade.

ratio of amplitude of fourth response to the first response provides the TOF ratio. It is a sensitive method to distinguish blockade of depolarizer and nondepolarizers. In depolarizers, there is no fade and response to all four twitches[Q] is low amplitude contraction, creating a TOF ratio of 1. Fade in the TOF response after injection of succinylcholine signifies the development of a phase II block.[Q] TOF ratio is an indicator of adequate reversal too, T4:T1 response ratio of 0.7 represents complete recovery of neuromuscular function. Main limitation of TOF is that it is painful and fade is difficult to interpret visually.

Tetany

Tetanic stimulation consists of very rapid (e.g., 30, 50, or 100-Hz) delivery of electrical stimuli. The most commonly used pattern in clinical practice is 50-Hz stimulation given for 5 seconds. Sustained contraction for 5 second indicates adequate neuromuscular transmission. In nondepolarizing block and phase II block (after the succinylcholine), the response is fade, i.e., gradual decrease in contractile response. Moreover, if a stimulus is applied after tetanic[Q] stimulation (*post-tetanic twitch stimulation*), there is facilitation of transmission during nondepolarizing blockade, seen as high amplitude contractile response. During depolarizing blockade, the tetanic response is well-sustained contraction, and no post-tetanic facilitation of transmission.

Post-tetanic Count Stimulation

In intubating doses, muscle relaxants produces neuromuscular blockade which is so intense that there is no response to TOF and single-twitch stimulation.[Q] Thus during intense blockade, these modes of stimulation cannot be used to determine the degree of blockade. It is possible, however, to quantify intense neuromuscular blockade of the peripheral muscles by applying tetanic stimulation (50 Hz for 5 seconds) and observing the post-tetanic response to single-twitch stimulation given at 1 Hz starting 3 seconds after the end of tetanic stimulation. When the intense neuromuscular blockade dissipates response to post-tetanic twitch stimulation is first to appear and other responses appear afterwards.

Post-tetanic count[Q] acts as a guide for further doses of relaxant when intense relaxation has to be maintained as in ophthalmic surgery where even a minor movement can produce devastating sequelae.[2]

Double Burst Stimulation

Double burst stimulation (DBS) consists of two short bursts of 50-Hz tetanic stimulation separated by 750 msec. The duration of each square wave impulse in the burst is 0.2 msec. Responses are same as of TOF, but DBS is more sensitive for visual interpretation of fade.

Equipment and Technique (Fig. 16.8)

Nerve stimulator is the equipment used for neuromuscular monitoring. Ideal nerve stimulator should produce a monophasic and rectangular waveform, and the length of the pulse should not exceed 0.2–0.3 msec as the pulse exceeding 0.5 msec may stimulate the muscle directly or cause repetitive firing. Electrical impulses are transmitted from stimulator to nerve by means of surface or needle electrodes, the former being more common.

Selection of Nerve

Any superficially located peripheral motor nerve may be stimulated. Clinically, the ulnar nerve is the most popular site;[Q] the median, posterior tibial, common peroneal, and facial nerves are also sometimes used. For stimulation of the ulnar

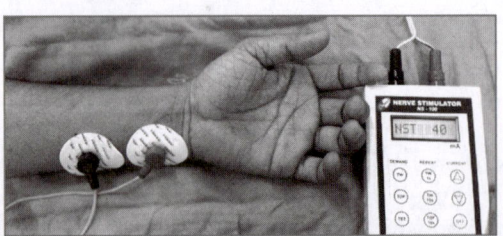

Fig. 16.8: Nerve stimulator equipment and technique for ulnar nerve monitoring.

nerve, the electrodes are placed over the volar side of the wrist. The negative electrode is placed distally over the tendon of flexor carpi ulnaris about 1 cm proximal to the proximal flexion crease of the wrist. With this placement, electrical stimulation normally elicits only finger flexion and thumb adduction.

It must be noted that different muscle groups have different sensitivities to neuromuscular blocking agents, thus results obtained for one muscle cannot be automatically extrapolated to other muscles. The diaphragm is among the most resistant of all muscles to both depolarizing and nondepolarizing neuromuscular blocking drugs. In general, the diaphragm requires 1.4^Q to 2.0 times as much muscle relaxant as the adductor pollicis muscle for same degree of blockade. Other respiratory muscles like laryngeal muscles are less resistant than the diaphragm. It must be noted that, upper airway muscles are more sensitive than the peripheral muscles, thus paralysis of adductor pollicis is a confirmatory sign of paralysis of upper airway muscles, which are of concern during intubation. Moreover during reversal, when adductor pollicis has recovered sufficiently, it can be assumed that no residual neuromuscular blockade exists in the diaphragm or in other resistant muscles. It is worthnoting that the response of the corrugator supercilii to facial nerve stimulation reflects the extent of neuromuscular blockade of respiratory muscles better than the response of the adductor pollicis to ulnar nerve stimulation does. But corrugator supercilii contractions are sometimes difficult to interpret.

TEMPERATURE MONITORING

Anesthesia is associated with impairment of thermoregulatory center. Core temperature or at least surface temperature should be monitored, so as to prevent inadvertent hypo- or hyperthermia. Both hypothermia and hyperthermia can alter drug metabolism and other physiologic parameters, thereby affecting anesthetic management.

Indications

American Society of Anesthesiology (ASA) recommends temperature monitoring in:
- All adult patients requiring general anesthesia of duration more than 30 minutes.
- In regional anesthesia when changes in body temperature are intended or suspected.
- All pediatric patients irrespective of anesthetic technique.

Technique

Mercury thermometers have been replaced by electronic thermometers, they are small, disposable and gives accurate reading. Electronic thermometers contain either thermostats or thermocouples.

Site

One can measure surface temperature, rectal temperature and core temperature. Core temperature is usually higher and is most important. Core temperature can be measured at lower end of esophagus (most frequently used site),^{Q} pulmonary artery (most accurate).^{Q} Nasopharynx, tympanic membrane can be used in the awake patient. Depending on the temperature, patient can have hypothermia or hyperthermia. Hypothermia is the most common thermal perturbation in perianesthetic period. Hyperthermia though less common is more dangerous.

Mechanism of Heat Loss

- Radiation, convection, conduction, evaporation.
- Radiation and convection^Q are the most common mechanism of perioperative heat loss.

> **Hypothermia**
> Core temperature less than 35°C. Based on the core temperature hypothermia can be:
> - **Mild:** 28–35°C [reduce basal metabolic rate (BMR) by 25%]
> - **Moderate:** 21–27°C (reduce BMR by 50%)
> - **Severe:** <20°C (reduce BMR by 80%)

Causes (Table 16.3)
Perioperatively cold surroundings are the most common causes of hypothermia.

Treatment and Prevention
- **Ambient OT temperature:** For surgery in an adult patient OT, temperature should be around 21°C,[Q] while for pediatric patients an OT temperature of 28°C is considered optimal.
- Warm IV fluids
- Hot air blanket
- Hot mattress.

MONITORING THE DEPTH OF ANESTHESIA

Due to long-term ill effect of awareness during anesthesia many studies are going on monitoring depth of anesthesia effect.

Till the invention of specific devices/monitors depth of anesthesia is monitored clinically.

Clinical signs of light anesthesia include:
- Tachycardia
- Hypertension
- Lacrimation (tears in eye) (sensitive)
- Perspiration
- Eye movement
- Intact reflexes.

Specific Monitors

Most monitors use complex electroencephalography (EEG) signals, to provide simple mathematical value of anesthetic depth:

Bispectral Index

First commercially available monitor for depth of anesthesia. A score ranging from 100 (fully awake) to 0 (brain dead) can be seen. Bispectral index (BIS) analyze EEG data by three different approaches: Fourier spectral analysis; bispectral analysis and time domain analysis. A BIS score of 40–60[Q] is suggestive of adequate depth.

Patient State Index

In addition to approaches used in BIS, patient state index (PSI) also uses spatial information to detect EEG changes. A PSI range of 25–50 suggest adequate depth.

Narcotrend

Narcotrend monitor uses sleep categorization approaches for EEG analysis to derive narcotrend stage which is indicated by capital letter ranging from A to E.

Evoked Responses

Evoked responses monitor the functional integrity of the pathways between the sensory receptor and the neural generator. As they are sensitive to anesthetic drugs, they are now being used to measure depth of anesthesia too.

Mid-latency auditory evoked potential is most sensitive evoked response for measuring depth of anesthesia.

MONITORING BLOOD LOSS

Following methods are used:

Gravimetric Methods

Blood-socked swabs and sponges are weighed to estimate blood loss. A standard swab absorbs 20 mL blood, while standard sponge absorbs 100 mL blood. A fist of 100 mL clot is suggestive of 300 mL blood loss.

Gravimetric method underestimate blood loss by 25%.

Calorimetric Method

Accurate but complex method in which swabs and sponges are mixed in known volume of water which is then estimated calorimetrically.

Table 16.3: Causes of hypothermia.

Accidental	Iatrogenic (induced hypothermia)
Impaired thermoregulation	Fall in core temperature by each degree Celsius reduce BMR by 6–7%
Cold IV fluids	Body is cooled with the target core temperature of 32–34°C
Cool surrounding	Used in neurosurgery for cerebral protection and cardiac surgery

(BMR: basal metabolic rate; IV: intravenous)

Arterial Blood Sampling

Sensitive Method

Intraoperative hemoglobin and hematocrit are estimated by blood sampling. If preoperative hematocrit is known blood loss can be estimated by following formula:

$$\text{Blood lost} = \text{EBV} \times \frac{\text{(Preoperative hematocrit} - \text{present hematocrit)}}{\text{Preoperative hematocrit}}$$

EBV = Estimated blood volume. EBV is usually 75 mL/kg for males and 65 mL/kg for females.

MONITORING COAGULATION

Perioperative coagulation monitoring has application in major surgeries where huge blood loss is expected, (e.g., cardiac surgeries, lung and liver transplants) and patients with coagulopathy. Commercially available coagulation monitors can be divided into four categories:

1. **Functional measures of coagulation**: The activated coagulation time (ACT), employs a contact activation initiator (celite or kaolin), to accelerate clot formation and reduce time for assay. The ACT in normal individuals is 107 ± 13 seconds. ACT testing remains a popular perioperative coagulation monitor because of its simplicity, low cost. Limitations of ACT monitoring include lack of sensitivity at low heparin concentrations and poor reproducibility.

2. **Heparin concentration measurement**: Protamine, a strongly basic protein, directly inhibits heparin in a stoichiometric manner, i.e., 1 mg of protamine will inhibit 1 mg (approximately 100 U) of heparin, thereby forming the basis for protamine titration as a measure of heparin concentration. As increasing concentrations of protamine are added to a sample of heparin-containing blood, time to clot formation decreases. If a series of blood samples with incremental doses of protamine are analyzed, the sample in which the protamine and heparin concentrations are most closely matched will clot first. In this manner, protamine titration methodology allows for heparin concentration estimation.
   - Advantages of heparin concentration measurement include sensitivity for low heparin concentrations as well as relative insensitivity to hemodilution and hypothermia. Limitation is failure to assess directly for an anticoagulant effect.

3. **Viscoelastic measures of coagulation**: Viscoelastic monitors measures the entire spectrum of clot formation from early fibrin strand generation through clot retraction and fibrinolysis. It includes:
   - *Thromboelastograph (Fig. 16.9)*: The thromboelastograph (TEG) uses a 0.35-mL blood sample placed into a disposable cuvette within the instrument. The cuvette is maintained at a temperature of 37°C and continuously rotates around an axis of approximately 5° to imitate sluggish venous flow and activate coagulation. A metal piston attached by a torsion wire to an electronic recorder is lowered into the blood within the cuvette. As clot formation occurs, the piston becomes enmeshed within the clot and rotation of the cuvette is transferred to the piston, torsion wire, and electronic recorder.
   - Various parameters describing clot formation and lysis are identified. "R value" (reaction time), which is time required for initial clot formation (normal, 7.5–15 minutes), it is comparable to the whole blood clotting time and may be prolonged by a deficiency of one or

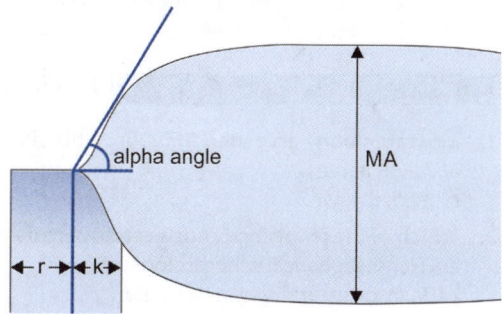

Fig. 16.9: Thromboelastograph.
(r: reaction time; k: rate of clot formation; MA: maximum amplitude)

more plasma coagulation factors or inhibitors such as heparin. Maximum amplitude (MA) provides a measure of clot strength and may be decreased by either qualitative or quantitative platelet dysfunction or decreased fibrinogen concentration. The alpha angle and K values measure rate of clot formation.
- Thromboelastograph is being used for real-time detection of excess fibrinolysis during liver transplantation and is beneficial in differentiating surgical bleeding from that of a coagulopathy.
- *Sonoclot*: In sonoclot, a rapidly vibrating probe is immersed into a 0.4 mL sample of blood. As clot formation occurs, impedance to probe movement through the blood increases and generates an electrical signal and characteristic clot "signature." The Sonoclot provide information regarding ACT, clot strength and fibrinolysis.

4. **Platelet function monitor**: Platelet function analyzer, HemoSTATUS, platelet works are the devices available for monitoring platelet functions.

LAST-MINUTE REVISION

- **Gold standard of BP monitoring:** Invasive BP monitoring by catheterization of artery.
- In continuous ECG monitoring, L-II is best for dysrhythmias and inferior wall ischemia. Lead V5 is sensitive for anterior and lateral wall.
- **Diagnosing intraoperative ischemia:** Flat and down sloping ST segment depression 60 or 80 millisec after the J Point exceeding 1 mm.
- Normal CVP is 3–10 cm of H_2O, subclavian vein is an ideal vein for CVP monitoring.
- Mixed venous oxygen saturation is best measured through pulmonary artery.
- Transesophageal echocardiography is the technique of choice for determining cardiac output, detecting air embolism.
- Pulse oximetry measures oxygen saturation through differential absorption of wavelength of oxygenated and deoxygenated Hb.
- Capnography continuous analysis of $ETCO_2$, normal value 35–45 mm Hg. Abrupt reduction is seen in cardiac arrest, massive pulmonary embolism.
- For neuromuscular monitoring, ulnar nerve is most frequently used.
- Bispectral index (BIS) is the most frequently used parameter for monitoring depth of anesthesia. BIS score of 100 suggest awake patients, 40–60 suggest adequate depth.

REFERENCES

1. Mack E. Focus on diagnosis: co-oximetry. Pediatr Rev. 2007;28(2):73-4. doi: 10.1542/pir.28-2-73. PMID: 17272524.
2. Duțu M, Ivașcu R, Tudorache O, Morlova D, Stanca A, Negoiță S, et al. Neuromuscular monitoring: an update. Rom J Anaesth Intensive Care. 2018;25(1):55-60.

REVIEW QUESTIONS

1. Most common nerve used for neuromuscular monitoring during anesthesia:
    a. Ulnar nerve
    b. Facial nerve
    c. Radial nerve
    d. Median nerve
2. Which of the following is not a cardiovascular monitoring technique?
    a. Transesophageal echocardiography
    b. Central venous pressure monitoring
    c. Pulmonary artery catheterization
    d. Capnography
3. Flat capnogram found in A/E:
    a. Disconnection of anesthetic tubing
    b. Accidental extubation
    c. Mechanical ventilation failure
    d. Bronchospasm

4. Placement of a double lumen tube DLT is best confirmed by:
   a. Clinically by auscultation
   b. Fiberoptic bronchoscopy
   c. Capnography
   d. Chest radiography
   e. Chest inflation on positive pressure
5. All of the following interfere with the SpO_2 measurement, *except*:
   a. Nail paint
   b. Black Henna
   c. Anemia
   d. Methemoglobinemia
6. The most sensitive and practical technique for detection of myocardial ischemia in the perioperative period is:
   a. Magnetic resonance spectroscopy
   b. Radiolabeled lactate determination
   c. Direct measurement of end diastolic pressure
   d. Regional wall motion abnormality detected with the help of 2D transesophageal echocardiography
7. Thromboelastography measures all, *except*:
   a. Time required for clot formation
   b. Strength of clot
   c. Extent of fibrinolysis
   d. Status of vessel wall
8. While introducing the Swan-Ganz catheter, its placement in the pulmonary artery can be identified by the following pressure tracing:
   a. Diastolic pressure is lower in PA than in RV
   b. Diastolic pressure is higher in PA than in RV
   c. PA pressure tracing has dicrotic notch from closure of pulmonary valve
   d. RV pressure tracing for plateau and sharp drop in early diastole
9. Swan-Ganz catheter measures all, *except*:
   a. PCWP
   b. Cardiac output
   c. Mixed venous O_2 saturation
   d. Right atrial pressure
10. By definition, core body temperature is measured at:
    a. Tympanic membrane
    b. Pulmonary artery
    c. Esophagus
    d. Anal area

ANSWERS

| 1. a | 2. d | 3. d | 4. b | 5. c | 6. d |
| 7. d | 8. c | 9. d | 10. b | | |

CHAPTER 17

Perioperative Fluid Therapy and Blood Transfusion

Anshul Jain

INTRODUCTION

All patients undergoing surgical procedures loose fluid in the form of blood, interstitial fluid, etc. So fluid has to be administered from outside to maintain homeostasis. Intravenous fluid therapy is preferred because oral fluid has got erratic absorption, enhances the chances of nausea and vomiting and aspiration. Some patients may require transfusion of blood or blood components too. Errors in fluid replacement or transfusion may result in considerable morbidity and even death.

FLUID COMPARTMENTS (FIG. 17.1)

Water constitute 60% weight of an average adult male, whereas 50% in an adult female. This water is distributed between two major fluid compartments separated by cell membranes: intracellular fluid (ICF) and extracellular fluid (ECF). Extracellular fluid can be further subdivided into intravascular and interstitial compartments. The interstitium includes fluid that is both outside cells and outside the vascular endothelium.

Different medical conditions produce alteration in these compartments, for proper management a basic knowledge of these compartments is must.

Intracellular Fluid

Potassium is the most important cation of ICF. The impermeability of cell membranes to most proteins results in a high intracellular protein concentration and they are the prominent intracellular anion.

Extracellular Fluid

Extracellular fluid provides a medium for exchange of nutrients and electrolytes and removal of intracellular waste products from cell. Maintenance of a normal extracellular

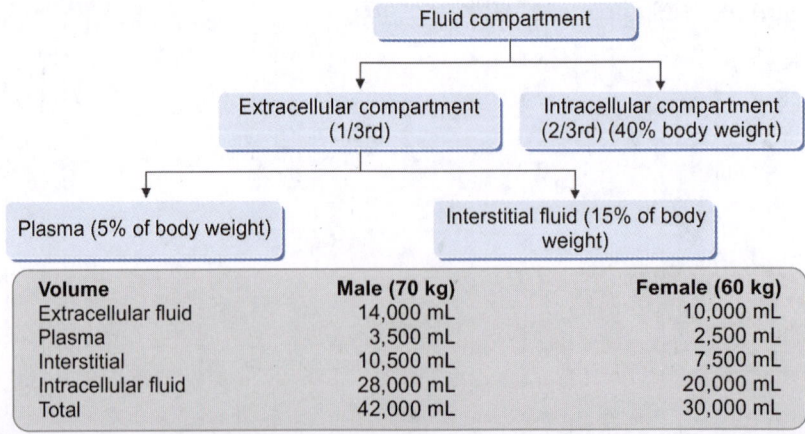

Fig. 17.1: Fluid compartment of the body.

volume—particularly the circulating component (intravascular volume)—is critical. "Sodium^Q is the most important extracellular cation," and the "major" determinant of extracellular osmotic pressure and volume. Changes in ECF volume therefore reflect changes in total body sodium content.

Extracellular fluid includes:
- **Interstitial fluid**: A healthy body contains very little free fluid in interstitial compartment. Most interstitial water is complexed with extracellular proteoglycans, forming a gel. Increased free water in interstitial compartment appears clinically as edema.
- **Intravascular fluid**: Intravascular fluid, commonly referred to as plasma, is restricted to the intravascular space and has electrolyte composition nearly identical to interstitium.

INTRAVENOUS FLUIDS

Broadly intravenous fluids are of two types:

Crystalloids (Table 17.1)

Crystalloids are fluids that contain water and electrolytes. They can be isotonic, hypertonic and hypotonic. They are used to provide water and electrolytes and to expand intravascular fluid compartment. The replacement requirement is three-fold^Q or four-fold the volume of blood lost because administered crystalloid is distributed in 1:4 ratios in to intracellular compartment.

Crystalloids are the initial resuscitation fluid in patients with:
- Hemorrhagic and septic shock
- Burn patients
- Patients with head injury
- Patients undergoing massive surgery

Important Crystalloids

Ringer Lactate Solution

- Most physiologic of all intravenous fluid, as its composition is almost same as that of plasma.
- Slightly hypotonic
- Lactate is metabolized in liver to form glucose and bicarbonate, so it is relatively contraindicated in diabetic patients and metabolic alkalosis.
- Fluid of choice for replacement therapy. However, due to high sodium content and low potassium content, it is less suitable for maintenance.

Normal Saline

- Available as 0.9% isotonic solution
- Second most frequently used fluid during perioperative period.
- Rapid infusion produces hyperchloremic acidosis.
- It is preferred over Ringer's lactate (RL) in craniocerebral injury; diabetic patients.
- Fluid of choice in upper gastrointestinal (GI) obstruction.
- It is the preferred solution for hypochloremic metabolic alkalosis and for diluting packed red blood cells (PRBCs) prior to transfusion.
- Normal saline (0.9% NaCl) contains more chloride than ECF. So when used in large volumes, can produce non-anion gap metabolic acidosis due to hyperchloremia.^{Q}

Table 17.1: Crystalloids fluids.

Crystalloids solution	Electrolyte composition (mEq/L)						
	Na$^+$	Cl$^-$	K$^+$	HCO$_3^-$	Ca^{2+}	Mg^{2+}	mOsm
Lactated Ringer's	130	109	4	28	3		273
0.9% sodium chloride	154	154					308
D$_5$ 0.45% sodium chloride	77	77					407
D$_5$W							253
3% sodium chloride	513	513					1,026

D_5W (Dextrose 5%)

- About 5% dextrose in water provides glucose and free water.
- Glucose enters cell, so the fluid behaves as hypotonic and provides only free water.
- In perioperative period indications are very few. Most common indication is in diabetic patients (for treating hypoglycemia).
- It is also used for replacement of pure water deficits and as a maintenance fluid for patients on sodium restriction.

Dextrose Normal Saline

- Hypertonic fluid primarily used for maintenance.
- Contains 5% dextrose and 0.9% sodium chloride.
- Fluid of choice in conditions like diarrhea, vomiting.

Other Crystalloids

- **IsoP**: For pediatric patient
- **IsoG**: For gastric fluid replacement (as in gastric outlet obstruction) (contains NH_4^+ to correct alkalosis).
- **IsoM**: For maintenance fluid (rich in potassium)
- **IsoE**: For ECF replacement.

Among the variety of crystalloids available, solutions are chosen according to the type of fluid loss being replaced.

Colloid (Table 17.2)

Solutions containing high molecular weight substances like proteins or large glucose polymers. The tight intercellular junctions between adjacent endothelial cells impede the passage of these high molecular weight substances. As a result, colloid solutions remain in intravascular compartment and maintain plasma colloid oncotic pressure. Intravascular half-life of most colloid solutions is between 3 and 6 hours in contrary to 20–30 minutes the half-life of crystalloid solution. However, the cost and occasional complications associated with colloids tend to limit their use **(Table 17.3)**.

> **KEY POINTS**
>
> **Plasma-Lyte:** Family of balanced crystalloid solutions with multiple different formulations. It closely mimics human plasma in its content of electrolytes, osmolality and pH. These solutions also have additional buffer capacity and contain anions like acetate and gluconate in addition to lactate. Plasma-Lyte corrects volume and electrolytes along with acidosis correction.

Important Colloids

Albumin

- Albumin is available in 5% and 25% concentration. They are heated to 60°C for at least 10 hours to minimize the risk of infectious diseases. Albumin occasionally results in hypotensive allergic reactions due to presence of globulin.
- These solutions are most appropriate when there is an abnormal loss of protein from the vascular space, as in cases of peritonitis or extensive burns.[1]

Table 17.2: Important colloids.

Colloids	
Albumin	Only natural colloid
	Available in 25 and 5% solution
Dextran	Polysaccharides, available as dextran 70, dextran 150, dextran 40
Gelatins	Can be urea-linked (Haemaccel®: 3.5% urea-linked) or succinylated (gelofusine: 4% succinylated)
Hydroxyethyl starch	Available as 6 and 10% solution
Hextend	Hydroxyethyl starch which containing glucose and lactate too

Table 17.3: Comparison between crystalloids versus colloids.

Features	Crystalloids	Colloids
Definition	Electrolyte solutions	Solution containing high molecular weight substances
Expansion	1/3 to 1/4 times of the volume infused	1–1.15 times the volume infused
Intravenous half-life	30 minutes	3–24 hours
Effect on interstitium	Edema	Dehydration
Effect on clotting factors	–	+ clotting abnormalities seen
Risk of pulmonary edema	+	+
Risk of peripheral edema	+	–
Interference with blood grouping	–	+
Allergic reactions	–	+
Cost	Cheap	Expensive

6% Dextran 70

- The dextran solutions are water-soluble glucose polymers synthesized by bacteria from sucrose. They are available as dextran 40 or dextran 70 with molecular weight of 40,000 Da and 70,000 Da respectively.
- Dextran 70 is a better volume expander than dextran 40, the latter, however also improves blood flow through the microcirculation by decreasing blood viscosity. Dextran 40 is primarily used in vascular surgery to prevent thrombosis and is rarely used as a volume expander.

Side Effects

- Anaphylactic reactions, increased bleeding time due to decreased platelet adhesiveness.
- Infusions exceeding 20 mL/kg/day can interfere with blood typing.
- Noncardiogenic pulmonary edema and renal failure (due to renal tubule blockage) are other rare complications.

Gelatins

Gelatins are produced by hydrolysis of gelatins. Haemaccel® is 3.5% urea-linked gelatin with molecular weight 35,000. Gelofusine is 4% succinylated gelatin[Q] with molecular weight 30,000. Gelatins do not affect blood cross matching and platelet adhesiveness. However, incidence of allergic reactions is quite high.

Hydroxyethyl Starch

Synthetic colloid, with molecular mass ranging from 10,000 Da to 2,000,000 Da. This colloid remains intravascular for more than 6 hours, and thus maintains intravascular volume for long periods. These solutions improve oxygen delivery by improving microcirculation. However, infusion in large quantities produces dilutional effects on coagulation factors and reduces factor VIII and von Willebrand factor (vWF) levels.

Further, these solutions are hyperoncotic and cause intravascular expansion by withdrawing fluid from interstitial space. Dehydration of interstitial space may occur.

Interferes with monocytic macrophage system. **Dose:** 20 mL/kg/hour up to a maximum of 50 mL/kg/day. Tetra starch is the newer HES with molecular weight of 130000 Dalton, a molar substitution of 0.4 (130/0.4) and a c2/c6 ratio greater among the HES group. These molecular character provide shorter elimination time (**Table 17.4**).

Hextend®

This is the newer colloid containing 6% hetastarch[Q] in a solution that approaches physiologic concentrations of the major electrolytes. It also

Table 17.4: Comparison of tetrastarch versus pentastarch.

Parameters	Tetrastarch (voluven)	Pentastarch (Haes-steril 6%)
Volume effect	100% for 4–6 hours	72% for 2–3 hours
Molecular weight	130000 Daltons	200000 Daltons
Molar substitution	0.4	0.5
Substitution pattern	C2:C6 ratio is 9:1	C2:C6 ratio is 5:1
Dosage	50 mL/kgwt/day	33 mL/kgwt/day
Usage in renal failure	Advocated	Contraindicated
Interference with coagulation	Nil	Rarely observed

contains physiologic levels of glucose and lactate as a buffer. Hetastarch[Q] is highly effective as a plasma expander, less expensive than albumin but possess a shorter intravascular half-life. Coagulation studies and bleeding times are generally not significantly affected following infusions of up to 0.5–1.0 L.[2]

Choice of Fluid (Colloid versus Crystalloids)

From the above discussion one must be thinking that there is controversy regarding the use of colloid or crystalloid fluids for surgical patients. Colloids by maintaining plasma oncotic pressure are more effective in restoring normal intravascular volume and cardiac output. However, they increase the chance of pulmonary edema in patients of congestive cardiac failure. Crystalloids are also equally effective when given in sufficient amounts. Generalized guidelines include:
- Replacing an intravascular volume deficit with crystalloids generally requires three to four times the volume needed when using colloids.
- Severe intravascular fluid deficits can be more rapidly corrected using colloid solutions.
- The rapid administration of large amounts of crystalloids (>4–5 L) should be avoided. If 3–4 L of crystalloid has been given, and the hemodynamic response is inadequate, colloids may be added.
- For losses up to 10% crystalloids are preferred over colloids as they are cheap, easily available, do not produce dilutional coagulopathy, no risk of allergy. Among crystalloids, normal saline and RL are the preferred one, further RL is preferred over NS in conditions where both fluids can be used.[3]
- **Amount**: For each mL of blood lost 3–4 mL of crystalloid should be infused.
- If both water and electrolytes are being lost as in diarrhea, replacement is with isotonic electrolyte solution (replacement-type solutions).
- Glucose present in many intravenous solutions maintains tonicity and prevents ketosis and hypoglycemia due to fasting. Children and women are more prone for this.
- For losses exceeding 10% colloids are preferred over crystalloids as large amount of crystalloid infusion can lead to electrolyte abnormality.
- For each mL of blood lost 1 mL of colloid should be infused.
- When blood loss exceed 30% or hemoglobin (Hb) falls below 7 g/dL (or a hematocrit < 21–24%), blood should be replace with blood (preferably with PRBCs). So, the final sequence is:

$$\frac{\text{Crystalloid} \rightarrow \text{Colloid} \rightarrow \text{Blood}}{\text{Blood lost}}$$

PERIOPERATIVE FLUID THERAPY

Intraoperatively fluids are required for two purposes:
1. **Replacement of ongoing losses:** Losses to be replaced by replacement type of fluid.

2. **Replacement of physiological losses (maintenance requirement):** Losses to be replaced by maintenance type of fluid.

Assessment of Surgical Fluid Losses

Blood Loss

Anesthesiologist must monitor blood loss by counting sponges (each sponge soak 4 mL), laps (each lap soak 150 mL of blood) and checking amount in suction apparatus.

Other Losses

In addition to blood, surgical procedures are associated with obligatory losses of other fluids through evaporation and internal redistribution (third space loss). This is particularly important in abdominal surgeries, as in exposed bowel evaporative fluid loss is very high.

Normal Maintenance Fluid Requirements

In the absence of oral intake, fluid and electrolyte deficits develops rapidly as a result of continued urine formation, GI secretions, sweating and insensible losses from the skin and lungs. Body requires an amount of fluid for these metabolic functions; this requirement is called as maintenance requirement.^Q It depends largely on patient body weight and is calculated by Holliday-Segar method:
Example: For a patient weighing 60 kg hourly maintenance requirement is:

- For first 10 kg—40 mL/hour
- For 10–20 kg—20 mL/hour
- For 20–60 kg—40 mL/hour
- Total is 100 mL/hour.

Weight	Rate
For the first 10 kg	4 mL/kg/hour
For the next 10–20 kg	Add 2 mL/kg/hour
For each kg above 20 kg	Add 1 mL/kg/hour

Pre-existing Deficits

Almost all patients undergo fasting prior to surgery, so at the time of surgery patients have a pre-existing deficit proportionate to the duration of the fasting. The deficit can be estimated by multiplying the normal maintenance rate by the duration of the fast. For the average 50 kg person fasting for 8 hours, the fluid deficit is (40 + 20 + 30) mL/hour × 8 hour, or 720 mL. 50% of this deficit has to be replaced in first hour.

Ringer's lactate and NS (RL preferred over NS) are most commonly used fluid.

Some patients presents with dehydration (diarrhea, vomiting) in such cases it is essential to quantity the degree of dehydration. In emergency situation it can be estimated roughly by bedside physical examination (**Table 17.5**). Patients should preferably be rehydrated before administration of anesthesia.

Table 17.5: Quantification of degree of dehydration through bedside clinical examination.

Features	Fluid loss (expressed as percentage of body weight)		
	5%	10%	15%
Mucous membranes	Dry	Very dry	Parched
Eyeball	Normal	Sunken	Sunken
Sensorium	Normal	Lethargic	Obtunded
Orthostatic changes	None	Present	Marked
Urinary flow rate	Mildly decreased	Decreased	Markedly decreased
Pulse rate	Normal or increased	Increased >100 bpm	Markedly increased >120 bpm
Blood pressure	Normal	Mildly decreased with exaggerated respiratory variation	Decreased

Calculating Fluid Requirement

Calculating amount of fluid during surgery is a complex process. Goal of perioperative fluid therapy is to replace:
- **Normal physiological losses**: Urine; water vapor in expired air
- Pre-existing fluid deficits
- Surgical wound losses including blood loss and simultaneous by present over infusion.

Intraoperative Fluid Replacement

Intraoperative fluid therapy should include supplying basic fluid requirements and replacing residual preoperative deficits as well as intraoperative losses (blood, fluid redistribution and evaporation). Selection of the type of intravenous solution depends upon the surgical procedure and the expected blood loss. For procedures involving minimal blood loss and fluid shifts, maintenance solutions can be used. For all other procedures, lactated Ringer's solution is the fluid of choice.

Replacing Blood Loss

Blood loss can be replaced with crystalloid (four times the volume of blood lost) or colloid (in amount equal to blood lost) solutions to maintain intravascular volume. However, it must be noted that at any cost hemoglobin should not be allowed to fall below 7 g/dL (transfusion point).[Q] If there is more blood loss, blood is replaced by blood; mL for mL, with whole blood or reconstituted PRBCs.

Replacing Redistributive and Evaporative Losses

Replacement of these losses depends upon degree of tissue trauma; surgical procedure. Recommendations include:

Degree of tissue trauma	Additional requirement
Minimal (e.g., herniorrhaphy)	0–2 mL/kg/hour
Moderate (e.g., cholecystectomy)	2–4 mL/kg/hour
Severe (e.g., bowel resection)	4–8 mL/kg/hour

For total amount, all requirements are added.

> **Example:** A patient weighing 50 kg posted for herniorrhaphy comes in OT after 8 hours fasting (calculate the fluid requirement)
> - **Pre-existing deficit**: 720 mL (as calculated above)
> - **Surgical loss**: 2 mL/kg/hour fluid loss
> - **Blood loss** (~ 1 mL/minute).
>
> Average duration of hernia surgery is 1 hour.
> Total fluid for first hour = 360 mL (50% of pre-existing deficit) +120 mL (surgical fluid loss) +180 mL (for 60 mL blood lost in 1 hour) +90 mL (maintenance requirement)
> Total = 750 mL in 1st hour

> **Note:** As a rough estimation, fluid is administered at rate of 10–15 mL/kg in first hour and 5–10 mL/kg/hour afterward.

Prevention of Over Infusion

Hypervolemia is as dangerous as hypovolemia. Pediatric and geriatric populations are especially vulnerable for fluid overload. Signs of hypervolemia are given in **Table 17.6**.

Table 17.6: Signs of hypervolemia (fluid excess).

Early	Late
Pitting edema	Tachycardia
Increased urinary flow	Pulmonary crackles, pink, frothy pulmonary secretions, cyanosis

BLOOD TRANSFUSION

- Main role of blood transfusion is to increase oxygen carrying capacity; increase in intravascular volume is an added advantage.
- In modern transfusion medicine, transfusion of whole blood is rarely indicated. However, in developing countries (where blood components are not available readily), transfusion of whole blood is indicated in situations like:
  - Acute blood loss >20% of blood volume (10% in pediatric patients)
  - Hemoglobin level <8 g/dL[Q]
  - Hemoglobin level <10 g/dL with major disease (e.g., emphysema, ischemic heart disease)
  - Hemoglobin level <12 g/dL and ventilator dependent.

Storage of Blood

- Using citrate phosphate dextrose (CPD) as preservative, blood can be stored for 21 days at 1 to 6°C.
- Citrate acts as anticoagulant, phosphate serves as buffer and dextrose acts as RBC energy source.
- The addition of adenine to CPD solution allows RBC to resynthesize adenosine triphosphate (ATP) which extends the storage time to 35 days.
- Shelf-life can be extended to 42 days when AS-1 (Adsol®), AS-3 (Nutricel®), AS-5 (Optisol) are used as preservative.

KEY POINTS
- One unit of blood rise hemoglobin by 0.8 g%.
- In India, one unit blood (350 mL total) has 301 mL blood and 49 mL anticoagulant.
- In western countries, 1 unit blood (450 mL total) has 387 mL blood and 67 mL anticoagulant.
- Patient with blood group O is called as universal donor.
- Patient with blood group AB is called as universal recipient.
- In case of dire emergence emergency O (-)ve packed red cells can be transfused without blood grouping.

Effect of Storage on Whole Blood

- Reduction in pH
- Rise in plasma potassium concentration
- Progressive reduction in the 2,3-diphosphoglycerate (2,3-DPG) content of RBC, as a result there is reduction in the release of oxygen at tissue level.^{Q}
- Loss of platelet functions in whole blood within 48 hours of donation.
- Reduction in factor VIII to 10–20% of normal within 48 hours of donation.
- Coagulation factors such as VII and IX remain relatively same in storage.

Massive blood transfusion
Massive transfusion can be defined as the replacement of blood loss equivalent to or greater than the patients total blood volume with stored blood in less than 24 hours or at a rate more than 1 mL/kg/minute.

Complications of massive blood transfusion
- Acidosis
- Hyperkalemia
- Hypocalcemia
- Citrate toxicity
- Fibrinogen depletion
- Platelet depletion
- Disseminated intravascular coagulation (DIC)
- Hypothermia
- Reduced 2,3-DPG
- Microaggregates
- Iron overload

Blood Components (Tables 17.7 and 17.8)

Blood is separated into its individual component (packed RBC, plasma, platelet), this strategy maximize the benefits while minimizing the risk to recipient.

KEY POINTS
Why is blood administration called transfusion (not infusion)?
Because blood is a living tissue.

Blood components used for transfusion are:

Packed Red Blood Cells

- Packed RBCs include RBCs only and much of the plasma has been removed.
- One unit of PBRC contains same amount of Hb as 1 unit of blood but in 250 mL. Hematocrit of PBRC is 70%.
- Packed red blood cells are indicated in cases where there is anemia but intravascular volume is maintained.
- One unit of PBRC raise Hb concentration by 1.5–2 g%.
- Packed red blood cells should not be administered with RL and dextrose 5%; however, 5% dextrose in 0.9% saline can be very well used.

Frozen RBC

Expensive, but 2,3-DPG concentration does not decrease for years.

Table 17.7: Transfusion guidelines for blood component (PRBC and platelet).

Transfusion guidelines for PRBCs indications	Transfusion guidelines for platelets indications

Indications:
• Hemoglobin <8 g/dL or acute blood loss in an otherwise healthy patient with signs and symptoms of reduced oxygen delivery and two or more of the following:
  – Estimated or anticipated acute blood loss of >15% of total volume
  – Diastolic blood pressure <60 mm Hg
  – Systolic blood pressure drop >30 mm Hg from baseline
  – Tachycardia (>100 beats/minute)
  – Oliguria/anuria
  – Mental status changes
• Hemoglobin <10 g/dL in patient known with coronary artery disease or pulmonary insufficiency
• Symptomatic anemia with any of the following:
  – Tachycardia (>100 beats/minute)
  – Mental status changes
  – Evidence of myocardial of ischemia, including angina
  – Shortness of breath or dizziness with mild exertion
  – Orthostatic hypotension
	Indications:
	• Recent (within 24 hours) platelets count <10,000 mm^3 (for prophylaxis)
	• Recent (within 24 hours) platelets <50,000 mm^3 with demonstrated bleeding (oozing) or a planned surgical/invasive microvascular procedure
	• Demonstrated microvascular bleeding and a precipitous fall in the platelet count
	• Adult patient in the operating room who have required more than 10 units of blood and have microvascular bleeding
	• Documented platelet dysfunction (e.g., bleeding time >15 minutes; abnormal platelets function tests) with petechiae, purpura, microvascular bleeding
	• Trigger for platelets transfusion
	  – *DIC*: 20,000–50,000 mm^3
	  – *Major surgery in leukemia*: <50,000/mm^3
	  – *Cardiopulmonary bypass*: <50,000–60,000/mm^3
	  – *Neurosurgery*: <1 lakh/mm^3

Some facts: • PRBC have slightly lower survival than whole blood • Each unit PRBC raises the HCT of recipient by 2–3% • PRBC should not be mixed with Ringer's lactate (blood may clot), D-5 (hemolysis). It can be safely reconstituted with 5% dextrose in 0.4% saline, DNS, NS	**Some facts:** • Bacterial contamination of blood products is leading cause of blood transfusion related infections of which contaminated platelet is most frequent • Each platelet unit transfused increase platelet count by 8,000 within 1 hour

(PRBC: packed red blood cells; NS: normal saline; DIC: disseminated intravascular coagulation)

Table 17.8: Transfusion guidelines for blood component (plasma and cryoprecipitate).

Transfusion guidelines for plasma	Transfusion guidelines for cryoprecipitate

Indications:
• Treatment of multiple or specific coagulation factor deficiency with an abnormal PT or APTT
• Abnormal specific factor deficiency in the presence of one of the following:
  – Congenital deficiency of antithrombin III, prothrombin; factor V, VII, IX, XI; protein C or S; plasminogen or antiplasmin
  – Acquired deficiency related to warfarin therapy, liver disease, vitamin K deficiency, massive transfusion, DIC
  – As a prophylaxis for the above conditions if surgical procedure is planned
• For urgent reversal of warfarin therapy
• It should not be used as plasma expander
	Indications:
	• Factor VIII deficiency or hemophilia A
	• Treatment of fibrinogen deficiency
	Some facts:
	• It can be administered without taking ABO compatibility into consideration
	• Rate of administration should be at least 200 mL/hour and infusion should be completed within 6 hours of thawing

(DIC: disseminated intravascular coagulation; PT: prothrombin test; APTT: activated partial thromboplastin time)

Note: Chances of transmission of blood born diseases are very rare in packed red blood cells (PBRCs) and frozen red blood cells (RBCs), chances of allergic reactions are also fewer.

Platelet Concentrates

- Prepared by differential centrifugation of freshly drawn units of blood.
- Only blood component which is stored at room temperature (survival at room temperature is up to 7 days, whereas survival at 4°C is 2 days only).
- However storage at room temperature enhances the risk of bacterial contamination, and this makes platelet concentrate, the most infectious blood component.
- One unit of platelet concentrate raise platelet concentration by 7,000–10,000/mm^3.
- When possible, ABO computable platelets should be used; however, ABO incompatible platelets are not contraindicated in urgency.

Note: One unit platelet concentrate = 50 mL.

Fresh Frozen Plasma (FFP)

- Plasma frozen within 6 hours of collection.
- It contains all the plasma proteins, factors V and factor VIII.
- One unit carries 225 mL of FFP.
- It should not be administered to augment plasma volume or albumin concentration, due to better and safer alternatives.
- Each unit of FFP raises the level of each clotting factor by 2–3%.

Cryoprecipitate

- Carries significant amount of factor VIII and fibrinogen, it also contains vWF and fibronectin.
- Should be administered as ABO compatible.

Prothrombin Complex

- Prothrombin recovered from plasma or plasma fractions by absorption with ion exchanges.
- Main indication is treatment of factor IV deficiency.
- Risk of infectious complications is similar to other products.

Fluid Therapy in Special Situations

- **Pediatric age group:**
  - Pediatric patients, due to lack of glycogen storage are always at risk for hypoglycemia, so glucose containing solutions are preferred with isotype P as fluid of choice.
  - In case of nonavailability of IsoP, 5% dextrose + 1/4 NS is the preferred fluid as it is isotonic.
  –

LAST-MINUTE REVISION

- Ringer lactate is the most physiologic of all IV fluids and is the preferred replacement fluid.
- Blood losses up to 10% are replaced by crystalloids; 10–30% are replaced by colloids. If loss exceeds 30% or Hct falls below 25%, it has to be replaced by blood (PBRCs) or fresh whole blood .
- Maintenance requirement is calculated by Holliday-Segar method: (4-2-1 rule).

REFERENCES

1. Schaefer TJ, Szymanski KD. Burn Evaluation and Management. [Updated 2022 Aug 23]. In: StatPearls [Internet]. Treasure Island (FL): StatPearls Publishing; 2022 Jan-. Available from: https://www.ncbi.nlm.nih.gov/books/NBK430741/
2. Weeks DL, Jahr JS, Lim JC, Butch AW, Driessen B. Does Hextend impair coagulation compared to 6% hetastarch? An ex vivo thromboelastography study. Am J Ther. 2008;15(3):225-30.
3. Myburgh JA, Finfer S, Bellomo R, Billot L, Cass A, Gattas D, et al; CHEST Investigators; Australian and New Zealand Intensive Care Society Clinical Trials Group. Hydroxyethyl starch or saline for fluid resuscitation in intensive care. N Engl J Med. 2012;367(20):1901-11.

REVIEW QUESTIONS

1. The outcome following resuscitation of cardiac arrest is worsened if during resuscitation patient is given:
   a. Ringer's lactate
   b. Colloids
   c. 5% dextrose
   d. Whole blood
2. IsoG is a suitable fluid for:
   a. Acquired pyloric stenosis
   b. Geriatric patients
   c. Burn patients
   d. Postoperative patients
3. Colloid includes all, *except*:
   a. Albumin
   b. Hartmann solution
   c. Dextron
   d. Hetastarch
4. Effect of storage on blood includes all, *except*:
   a. Reduced 2,3-DP G
   b. Reduction in pH
   c. Reduced coagulability
   d. Reduction in hemoglobin
5. The term massive blood transfusion signifies:
   a. Transfusion at a rate >1 mL/kg/hour
   b. Transfusion of volume equal or greater than patients' blood volume is less than 24 hours
   c. Both a and b
   d. Neither a nor b
6. One unit of platelet raises the platelet count by:
   a. 5,000
   b. 10,000
   c. 20,000
   d. 50,000
7. Most suitable fluid for the replacement of maintenance requirements in perioperative period:
   a. Dextrose normal saline
   b. Normal saline
   c. Ringer's lactate
   d. Dextrose 5%

8. True statement regarding colloid includes all, *except*:
    a. Albumin is a natural colloid
    b. Hetastarch lacks effect on coagulation profile
    c. Gelatins interfere with blood cross-matching
    d. Gelatins never show allergic reaction
9. **During surgery water is lost as:**
    a. Blood loss
    b. Direct evaporation from exposed surgical site
    c. Respiratory loss
    d. All of the above

ANSWERS

| 1. c | 2. | 3. b | 4. d | 5. b | 6. a |
| 7. c | 8. d | 9. d | | | |

CHAPTER 18

Blood Salvage Techniques

Sadik Mohammed, Pradeep Bhatia, Kamlesh Kumari

"Cell Salvage: The tech at the cutting edge of the blood management".

INTRODUCTION

Allogenic packed red cell transfusion has been generously used to treat perioperative anemia and blood loss, which is known to has its own associated risks and complications **(Table 18.1)**. Moreover, for some patients (Jehovah's Witnesses), the transfusion of allogenic blood is specifically prohibited. Therefore, patient blood management (PBM), "a multimodal, multidisciplinary patient-centered strategy aimed at minimizing the use of blood products and improving patient's outcomes", may be considered to avoid the transfusion associated complications and when its use is prohibited.[1] In 2010, the WHO (WHA63.12) adopted the PBM as a principle to target avoidable transfusion which includes three pillars of care **(Fig. 18.1)**.[1] It has been demonstrated that using a pillar of care or their combination, depending on the specific needs of each patient and the proposed surgery, can lower the prevalence of anemia at the time of surgery, perioperative blood loss, and the transfusion rate.[2] This chapter will discuss the perioperative blood salvage techniques as a part of PBM.

PERIOPERATIVE BLOOD SALVAGE

Perioperative blood salvage has been suggested for surgical procedures having a high likelihood of significant blood loss. According to the American Association of Blood Banks, cell salvage is recommended in surgical situations where blood would ordinarily be cross-matched or where more than 10% of patients need transfusions. **Table 18.2** describes indications and contraindications

Table 18.1: Risk and complications associated with blood transfusion.

Immune mediated	Nonimmune mediated

<ul><li>Allergic reactions</li><li>Anaphylactic reactions</li><li>Transfusion-associated lung injury</li><li>Hemolytic reaction acute or delayed</li><li>Febrile nonhemolytic</li><li>Graft vs. host disease</li><li>Post-transfusion purpura</li></ul>	1. **Infectious:** Transfusion-transmitted infection (e.g., hepatitis, bacterial infection, parasites)
	2. **Noninfectious:**
	   - Coagulopathy (after massive transfusion)
	   - Circulatory overload
	   - Metabolic derangements (e.g., hyperkalemia, hypocalcemia)
	   - Errors handling/storage of blood
	   - Delayed wound healing
	   - Hypothermia
	   - Thrombophlebitis
	   - Citrate toxicity
	   - Iron overload

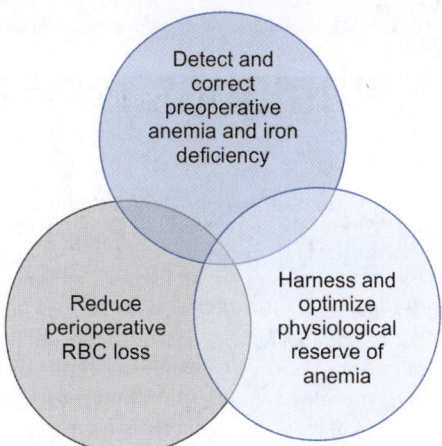

Fig. 18.1: The three pillars of care in safe patient blood management.

Table 18.2: Indications and contraindications of perioperative blood salvage.

Indications	Contraindications
• Anticipated intraoperative blood loss 1L or 20% of blood volume • Patients with preoperative anemia, increased risk factors for bleeding, rare blood group or antibodies • Avoiding or minimizing allogeneic transfusion • Patients who will not accept allogeneic blood (Jehovah's witnesses)	• Relative: Bacterial infections, active malignancy • Uncertain: Obstetrics, hemoglobinopathies and cold agglutinin disease

of perioperative blood salvage. There are various methods/strategies of perioperative blood conservation, which can be divided into three broad categories: preoperative, intraoperative and postoperative blood salvage strategies.

Preoperative Strategies

This include preoperative autologous blood donation (PAD),[3,4] i.e., repeated blood donation of approximately 450 mL of patients own blood per week starting about five weeks prior to scheduled surgery and continuing as long as their hematocrit is at least 34% or hemoglobin at least 11 g/dL, with last donation at least 72 hours prior to surgery to ensure patients plasma volume returns to normal. The blood must be collected in clearly marked citrated phosphate dextrose blood bags before being customarily kept in the blood bank where it is then made accessible for transfusion if necessary during or after surgery. The risks of viral transmission (HIV and hepatitis C), immune-mediated hemolysis, and fever or allergic responses are reduced with PAD in comparison to allogenic transfusion. There is immune modulation, which can lower the chances of infection following surgery and cancer recurrence.

The main drawbacks of PAD include benefits only available in elective patients, increased logistic requirements and preparation well in advance of surgery, as well as frequent phlebotomy prior to surgery. It is associated with risk of immunological reactions due to errors in collection, labeling, and administration; improper storage and bacterial contamination. Moreover, more than 50% of donated autologous blood is unused thereby increasing the cost compared to allogeneic blood.[5] Despite its drawbacks, PAD can be helpful for patients with rare blood types, those who have trouble cross-matching, or in situations when there is not enough blood available.[6]

Intraoperative Strategies

Hemodilution

Hemodilution may be either normovolumic or hypervolumic. Acute normovolumic hemodilution (ANH)[7] is an autologous blood collection technique in which one or two units of whole blood are removed from the patient immediately prior to surgery via a large-bore intravenous catheter and replaced with crystalloid or colloids for maintaining normovolemia and stable hemodynamics. Autologous blood is collected in standard bags containing citrate anticoagulant and stored in the operating room at room temperature for 8 hours or at 4°C for 24 hours and is reinfused at the end of surgery after cessation of major blood loss. The basic principle of ANH is that dilution of patients circulating blood volume reduces the percentage of red blood cells lost per unit of total blood volume lost during surgical bleeding and also cardiac output is maintained because of normal intravascular volume. Compared to PAD, ANH has advantages of its use in nonelective surgery, prevention of blood storage problems and clerical errors.

Hypervolemic hemodilution involves diluting blood volume without extracting blood, with the goal of achieving a reduced hematocrit to reduce the loss of RBCs as a whole in the case of bleeding and to keep tissue perfusion intact. It is important to take precautions to prevent circulatory overload, especially in patients with impaired heart function.

Cell Salvage

Cell salvage[8] is the process wherein blood from the surgical field (during surgery) or drains (postoperatively) is collected to produce autologous blood for transfusion back to the patient after filtration and washing. This allows maintenance of circulating RBCs however, plasma, platelets, heparin, free hemoglobin, and inflammatory mediators are discarded along with a washing solution. Compared with stored RBCs, salvaged blood has normal levels of 2, 3-DPG (no left shift in the hemoglobin-oxygen dissociation curve) and better cell membrane deformability. **Table 18.3** describes various advantages and disadvantages of the cell salvage technique. The technique has become a standard of care in cardiac surgery which is evident by the fact that various societies like European Society of Cardiology (ESC)/EACTS), Society of Thoracic Surgeons (STS) and the Society of Cardiovascular Anesthesiologists (SCA) recommended red cell salvage as a routine procedure. (Class I, Level of Evidence A).[9,10]

Procedural Steps

The blood salvage machine "cell saver" or "cell recovery" separates, washes, and concentrates salvaged RBCs. The steps involved include suctioning of blood from the surgical field,

Table 18.3: Advantages and disadvantages of the use of cell salvage.

Indications	Contraindications
• By reducing the requirements for allogeneic transfusion by 40%, cell salvage reduces the risk of infection transmission and also there is no risk of ABO incompatibility • For cell salvage no preoperative preparation of the patients is required which makes it ideal option for unexpected massive blood loss • Cell salvage is a good option in case of rare blood group and antibodies and is acceptable for some Jehovah's witnesses	• Initial high cost of the machinery and cost of disposables • Complex device which requires staff training and competencies • Adverse reactions like bacterial contamination, immune and nonimmune hemolysis, febrile and reactions, coagulopathies, DIC, electrolyte imbalance, air and fat embolism • Use of cell salvage is relatively contraindicated in cancer, obstetric and contaminated bowel surgeries

addition of an anticoagulant, separation and washing of RBCs, concentration of the blood, and reinfusion to the patient **(Fig. 18.2)**.

1. **Collection of blood**: The first step in the process of cell salvage is the suctioning of the blood collected in the surgical field or squeezing the blood-soaked surgical gauze pads. An anticoagulant preferably heparin (30,000U/L @ 15 mL/100 mL of collected blood) is slowly and automatically added to the collected blood to prevent coagulation which is subsequently removed during washing of the collected blood. Citrate-based anticoagulant (15 mL/100 mL of collected blood) may be preferred when there is risk of heparin induced thrombocytopenia.
2. **Treatment of collected blood**: The blood collection is continued until a sufficient amount around 500 mL is collected in sterile reservoir. The blood then undergo centrifugation to separate and concentrate the higher density RBCs. The other content like plasma, platelets, and waste are diverted to the waste bag.

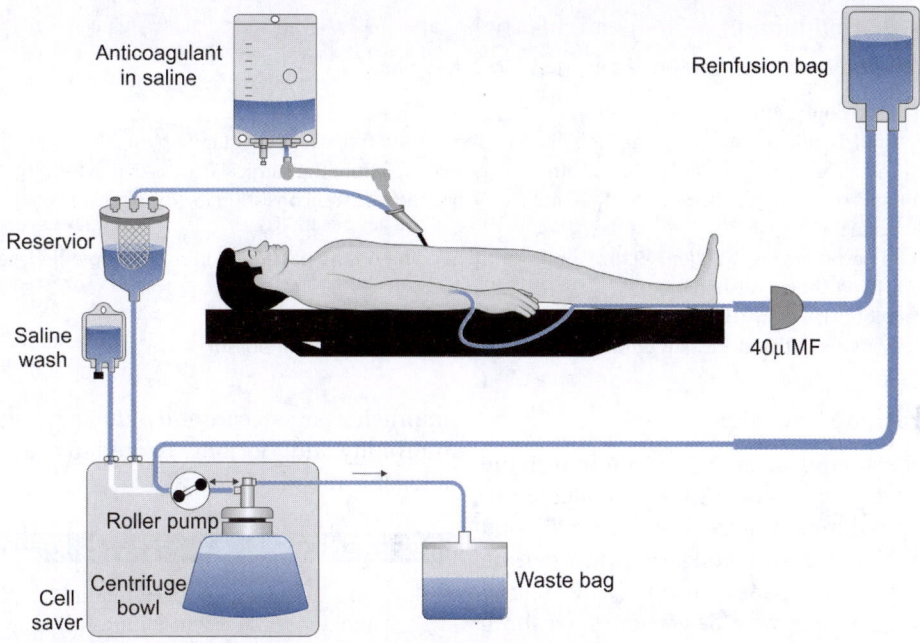

Fig. 18.2: Schematic diagram demonstrating the components of a blood salvage system.

After centrifugation, the salvaged RBCs undergo washing with normal saline to remove free hemoglobin, inflammatory mediators, and other cellular debris. Other solutions like balanced bicarbonate buffered solution (Balsol) and balanced electrolyte solution (e.g., PlasmaLyte-A) can be used for washing which are reported to be associated with fewer acid-base and electrolyte derangements compared with the use of normal saline. A full reservoir of blood can be processed in approximately three minutes with recovery of 55–250 mL of RBCs with hemoglobin concentration as high as 17 g/dL. The processed RBCs are then collected in a blood salvage bag for reinfusion.

3. **Reinfusion:** The salvaged blood reinfusion can be instituted using a microaggregate filter (40-micron) installed between the blood salvage bag and the patient within six hours after its collection in blood salvage bag. A leukocyte depletion filters can be used to achieve optimal removal of bacteria, cancer cells, fat particles, or amniotic fluid.

Salvaged Washed Red Cells

The process of washing removes anticoagulant (heparin or citrate), free hemoglobin, platelets, white blood cells, and cellular stroma products (which are potentially thrombogenic) along with the fibrinogen and other coagulation factors (II, VII, X, and XIII). Therefore, after infusion of large amount of washed RBCs patient may develop dilutional coagulopathy and may require replacement with transfusion of plasma and/or platelet.

Salvaged Unwashed Red Cells

In cases with extreme blood loss (>500 mL/min), returning of salvaged unwashed blood may be lifesaving until the control of bleeding is achieved, but there is associated significant risk and disadvantage of infusing unwashed blood **(Box 18.1)**. In view of these associated risk, it is particularly important to use a microaggregate filter for reinfusion.

BOX 18.1

Risk and complications of reinfusion of salvaged unwashed blood.

Unwashed blood reinfusion
- The anticoagulant that was added to the blood is not removed and may cause coagulopathy.
- The reinfused platelets may be dysfunctional after being suctioned from the surgical field.
- Thrombogenic substances (inflammatory mediators and microaggregates consisting of white cell and platelet debris) may be introduced.
- Hemoglobin levels are low [range: 7–9 g/dL or lower (depending on the patient's current hemoglobin level), versus 16–18 g/dL in processed washed blood].
- Free hemoglobin levels may be very high due to hemolysis.
- Fat may be present in the unwashed product, which increases the risk of fat embolism.

Postoperative Strategies

After major surgeries, bleeding can continue in the postoperative period which may be collected in the drains put during surgery. The collected blood is anticoagulated during collection and can be reinfused back to the patient through a 40-micron microaggregate filter, with or without a washing process. This technique has been shown to be effective in reducing perioperative allogenic blood transfusion particularly after major orthopedic surgery. However, mediastinal blood from chest drain after cardiac surgery contains fibrinogen degradation products, tissue-type plasminogen activators, inflammatory cytokines, complements and endotoxins therefore, reinfusion of this should be avoided in view of increased risk of postoperative bleeding tendency and sternal or systemic infections.[11]

KEY POINTS

- There is a need to reduce allogenic blood transfusion due to associated complications and scarcity.
- Autologous blood transfusion is a good and safe alternative to allogenic blood transfusion.
- Blood salvage strategies plays an important role in improving patient care and reducing perioperative morbidity and mortality by reducing allogenic blood transfusion requirement.
- Blood salvage strategies should include a multidisciplinary and individualized approach throughout the patient's perioperative period.

To summarize, blood salvage strategies as a part of patient blood management are important for improving patient care and reducing perioperative morbidity and mortality related to transfusion of allogenic blood.

REFERENCES

1. Spahn D, Theusinger O, Hofmann A. Patient blood management is a win win: a wake-up call. Br J Anaesth. 2012;108(6):889-92.
2. Kotze´ A, Carter LA, Scally AJ. Effect of a patient blood management programme on preoperative anaemia, transfusion rate, and outcome after primary hip or knee arthroplasty: a quality improvement cycle. Br J Anaesth. 2012;108:943-52.
3. Singbartl G. Preoperative autologous blood donation: Clinical parameters and efficacy. Blood Transfus, 2011;9:10-8.
4. Henry DA, Careless PA, Moxey AJ, et al. Preoperative autologous donation for minimising perioperative allogeneic blood transfusion [review]. Cochrane Database Syst Rev. 2001; CD003602.
5. Kozek-Langenecker SA. Perioperative coagulation monitoring. Best Pract Res Clin Anaesthesiol. 2010;24:27-40.
6. Muirhead B. Con: Preoperative autologous donation has no role in cardiac surgery . J Cardiothorac Vasc Anesth. 2003;17:126-8.
7. Jamnicki M, Kocian R, van der Linden P, et al. Acute normovolaemic haemodilution: physiology, limitations, and clinical use. J Cardiothorac Vasc Anesth. 2003; 17:747-54.
8. Blood transfusion and the anaesthetist: intra-operative cell salvage. AAGBI safety guideline. https://www.aagbi.org/sites/default/files/cell%20_salvage_2009_amended.pdf.
9. Windecker S, Kolh P, Alfonso F, et al. 2014 ESC/EACTS guidelines on myocardial revascularization: the task

force on myocardial revascularization of the European Society of Cardiology (ESC) and the European Association for Cardio-Thoracic Surgery (EACTS) developed with the special contribution of the European Association of Percutaneous Cardiovascular Interventions (EAPCI). Eur Heart J. 2014, 35:2541-619.
10. Ferraris VA, Brown JR, Despotis GJ, et al. 2011 update to the Society of Thoracic Surgeons and the Society of Cardiovascular Anesthesiologists blood conservation clinical practice guidelines. Ann Thorac Surg. 2011;91:944-82.
11. Society of Thoracic Surgeons Blood Conservation Guideline Task Force, Ferraris VA, Ferraris SP, et al. Perioperative blood transfusion and blood conservation in cardiac surgery: the Society of Thoracic Surgeons and The Society of Cardiovascular Anesthesiologists clinical practice guideline. Ann Thorac Surg. 2007;83:S27.

REVIEW QUESTIONS

1. Which of the following is not an immune mediated reactions of allogenic blood transfusion?
   a. Transfusion associated lung injury
   b. Thrombophlebitis
   c. Post-transfusion purpura
   d. Allergic reactions

2. All of the following are techniques for autologous blood donation, *except*:
   a. Donor directed transfusion
   b. Preoperative autologous blood donation
   c. Acute normovolaemic hemodilution
   d. Postoperative blood salvage

3. Drawbacks of preoperative autologous blood donation (PAD) are all of the following, *except*:
   a. Requires frequent phlebotomy prior to surgery
   b. Beneficial only for elective surgeries
   c. Associated with risks of transmission of infection
   d. Associated with risk of immunological reactions

4. For preoperative autologous blood donation, minimum time between last donation and planned surgery should be at least:
   a. 24 hours
   b. 36 hours
   c. 48 hours
   d. 72 hours

5. Which of the following statement is true regarding perioperative use of processed salvaged red blood cells?
   a. All malignant cells are removed by washing process
   b. The salvaged cells have lower oxygen carrying capacity than allogenic blood
   c. The salvaged RBCs have hemoglobin concentration as high as 17 g/dL
   d. The survival of the salvaged RBCs is significantly impaired

6. Cell salvage is relatively contraindicated in all of the following surgeriea, *except*:
   a. Oncosurgeries
   b. Obstetric surgeries
   c. Neurosurgeries
   d. Contaminated bowel surgeries

7. Which of the following statement is not correct regarding red blood cell salvage technique?
   a. Cell salvage increases the risk of transmission of infection
   b. Cell salvage is a good option in case of rare blood group and antibodies
   c. There is no risk of ABO incompatibility.
   d. No preoperative preparation of the patients is required

8. Adverse reaction associated with cell salvage:
    a. Disseminated intravascular coagulation
    b. Electrolyte imbalance
    c. Air embolism
    d. All of the above
9. Postoperative cell salvage is most effective for:
    a. Cardiac surgeries
    b. Oncosurgeries
    c. Orthopedic surgeries
    d. Neurosurgeries
10. Which of the following statement is not true for salvaged unwashed red cells?
    a. Free hemoglobin levels may be very high due to hemolysis
    b. Associated with increased risk of fat embolism
    c. Associated with increased risk of coagulopathy
    d. Hemoglobin levels are in range of 16–18 g/dL

ANSWERS

| 1. b | 2. a | 3. c | 4. d | 5. c | 6. c |
| 7. a | 8. d | 9. c | 10. d | | |

CHAPTER 19

Anesthesiologist as a Perioperative Physician

Manbir Kaur, Bharat Paliwal, Ankur Sharma

"The Good Physician treats the disease; The Great Physician treats the patient who has the disease."

The Great physician in this quote by **William Osler** completely describes the quintessence of anesthesiologists. With increasing knowledge and awareness, the value of an anesthesiologist as a perioperative physician becomes more intelligible among the general population. The perioperative physician, by definition, provides medical care to the patients who must undergo surgical procedures and evaluates the patient's status before, during, and after surgery.[1] Anesthesiologists accurately fit in this definition as they do a thorough evaluation of the patient before surgery by not only dealing with the various critical issues of the patient like hypertension, diabetes, myocardial ischemia, arrhythmias, abnormal serum electrolytes and other metabolic derangements (alkalosis/acidosis) but also optimizing such patient with multiple comorbidities before surgery.

Before surgery, they establish a good rapport with the patient and help them relieve anxiety. Intraoperatively, they not only provide anesthesia and analgesia but closely monitor hemodynamics and all the vital body functions. For adequate depth of anesthesia and muscle relaxation, bispectral index (BIS) and neuromuscular transmission (NMT) monitors, respectively prevent awareness during anesthesia. Anesthesiologists also manage the perioperative challenges like hemodynamic disturbances due to the surgical blood loss as well as fluids and electrolyte disturbances due to third space losses intraoperatively. They monitor and manage the respiratory parameters like oxygen, carbon-dioxide levels; along with metabolic parameters like bicarbonates and lactates level perioperatively. They control the respiration (tidal volume, rate, pressures, etc.) with ventilators, incorporated with anesthesia workstations. They have vast knowledge of effects of various anesthesia drugs on different organ systems of the body. They confirm adequate recovery parameters including consciousness level, and protective airway reflexes before shifting the patient in the postanesthesia care unit. Further, in the postoperative period, they monitor the patient's recovery as well as hemodynamic parameters and provide adequate pain management. They also manage the postoperative issues like nausea, vomiting, pain, shivering, delirium or any postoperative respiratory or cardiac dysfunction requiring ventilatory or hemodynamic support in the high dependency units and intensive care units.

Gone is the time when the identity of the anesthesiologist was obscure. With increasing awareness, people started acknowledging anesthesia and the anesthesiologists. Nowadays, this field is not only limited to providing only general or regional anesthesia but also includes critical care and pain and palliative care, which are the greatest achievements of this field. The recent COVID-19 pandemic[2] has made the world realize about the role of anesthesiologists as critical care intensivists. They are the forefront warriors in dealing with critically ill patients requiring intensive care and ventilatory support.[3] They diagnose and manage all sorts of respiratory problems, deal with ventilators, and perform bronchoscopy procedures as pulmonologists. From a cardiac point of view, performing bedside echocardiography, dealing with all cardiac issues, and managing cardiac patients by anesthesiologists has decreased the burden on cardiologists.

Anesthesiologists are further specialized in neuroanesthesia, cardiac anesthesia, pediatric anesthesia, obstetric anesthesia, oncoanesthesia and transplant anesthesia.

Cardiac anesthesiologists enhanced this field of anesthesia by developing knowledge and nuances in patients with heart diseases undergoing cardiac or noncardiac surgeries. Their expertise in transesophageal echocardiography (TEE), its use intraoperatively has contributed a lot to the diagnosis and management of cardiac abnormalities in the patients. Likewise, providing anesthesia to newborns and infants not only requires expertise but also a vast understanding of the pharmacology of anesthesia drugs which is different from adults.

Labor analgesia, also known as painless vaginal deliveries, is one of the major contributions of anesthesiologists in the obstetric field. They guide in the safe, smooth, and painless delivery of pregnant females, thus defying the general notion that childbirth is not without bearing pain. The anesthesiologists also provide resuscitation to the newborns with respiratory failure or congenital heart conditions along with pediatricians after the delivery of the babies.

Transplant anesthesia is the recent developed specialty involved in providing anesthesia to both the donor and recipients of organ transplantations. These mainly includes kidney, liver, lung, and heart transplantation. Oncoanesthesiologists are full-time physicians dealing with cancer patients. They know the impact of anesthesia drugs on malignancy and deal with the perioperative complications associated with these drugs. They have knowledge of the effects and adverse effects of various chemotherapeutic agents and the impact of other modalities like radiotherapy and immunotherapy.

As emergency physicians, the anesthesiologists provide basic life support (BLS) and advanced cardiac life support (ACLS). Thus, they are more valuable in trauma and emergency services. Their role in trauma is far more important than any other physicians because of their early and effective airway management and resuscitation of the patients. They are experienced in securing intravenous lines and inserting central venous catheters. They are more calculated in providing accurate doses of drugs. This can be attributed to their knowledge of the physiology and pharmacology of drugs. Also, anesthesiologists are fundamentally strong in managing the airway, breathing, and circulation in emergency services. With the advancement of point-of-care ultrasonography, anesthesiologists are nowadays trained in the focused assessment with sonography in trauma (FAST) to rule out blood in the peritoneum cavity, hemopericardium, or hemothorax.

It is not wrong to say that anesthesiologists are just like the medicines of pain or more accurately to say, pain physicians. Thinking of the time when the surgery was performed on an awake patient without providing anesthesia, still, gives us goosebumps. Anesthesiologists can deal with all sorts of acute and chronic pain. Pain is a very distressing symptom and inadequate pain relief causes more harm than good. Acute pain services include perioperative pain relief as well as pain relief in traumatic injuries. Adequate pain relief leads to early ambulation of the postoperative patients leading to early recovery and less hospital stay. Anesthesiologists are proficient in various nerve and plane block techniques thus providing adequate analgesia using local anesthetic drugs. In chronic pain, anesthesiologists can deal with all types of cancer pain, including but not limited to the radicular pain in neuropathies. As physicians, they incorporate the concept of multimodal analgesia by judicious use of different analgesic agents both in acute and chronic pain.

Anesthesiologists are also palliative care physicians. Palliative care is a relatively new approach to the healthcare delivery system. It improves the quality of life of the patients having life-threatening illness by preventing suffering from pain.[4] Anesthesiologists not only help in providing pain relief to terminally ill patients but also integrate psychological and spiritual aspects of patient care along with hospice and supportive care to the patients and their family members through effective communication skills.

🔑 KEY POINTS

- Anesthesiologist, as a perioperative physician provides medical care to the surgical patients before, during, and after surgery.
- Anesthesiologist covers preoperative clinic, operating room, postanesthesia care unit, respiratory care, intensive care unit, pain and palliative care clinic and trauma and emergency services.
- Anesthesiologists are specialized in the various fields, including neuroanesthesia, cardiac anesthesia, pediatric anesthesia, obstetric anesthesia, oncoanesthesia and transplant anesthesia.

REFERENCES

1. Lande-Marghade P. Anesthetist as a perioperative physician: A new perspective. Journal of Anaesthesia and Critical Care Case Reports. 2017;3:1-2.
2. Muralidar S, Ambi SV, Sekaran S, Krishnan UM. The emergence of COVID-19 as a global pandemic: Understanding the epidemiology, immune response and potential therapeutic targets of SARS-CoV-2. Biochimie. 2020;179:85-100.
3. Singh A, Khanna P. Anesthetist and pandemic: Past and present. Trends in Anaesthesia & Critical Care. 2021;36:5-8.
4. Rome RB, Luminais HH, Bourgeois DA, Blais CM. The role of palliative care at the end of life. Ochsner J. 2011;11:348-352.

REVIEW QUESTIONS

1. Perioperative physician is the person who provides medical care to the patients:
   a. Before the surgical procedure
   b. During the surgical procedure
   c. After the surgical procedure
   d. All of the above
2. Anesthesia includes:
   a. Amnesia
   b. Analgesia
   c. Muscle relaxation
   d. All of the above
3. Anesthesiologists are trained in:
   a. Inducing pain
   b. Providing good patient doctor communication
   c. Irreversible muscle relaxation
   d. None of the above
4. Anesthesia covers:
   a. Preoperative clinic
   b. Operating room
   c. Postanesthesia care unit
   d. All of the above
5. Anesthesiologists provide pain relief to:
   a. Patients undergoing surgery
   b. Cancer patients
   c. Both (a) and (b) are correct
   d. Both (a) and (b) are incorrect
6. Drugs relieving anxiety includes:
   a. Benzodiazepines
   b. Opioids
   c. Muscle relaxants
   d. Barbiturates
7. Monitor used for assessing adequate depth of anesthesia is:
   a. Neuromuscular transmission (NMT)
   b. Bispectral Index (BIS)
   c. Transesophageal echocardiography (TEE)
   d. All of the above

ANSWERS

1. d	2. d	3. b	4. d	5. c	6. a
7. b					

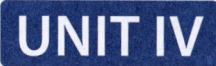

Regional Anesthesia: Techniques and Complications

Unit Outline

20. Central Neuraxial Blockade
21. Nerve Blocks

COMPETENCIES COVERED IN UNIT IV

Competency Number	Competency Name	Chapter Number
AS5.1	Enumerate the indications for and describe the principles of regional anaesthesia (including spinal, epidural and combined).	20
AS5.2	Describe the correlative anatomy of the brachial plexus, subarachnoid and epidural spaces.	21
AS5.3	Observe and describe the principles and steps/techniques involved in peripheral nerve blocks.	21
AS5.4	Observe and describe the pharmacology and correct use of commonly used drugs and adjuvant agents in regional anesthesia.	13, 19, 20
AS5.5	Observe and describe the principles and steps/techniques involved in caudal epidural in adults and children.	20
AS5.6	Observe and describe the principles and steps/ techniques involved in common blocks used in surgery (including brachial plexus blocks).	21

CHAPTER 20

Central Neuraxial Blockade

Jitendra Agarwal, Anshul Jain

INTRODUCTION

Central neuraxial blockade[Q] (CNB[Q]) is the term used for procedures in which local anesthetic is injected in the vicinity of spinal cord through vertebral column, so as to block both afferent and efferent fibers at the level of spinal cord. It includes:
- Subarachnoid block [spinal anesthesia (SA)] or intrathecal block
- Epidural block
- Caudal block[Q]

APPLIED ANATOMY (FIGS. 20.1 AND 20.2)

Vertebral Column

Spine is made up of *33[Q] vertebral bones (7 cervical, 12 thoracic, and 5 lumbar, 5 fused sacral and 4 fused coccygeal vertebrae)* connected by fibrocartilaginous intervertebral disks. The spine as a whole provides structural support for the body and protection for the spinal cord and nerves, and acts as a conduit connecting peripheral and central nervous system. At each vertebral level, paired spinal nerves exit the central nervous system. The anterior and posterior nerve roots at each spinal level join one another and *exit the intervertebral foramina forming spinal nerves from C1 to S5*. At the cervical level, the nerves arise above their respective vertebrae, but starting at T1 they exit below their vertebrae. As a result, there are *eight cervical nerve roots* in seven cervical vertebrae.

Curves: The spinal column normally forms a double C, being *convex anteriorly (lordosis)* in the *cervical*[Q] and *lumbar regions* while *concave anteriorly (kyphosis)* in *thoracic and sacral region* (Fig. 20.1).

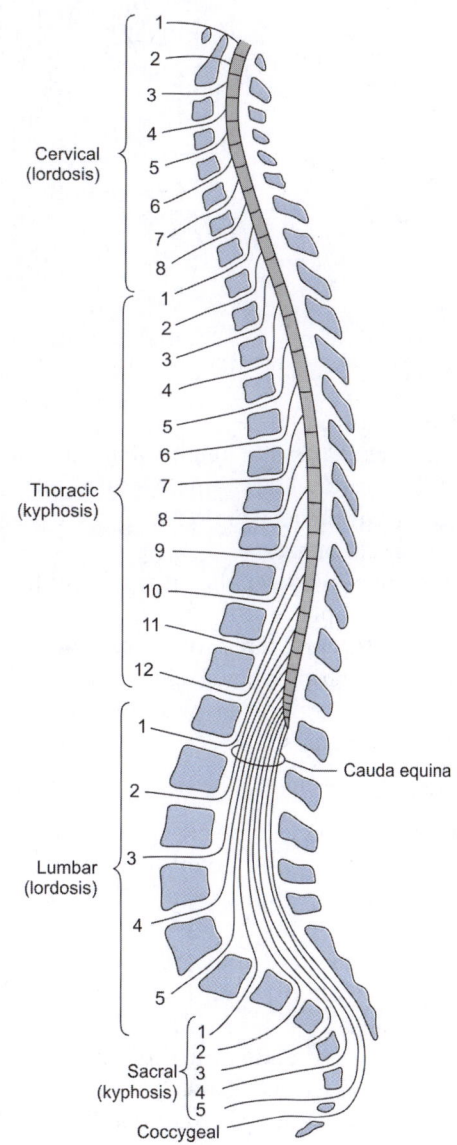

Fig. 20.1: Vertebral column.

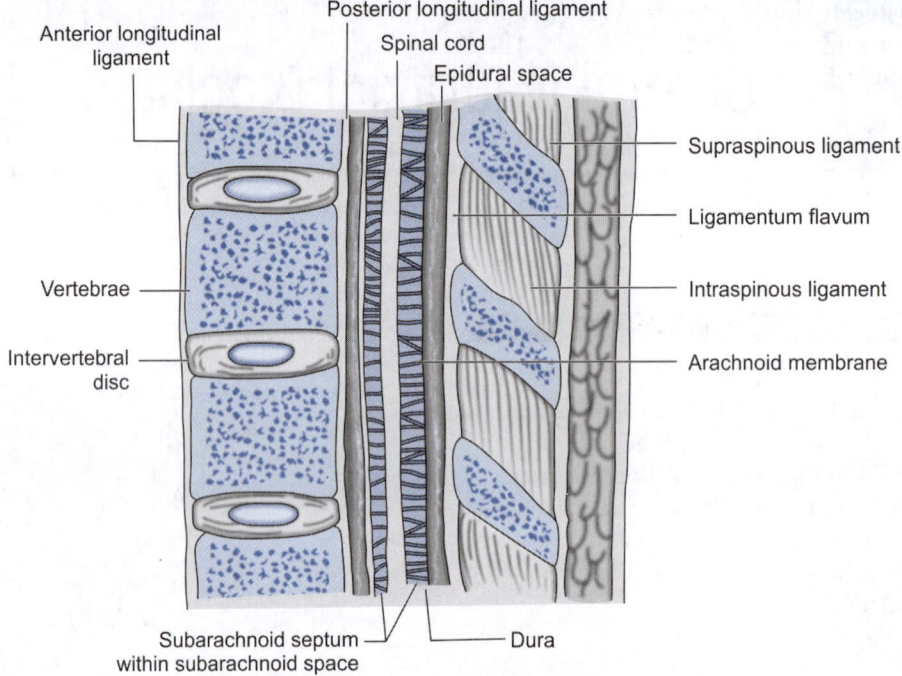

Fig. 20.2: Relations of epidural space in sagittal section.

Primary curvature: The thoracic and sacral (pelvic) curvatures are concave anteriorly and appear during the fetal period so they are referred as primary curvature.

Secondary curvature: The cervical and lumbar curvatures appears after birth as baby start walking, these curvatures are concave posteriorly and convex anteriorly, being referred to as lordosis. These curvatures are termed as secondary or acquired curvatures.

Spinal Cord

Spinal cord along with its coverings (the meninges), fatty tissue, and a venous plexus lies in spinal canal. The spinal cord extends from the foramen magnum to the lower border of L1[Q] in adults. In children, it ends at L3[Q] and moves up as they grow older (adult level is achieved by 2 years).[Q]

As spinal cord ends at L1, lower nerve roots have to course some distance before exiting their respective intervertebral foramina. These lower spinal nerves form the cauda equina.[Q] Therefore, performing a lumbar (subarachnoid) puncture below *L1*[Q] in an adult (*L3*[Q] in a child) avoids potential needle trauma to the cord. Damage to the cauda equina is unlikely as these nerve roots float in the dural sac below L1 and tend to be pushed away (rather than pierced) by an advancing needle. However, injury to cauda equina has been reported in spinal catheters because of which they had been withdrawn.

The meninges include *pia mater* which is closely adherent to the spinal cord; the *arachnoid mater* which is usually closely adherent to the outer thicker and denser *dura mater*.

Note: During development, vertebral column elongates more rapidly than the spinal cord. So, there is an increasing disparency between anatomical level of spinal cord and their corresponding vertebral column.

Blood Supply of Spinal Cord

Spinal cord derives its blood supply from:
- **Anterior spinal artery**[Q]: *Single* artery derived from vertebral artery at the base of the skull. It supplies the *anterior two-thirds*[Q] of the cord.

- **Two posterior spinal arteries**: Arise from the posterior inferior cerebellar arteries[Q]. They supply the *posterior one-third*.[Q]
- **Additional radicular arteries**: Arise from the intercostal arteries in the thorax and the lumbar arteries in the abdomen. One of these radicular arteries, the artery of *Adamkiewicz, or arteria radicularis magna*, is a unilateral artery on the left side, which directly arise from the aorta somewhere between T5 and L2 (origin vary individual to individual). It provides the major blood supply to the anterior aspect of *lower two-thirds of the spinal cord*. Injury to this artery can result in the *anterior spinal artery syndrome*.[1]

Subarachnoid Space

Between the *pia* and *arachnoid mater* lies subarachnoid space which contains cerebrospinal fluid (CSF). Though the spinal cord ends at the lower border of L1, the subarachnoid space ends at S2.[Q] In SA, drug is injected in this space.

✏ KEY POINTS

Spinal cord	: Ends at L1 in adult; L3 in child
Subarachnoid space	: Ends at S2
Epidural space	: Ends at sacral hiatus
Ligamentum flavum	: Extends from foramen magnum to sacral hiatus

✏ KEY POINTS

Common causes of anterior spinal artery syndrome
- Aortic aneurysm, dissection, atherosclerosis
- Disk herniaiton, cervical spondylosis
- Neoplasia

Subdural Space

Subdural space is a poorly demarcated, potential space that exists between the dura and arachnoid membranes. There is no established method to identify this space clinically, so till now it has not been explored for clinical purpose, although injection into subdural space during SA may explain the occasional failed/partial spinal anesthesia and the rare "total spinal" after epidural anesthesia.

Epidural Space

Surrounding dura mater, lies better defined potential space known as epidural space. The spinal epidural space extends from the foramen magnum to the sacral hiatus. This space is utilized in epidural and caudal anesthesia where drug is injected into this space.

Boundaries (Fig. 20.2)

- **Anterior:** Posterior longitudinal ligaments
- **Lateral:** Pedicles and intervertebral foramina
- **Posterior:** Ligamentum flavum

Contents[Q]

- **Spinal nerve roots**: They traverse epidural space, before exiting from vertebral foramina
- Fat
- Areolar tissue
- Lymphatics
- Blood vessels, including the well-organized *Batson venous plexus* and spinal arteries.

Batson venous plexus[Q] is a valveless[Q] communication between pelvic veins and intracranial veins. So, accidental injection of air or local anesthetic into these veins can lead to direct CNS toxicity. *In presence of pregnancy, abdominal tumor, and inferior vena cava obstruction, veins of Batson plexus get engorged which reduces the size of epidural space*. Thus, in such conditions lesser drug is required to achieve desired level and there is increased chance of venous puncture.

Lumbar Puncture (Fig. 20.3)

In SA, local anesthetic is injected into subarachnoid space, by lumbar puncture. Following structures has to be pierced[Q] while performing lumbar puncture:
- Skin
- Subcutaneous tissue
- Supraspinous ligament (which connects the tips of spinous process)

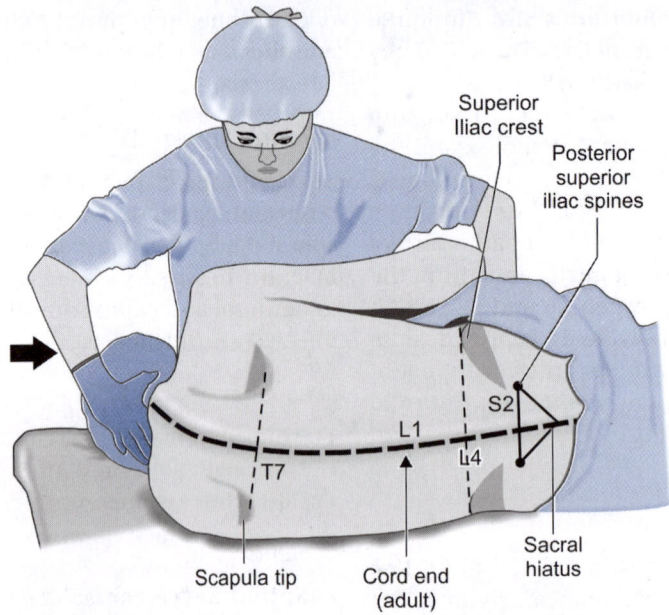

Fig. 20.3: Lateral position for spinal and epidural blocks.

- Interspinous ligament (which joins the spinous process together)
- **Ligamentum flavum (yellow ligament):** This also extends from sacral hiatus to S2[Q]
- Dura mater
- Arachnoid mater.

Mnemonic: S3IFDA

Surface Landmarks[Q]

While administrating anesthesia, it is important to know the level of spine, there are some landmarks which can be used to delineate level.
- **C7**: Spinous process of C7 is most prominent and is easily palpable.
- **T7**: Lies opposite to inferior angle of scapula
- **L4**: A line drawn between the highest points of both iliac crests *(Tuffier's line)* usually crosses either the body of L4 or the L4-L5[Q] interspace.

CENTRAL NEURAXIAL BLOCKADE

Both spinal and epidural anesthesia shares many thing in common like mechanisms of action, physiologic effects, etc.

Mechanism of Action

The principal site of action for CNB is the nerve root.[Q]

In SA, drug is injected directly in to CSF[Q] where it acts on nerve roots. Thus, SA requires a relatively small dose and volume.

> **KEY POINTS**
>
> **Cerebrospinal fluid**
> - **Produced by:** Ependymal cell in choroid plexus (500 mL per day)
> - **Absorbed by:** Arachnoid granulation in superior sagittal sinus
> - **Volume:** 135–150 mL
> - **Content:** Glucose 50–80 mg/dL; Protein 15–40 mg/dL, No RBC, No WBC.

In epidural and caudal blockade, three principal mechanisms are suggested:
1. Diffusion across the dura into subarachnoid space where it acts on nerve roots.
2. Diffusion to paravertebral areas where they blocks nerve distal to their dural sheath.

3. After diffusion across the dura, local anesthetic may act directly on spinal cord.

SYSTEMIC EFFECTS OF NEURAXIAL BLOCKADE

Cardiovascular Manifestations

Hypotension

This is the most prominent effect of CNB on CVS. Hypotension vary in intensity, *maximum decrease in BP is seen with SA.*[Q] In SA, the intensity of hypotension is proportional to the degree (level of block) of the sympathectomy.

Reason: Vasomotor tone is maintained by sympathetic fibers arising from T5 to L1. Blocking these nerves causes dilation of the venous capacitance vessels, and consequently pooling of blood. *Pumping action of lower limb muscles (soleus) is also lost due to motor paralysis.* Overall result is decreased venous return to the heart[Q] and hence hypotension **(Fig. 20.4)**.

Bradycardia

Hypotension may be accompanied by a decrease in heart rate and cardiac contractility, if the level of block is very high. This is due to blockade of sympathetic cardiac accelerator fibers that arise at T1–T4. The unopposed vagal tone can rarely lead to sudden cardiac arrest too.

Nervous System (Fig. 20.5)

Different types of nerve fibers have different sensitivity thresholds to local anesthetic blockade. After neuraxial block order of blocking nerve fiber is as follows:

- Autonomic preganglionic B fibers *(most sensitive)*[Q]
- Temperature fibers (cold before warm)
- Pinprick fibers
- Pain fibers
- Touch fibers
- Deep pressure fibers
- Somatic motor fibers
- Fibers carrying vibratory and proprioceptive impulses *(most resistant).*[Q]

> **KEY POINTS**
>
> **What do we mean by level of block?**
> Well, this question must be arising in your brain, so here comes the answer. Suppose after injecting drug in subarachnoid space analgesia up to the level of umbilicus is obtained. Cutaneous supply of umbilicus level is derived from T10 spinal nerve, so the sensory level of block is T10 in this hypothetical case. Sympathetic block is usually two segments higher than sensory block (T8 in this case).

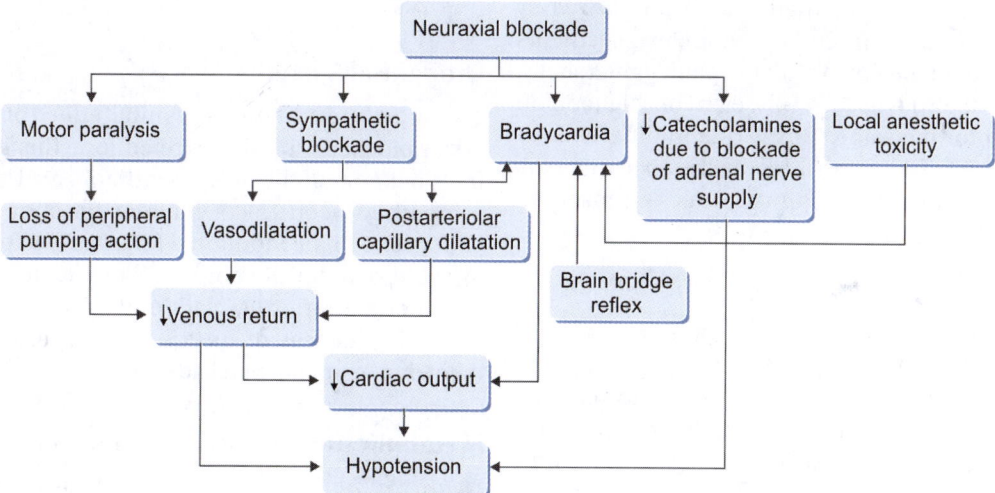

Fig. 20.4: Mechanism of hypotension in central neuraxial blockade.

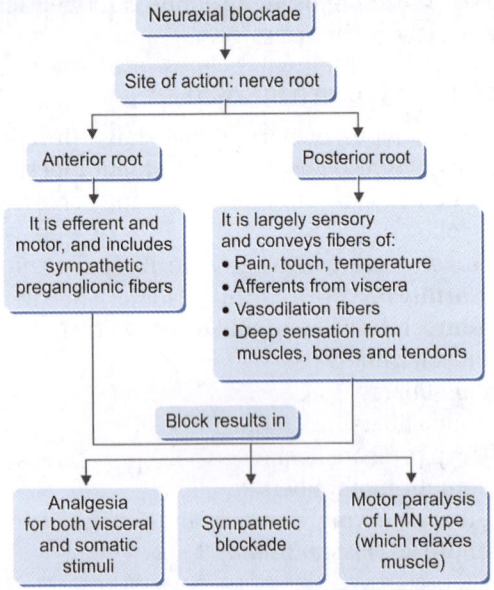

Fig. 20.5: Effect of neuraxial blockade.

Interruption of efferent autonomic transmission produces more sympathetic in comparison to parasympathetic blockade. This can be explained by the fact that sympathetic outflow is via thoracolumbar spinal nerves (T1-L2), whereas parasympathetic outflow is craniosacral, out of which cranial nerves always remain spared in CNB.

An important aspect of SA is differential blockade, i.e., sympathetic blockade *(judged by temperature sensitivity)* is usually two segments higher than the sensory block (pain, light, touch), which in turn is usually two segments higher than the motor blockade. This is due to difference in sensitivity of different fibers (as shown earlier). So, the sequence of block is Autonomic → Sensory → Motor[Q].

Respiratory System

In normal individual, lung function is well-maintained except slight reduction in vital capacity in case of high block, which is due to reduced contribution of abdominal muscles in expiration.

In patients with severe lung diseases who rely on accessory muscles (abdominal muscles, intercostals) for breathing, high level of neural blockade results in marked impairment in ventilation due to blockade of these muscles.

Apnea though very rare in neuraxial blockade can be caused by:
- Medullary ischemia due to severe hypotension (most common cause)
- Ischemia to respiratory muscles due to severe hypotension
- **Total spinal**: Due to accidental intrathecal injection in epidural anesthesia
- **Systemic toxicity of local anesthetic**: Due to accidental intravascular injection in epidural anesthesia.

Gastrointestinal System

Sympathetic supply of gastrointestinal tract originates from T5-L1 spinal nerves, whereas parasympathetic supply comes from vagus. *Neuraxial block-induced sympathectomy allows uninterrupted vagal action* which results in a small, contracted[Q] gut with active peristalsis, thus providing the excellent operative conditions.

Some patients complaints of nausea after CNB (maximum in SA) due to following reasons:
- Hypotension leading to hypoxia of chemo-receptor trigger zone
- Uninterrupted vagal activity
- Bile in stomach (due to relaxed pyloric sphincter)
- Psychological

Urogenital System

The most prominent urogenital effect of neuraxial blockade is urinary retention. This is due to blockade of both sympathetic and parasympathetic control of bladder function. The patient should be monitored for urinary retention to avoid bladder distention following neuraxial anesthesia. Moreover, bladder distension is one of the few causes of unexpected hypertension following neuraxial blockade.

Metabolic and Endocrine Manifestations

Neuraxial blockade suppresses stress response by *blocking catecholamine[Q] release from adrenal* glands. Thereby neuraxial blocks may decrease perioperative arrhythmias and possibly reduce the incidence of ischemia.

The ADH increase which is a normal response to surgery is abolished by neuraxial blockade.

Thermoregulation

As there is vasodilatation below the level of block heat loss is accelerated.^Q As a compensatory mechanism, there is vasoconstriction above the block which may be accompanied by *shivering* (*a common complication of SA*).

SPINAL ANESTHESIA

This is the cheapest and one of the most common anesthetic technique. In SA, local anesthetic is injected directly into CSF.

Indications

- **General surgery**: Lower abdominal, inguinal, urogenital, rectal surgery
- **Orthopedic surgery**: All lower limb surgeries, few pelvic surgeries
- **Gynecologic and obstetrics surgery**: SA is an *anesthetic technique of choice*^Q for cesarean section. All common gynecologic surgeries can be performed under SA.
- **Urologic surgery**: Prostate surgery, bladder and ureteric surgery.

In general, all surgery below diaphragm can be performed under SA.

Contraindications

- Patient refusal
- Fixed cardiac output lesion
- Shock
- Infection at injection site
- Increased intracranial tension
- Overt coagulopathy.

Technique

Patient's Position (Fig. 20.3)

Spinal anesthesia can be achieved in lateral (most common), sitting and prone (using hypobaric drug) position. *Sitting position*^Q is preferred in obese patients due to better appreciation of anatomic midline where flexion of the spine (arching the back) maximizes the space between adjacent spinous processes and brings the spine closer to the skin surface.

Spinal Needles (Figs. 20.6A to C)

Broadly, spinal needles are of two types:
1. **Cutting tip (dura cutting):** Quincke needle
2. **Blunt tip (dura separating):** This includes Whitacre and Sprotte needles. The *incidence of postdural puncture headache* (PDPH) *is less with these needles.*

Both cutting and blunt tip needles are available in sizes ranging from 16–30 gauge.

Approach

Approach to subarachnoid space can be through midline (*most common*), lateral (*paramedian*) and lateral at S1-S2 *(Taylor's approach)*.

Midline Approach

Needle is introduced in the midline and directed slightly cephalad. If bone is contacted superficially, needle is likely hitting the lower spinous process. Contact with bone at a deeper depth usually indicates the upper spinous process or it is lateral to the midline and hitting a lamina.

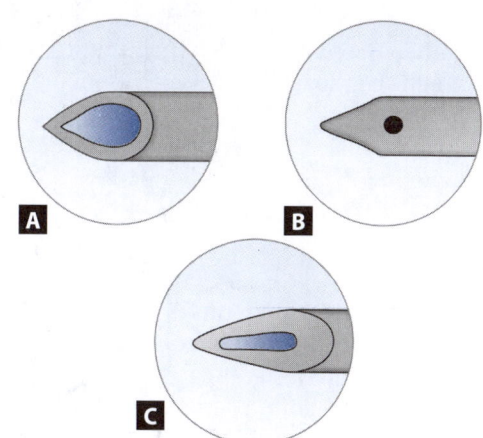

Figs. 20.6A to C: Lumbar puncture needles: (A) Quincke; (B) Whitacre; (C) Sprotte.

In either case, the needle must be redirected. As the needle penetrates the ligamentum flavum an obvious increase in resistance is usually felt. The needle is advanced further to penetrate the dura-subarachnoid membranes as signaled by free flowing CSF. *Free flowing CSF is the best sign*[Q] *of correct lumbar puncture* **(Fig. 20.3)**.

Lateral Approach (Paramedian Approach)

Paramedian technique is indicated in patients with positioning difficulty (e.g., severe arthritis, kyphoscoliosis). The site of needle entry is 1 cm lateral and 1 cm caudal to the inferior aspect of the spinous process of the desired level. The needle is directed and advanced at a 10–25° angle with sagittal plane toward the midline **(Fig. 20.7A)**.

Taylor's Approach

Paramedian approach at the L5-S1 interspace, the largest interlaminar interspace of the vertebral column. Used in conditions of spinal deformity involving lumbar spine **(Fig. 20.7B)**.

Saddle Block

Saddle block is the technique of SA by *which only sacral segments are blocked.*[Q] Usually, there is no hypotension which makes it extremely useful for anal and perineal surgery. Lumbar puncture is done in sitting position in L4-L5 space and hyperbaric lignocaine or bupivacaine is injected in low volume. Patient remains seated for 5 minutes *(lignocaine)* or 10 minutes *(bupivacaine)*, which, allows drug to settle down along the gravity, afterward patient can be placed in surgical position.

SEGMENTAL SPINAL ANESTHESIA

Pharmacology

Injection of low concentration of local anesthetics into the subarachnoid space anesthetize only the small nmber of nerve roots, sparing rest.

Segmental spinal anesthesia is now being explored in cervical and thoracic area. Segment spinal nesthesia is being successfully used in laparoscopic cholecystectomy particularly in high risk patients.

Drugs

Bupivacaine (0.5%)[Q] *hyperbaric and lignocaine 5% hyperbaric* are the most commonly used drug for SA. Ropivacaine, levobupivacaine are other newer drugs **(Table 20.1)**.

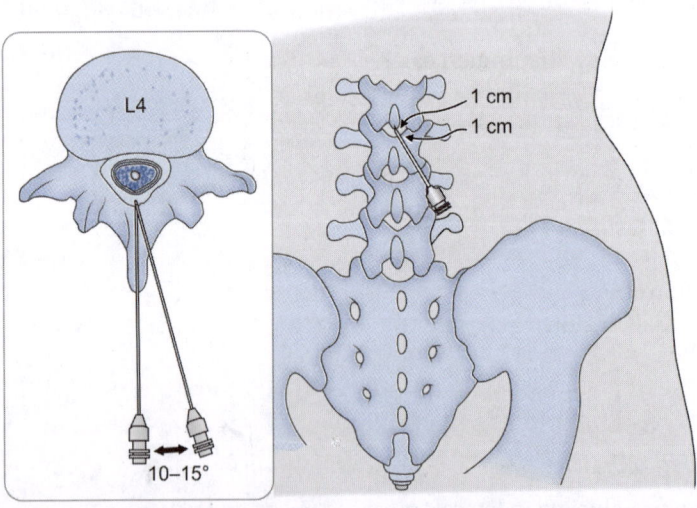

Fig. 20.7A: Paramedian approach for spinal anesthesia.

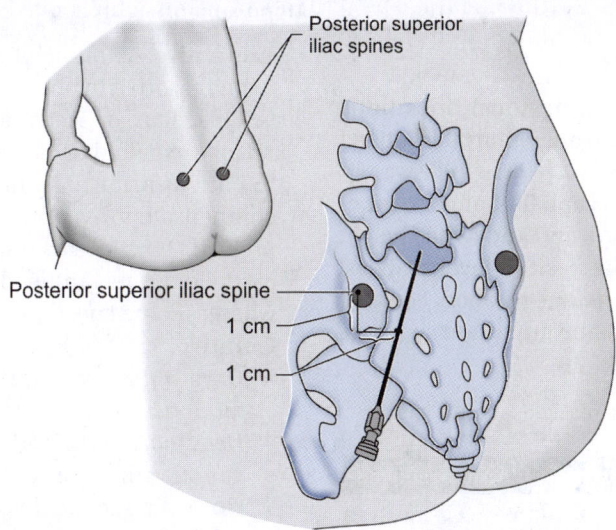

Fig. 20.7B: Paramedian approach for spinal anesthesia (Taylor's approach).

Table 20.1: Drugs for spinal anesthesia.

Drug	Doses	Duration
Lignocaine 5%	1–2 mL	1–1.5 hour
Bupivacaine 0.5%	2–4 mL	2–4 hour
Ropivacaine	2–4 mL	2–4 hour

Baricity

Baricity refers to the specific gravity of local anesthetic solution in relation to CSF (specific gravity 1.0069). Hyperbaric solutions are heavier *(higher specific gravity)* than CSF, so they tend to move in dependent portion (along the gravity). Thus, after spinal, if patient is kept in head down position hyperbaric drug will move cephalad and a higher level can be achieved. Local anesthetic are being made hyperbaric by mixing dextrose 5–8% with the desired local anesthetic.

Level of Block

For same desired level of blockade, main determinant of drug dose is length of spine (in which drug has to be distributed), which in-turn is determined by the height of patient. Tall patients have long spine and require large dose when compared to dwarfs.

KEY POINTS

Bloody tap
Sometimes in spite of CSF, blood comes during lumbar puncture, the best way to deal is to remove needle, wash it with saline and reinsert in different space. Repeated bloody tap may represent some undiagnosed coagulopathy.

CSF volume is another important determinant. In conditions with increased intra-abdominal pressure (pregnancy, tumor), there is compression of intrathecal space and CSF volume decreases. So, the same volume of drug will result in higher level of block.

Factors Affecting Level of Block/Height of Block

As mentioned earlier, SA is administered at the level of L2-L3 or L3-L4 space usually. Added to this, even lower abdominal surgery require block at least up to T10. So, height of block has to be increased.

The factors affecting block height are:
Modifiable factors:
- Dose (volume and concentration)
- Site of injection
- Baricity of local anesthetic
- Posture of patient.

Nonmodifiable factors:
- Volume of CSF
- Density of CSF

In general, after injecting local anesthetic patient is turned supine and operation table is tilted downward (head-down position = Trendelenburg's position). This favors the cephalad movement of hyperbaric drug (due to gravity) and hence height of block increases. As the desired level reaches, operation table is reset to neutral position. For level of blockade required for some important surgeries (**Table 20.2**).

Table 20.2: Level of blockade required for some important surgeries.

Surgery	Level of sensory blockade required
Cesarean section	T6
TURP	T10
TURBt	T10
Knee surgery	L1
Lower limb	L1
Penis	S2–S4

(TURP: transurethral resection of the prostrate; TURBt: transurethral resection of bladder tumor)

Factors Affecting Duration of Block

Another most important aspect of spinal anesthesia is duration of block, the duration of spinal anesthesia depends upon the local anesthetic drug being used and amount being injected. Out of the two, drug is more important—bupivacaine. Ropivacaine provides long duration whereas lignocaine provides short duration.

Complications

Hypotension

Hypotension is the most common[Q] complication of SA. Severe hypotension (systolic blood pressure < 90 mm Hg) may be seen in up to 33% of cases.

Slight reduction in blood pressure is beneficial as this reduces bleeding, however, if systolic blood pressure falls below 80 mm Hg renal perfusion gets impaired. So it is recommended to take action, whenever systolic blood pressure falls below 90 mm Hg.[2]

Management

- **Preventive**: At this point, you all must know that main reason of hypotension after SA is reduced venous return or decreased preload. If 500–1,000 mL of crystalloid or 500 mL of colloid is infused to patient prior to spinal block, this tends to compensate for venous dilation and maintain preload. Thus, preloading with 10–20 mL/kg of crystalloid is recommended in high risk patient whereas some anesthesiologists use it routinely.
- **Curative**:
  - *Oxygen supplementation*: This is the first and foremost step.
  - *Head-down tilt*: Head-down tilt will augment venous return and thereby increases BP. However, tilt should not exceed 15% as this might increase the height of block (when hyperbaric drug has been used).
  - *Fluids*: Colloids are preferred over crystalloids for curative therapy as they remain in intravascular compartment thus less volume (or less time) is required.
  - *Vasopressors*: Ephedrine and mephentermine are preferred drugs. Both are given in bolus doses of 6 mg.
  - *Inotropes (dopamine and dobutamine)*: Used when other measure fails. They tend to increase blood pressure by increasing cardiac output, but simultaneously they increase myocardial oxygen demand too.
  - *Atropine*: It is indicated only when hypotension is associated with bradycardia.

Postdural Puncture Headache

Any breach of the dura may result in a PDPH. This may follow all procedures requiring lumbar puncture, e.g., myelogram, SA, lumbar tap.

Pathogenesis (Box 20.1)

Postdural puncture headache is a low pressure headache that results from leakage of CSF from the dural defect and thereby decreasing intracranial pressure. The *incidence of PDPH is strongly related*[Q] *to needle size, needle type, and patient population.* Thicker[Q], the needle more would be the CSF leak

> **BOX 20.1**
>
> **Factors affecting postdural puncture headache**
> - **Age:** Younger more frequent
> - **Gender:** Females > males
> - **Needle size:** Larger > smaller
> - **Needle type:** More with cutting type needle
> - **Pregnancy:** More when pregnant
> - **Dual punctures:** More with multiple punctures

or more would be the PDPH. Further risk is higher with *cutting* type needle (see above).

Clinical Presentation

Headache is usually seen *12–72 hours*[Q] following the procedure. PDPH[Q] is *typically bilateral, frontal or retro-orbital, and occipital and extends into the neck.* It may be throbbing or constant and associated with photophobia and nausea. The characteristic feature of PDPH is its association with body position. The pain is aggravated by sitting or standing and relieved or decreased by lying down flat.

Differential Diagnosis

The most common differential diagnosis is headache due to meningeal irritation. Meningeal irritation causes high pressure headache which is not related to posture. Queckenstedt's test is used to differentiate both.

Management

Preventive:
- Use fine noncutting type of needle
- Adequate hydration
- Avoid head up position
- Improve hydration with oral or IV fluids.

Curative:
- Analgesics, range from acetaminophen to nonsteroidal anti-inflammatory drugs.
- An *autologous epidural blood patch* is the most effective treatment for PDPH.[Q] It involves injecting 15–20 mL of autologous blood into the epidural space, at or one interspace below, the level of the dural puncture. Blood patch believed to stop further leakage of CSF by either mass effect or coagulation.

Historically, early ambulation was considered to be the risk factor and patient were advised strict bed rest; however, recent studies contradict it and shown that *early ambulation tends to decrease headache.*[Q]

Backache

Mild-to-moderate backache is one of the common complains after anesthesia (irrespective of regional or general) and is probably related to position. A small pillow under lumbar region reduces the incidence of backache.

Meningitis

Due to aseptic precaution, the septic meningitis has become rare sequelae. Aseptic meningitis may be seen rarely due to tracking of betadine or glove powder with needle. So before needle insertion, site must be thoroughly cleaned with spirit.

> **KEY POINTS**
>
> **Queckenstedt's test**[Q]**:** On application of pressure over jugular vein PDPH decreases while headache due to meningeal irritation increases.

Cranial Nerve Palsy

Cranial nerve palsy after spinal is a rare squeal. *All cranial nerve except (I, IX, X) may be involved. Sixth*[Q] *nerve is the most common nerve to be involved.*

The most common cause is decreased CSF pressure which results in traction and stretching over the nerve nucleus.

Paralysis appears after third postoperative day and is almost always associated with headache. Features include blurred vision, photophobia. Most of the cases respond spontaneously.

Neurological Injury

Neurological injury may occur due to injury to nerve roots or spinal cord. The latter can be avoided by performing neuraxial blockade below L1 in adults and L3 in children. Unexplained pain at the time of injection is the earliest sign and this alerts the clinician to redirect needle. Although most neurological injuries resolve spontaneously, some are permanent.

Cauda equina syndrome now rare was seen with spinal catheters (which were later withdrawn) and lidocaine. Cauda equina syndrome is characterized by bowel and bladder dysfunction with LMN type paresis of legs, along with evidence of multiple nerve root injury. Exact cause is not known. Animal studies suggest that pooling or "maldistribution" of hyperbaric solutions of lidocaine can lead to neurotoxicity of the nerve roots of the cauda equina. The *local anesthetics associated with neurotoxicity include: lidocaine*^{Q} = tetracaine > bupivacaine > ropivacaine.

Other Causes of Paraplegia after Central Neuraxial Blockade

- Epidural/spinal hematoma
- Epidural abscess
- Arachnoiditis
- Anterior spinal artery syndrome
- Prolong intraoperative hypotension resulting in spinal ischemia.

Transient Neurological Symptoms

Transient neurological symptoms are characterized by back pain radiating to the legs without sensory or motor deficits, occurring after the resolution of spinal block and resolving spontaneously within several days. *The most common associated agent is hyperbaric lidocaine.*^{Q} The incidence of this syndrome is highest among outpatients (early ambulation) and in those undergoing surgery in the lithotomy position.

Hypoventilation/Apnea

Hypoventilation or apnea is usually secondary-to-severe hypotension compromising medullary blood supply. Thus, it usually resolves as BP increases. Rarely, very high block or total spinal can lead to diaphragmatic paralysis; in such condition, intermittent positive pressure ventilation is indicated.

Nausea/Vomiting

This is also usually secondary to hypotension, management include correction of BP, oxygenation, antiemetics (*prokinetic agents like metoclopramide are preferred*).

Cardiac Arrest

One of the rarest, but serious complication, causes include severe hypotension, anaphylaxis, and very high block. Immediate CPR with ATLS guidelines is the management. *It is worth to note that cardiac arrest in this setting (after SA) has best prognosis.*

Urinary Retention

Retention usually resolves as the effect of spinal wears off. Prolonged retention suggests sphincter spasm, which mandates urinary catheterization.

EPIDURAL ANESTHESIA

Epidural anesthesia is most versatile neuraxial technique offering a range wider than the typical SA. An epidural block can be performed at the sacral lumbar, thoracic, or cervical level. *Sacral epidural anesthesia is referred as a caudal block.*^{Q}

Epidural techniques can be used for operative anesthesia, obstetric analgesia, postoperative pain control, and chronic pain management. It can be used as a *single shot technique* (in which whole drug is injected in one shot) or with a catheter that allows intermittent boluses and/or *continuous infusion*. The most advantageous factor is motor block which ranges from none to complete. The drug administered, its concentration and dose, control the degree of motor blockade.

Procedure

All initial steps are same as that of SA. Like spinal, it can be given in sitting or lateral positions. After puncturing ligamentum flavum, needle enters in epidural space, unlike spinal block needle is not advanced further. It is in this epidural space where one injects the drug for epidural anesthesia.

Thoracic Epidural

Thoracic epidural is indicated for pain control in rib fractures, post-thoracic surgery, postcardiac surgery.

For thoracic epidural, *paramedian approach*[Q] is preferred as the spinous processes of thoracic vertebrae are directed downward which makes median approach very difficult. Correctly speaking, thoracic epidural is most difficult to administer.

Cervical Epidural

Cervical epidural is given through catheter in C6-C7 or C7-T1[Q] space as C7 can be easily identified. *Median approach* is preferred and needle is kept horizontal. Dura is very thin in cervical area, so the chance of accidental dural puncture is high in cervical epidural.

Epidural Needles (Fig. 20.8)

Epidural needles are thicker stout in comparison to spinal needle. The most commonly used needle is *Tuohy needle*.[Q] Its tip is curved (called as *Hyber's tip*) at an angle of 15–30°. Curve helps in the advancement of catheter in desired direction. Crawford is another epidural needle which is appropriate for single-shot epidural technique.

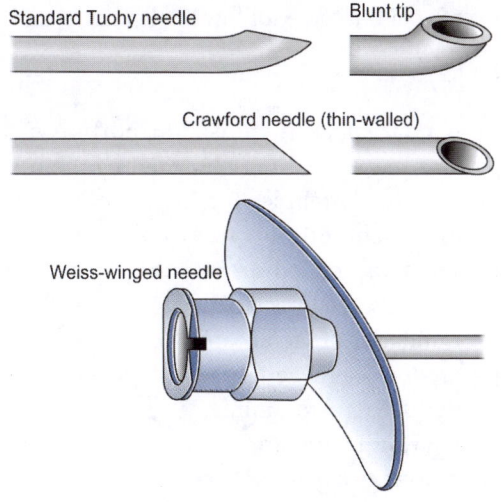

Fig. 20.8: Epidural needles.

Methods of Detecting Epidural Space

- **Loss of resistance technique**: In epidural space, there is negative pressure, which results in sudden loss of resistance as needle enters epidural space. In this technique, there are two choices regarding the type of syringe, i.e., glass versus plastic and Luer-Lok versus friction hub. *The theoretical ideal is a Luer-Lok, finely ground-glass syringe because it minimizes the chance of misidentification of the epidural space.* Loss of resistance can be accomplished through air or saline. Air carries risk of air embolism.
- **Technique**: Glass syringe or other loss of resistance syringe is filled with 2–4 mL of air or saline and attached to epidural needle. Needle is advanced slowly with one hand, while other hand applies pressure on the plunger, i.e., injecting air or saline with moderate pressure, as needle traverse various structures, saline or air remain in syringe. As needle enters epidural space, this saline or air get virtually sucked in.
- **Hanging drop method (Gutierrez's sign)**: In this method, a drop of saline is placed over the hub of needle. When needle enters epidural space, then the drop would be sucked in.
- Recently, few advanced techniques based on difference in light absorption pattern have also been used, but till now they are of experimental purposes only.

Test Dose

Epidural block carries increased risk of intravascular or intrathecal injection, so a small amount of drug is given initially as test dose[Q] to check any deleterious hemodynamic effect. For this purpose most commonly, *2 mL of lignocaine with adrenaline is injected* initially, with simultaneous monitoring of heart rate and lower limb movements. Intravascular injection is suggested by tachycardia while intrathecal injection is suggested by loss of toe movements in dependent lower limb. After ruling out both conditions, chosen drug is given at a rate not greater than 2 mL per second.

For continuous catheter technique after identification of epidural space, catheter is inserted through Touhy needle and advanced 2-6 cm in epidural space. Test dose is given through catheter.

Pharmacology

Epidural Anesthetic Agents

The epidural agent is chosen based on the desired clinical effect, whether it is to be used as a primary anesthetic, or for supplementation of general anesthesia, or for analgesia. Drugs can be categorized as:
- **Short-to-intermediate acting**: Lidocaine, chloroprocaine, and mepivacaine
- **Long-acting agents**: Bupivacaine, levobupivacaine, and ropivacaine. Etidocaine is used only rarely because of the reports that motor block is more profound than sensory block with the drug.
- **Additives**: There are few drugs which when mixed with local anesthetics increase the duration, improve the quality of blockade, or accelerate the onset of blockade. *Epinephrine is the most commonly used additive agent.*[Q] It increases the duration of all the agents, although the effect is greatest with lidocaine.
  - The addition of bicarbonate increases the speed of onset of the block. Clinically, the addition of 1 mEq of sodium bicarbonate to each 10 mL of commercially prepared 1.5% lidocaine solution produces a rapid and complete sensory block.
  - Other commonly used additives are opioids, clonidine and neostigmine. It is essential that additive should be preservative free.

Factors Affecting Level of Block

Factors affecting the level of epidural anesthesia are not as predictable as with SA. In adults, an accepted guideline is to inject 1.5–2 mL of local anesthetic per spinal segment to be blocked. For example, to achieve a T4 sensory level from an L4–L5 injection, 18–24 mL of LA solution would be required.

In elder patient, lesser dose is required to achieve the same level of anesthesia. Shorter and obese patients require only 1 mL of local anesthetic per segment to be blocked. Similarly, patients with increased intra-abdominal pressure (pregnancy, intra-abdominal tumor) require lesser volume of drug. Although less than with SA, spread of epidural local anesthetics is also affected by gravity and head-down tilt tends to increase the block height or level of block.

CAUDAL ANESTHESIA

Sacral epidural anesthesia is referred as a caudal block.[Q] But due to its different technique and applications, it is being discussed separately.

Indications

In children, caudal anesthesia is typically combined with general anesthesia for intraoperative supplementation and postoperative analgesia in urogenital, rectal, inguinal, and lower extremity surgery. *Caudal epidural is the most commonly used regional techniques in pediatric patients.*[Q]

In adults, it can also be used for anorectal surgeries, postoperative analgesia after abdominal surgery. Recently, steroids are being administered through caudal route for low back pain.[Q]

Anatomy

The caudal space is the sacral portion of the epidural space. Sacrum is formed by the fusion of five sacral vertebrae. The lamina of 5th sacral vertebrae (sometimes 4th) remain nonfused forming a gap called *sacral hiatus*. This gap is normally covered by sacrococcygeal ligament. So, the boundaries of sacral canal[Q] are:
- **Anterior**: Sacral vertebrae
- **Lateral**: Sacral foraminae
- **Posterior**: Laminae

The average capacity of sacral canal is 35 mL in males[Q] and 30 mL in females.

Technique (Fig. 20.9)

Caudal anesthesia requires penetration of sacrococcygeal ligament (an extension of ligamentum flavum) through sacral hiatus. The posterior superior iliac spines and the sacral hiatus define an equilateral triangle. Thus, by locating the posterior superior iliac spines, the position of the sacral hiatus can be approximated. After locating sacral hiatus, needle is inserted at an angle of approximately 45° to the sacrum. The needle is advanced until bone (i.e., dorsal aspect of the ventral plate of the sacrum) is contacted; needle is then withdrawn, and is redirected by decreasing the angle of insertion relative to the skin surface. In male patients, this angle is almost parallel to the coronal plane; female patients require a slightly steeper angle (15°). After redirection, needle is advanced to identify loss of resistance in a manner similar to epidural block.

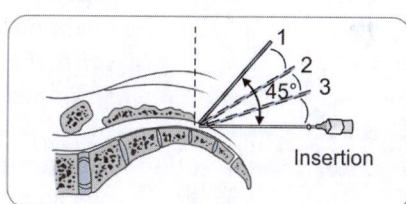

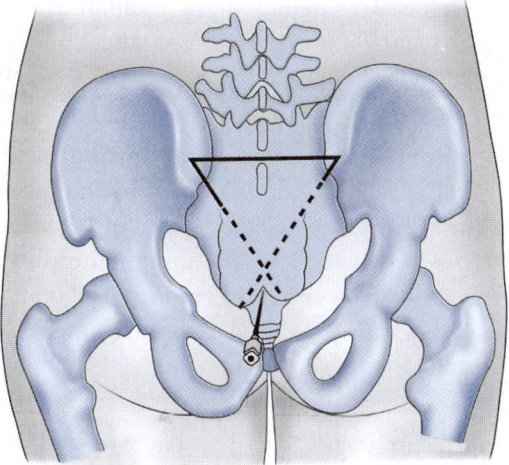

Fig. 20.9: Caudal block technique. Note the initial insertion and redirection of needle.

Complications of Epidural and Caudal Block

Intravascular Injection

Chances of intravascular injection are high in epidural anesthesia. The use of test doses, incremental dose, and aspiration minimize unintentional intravascular injections.

Even after all precautions intravascular injections are known and anesthetist must know the management of inadvertent intravascular injection.

Subarachnoid Injection (Total Spinal)

Accidental injection of epidural drug in subarachnoid space, results in a very high block sometimes total spinal. Again the best management is prevention. With small incremental doses, subarachnoid block can be identified early.

Management

As in any neuraxial block that reaches high levels, arterial blood pressure and heart rate should be supported. Patient should immediately be put in Trendelenburg position so as to maximize venous return. Ventilation should be supported, and if the entire dose (20–25 mL) of local anesthetic has been administered into the CSF, tracheal intubation and mechanical ventilation are indicated as patients may require approximately 1–2 hours to maintain adequate spontaneous ventilation consistently.

Neurologic Injury

Epidural anesthesia has not been linked to neurologic injury. Despite this, it is wise to avoid epidural anesthesia in patients in whom antiplatelet drugs or other anticoagulants have been used preoperatively, which theoretically increase incidence of neurologic injury caused by epidural bleeding (hematoma).

It is recommended to avoid epidural, if INR more than 1.2 and/or platelet count is below 50,000/mm³ **(Table 20.3)**.

Table 20.3: Spinal anesthesia versus epidural anesthesia.

Feature	Spinal anesthesia	Epidural anesthesia
Space utilized	Subarachnoid space	Epidural space
Site	Always lumbar	Can be lumbar, cervical, thoracic, sacral
Site of action	Spinal cord	Nerve roots
Ease of application	Easy	Difficult
Dose of local anesthetic required	Low	Large
Needles required	Fine (23–27)	Thick (16–18)
Onset	Fast	Gradual
Intensity of block	Intense	Variable
Duration	Depend on drug but cannot be prolonged	Duration can be increased by continuous epidural
Side effects		
• Hypotension	Frequent and severe	Infrequent and mild
• Vascular injection	Rare	High
• Total spinal	Very rare	Chances are there
• Postdural puncture headache	Seen	Rare, but chances are very high after accidental dural puncture
• Meningitis	Rare	Extremely rare
• Epidural hematoma/abscess	Extremely rare	Rare
Cost effectivity	Cheap	Expensive

KEY POINTS

Incremental dose
Most effective method, for prevention of serious complications after epidural and caudal block. Local anesthetic solution for epidural/caudal block is injected after negative aspiration in increments of 5 mL. Means inject 5 mL rule out any unwanted symptom or sign (numbness, tachycardia) aspirate again and inject 5 mL, repeat same cycle till the completion of administration of desired dose.

If any unwanted sign or symptom appear stop further injection and manage the patient accordingly.

LAST-MINUTE REVISION

- Central neuraxial block includes spinal, epidural and caudal blocks.
- In spinal anesthesia, a low dose of local anesthetic is injected in subarachnoid space.
- Saddle block is the type of spinal anesthesia, where only sacral nerve roots are blocked.
- In epidural and caudal block, a relatively large amount of drug is injected in epidural space, from where drug diffuses to act on nerve roots.

REFERENCES

1. Lindeire S, Hauser JM. Anatomy, Back, Artery of Adamkiewicz. 2022 Jul 25. In: StatPearls [Internet]. Treasure Island (FL): StatPearls Publishing; 2022 Jan-. PMID: 30422566.
2. Hofhuizen C, Lemson J, Snoeck M, Scheffer GJ. Spinal anesthesia-induced hypotension is caused by a decrease in stroke volume in elderly patients. Local Reg Anesth. 2019;12:19-26. doi: 10.2147/LRA.S193925. PMID: 30881108; PMCID: PMC6404676.

REVIEW QUESTIONS

1. Central neuraxial anesthesia is not contraindicated in:
   a. Platelets less than 80,000
   b. Patients on aspirin
   c. Patients on oral anticoagulants
   d. Patients on IV heparin

2. A lower segment cesarean section can be carried out under all of the following techniques of anesthesia, *except*:
   a. General anesthesia
   b. Spinal anesthesia
   c. Caudal anesthesia
   d. Combined spinal epidural anesthesia

3. Epidural anesthesia has been administered to a patient posted for hernia surgery with 15 mL of 0.5% lignocaine with adrenaline. He developed hypotension and respiratory depression within 3 minutes after administration of block. The most probable cause would be:
   a. Allergy to drug administered
   b. Systemic toxicity of drug
   c. Patient has got vasovagal shock
   d. Drug has entered subarachnoid space

4. Postdural puncture headache is commonly seen after:
   a. Epidural anesthesia
   b. Spinal anesthesia
   c. Caudal anesthesia
   d. General anesthesia

5. In an infant, spinal anesthesia is being planned. Which is the most suitable spinal interspace to accomplish this:
   a. L1–L2 space
   b. L2–L3 space
   c. L3–L4 space
   d. L4–L5 space

6. In caudal anesthesia, drug administered is:
   a. Epidural space
   b. Subdural space
   c. Subarachnoid space
   d. Lateral ventricles

7. Absolute contraindications to spinal anesthesia includes all, *except*:
   a. Patient refusal
   b. Coagulopathy
   c. Critical aortic stenosis
   d. Pre-existing neurologic deficit

8. Postspinal headache is usually secondary to:
   a. CSF leak
   b. Meningitis
   c. Increased ICT
   d. Periostitis of skull bones

9. Factors increasing postspinal headache are:
   a. Thicker spinal needle
   b. Pregnancy
   c. Cutting type needle
   d. All of the above

10. Complications of spinal anesthesia includes all of the following, *except*:
    a. Hypotensia
    b. Headache
    c. Urinary retention
    d. Paralytic ileus

11. In spinal anesthesia, the drug is deposited between:
    a. Pia and arachnoid
    b. Dura and arachnoid
    c. Dura and vertebrae
    d. Into spinal cord

12. **Complications of epidural anesthesia are all, *except*:**
    a. Headache
    b. Hypotension
    c. DIC
    d. Epidural hematoma

13. **In spinal anesthesia, which fibers are affected earliest?**
    a. Sensory
    b. Motor
    c. Sympathetic preganglionic
    d. Vibration

ANSWERS

1. a	2. c	3. d	4. b	5. d	6. a
7. d	8. a	9. d	10. d	11. a	12. c
13. c					

CHAPTER 21

Nerve Blocks

Anshul Jain, Sandeep Sahu

INTRODUCTION

A patient asks a question, my hand is being operated and you are anesthetizing me completely why? Historically, the answer of this question was nothing but a question mark. Now, nerve blocks a well-accepted component of comprehensive anesthetic care makes this possible. Indications of nerve blocks ranges from surgical anesthesia to cancer pain relief.

Nerve blocks are accomplished by administering LA selection in closed vicinity of respective nerve. Current chapter deals with the basic anatomy and technique of the blocks commonly administered by an anesthesiologist.

Techniques of Localizing Neural Structures

To accomplish nerve block it is necessary to localize the nerve that has to be blocked. This can be done either by visualizing the nerve or by localizing the nerve through stimulating which generated muscle contraction. Out of several methods available, elicitation of paresthesia[Q] (in the distribution of respective nerve) is most specific, while direct imaging by ultrasonography, computed tomography (CT) is more sensitive.

Electric nerve stimulation, to elicit motor response is another commonly employed technique, but this is less sensitive than ultrasound and/or CT where one can see the path of needle along with the neural bundle.

Broadly nerve blocks can be divided into four subgroups:
1. Blocks of head and neck
2. Blocks of upper extremity
3. Blocks of thorax and abdomen
4. Blocks of lower extremity

Common complications of all nerve blocks include inadvertent intravascular injection, injury to nerve and nearby structures.

BLOCKS OF HEAD AND NECK

Nerve blocks of the head and neck have become less popular as safer methods of general anesthesia are available. Presently, main application of these blocks is in chronic pain setting and to aid awake intubation. The commonly performed blocks are:

Trigeminal Nerve Block

Trigeminal nerve through its three branches—the ophthalmic, maxillary and mandibular nerves, provides sensation to eye and forehead, mid face and upper jaw, lower jaw respectively. With the exception of motor fibers to the muscles of mastication, carried by the mandibular nerve, these nerves are wholly sensory.

Indications

Gasserian ganglion (ganglia of trigeminal nerve) block was indicated in the past for the diagnosis and treatment of trigeminal neuralgia. The ganglion is approached through foramen ovale. The safety and popularity of thermocoagulation for ablation of the ganglion have made this block virtually out of practice.

Blocks of the second and third division of the trigeminal nerve are occasionally used for diagnosis and management of chronic pain syndromes and for minor facial surgery in selective patient.

Technique

Both maxillary and mandibular branches can be blocked through single entry by a 22 G, 8 cm long needle. Needle is inserted at the inferior edge of coronoid notch till lateral pterygoid plate is encountered. Maxillary nerve is anterior to lateral pterygoid plate while mandibular nerve is located posteriorly.

Side Effects and Complications

- Hematoma formation
- Temporary blindness (after maxillary nerve block) due to spread of LA solution to optic nerve.
- Rarely, subarachnoid spread of LA may occur which can result in brainstem anesthesia.

Cervical Plexus Blockade (Figs. 21.1A and B)

Cervical plexus blocks include blockade of:
- Superficial cervical plexus which is derived from the C1, C2, C3 and C4 spinal nerves, supplies the prevertebral muscles, strap muscles of the neck and phrenic nerve.
- Deep cervical plexus, which supplies the musculature of neck and carries cutaneous sensation of the neck.

Indications

This block can provide anesthesia for surgical procedure in the distribution of C2 to C4, e.g., cervical lymph node dissection, superficial procedures of neck. It is specifically indicated in carotid endarterectomy as patient remains awake which allows continuous monitoring of neurologic status.

Bilateral block can be used for tracheostomy and thyroidectomy.

Technique

Superficial cervical plexus is blocked at the midpoint of the posterior border of the sternocleidomastoid muscle.

Deep cervical plexus can be blocked either by a single injection at the transverse process of fourth cervical vertebrae or by three separate injection over the transverse process of C2, C3 and C4.

Complications

- Blockade of phrenic and superior laryngeal nerve (SLN), if bilateral this can compromise respiration.
- Spread of LA solution into epidural and subarachnoid space.

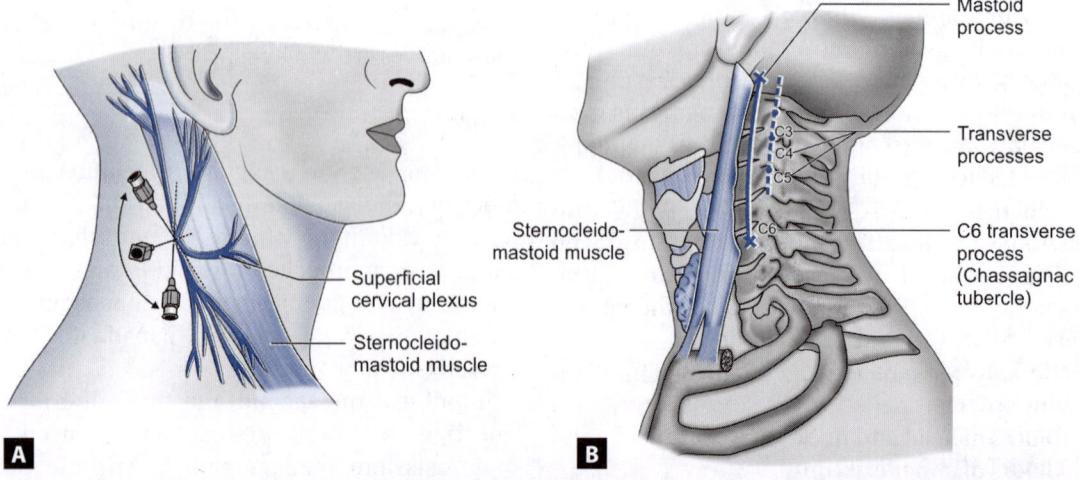

Figs. 21.1A and B: Cervical plexus blockade: (A) Superficial cervical plexus block; (B) Deep cervical plexus block.

Stellate Ganglion Block

A stellate ganglion is formed by the fusion of lower cervical and the first thoracic ganglion. Blockade of the stellate ganglion is used primarily for the treatment of upper extremity sympathetic dystrophy, so as to increase blood flow to the ischemic area.

Technique

Stellate ganglion is located anterior to the C6 transverse process (Chassaignac tubercle) which is the most prominent cervical transverse process. A 23 G needle is inserted perpendicular to skin after palpating Chassaignac tubercle, as needle strikes the tubercle, it is then withdrawn 3 mm and fixed. After careful aspiration, 8–12 mL of LA solution is injected. Signs of successful block^Q include Horner's syndrome (miosis, ptosis, enophthalmos)^Q conjuctival congestion, nasal stiffness (Guttman's sign), increased skin temperature, congestion of tympanic membrane (Mueller's syndrome) and anhydrosis over ipsilateral face and neck.

Side Effects and Complications

Due to close proximity of several neural and vascular structures, side effects and complications are common with this block. Complication includes:
- Hematoma formation
- Intrathecal or epidural injection
- Misplacement of needle in pleura which can lead to pneumothorax or pleural block
- Esophageal perforation
- Phrenic nerve block
- Brachial plexus block

Phrenic Nerve Block

Rarely indicated for intractable hiccups. Nerve is blocked just lateral to posterior border of sternomastoid at a point 3 cm above the midpoint of clavicle. Bilateral phrenic nerve block is contraindicated, as it may compromise respiration by paralyzing whole diaphragm.

LOCAL ANESTHESIA OF THE AIRWAY

Anesthetizing airway,^{Q} is the prerequisite for awake endotracheal intubation whether blind or fiberoptic guided.

Complete anesthesia of airway (oropharynx to trachea) requires topical application of LA to the oral and nasal mucosa, bilateral SLN block and translaryngeal injection of LA.

Superior Laryngeal Nerve Block (Fig. 21.2)

Superior laryngeal nerve lies behind thyrohyoid membrane. For block, the patient is placed supine with the neck extended. The hyoid bone is displaced laterally toward the side to be blocked, and a 25 G 2.5 cm needle is inserted perpendicular to skin of neck till it strikes greater cornu of hyoid bone. Needle is withdrawn slightly and walked off the greater cornu of the hyoid bone inferiorly and advanced 2–3 mm, as needle pierces thyrohyoid membrane a loss of resistance is felt. After negative aspiration, 3 mL of LA solution is injected. The block is then repeated on the opposite side. This block provides anesthesia from inferior aspect of epiglottis to the vocal cord.

Superior laryngeal nerve may also be blocked by application of lidocaine soaked gauze pads in piriform fossa (for at least a minute) through Krause angle forceps.

Translaryngeal block anesthetize the trachea below the vocal cord. With the patient in supine

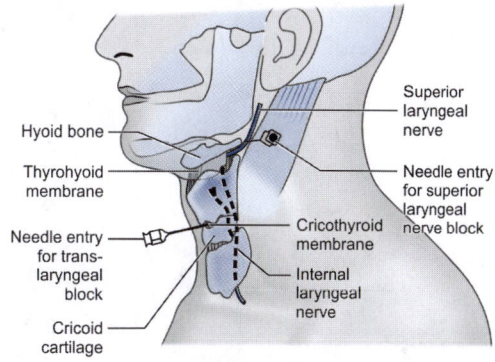

Fig. 21.2: Superior laryngeal nerve block and translaryngeal block.

position the cricothyroid membrane is located and a 20 G intravenous (IV) cannula is introduced in midline to pierce cricothyroid membrane. Inner steel stylet is withdrawn leaving catheter in place; aspiration of air confirms correct catheter placement. 2.5 mL of plain lignocaine solution is injected rapidly after full expiration. Injection is usually followed by vigorous cough which aids in spread of LA solution within the trachea. This block should be avoided in patients in whom coughing is undesirable.

BLOCKS OF UPPER EXTREMITY

Brachial plexus carries both sensory and motor supply to upper limb. So, surgical anesthesia of the upper extremity and shoulder can be obtained by neural blockade of brachial plexus (C5-T11) or its terminal branches.

Brachial Plexus Block

Brachial plexus block is the most commonly practiced peripheral nerve block. There are four approaches for blocking brachial plexus (**Figs. 21.3A and B**).

Interscalene Approach

Through this approach, blockade occurs at the level of upper and middle trunk. Blockade of inferior trunk (C8-T1) is often incomplete, thus ulnar nerve usually remains spared (a usual happening with this approach). Main application of this block is in shoulder and arm surgery.

Technique: Drug is injected through interscalene groove, which can be palpated easily posterolaterally to sternocleidomastoid.

Complications: Due to close proximity to vital structures, complication rate is high and is the reason because of which this approach is not practiced routinely. Common complications are:
- Ipsilateral phrenic nerve block (seen in all patients)
- Intravascular injection in carotid artery
- Horner's syndrome
- Intrathecal and epidural injection
- Severe hypotension and bradycardia (Bezold-Jarisch reflex)
- **Pneumothorax**: Though chances are low with this approach.

Supraclavicular Approach

This is the most commonly practiced approach. Through this approach blockade occurs at the level of distal trunk-proximal division.[Q] At this point, plexus is compact and a small volume of solution produces rapid and complete block.

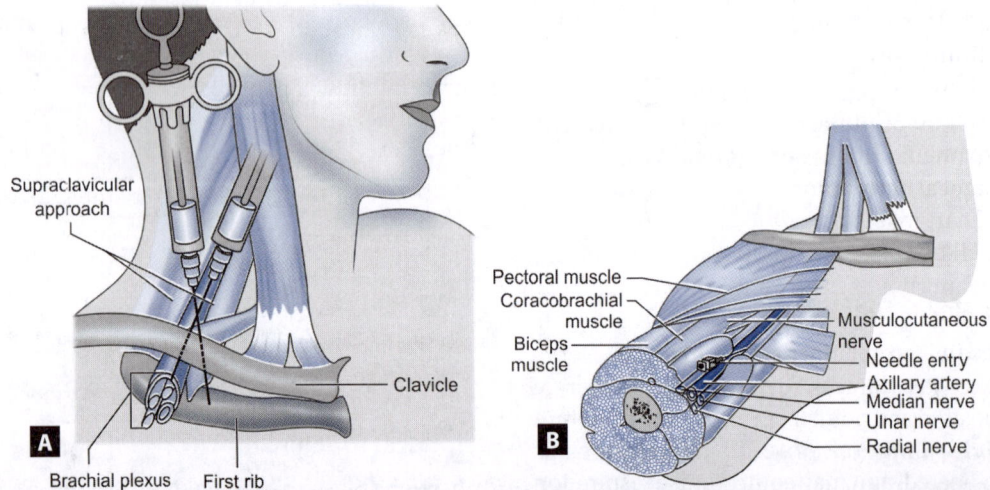

Figs. 21.3A and B: Brachial plexus block: (A) Supraclavicular approach; (B) Axillary approach.

Technique (Fig. 21.3A): Patient is positioned supine, with head turned away to the opposite side, the arm should be adducted. Supraclavicular pulsations of subclavian artery are identified. A 22 G needle is inserted 1 cm superior to clavicle just lateral to subclavian artery pulsation. Needle is advance in slightly medial, caudal and posterior direction, until paresthesia appears or first rib is encountered. If needle strikes first rib without elicitation of paresthesia, needle can be walked anteriorly and posteriorly along the rib until paresthesia appears. After eliciting paresthesia, 15–30 mL of LA solution is injected in incremental dose.

Complication: Pneumothorax: Incidence of pneumothorax is highest (1–6%) with this approach. In most cases pneumothorax are small and does not require any intervention. The best method of preventing pneumothorax is not to insert or direct needle too medially.

Horner's syndrome, hematoma formation, phrenic nerve block (40–60%) are other complications.

Infraclavicular Approach

This approach produce complete blockade of brachial plexus (similar to supraclavicular approach) with less chance of pneumothorax though chances of intravascular injection are more.[1]

Technique: Due to absence of perfect landmarks, nerve stimulator or ultrasound guidance is preferred to locate brachial plexus in infraclavicular area. Course of brachial plexus can be approximated by marking a line between C6 tubercle and axillary artery pulsation with the arm abducted. An insulated nerve stimulator needle is inserted 2 cm below the midpoint of clavicle and is advanced along the above mentioned line. After locating the plexus, 20–30 mL of LA solution is injected in incremental dose.

Axillary Approach

This is the second most commonly used approach, in this approach blockade occurs at the level of terminal nerves. Musculocutaneous nerve and intercostobrachial nerve usually remain spared through this approach and need to be blocked separately.

KEY POINTS

Branchial block approach	Level of blockade
Interscalene	Upper and middle trunk
Supraclavicular	Distal trunk, proximal division
Axillary	Terminal nerves

Indications: Indications for axillary block include surgery on the forearm and hand. Elbow procedures can also be successfully performed with the axillary approach. This approach is the ideal and most commonly used approach of brachial plexus block in pediatric patients and outpatients.^{Q} However, an axillary block is unsuitable for surgical procedures on the upper part of the arm or the shoulder, and the patient must be able to abduct the arm to perform the block.

Technique (Fig. 21.3B): Axillary artery pulsation is the landmark of this approach. With the arm abducted, the axillary artery is palpated, and a line is drawn tracing its course from the lower axilla as far proximally as possible. The artery is then fixed against the patient's humerus. Median nerve is superior to artery, ulnar nerve is inferior and radial nerve is posterior. These nerves can be blocked either by perivascular infiltration or transarterially.

Complication/disadvantages: Incomplete blockade is very common, and musculocutaneous and intercostobrachial nerve usually get spared.

Nerve injury and intravascular injection are the most prominent complications.

Note: This is the only approach of brachial block which possesses no risk of pneumothorax.

Peripheral Brachial Block

As the technique for brachial plexus block at root and trunk level is easy and provides complete blockade, indication for midhumeral and elbow block have diminished.

Wrist Block

Wrist block **(Figs. 21.4A and B)** can be used for surgical procedure of palm^Q which does not require tourniquets. Here median nerve is blocked between tendons of palmaris longus and flexor carpi radialis; for ulnar nerve blockade, drug is injected between pulsations of ulnar artery and flexure carpi ulnaris tendon. Radial nerve is blocked superficial to the tendon of externus pollicis longus (*which can be identified by asking the patient to extend the thumb*) additional 1 mL of LA is injected in the anatomic snuff box.

Intravenous Regional Anesthesia (Bier Block)

First described by German surgeon August Bier.^{Q}

Clinical Applications

Bier block has multiple advantages, including ease of administration, rapid onset (within 5 minutes), rapid recovery, muscle relaxation and controllable extent. It is indicated for short surgical procedures of extremities. Bier block in upper extremity is easier and more feasible than lower extremity Bier block.

Contraindications^Q

- Sickle cell disease
- Raynaud's disease
- Scleroderma
- Any condition that precludes the use of tourniquet.

Technique

An IV cannula is placed in the upper extremity to be blocked as far distally as possible (commonly on dorsal aspect of palm). A wide single or double tourniquet is applied proximal to the surgical site. After inflating the proximal tourniquet 150 mm Hg above systolic pressure; total dose of LA (3 mg/kg of 0.5% prilocaine or lidocaine, without epinephrine) is injected slowly. The onset of anesthesia usually occurs within 5 minutes.

Bupivacaine because of its high systemic toxicity is contraindicated in IV regional anesthesia.^{Q}

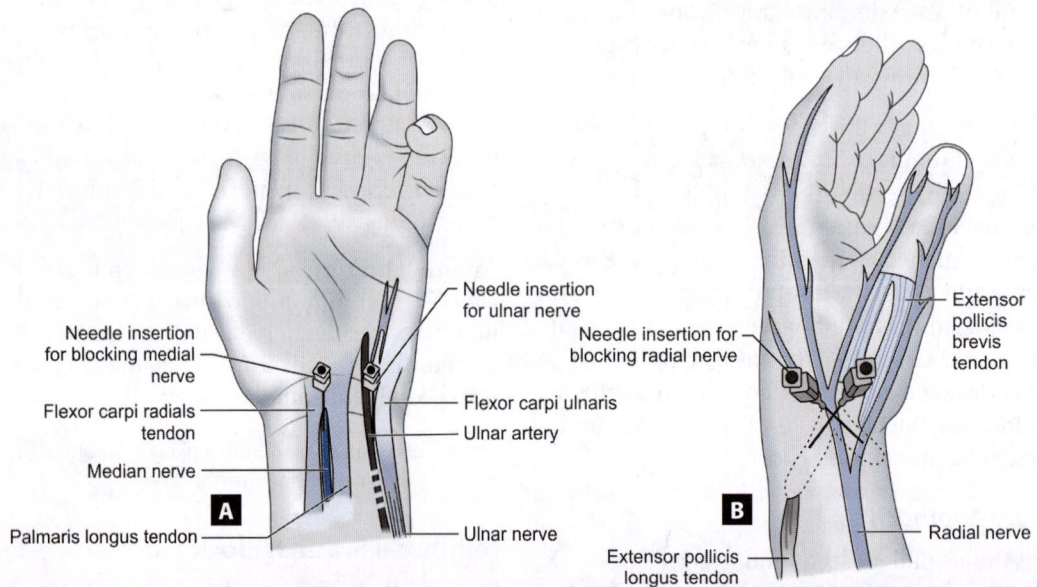

Figs. 21.4A and B: Wrist block (A) Anterior view; (B) Lateral view.

When the patient complains of tourniquet pain, the distal tourniquet, which overlies anesthetized skin is inflated and the proximal tourniquet is released. Proper tourniquet functioning is must for this block, as tourniquet failure or leak can cause systemic toxicity which may even progress to death. Use of a single wide cuff allows lower inflation pressures. The tourniquet may be safely released after 30 minutes of injection, but the patient should be closely observed for LA toxicity.

Complications and Side Effects

Common side effects include:
- Tourniquet discomfort, venous engorgement which increases surgical bleeding
- Rapid recovery leads to postoperative pain
- Tourniquet can, only be released after 30 minutes. Thus, if surgery is over before 30 minutes, tourniquet has to remain in place.

Bier block is associated with some serious complications also which limits its routine use:
- Accidental or early deflation of the tourniquet, transfers large doses of LAs into systemic circulation resulting in systemic toxicity which may even progress to death
- Compartment syndrome
- Tourniquet syndrome
- Tourniquet related nerve injury

BLOCKS OF THORAX AND ABDOMEN

Intercostal Nerve Blocks

Intercostal nerves are the primary rami of T1 through T11. Each intercostal nerve has four branches:
1. Gray ramus communicans, which passes anterior to the sympathetic ganglion.
2. Posterior cutaneous branch, which supplies the skin and muscle in the paravertebral area.
3. Lateral cutaneous branch, which sends subcutaneous branches anteriorly and posteriorly.
4. Anterior cutaneous branch, which is the termination of the nerve.

Though intercostal block provides anesthesia to thorax, the application of intercostal block has largely been supplanted by epidural block. In patient where thoracic epidural is contraindicated intercostal blocks are indicated for rib fractures, herpetic neuralgia, postoperative analgesia for thoracic surgery.

Technique

The intercostal nerve can be readily blocked at the angle of the rib just lateral to the sacrospinalis muscle group. Each intercostal nerve has to be blocked separately. 3–5 mL of LA solution is required per nerve.

Side Effects

- Pneumothorax
- As large volume of LA solution is being used and high vascularity of chest results in rapid absorption of LA in systemic circulation, chances of systemic toxicity are high.

Celiac Plexus Blocks

Celiac plexus (solar plexus) contains visceral afferent and efferent fibers derived from T5–T12 by means of greater-lesser and least splanchnic nerve. The plexus has provided autonomic supply to whole viscera. Its blockade reduces stress and endocrine response to surgery. The main application of this block is for pain relief in gastric and pancreatic malignancy. The plexus lies in close relation to the L1 vertebra. The left-sided ganglia are usually lower than those on the right.

Technique

Due to its deeper location, celiac plexus block is usually performed under CT guidance with the the patient in prone position.

Side Effects and Complications

- Immediately after celiac plexus block, there is postural hypotension due to blockade of lumbar sympathetic chain so, IV fluids should be administered prior to blockade and the patient should be advised to rest in lying down position.
- Intrathecal, epidural injection
- Retroperitoneal hematoma

- Pneumothorax, puncture of viscera, aortic perforation are rare but serious complications.

Ilioinguinal Block

Nerve supply of inguinal region is derived from iliohypogastric, ilioinguinal and genitofemoral nerve.

Indication of ilioinguinal block includes repair of inguinal hernia in elder poor-risk patient where central neuraxial blockade is risky, and for postoperative analgesia after hernia repair. Some surgeons use this block routinely for all cases of inguinal hernia, according to them, surgical bleeding is less when operation is being performed under ilioinguinal block.

Technique

- Ilioinguinal and iliohypogastric nerves are blocked by inserting needle 1 cm medial to anterior-superior iliac spine. Needle is advanced vertically downward until it pierces the aponeurosis of external oblique. After aspiration, 20-30 mL of diluted solution of LA is injected.
- Genitofemoral nerve is blocked 0.5 cm above the midinguinal point. After insertion, needle is advanced vertically downward until it pierces the aponeurosis of external oblique. After aspiration, 10-20 mL of diluted solution of LA is injected.

> **KEY POINTS**
> For some amount of local anesthetic injection of systemic concentration of local anesthetic raises most rapidly after intercostal block.

Complications

- Hematoma
- Femoral nerve block which can produce anesthesia of ipsilateral lower limb.

Penile Block

Nerve supply of penis is derived from the terminal branches of internal pudendal nerve (main), ilioinguinal nerve, genitofermoral nerve and perineal nerve. So, for penile surgery these four nerves have to be blocked.

Penile block is a satisfactory alternative to central neuraxial blockade for penile surgery like circumcision. In penile block, adrenaline is contraindicated as penile artery is an end artery and adrenaline containing LA can lead to penile necrosis by constricting penile artery.

Technique

A fan-shaped (triangular) field block with 10-15 mL of LA injected at the base of the penis and 2-4 cm lateral to the base on both sides of the penis.

BLOCKS OF LOWER EXTREMITY

Lower extremity blocks are not common as upper extremity blocks due to following reasons:
- Central, neuraxial blockade is easier and more feasible.
- Lower extremity derives nerve supply from two separate plexuses—lumbar plexus and sacral plexus.
- Unlike brachial plexus, there is no anatomic point where nerve supply of lower limb is clustered. Lower extremity block are indicated in high-risk patient where central neuraxial blocks are contraindicated or for postoperative analgesia. The commonly performed blocks are:

Psoas Compartment Block

Psoas compartment block results in blockade of lumbar plexus through single injection. This block provides anesthesia of the hip and anterolateral aspect of thigh.

Perivascular Three-in-One (Femoral) Nerve Block

Three-in-one block[Q] provides blockade of femoral nerve, lateral femoral cutaneous nerve, obturator nerve through single injection in femoral canal. Sciatic nerve always remains spared in this block.

Indications of this block include knee arthroscopy, surgical procedure of thigh and postoperative analgesia after knee surgery.

Modified Femoral (Fascial Iliaca) Nerve Block

This block is used in children for indications same as that of femoral nerve block.

Sciatic Nerve Block

Sciatic nerve provides cutaneous innervation to the posterior aspect of the thigh and whole of the leg. Sciatic nerve block, together with femoral nerve block can be used for any surgical procedure below the knee.

Sciatic nerve can be blocked through three approaches:
1. Classic (posterior) approach of Lobat
2. Subgluteal approach
3. Anterior approach.
As such indications are very few.

Ankle Block

Ankle block is an ideal block for surgery of foot that does not require tourniquet. The main limitation is the number of needle puncture required for this block. In ankle block, five nerves are blocked viz:
1. Posterior tibial nerve
2. Sural nerve
3. Deep peroneal nerve
4. Superficial peroneal
5. Saphenous nerve

This requires at least three needle punctures as shown in **Figures 21.5A and B**.

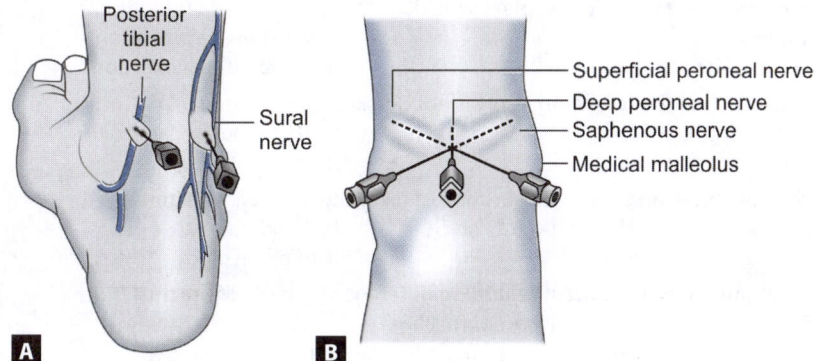

Figs. 21.5A and B: Needle Insertion for ankle block: (A) Posterior view (B) Anterior view.

LAST-MINUTE REVISION

- **Gasserian ganglion block**: Historic treatment of choice for trigeminal neuralgia (nowadays thermocoagulation is the treatment of choice).
- **Signs of successful stellate ganglion block**: Horner's syndrome, Guttman's sign, Mueller's syndrome
- **Anesthetizing airway**: Bilateral SLN block, translaryngeal injection of LA solution, topical applications over nasal and oral mucosa.
- **Brachial block**:
  - *Interscalene approach*: Spares ulnar nerve, best for shoulder surgery.
  - *Supraclavicular approach*: Maximum chance of pneumothorax, most common used approach.
  - *Axillary approach*: No chance of pneumothorax, but musculocutaneous, and intercostobrachial nerve usually remain spread.
  - *Three-in-one block*: Blocks femoral nerve, obturator nerve and lateral cutaneous nerve to thigh.

Unit IV: Regional Anesthesia: Techniques and Complications

REFERENCE

1. Gauss A, Tugtekin I, Georgieff M, Dinse-Lambracht A, Keipke D, Gorsewski G. Incidence of clinically symptomatic pneumothorax in ultrasound-guided infraclavicular and supraclavicular brachial plexus block. Anaesthesia. 2014;69(4):327-36.

REVIEW QUESTIONS

1. All of the following nerves need to be blocked for awake intubation, *except*:
   a. Facial nerve
   b. Glossopharyngeal nerve
   c. Superior laryngeal nerve
   d. Vagus nerve partially

2. Three-in-one femoral nerve blocks which of the following to nerve combination:
   a. Femoral nerve, sciatic nerve and obturator nerve
   b. Femoral nerve, lateral cutaneous nerve and obturator nerve
   c. Femoral nerve, sciatic nerve and common peroneal nerve
   d. Femoral nerve, lateral cutaneous nerve and sciatic nerve

3. Which of the following is not a sign of successful stellate ganglion block?
   a. Nasal stuffiness
   b. Guttman's sign
   c. Horner's syndrome
   d. Bradycardia

4. Most common complication of celiac plexus block:
   a. Pneumothorax
   b. Postural hypotension
   c. Retroperitoneal hemorrhage
   d. Intra-arterial injection

5. In ankle block which of the following nerve is not blocked:
   a. Sural nerve
   b. Deep perioneal nerve
   c. Saphenous nerve
   d. Sciatic nerve

6. From which of the following routes absorption of local anesthetic is maximum:
   a. Intercoastal
   b. Epidural
   c. Brachial block
   d. Caudal block

7. Following statement is not incorrect regarding different approach of brachial block:
   a. Pneumothorax is highest after axillary approach
   b. Supraclavicular approach usually spares musculocutaneous nerve
   c. Interscalene approach usually paralyze ipsilateral phrenic nerve
   d. Infraclavicular approach is associated with lesser chances of intravascular injection in comparison to supraclavicular approach

8. Contraindications for Bier block include all, *except*:
   a. Sickle cell anemia
   b. Megaloblastic anemia
   c. Raynaud's disease
   d. Surgery expected to last more than 3 hours

9. Anesthetic agent of choice for intravenous regional anesthesia of upper extremity:
   a. Prilocaine
   b. Bupivacaine
   c. Lignocaine
   d. Procaine

10. Adrenaline containing local anesthetics is contraindicated in:
    a. Wrist block
    b. Penile block
    c. Digital block
    d. Brachial plexus block

ANSWERS

1. a	2. B	3. d	4. b	5. d	6. a
7. c	8. b	9. c	10. b and c		

UNIT V
Anesthesia and Associated Diseases

Unit Outline

22. Anesthesia for Patients with Cardiovascular Disease
23. Anesthesia for Patients with Respiratory Disease
24. Anesthesia for Patients with Hematological Disorders
25. Anesthesia for Patients with Hepatobiliary Disorders
26. Anesthesia for Patients with Neuropsychiatric Disease
27. Anesthesia for Patients with Musculoskeletal Disease
28. Anesthesia for Patients with Endocrinal Disease
29. Anesthesia for Patients with Renal Disease
30. Anesthesia for Obese Patients

COMPETENCIES COVERED IN UNIT V

Competency Number	Competency Name	Chapter Number
AS6.3	Describe the common complications encountered by patients in the recovery room, their recognition and principles of management.	22-30
AS10.1	Enumerate the hazards of incorrect patient positioning.	30
AS10.2	Enumerate the hazards encountered in the perioperative period and steps/techniques taken to prevent them.	22-30

CHAPTER 22

Anesthesia for Patients with Cardiovascular Disease

Anshul Jain, Manish Kumar Singh

INTRODUCTION

Internationally, cardiovascular diseases are the most frequently encountered medical disease in anesthetic practice and are major cause of perioperative morbidity and mortality.

Broadly cardiovascular diseases are classified into:
1. Hypertension
2. Congenital heart disease
3. Valvular heart disease
4. Ischemic heart disease (IHD)

Risk Factors for Patients with Cardiac Disease (Box 22.1)

American Heart Association (AHA) has classified clinical markers of increased cardiovascular risk into major, intermediate, and minor predictors. Patients with major predictors require intensive management and should undergo noninvasive cardiac evaluation. These patients have enhanced risk for perioperative morbidity. The two most important risk factors are an unstable coronary syndrome and evidence of congestive heart failure (CHF).

SYSTEMIC HYPERTENSION

The current definition of hypertension (HTN) is systolic blood pressure (SBP) values of 130 mm Hg or more and/or diastolic blood pressure (DBP) >80 mm Hg[1] **(Table 22.1)**.

BOX 22.1

Markers of increased perioperative cardiovascular risk

Major
- Unstable coronary syndromes
- Acute or recent myocardial infarction (MI)
- Unstable or severe angina
- Decompensated heart failure
- Significant arrhythmias with uncontrolled ventricular rate
- High-grade atrioventricular block
- Severe valvular disease

Intermediate
- Mild angina pectoris (Canadian class I or II)
- Previous MI by history or pathological Q waves
- Compensated or prior heart failure
- Diabetes mellitus (particularly insulin-dependent)
- Renal insufficiency

Minor
- Advanced age
- Abnormal electrocardiogram (ECG) in an asymptomatic patient
- Rhythm other than sinus (e.g., atrial fibrillation)
- Low functional capacity
- History of stroke
- Uncontrolled systemic hypertension

Table 22.1: Stages of hypertension.

Classification	Systolic blood pressure	Diastolic blood pressure
Pressure	120–139	80–89
Normal	<120 mm Hg	<80 mm Hg
Elevated	120–129	<80 mm Hg
Stage 1	130–139	80–89
Stage 2	≥140	90

Anesthetic Management

Preoperative Evaluation

Goal is to determine the adequacy of BP control, and side effects of antihypertensive drug therapy. All patients should be rendered normotensive prior to elective surgery.

It is useful to review the pharmacology and potential side effects of the drugs being used for antihypertensive therapy. In addition to routine investigations, electrolytes are indicated in all cases.

Premedication

Premedication with anxiolytic agent such as midazolam reduces preoperative anxiety which is highly desirable in hypertensive patients.

Antihypertensive agents [except angiotensin-converting enzyme (ACE) inhibitors and angiotensin II antagonist] should be continued as per schedule and can be given with a small sip of water on the day of surgery. Current chapter deals with the anesthetic management of patients with common cardiovascular disease posted for noncardiac surgery.

Intraoperative Blood Pressure Management

Goal is to maintain an appropriate stable BP range. Arterial BP should generally be kept within 10–20% of preoperative levels. If marked hypertension (>180/120 mm Hg) is present preoperatively, arterial BP should be maintained in the high-normal range (150–140/90–80 mm Hg).

Choice of Anesthesia

General anesthesia is usually preferred as these patients show exaggerated hypotension after spinal and epidural anesthesia. Peripheral nerve blocks can also be used safely.

Induction

Induction of anesthesia carries risk of hemodynamic instability in hypertensive patients. Most hypertensive patients exhibit an accentuated hypotensive response *(due to depressant effects of inducing agents)* to induction followed by an exaggerated hypertensive response to intubation.

To reduce the hypertensive response following techniques are employed:
- Minimize the duration of laryngoscopy
- Deepening anesthesia with a potent volatile agent for 5–10 minutes
- Administering a bolus of an opioid (fentanyl, alfentanil, sufentanil, remifentanil)
- Administering lidocaine, 1.5 mg/kg intravenously or intratracheally
- Achieving alpha-adrenergic blockade with esmolol.

> **KEY POINTS**
>
> **Why hypertension is risky?**
> - It is a significant risk factor for the development of IHD and a predisposing factor for congestive heart failure, cerebral vascular accident (stroke), arterial aneurysm, and end-stage renal disease.
> - Hypertension by increasing afterload, increase myocardial oxygen demand.[Q]

Choice of Drugs

- **Induction agents**: Propofol, barbiturates, benzodiazepines, and etomidate are most suited. Ketamine is contraindicated[Q] because its sympathetic stimulation can precipitate marked hypertension.
- In opioids, sufentanil[Q] provide the greatest control over BP.
- **Muscle relaxants**: Except pancuronium[Q] (increases BP) all agents can be used. Agent of choice is vecuronium[Q] (due to its cardiac stability).
- **Vasopressors**: Patients in whom hypotensive response is very severe, vasopressor are indicated. Here direct-acting agent, such as phenylephrine is preferred over indirect one.

Monitoring

Properly controlled hypertensives require routine monitoring only. Direct intra-arterial pressure and pulmonary capillary wedge pressure monitoring should be reserved only for patients with uncontrolled BP and underlying severe cardiac disease.

In patients with renal impairment who are undergoing procedures expected to last more than 2 hours, urine output should be closely monitored.

Postoperative Management

Postoperative hypertension is common and BP monitoring should be continued in postoperative period.

For treatment labetalol^Q is the agent of choice when tachycardia is present while nicardipine is useful in controlling BP when heart rate is low.

ISCHEMIC HEART DISEASE

It is not uncommon to have a patient with history of myocardial infarction (MI) or angina posted for incidental surgery. These patients, due to their compromised cardiovascular status need special care. Elective surgery must be deferred for at least 6 weeks^Q following an acute MI or any other coronary intervention [angioplasty, percutaneous coronary intervention (PCI)].

Note: Previous recommendation of differing surgery for 6 months is not followed now.

In patients with IHD, morbidity is directly proportional to duration of surgery. If duration of surgery more than 3 hours, then chances of re-infarction increase significantly.

Anesthetic Management

Preoperative Evaluation

- Patients should be evaluated to find the functional cardiac reserve. Most of these patients are on some sort of medical treatment which decrease myocardial oxygen requirements and improve coronary blood flow. Commonly used drugs are beta-blockers, nitrates, antiplatelet drugs and ACE inhibitors.
- Effective beta-blockade is suggested by a resting heart rate of 50–60 beats per minute.
- Patients on ACE inhibitors show exaggerated hypotensive response to general anesthetics. So, many authorities recommend withdrawal of ACE inhibitors 24 hours before major surgical procedures.
- In addition to routine investigations transthoracic echocardiography to detect wall motion abnormality and ejection fraction is indicated in all cases. *Ejection fraction below 50% carries high risk.*

Choice of Anesthesia

General anesthesia is preferred over spinal anesthesia due to better hemodynamic control. Epidural and other peripheral nerve blocks can be used safely with adrenaline-free local anesthetic solution.

Perioperative Management

- Short-acting benzodiazepines are administered night before surgery to allay anxiety. Anticholinergic agents (atropine or glycopyrrolate) should be avoided.
- Goal is to avoid tachycardia and hypertension as both of them increase myocardial oxygen demand. Technique and drug choice are same as that in hypertensive patient. *In cases with severe IHD, opioid induction^Q is preferred.*
- Anesthesia is usually maintained on $O_2 + N_2O$ along with an opioid and/or volatile agent.
- Initial thinking that myocardial depression of volatile agents is deleterious in IHD patient is wrong. Volatile anesthetics decrease myocardial oxygen requirements and precondition the myocardium to tolerate ischemic events. *Desflurane less than 6% is the agent of choice^Q* (above 6% it produces sympathetic stimulation); although isoflurane can also be used safely, in fact isoflurane is the most commonly used volatile agent in cardiac patients.
- Heart rate should be maintained below 80 beats per minute. Hyperventilation must be avoided because hypocapnia constricts the coronary artery.
- Vecuronium (best), rocuronium, cisatracurium are the preferred muscle relaxant because of their minimal effect on heart rate and systemic BP.

Note: Halothane and ketamine are contraindicated in IHD patients.^Q

- The timing of tracheal extubation is extremely important *as most perioperative MI occurs immediately after extubation.*^Q Emergence from anesthesia and/or weaning is usually associated with an increased heart rate and BP. These hemodynamic alterations can precipitate MI. Beta-blocker or combined alpha and beta-blockers such as labetalol can reduce this hemodynamic alteration.

Monitoring

The goal is to detect ischemia before its clinical manifestation appears. Electrocardiogram (ECG) monitoring should be the integral part of monitoring.

Electrocardiography

It is the simplest and cost-effective method for detecting perioperative MI. Minimum two leads should be monitored *V5 is the best for detecting left ventricular (LV) ischemia,*^Q i.e., in the distribution of left anterior descending coronary artery, *lead II (LII) is ideal for detecting arrhythmias and ischemia in distribution of right coronary artery.*^Q Monitoring three leads improves the ability to detect ischemia. LII, V4 and V5 are the recommended three leads.

Modified Chest Lead V (CM5) is the single lead which can detect both arrhythmias and ischemia with equal sensitivity.

ST-segment depression or elevation of at least 1 mm with T-wave inversion suggests myocardial strain.^Q The degree of ST-segment depression is proportional to the severity of myocardial ischemia. Computerized ST-segment analysis improves diagnostic capability.

Echocardiography

Echo is more sensitive but less specific than ECG.^Q Regional wall motion abnormalities detected by echo occur before an ECG change appears and represent the first clinically detectable abnormality in perioperative period. Transesophageal echo is more sensitive than transthoracic echo.

Pulmonary Artery Pressure

In patients undergoing major surgery, central venous line with pulmonary artery catheter should be inserted. Intraoperative MI can manifest as an acute increase in pulmonary artery occlusion pressure due to changes in LV compliance and systolic performance. Beside this, pulmonary artery pressure can also be used as a guide to fluid replacement.

Intraoperative management of myocardial ischemia
Whenever there is 1-mm ST-segment changes on the ECG. Prompt, aggressive pharmacologic treatment of MI should be started on the following basis:
- **Tachycardia:** Intravenous (IV) esmolol
- **Hypertension:** Nitroglycerin
- **Hypotension:** Sympathomimetic drugs, fluid infusion
- **Unstable hemodynamics:** Inotropes ± intra-aortic balloon pump.

Intra-aortic balloon pump should be considered in ischemia refractory to medical treatment.

Postoperative Care

Prevent and treat myocardial ischemia or infarction, monitor for myocardial injury. Pain, hypoxemia, hypercarbia, sepsis increase myocardial oxygen demand, so should be avoided.

Continuous ECG monitoring is useful in detecting postoperative MI, as they are often silent.

VALVULAR HEART DISEASE

Mitral Stenosis

Mitral stenosis (MS) is the *most common valvular lesion* and is almost always rheumatic in origin. MS is characterized by progressive decrease in the mitral valve (MV) orifice. As valvular diameter decreases obstruction increases.

Pathophysiology

Mitral valve obstruction produces the increases in left atrial (LA) volumes and pressures, when severe this can lead to pulmonary hypertension and right ventricular failure (RVF).

As ventricular filling occurs in diastole, any event which decrease diastolic phase tends to decrease ventricular filling. So, slight reduction in heart rate is beneficial as this improves ventricular filling by increasing the diastolic period.

> **KEY POINTS**
>
> Area of normal MV is more than 4.0 cm². MS can be:
> - **Mild**: Mitral valve area is between 1 cm² and 2 cm²
> - **Critical**: Mitral valve area less than 1.0 cm²
>
> In critical, MS a transvalvular pressure gradient of 20 mm Hg is required to maintain normal cardiac output.

Anesthetic Management (Table 22.3)

The goals include maintenance of sinus rhythm and normovolemia (by judicious fluid therapy) with following precautions:
- Avoid tachycardia or rapid ventricular response rate during atrial fibrillation (AF).
- Avoid marked increases in central blood volume as associated with over infusion or head-down position. This may precipitate acute RVF.
- Avoid any abrupt decreases in systemic vascular resistance (SVR).
- Avoid events such as arterial hypoxemia or hypoventilation that may exacerbate pulmonary hypertension and can precipitate RVF.

Mitral Regurgitation

Mitral regurgitation (MR) can be acute or chronic. *Chronic MR is usually rheumatic in origin while acute MR is often seen after acute MI.* The principal derangement is a reduction in forward stroke volume due to backward flow of blood into the left atrium during systole.

This regurgitant fraction depends on:
- The size of the MV orifice
- Heart rate (systolic time)
- Pressure gradients across the MV.

A decrease in SVR or an increase in mean LA pressure will reduce the regurgitation and vice versa.

Patients with regurgitation fractions of more than 0.6% are considered to have severe MR.

Anesthetic Management

The goal is to avoid factors that exacerbate the regurgitation, such as slow heart rates (long systole) and an increased afterload. Bradycardia can increase the regurgitant volume by increasing LV end-diastolic volume and acutely dilating the mitral orifice. The heart rate should ideally be kept between 80 and 100 beats/minute. In severe MR, *magnitude of regurgitation flow should be continuously monitored with echocardiography and/or a pulmonary artery catheter.*

Spinal and epidural anesthesias are well tolerated, provided bradycardia is avoided.

Choice of Drugs

Isoflurane, desflurane, sevoflurane are volatile agents of choice while halothane is contra-indicated. Among IV agents, all except ketamine can be used. Pancuronium (if available) is the preferred muscle relaxant. Atracurium is the second choice.[Q]

Aortic Stenosis

Aortic stenosis (AS) results from degeneration and calcification of the aortic valve leaflets. Among all valvular lesions incidence of sudden death is highest in patients with AS.

Aortic stenosis is said to be critical if transvalvular pressure gradients is higher than 50 mm Hg and/or aortic valve orifice area less than 0.8 cm² (normal aortic valve area is 2.5–3.5 cm²).

Table 22.2: Choice of agents in mitral stenosis.

Class	Preferred	Avoided
Anticholinergics	Glycopyrrolate	Atropine
Opioid	Fentanyl morphine	Pethidine pentazocine
Inducing agent	Etomidate > propofol	Ketamine
Muscle relaxant	Vecuronium	Pancuronium
Volatile agent	Halothane	Desflurane >6%
Vasopressors	Phenylephrine	Ephedrine

Choice of Anesthesia

General anesthesia is usually preferred over spinal and epidural anesthesia as reduced preload in central neuraxial blockade can lead to severe hypotension. Further epidural is preferred over spinal anesthesia, when necessary. Peripheral nerve blocks can be used safely. Adrenaline containing local anesthetics should be avoided in peripheral nerve blocks.

Management of Anesthesia

Protocols of anesthetic management for noncardiac surgery are based on the following principles:
- Maintain normal sinus rhythm
- Avoid bradycardia
- Avoid sudden increases or decreases in SVR
- Optimize intravascular fluid volume to maintain venous return
- Preservation of normal sinus rhythm is critical because LV outflow is dependent on properly timed atrial contractions which ensure an optimal LV filling and stroke volume.

Marked increases in heart rate (>100/minute) can decrease the time for LV filling and ejection, whereas bradycardia (<60/minute) can acutely over distend LV.

Choice of Drugs

For induction *etomidate is drug of choice* in mild to moderate cases. In *severe AS, opioid based induction is preferred.* Among volatile agents halothane is relatively contraindicated.

Aortic Regurgitation

Aortic regurgitation (AR) results from disease of aortic leaflets or of aortic root that distorts the leaflets. Infective endocarditis and rheumatic fever are the most common cause.

The basic derangement in patients with AR is a decrease in forward LV stroke volume because part of the ejected stroke volume regurgitate back into the LV during diastole. The magnitude of the regurgitant volume depends on:
- The time available for regurgitant flow to occur, which is determined by heart rate.
- The pressure gradient across the aortic valve, which depends on SVR.

The magnitude of AR is decreased by tachycardia and peripheral vasodilatation and vice versa.

Management of Anesthesia

Goal is to maintain the forward LV stroke volume. Principles include:
- Avoid sudden decreases in heart rate.
- Avoid sudden increases in SVR.
- Minimize drug-induced myocardial depression.
- **General anesthesia** is preferred over spinal or epidural anesthesia as later may produce uncontrollable and unpredictable hypotension.
- **Induction** should be smooth *ketamine* may be advantageous by virtue of its ability to increase the heart rate, but it may cause excessive increase in SVR which is undesirable.
- **Succinylcholine** may cause bradycardia and should better be avoided. *Muscle relaxant* with minimal cardiovascular effect should be used.
- **Halothane** and **enflurane are** contraindicated as they may reduce stroke volume and cardiac output markedly. *Isoflurane is the preferred agent* due to its favorable hemodynamic effects.
- Sympathomimetic drugs can increase regurgitant fraction by increasing SVR, so they should be used with sensible precautions.

Tricuspid Regurgitation

Tricuspid regurgitation (TR) is usually functional, reflecting dilatation of right ventricle due to pulmonary hypertension.

Management of Anesthesia

The goal is to:
- **Maintain intravascular fluid volume** and **central venous pressure (CVP)** in high normal ranges to facilitate adequate RV stroke volume and LV filling.
- Avoid factors increasing pulmonary vascular resistance (PVR).

Intraoperative monitoring should include the measurement of right atrium (RA) filling pressures which acts as a guide for intravascular fluid replacement and detects the adverse effects of the anesthetic technique on the amount of TR.

Choice of Agents

A volatile anesthetic that could produce pulmonary vasodilatation should be preferred. *Ketamine* is useful by virtue of its ability to maintain venous return. N_2O increases pulmonary vascular resistance and should be avoided.

CONGENITAL HEART DISEASE

Due to better treatment increasing number of patients with congenital heart disease are being encountered for noncardiac surgery in later childhood or adulthood. Broadly congenital heart disease are classified into cyanotic and acyanotic heart disease.

In acyanotic heart disease, there are more chances of LV hypertrophy and congestive heart failure.

Patients with cyanotic heart disease have chronic hypoxemia which often results in erythrocytosis and hyperviscosity. Coagulation abnormalities are also common in patients with cyanotic heart disease.

Acyanotic Lesion

Atrial septal defect (ASD) is the most common congenital heart disease detected in adults. Anatomically, ASD is of two types: (1) ostium secundum and (2) ostium primum. Ostium secundum is common and mild form.

Ventricular septal defect (VSD) is the most common congenital cardiac abnormality in infants and children. In patent ductus arteriosus (PDA), there is moderate left-to-right shunt. If the left-to-right shunt is large, LV hypertrophy may be there.

KEY POINTS

Conditions where ketamine is inducing agent of choice:
- Tetralogy of Fallot
- Asthmatic patient

Anesthetic Management

Anesthetic protocols are common for ASD, VSD, PDA and include:
- Avoid any change in systemic or PVR during the perioperative period. Any increases in SVR or decrease in PVR would increase left-to-right shunt.
- High FIO_2 should be avoided as it will decrease PVR and will increase shunt. Decreases in SVR or increases in PVR due to positive-pressure ventilation of the lungs, tend to decrease the magnitude of the left-to-right shunt but marked increase in PVR can lead to reversal of shunt.
- Administer prophylactic antibiotics so as to prevent infective endocarditis.

Cyanotic Disease

Cyanotic heart diseases are characterized by a right-to-left intracardiac shunt which reduces pulmonary blood flow and leads to the development of arterial hypoxemia. This chronic arterial hypoxemia results in erythrocytosis. Patients with secondary erythrocytosis may exhibit defects in coagulation and platelet aggregation. Tetralogy of Fallot is the most common and prototype of these defects.

Management of Anesthesia

Principles for the management of anesthesia are same for all cyanotic congenital cardiac defects and include avoidance of all those events and drugs that can alter the magnitude of the right-to-left intracardiac shunt.

The magnitude of a right-to-left intracardiac shunt can be increased by:
- Decreased SVR
- Increased PVR
- Increased myocardial contractility

Out of these, it is SVR which is most variable and hence the magnitude of the shunt is inversely proportional to the SVR. Thus, drugs that decrease SVR (volatile anesthetics, propofol) can increase the magnitude of the right-to-left shunt and accentuate arterial hypoxemia.

Ketamine[Q] (as it increases SVR) is the inducing agent of choice. Among volatile agents desflurane and halothane (as they reduces contractility) are the agents of choice. Histamine-releasing muscle relaxants must be avoided, pancuronium[Q] (as it increases SVR) is the muscle relaxant of choice. N_2O must be avoided as it increases PVR.

The onset of action of IV agents is rapid in the presence of right-to-left shunts as first pass metabolism through lung is not there.

Crying in perioperative period must be prevented as this may precipitate hypercyanotic attacks.

Intravascular fluid volume must be maintained because acute hypovolemia can increase the magnitude of the right-to-left intracardiac shunt.

LAST-MINUTE REVISION

- **In hypertensive patient posted for surgery**, all antihypertensives should be continued except ACE inhibitors and angiotensin II antagonist.
- **In hypertensive patient, agents of choice are:** Etomidate, propofol, sufentanil, vecuronium.
- **Agents contraindicated are:** Ketamine, pethidine, pentazocine, pancuronium.
- **Valvular heart disease:**
  - **MS:** Heart rate should be kept toward lower side
  - **MR:** Heart rate should be kept toward higher sides
  - **AS:** Heart rate should be kept around preoperative value
- **For congenital heart disease:** Ketamine is induction agent of choice in cyanotic heart disease.

REFERENCE

1. Iqbal AM, Jamal SF. Essential hypertension. 2023 Jul 20. In: StatPearls [Internet]. Treasure Island (FL): StatPearls Publishing; 2023 Jan–. PMID: 30969681.

REVIEW QUESTIONS

1. A 30-year-old woman with coarctation of aorta is admitted to the labor room for elective cesarean section. Which of the following is the anesthesia technique of choice?
   a. Spinal anesthesia
   b. Epidural anesthesia
   c. General anesthesia
   d. Local anesthesia with nerve block

2. A 5-year-old child is suffering from cyanotic heart disease. He is planned for corrective surgery. The induction agent of the choice would be:
   a. Thiopentone
   b. Ketamine
   c. Halothane
   d. Midazolam

3. The most common cause of morbidity and mortality in patients undergoing major vascular surgery is:
   a. Renal complications
   b. Thromboembolic phenomenon
   c. Coagulopathies
   d. Cardiac complications

4. A patient of mitral stenosis has been posted for emergency cesarean section due to severe fetal distress. Which of the following agent needs to be avoided?
   a. Ketamine
   b. Etomidate
   c. Propofol
   d. Halothane

ANSWERS

1. c   2. b   3. d   4. a

CHAPTER 23

Anesthesia for Patients with Respiratory Disease

Anshul Jain

INTRODUCTION

Pulmonary dysfunction[Q] is the most common postoperative complication worldwide. The severity of perioperative pulmonary complication is directly proportional to the degree of pre-existing pulmonary dysfunction. *The two strongest predictors* are history of dyspnea and surgical site as thorax. Respiratory disease should be suspected in smokers and those with complaints of dyspnea or cough. Current chapter deals with the general principles of anesthesia in the patients with respiratory diseases.

GENERAL CONSIDERATIONS

Preoperative Evaluation

All patients with respiratory disease should undergo pulmonary function testing (PFT). Based on PFT findings, respiratory disease can be classified into obstructive or restrictive lung diseases. Chest radiograph is also mandatory in all cases.

Any complain of dyspnea has to be taken seriously and requires further evaluation. Dyspnea is graded according to the degree of physical activity that produces breathlessness **(Table 23.1)**.

🔑 KEY POINTS

Criteria suggestive of severe pulmonary disease
- Dyspnea grade ≥III
- FEV_1 <15 mL/kg
- PaO_2 <60 mm Hg, i.e., presence of hypoxemia or oxygen saturation <90% at room air

(FEV_1: forced expiratory volume in 1 second)

Preoperative Preparation

Preoperative preparation with respiratory disease revolves around five elements (5S):

1. **Stop smoking**: Though it takes weeks for full reversal of respiratory effects, abstinence for as short as 12–48 hours decrease carboxyhemoglobin level in blood **(Table 23.2)**.[1]
2. **Dilating the airways (relieve spasm)**: Patients with increased airways resistance [chronic obstructive pulmonary disease (COPD), asthma] are candidates for preoperative bronchodilator therapy. β_2-agonists are the preferred agents.
3. **Loosening the secretions**: In this third step, thick adherent secretions are loosened, so they can be coughed out. The most efficient and commonly used method is steam inhalation. Steam loosens the secretion by increasing the water content.

Table 23.1: Grading of dyspnea in terms of physical activity.

Category	Description
0	No dyspnea
I	Dyspnea while performing abnormal activity which a normal person can perform, e.g., running
II	Specific (street) block limitation ("I have to stop for a while after one or two blocks")
III	Dyspnea on mild exertion
IV	Dyspnea at rest

Table 23.2: Beneficial effects of smoking cessation and time course.

Time course	Beneficial effects
12–24 hours	Decreased blood carbon monoxide and nicotine level
48–72 hours	Normalization of carboxyhemoglobin Improvement of ciliary function
1–2 weeks	Decreased sputum production
4–6 weeks	Improved pulmonary function
6–8 weeks	Normalization of immune function and metabolism
8–12 weeks	Decreased overall postoperative morbidity and mortality

4. **Removing the secretions**: This can be accomplished by combination of postural drainage, coughing, percussion and vibrations.
5. **Support**: Rather neglected but very important aspect in respiratory patients.

Premedication

If patient is receiving bronchodilators or steroids, then they should be continued. Benzodiazepines and opioids are best avoided, as these patients are prone for respiratory depression.

Anticholinergics (atropine), by virtue of their bronchodilating properties, are usually administered.

Choice of Anesthesia

Regional anesthesia is preferred choice,[Q] provided, level of the block remains below T8. The block above T8 level can paralyze intercostal muscle, which may be detrimental in COPD patients, who depends on these muscles for expiration. *Epidural anesthesia* produces reflex bronchodilation and provides better control of postoperative pain, thus it is *preferred*[Q] over *spinal anesthesia*.

General anesthesia has got following disadvantages:
- Increased dead space and ventilation/perfusion (V/Q) mismatch
- Dry gases and all inhalational agents inhibit ciliary activity of respiratory tract
- All commonly used anesthetic agents produce respiratory depression of variable intensity.
- Respiratory drive of COPD patients depends on the high CO_2 level, thus any effort to produce normocapnia in these patients, can lead to apnea.

Wherever essential, the preferred drugs for general anesthesia are:
- **Inducing agents**: Ketamine[Q] more than propofol, because of their bronchodilating properties
- **Volatile agent**: Halothane (bronchodilation).
- **Muscle relaxants**: Vecuronium and rocuronium, as they do not release histamine.
- **Gases should be humidified before administration.**

Postoperative Care

Proper pain control carries highest priority. Pain particularly after upper abdominal surgery, compromises respiratory movements and impair ventilation, which can progress to atelectasis. Epidural analgesia is preferred for postoperative analgesia.

SPECIFIC DISEASE

Asthma

Preoperative Preparation

Active bronchospasm must be ruled out before any elective procedure. Patients who have been receiving long-term steroid therapy should be given supplemental doses (hydrocortisone 50–100 mg) to compensate adrenal suppression.

Intraoperative Management

The most critical time for asthmatic patient is during intubation. Asthmatic patients have irritable airway and any instrumentation (e.g., endotracheal tube insertion) can precipitate severe bronchospasm, that is why general anesthesia by mask or regional anesthesia is preferred, whenever possible.

Intraoperative bronchospasm can be treated by increasing the concentration of volatile agent and aerosolized β-adrenergic agonist.

Note: Though halothane is the preferred volatile agent, it should not be used in the patients receiving aminophylline, as halothane sensitizes the heart to arrhythmogenic effects of aminophylline.ᵠ Sevoflurane can be used safely.

Chronic Obstructive Pulmonary Disease

General guidelines are same as discussed earlier. Points of special interest are:
- Nitrous oxide is contraindicated in emphysematous patients with bullae. N_2O increases the size of bullae to such an extent that they may rupture, which can lead to pneumothorax.
- In contrary to the historic practice of using large tidal volumes, present guidelines recommend *small to moderate tidal volume*ᵠ *(10 mL/kg) with low respiratory rate*. This prevents air-trapping and allows more uniform distribution to gases. Arterial CO_2 measurement can be used to guide ventilation.
- **Permissive hypercapnia:**ᵠ COPD patient has hypercapnic respiratory drive means their respiratory center works only when CO_2 level is high in blood. So, it is recommended to keep their intraoperative CO_2 level same as their preoperative level which is usually above 40 mm Hg.

Restrictive Lung Disease

Preoperative Evaluation
Focus on determining the degree of pulmonary impairment. Vital capacity <15 mL/kg signifies severe dysfunction.

Intraoperative Management
Intraoperative management of restrictive lung disease patients is based on the following principles:
- The initial concentration of inhalational anesthetic should be kept low, as these patient exhibits accelerated uptake.
- As these patients are susceptible to oxygen toxicity, FiO_2 (fraction of inspired O_2) should be kept below 0.5.
- Ventilate the patient with a smaller tidal volume at rapid respiratory rate, so as to keep peak inspiratory pressure low. This is to avoid pneumothorax secondary to high peak inspiratory pressure.

Tuberculosis

The most commonly encountered respiratory disease in India is none other than pulmonary tuberculosis.

Anesthetic management of tubercular patients is based on following points:
- In case of active (open) pulmonary tuberculosis, elective surgery should be deferred and the patients should be treated with antituberculous therapy (ATT) (proved by three consecutive negative acid-fast bacilli samples).
- For the patient taking ATT, liver function test should be advised; chest X-ray is indicated in all patients to assess pulmonary damage and to rule out pleural effusion.
- Disposable equipment should be used for emergency surgery in an active case.

Respiratory Tract Infection

Concurrent respiratory tract infection (RTI) is the most common coexisting condition in pediatric patients posted for surgery.

Respiratory tract infection in patients undergoing surgery enhance the chances of:
- Bronchospasm
- Laryngospasm
- Postintubation croup
- Postoperative atelectasis

Guidelines for patients with RTI posted for surgery are as follows:
- In the patients with (any two of the following) active cough, fever, crepitation, dyspnea and rhonchi, postpone elective surgery for 6 weeks.
- Patients with only running nose and occasional cough can undergo elective surgery.

Unit V: Anesthesia and Associated Diseases

- All patients must be undertaken for life-saving surgery, irrespective of severity of RTI. Anesthetic management is based on following guidelines:
- Prefer regional anesthesia, wherever possible.
- In general anesthesia, LMA is preferred over endotracheal tube for airway management.
- Administer humidified gases.
- Among anesthetic agents, avoid thiopental, isoflurane and desflurane.

LAST-MINUTE REVISION

- Criteria suggestive of severe pulmonary disease (dyspnea ≥III grade, FEV_1 <15 mL/kg, PaO_2 <60 mm Hg).
- Regional anesthesia is preferred over general anesthesia.
- In asthmatic patients, ketamine is the induction agent of choice and halothane is the volatile agent of choice
- In emphysematous patient, N_2O is contraindicated.
- In respiratory tract infection, elective surgery is contraindicated for 4 weeks.

REFERENCE

1. Carrick MA, Robson JM, Thomas C. Smoking and anaesthesia. BJA Educ. 2019;19(1):1-6. doi: 10.1016/j.bjae.2018.09.005.

REVIEW QUESTIONS

1. During preoperative check-up, all of the following signifies severe of respiratory disease, *except*:
   a. FEV_1 <15 mL/kg
   b. Dyspnea on climbing stairs
   c. Oxygen saturation <90%
   d. Vital capacity <15 mL/kg
2. Drug of choice for administering anesthesia to an asthmatic patient, posted for exploratory laparotomy:
   a. Ketamine
   b. Propofol
   c. Thiopental
   d. Etomidate
3. All of the following drugs are contraindicated in the asthmatic patient, *except*:
   a. Sodium Pentothal
   b. Rapacuronium
   c. Propofol
   d. Pancuronium
4. Regarding anesthetic management of COPD patients, all of the following statements are correct, *except*:
   a. $PaCO_2$ is maintained around 45 mm Hg
   b. Anesthesia is maintained on N_2O, O_2 mixture in ratio of 2:1
   c. Halothane is preferred over isoflurane
   d. For lower limb surgery, epidural anesthesia can be used
5. Volatile agent of choice for status asthmaticus:
   a. Halothane
   b. Isoflurane
   c. Sevoflurane
   d. Enflurane
6. In the emphysematous patient with bullae, which of the following anesthetic agent is contraindicated?
   a. Nitrous oxide
   b. Propofol
   c. Etomidate
   d. Halothane
   (N_2O distends the air bullae and may rupture them)

ANSWERS

| 1. b | 2. a | 3. c | 4. b | 5. a | 6. a |

CHAPTER 24

Anesthesia for Patients with Hematological Disorders

Avtar Singh, Anshul Jain

INTRODUCTION

Hematological disorders ranges from highly prevalent iron deficiency anemia to rare genetic disorders like hemophilia that may remain hidden till surgery. In current chapter authors will discuss about the basic principles of anesthesia in a patient with hematological disorder posted for surgery.

ANEMIA

Anemia is the most common coexisting condition[Q] in surgical patients of India (in world it is hypertension). Anemia is usually defined as hemoglobin (Hb) concentration <11.5 g/dL in females and <12.5 g/dL in males. Anemia like fever is the sign of an underlying disease. In India, most common causes are iron deficiency and worm infestation.

> ### ★ KEY POINTS
>
> **Why anemia is dangerous?**
> Due to reduced hemoglobin, oxygen carrying capacity of blood decreases resulting in decreased tissue oxygen delivery. To compensate this reduced delivery cardiac output increases and oxygen dissociation curve shift to right. Increase cardiac output means increase myocardial oxygen requirement; this coupled with reduced blood oxygen content, render anemic patients susceptible to congestive cardiac failure and myocardial ischemia.

Preoperative Preparation[Q]

The goal is to optimize the Hb level and find out the cause of anemia. If anemia is due to blood loss begin (e.g., dysfunctional uterine bleeding) and surgery is the only treatment then patient should be taken for surgery irrespective of Hb level. Blood transfusion can be performed intraoperatively or postoperatively.

Historically, 10 g/dL is considered as minimum acceptable Hb concentration for patients posted for elective surgery. But recently Hb level of 7 g/dL (below which transfusion is mandatory) has been suggested as transfusion trigger by American Association of Blood Bank (**Table 24.1**).

If transfusion is indicated, then it should be performed atleast 24 hours before surgery.[1,2] Packed red cells should be preferred over whole blood.

Table 24.1: Indications and target of Intraoperative blood transfusion.

A. **Hemoglobin (g/dL) concentration**	
Trigger	• <6.0–≤7.5 without increased risk end-organ ischemia • <7.0–<10.0 with increased risk end-organ ischemia
Target	7.0–9.0
Other	Restrictive transfusion strategy may be safe, decision to transfuse between 6.0–10.0 is subjective
Transfusion contraindicated	>8.5–>10.0
B. **Hematocrit concentration**	
Trigger	<30%
C. **Blood loss**	
Trigger	≥1500 mL

Anesthetic Considerations

Principles of anesthetic management are:
- Avoid any drug that can reduce cardiac output.
- Avoid any event that produces leftward shift of dissociation curve, e.g., hypothermia, hyperventilation.
- Minimize surgical blood loss.
- Minimize surgical stress and acute sympathetic stimulation.

Note: Most dangerous period in anemia patients is immediately after extubation.

Maximum Allowable Blood Loss

In all surgical patients, it is essential to calculate maximum allowable blood loss (MABL). If blood loss exceed this value or hematocrit (Hct) is already <24, then perioperative transfusion is mandatory.

$$MABL = EBV \times \frac{Hcti - Hctt}{Hcti}$$

Hcti = Preoperative hematocrit
Hctt = Targeted hematocrit
EBV = Estimated blood volume

In patient with megaloblastic anemia due to vitamin B_{12} deficiency, nitrous oxide should be avoided, and if neurologic deficit is there, regional anesthetic techniques should also be avoided.

SICKLE CELL ANEMIA

In this condition, lifespan of red blood cell (RBC) is reduced. Anemia should be corrected preoperatively to a target Hct of 30%. Goal of anesthesia is to avoid any event that can lead to sickling crises[Q]:
- Hypoxia
- Dehydration
- Acidosis
- Hypothermia
- Stress
- Shock

Tourniquet produces local stasis, hypoxia, acidosis and may precipitate sickling crisis. Hence, tourniquet should be avoided (not contraindicated) unless benefit outweighs risk. IV regional anesthesia or Bier block (*which requires tourniquet*) is also contraindicated in sickle cell anemia.

PLATELET DISORDERS

Normal platelet count is 1.5–4.5 lakh/µL. Only 30,000–50,000/µL normal functioning platelets are required for adequate clotting.

A platelet count of atleast 30,000/µL[Q] is prerequisite for minor procedures like lumbar puncture, catheter insertion; while 80,000/µL is required for major surgery. In patients with platelet count below above-mentioned level, platelet transfusion is indicated **(Fig. 24.1).**

Bleeding time provides rough estimate of platelet count, however, it has not been found to predict bleeding risk with surgery.

For emergency surgery, when platelets are not available, *regional anesthesia is contraindicated; in general anesthesia, laryngoscopy must be non-traumatic.*[3]

KEY POINTS

1 µL = 1 mm³
1 Liter = 10^6 µL
1 Liter = 10 dL

COAGULATION FACTOR DISORDERS

Coagulation disorders can be hereditary, e.g., hemophilia or acquired which also include iatrogenic conditions.

Hereditary Conditions
Preoperative Evaluation

All patients with suspected coagulopathy should be advised activated partial thromboplastin time (APTT) and prothrombin time (PT) in addition to routine investigations.

Prothrombin Time

The PT assesses integrity of the extrinsic[Q] and common pathways of plasma-mediated hemostasis.

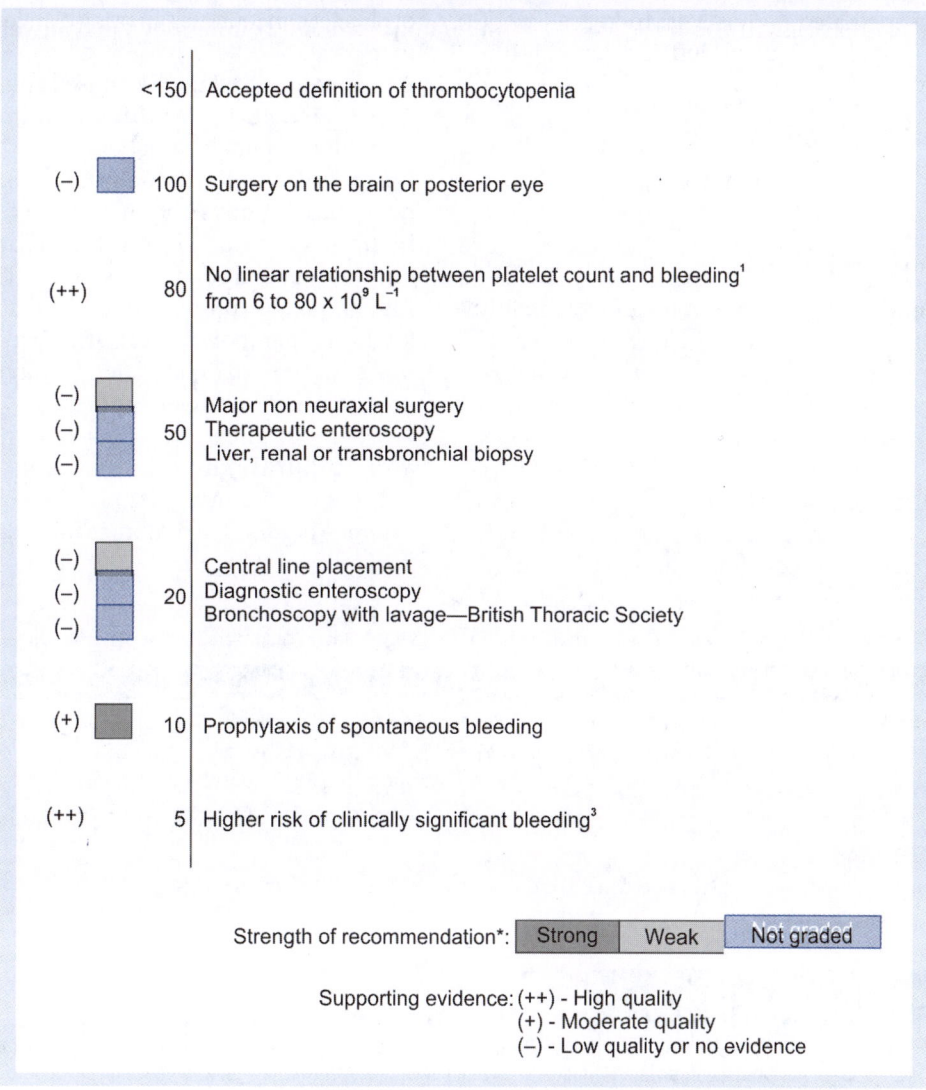

Fig. 24.1: Clinically significant platelet count thresholds in patients undergoing elective surgery or invasive procedures.

It measures time required in seconds for clot formation after mixing a sample of patient plasma with tissue factor (thromboplastin) and calcium.

There is wide variability among different laboratory, regarding normal ranges of APTT and PT, limiting the ability to compare results between laboratories. Due to this, international normalized ratio (INR) was introduced as a means of normalizing PT results among different laboratories. The INR is calculated as:

$$INR = \frac{Patient\ PT}{Standard\ PT\ of\ that\ laboratory}$$

Activated Partial Thromboplastin Time

Activated partial thromboplastin time assesses integrity of the intrinsic[Q] and common pathways of plasma-mediated hemostasis. Increased aPTT suggests coagulation factor deficiencies >30–40% of normal.

Anesthetic Considerations

Anesthetic considerations have been discussed in **Table 24.2**.

Iatrogenic Conditions

- **Patients taking aspirin**: Aspirin irreversibly inhibits cyclooxygenase, the enzyme essential for aggregation of platelet. Cyclooxygenase cannot be regenerated within the life span of platelet, so one aspirin tablet may affect platelet function for a week (turn over time of platelet). Thus aspirin should be stopped 7 days prior to major elective surgery. In situation, where it is not possible to wait; administration of 2–5 units of platelet concentrate can bring platelet function to normal.

  For patients taking low dose aspirin (< 650 mg/day), a 48-hour period is sufficient for normalizing platelet function.

- **Patients taking anticoagulants**: Stop anticoagulants 3 days[Q] before surgery, so as to bring INR <1.5. The oral anticoagulants can be resumed on postoperative day. An alternative approach in patient at high-risk for thromboembolism is to start heparin in place of warfarin; heparin can then be discontinued 4–6 hours before surgery.

  Regional anesthesia (particularly spinal and epidural) should only be used when INR is <1.5 as central neuraxial blockade can produce epidural hematoma which can lead to paraplegia.

Table 24.2: Perioperative management of commonly encountered coagulation disorders.

Coagulaton disorder	Postoperative management
Hemophilia A (defect in factor VIII)	Restore factor VIII level to 40% of normal prior to surgery. This can be accomplished by administering factor VIII as an initial bolus of 20 U/kg followed by 1.5 U/hr/kg. For dental extraction and tonsillectomy level should be restored to 100%
Hemophilia B (defect in factor IX)	Same guideline as hemophilia A, except follow-up dose in hemophilia B is 1 U/hr/kg
von Willebrand disease (defect in platelet function)	Desmopressin is the drug of choice. DDAVP stimulates release of vWF

LAST-MINUTE REVISION

In sickle cell anemia, Bier's block and tourniquets are contraindicated. Elective surgery are C/I when platelet count is <30,000/μL. For patients on aspirin an abstinence of 1 week is required prior to surgery, in case of low-dose aspirin, a 48-hour period is sufficient.

REFERENCES

1. Unal D, et al. Peri-operative blood transfusion in elective major surgery: incidence, indications and outcome-an observational multicentre study. Blood Transfus. 2020;18(4):261-279. doi:10.2450/2020.0011-20. PMID: 32697928; PMCID: PMC7375885.
2. Practice Guidelines for Perioperative Blood Management: An Updated Report by the American Society of Anesthesiologists Task Force on Perioperative Blood Management. Anesthesiology 2015; 122:241–275 doi: https://doi.org/10.1097/ALN.0000000000000463
3. Nagrebetsky A, et aL. Perioperative thrombocytopenia: evidence, evaluation, and emerging therapies. Br J Anaesth. 2019;122(1):19-31. doi: 10.1016/j.bja.2018.09.010. Epub 2018 Oct 25. PMID: 30579402.

Chapter 24: Anesthesia for Patients with Hematological Disorders

REVIEW QUESTIONS

1. Hemoglobin level below which patient would not be accepted for surgery:
   a. 8 g/dL
   b. 1 g/dL
   c. 12 g/dL
   d. No such dead line

   Note: If there is bleeding, surgery is the only option to control bleeding, In such a situation the patient can be accepted even at Hb level of 2 g% (e.g., bleeding hemorrhoids). Blood transfusion can be performed intraoperatively or in postoperative period.

2. Regarding aspirin and surgery, what holds true?
   a. Aspirin can be continued at the time of surgery
   b. Aspirin must be stopped 10 days before surgery
   c. Aspirin must be stopped 1 month before surgery
   d. Aspirin must be stopped 1 week before surgery

3. In sickle cell anemia, which anesthesia technique is contraindicated in a patient posted for surgery over wrist:
   a. Brachial plexus black
   b. General anesthesia
   c. Bier's block
   d. Axillary block

ANSWERS

1. d   2. a   3. c

CHAPTER 25

Anesthesia for Patients with Hepatobiliary Disorders

Anshul Jain

INTRODUCTION

Liver, the largest internal organ in the body, plays a crucial role in the homeostasis of many physiologic systems, including drug metabolism, synthesis of plasma proteins, and detoxification and elimination of many endogenous and exogenous substances.

Acute or chronic hepatobiliary dysfunction can impair the response to anesthesia and surgery in several critical ways. In addition to this certain anesthetics and hemodynamic disturbances can produce serious alterations in already compromised hepatic function. Current chapter provides the brief concepts of anesthetic management in a patient with hepatobiliary disorder.

EFFECT OF ANESTHETIC AGENTS ON HEPATIC FUNCTION

Volatile Agents

All volatile agents tend to decrease hepatic blood flow. Portal blood flow is affected more than hepatic arterial flow. Maximum reduction is seen with halothaneQ, while desflurane and sevoflurane have minimal effect. Thus, sevoflurane and desflurane are the most suited volatile agents for patients with hepatocellular disease **(Table 25.1)**.

Intravenous Anesthetics

Less information is available regarding the impact of intravenous anesthetics on hepatic function, etomidate and thiopental reduce hepatic blood flow, whereas ketamine has not much impact on hepatic blood flow. *PropofolQ tends to increase total hepatic blood flow by dilating splanchnic vesselsQ.*[1]

Table 25.1: Anesthetic drugs and their effects on hepatic function.

Anesthetic drug	Hepatic arterial blood flow	Portal venous blood flow	Total HBF
Halothane	↓	↓	↓↓
Isoflurane	–	↓	–/↓
Sevoflurane	↑/–	↓	–/↓
Desflurane	↑/–	↓	–/↓
Propofol	↑	↑	↑
Thiopentone	↓		↓
Ketamine	↑	–	↑

(HBF: hepatic blood flow)

Central Neuraxial Blockade

There is reduction in hepatic blood flow after high spinal and epidural anesthesia due to reductions in systemic arterial blood pressure. This reduction can be reversed by vasopressor drugs or fluid administration.

ANESTHETIC MANAGEMENT

Risk Assessment

Child-Pugh scoreQ is the gold standard for evaluating hepatic reserve in patient with liver disease **(Table 25.2)**.

Preoperative Considerations

In addition to routine investigations, all patients with hepatic disease should be assessed and managed accordingly for:
- **Liver function test**: Liver function tests are indicated in all cases.

Table 25.2: Child-Pugh criteria.

Factor	Units	1	2	3
Serum bilirubin	μmol/L	< 34	34–51	> 51
	mg/dL	< 2.0	2.0–3.0	> 3.0
Serum albumin	g/L	> 35	30–35	< 30
	g/dL	> 3.5	3.0–3.5	< 3.0
Prothrombin time	Seconds prolonged	0–4	4–6	> 6
	INR	< 1.7	1.7–2.3	> 2.3
Ascites		None	Easily controlled	Poorly controlled
Hepatic encephalopathy		None	Minimal	Advanced

(INR: international normalized ratio)

Note: The Child-Pugh score is calculated by adding the scores of the five factors and can range from 5 to 15. Child-Pugh class is either A (a score of 5–6), B (7–9), or C (10 or above). Decompensation indicates cirrhosis with a Child-Pugh score of 7 or more (Class B).

- **Coagulation abnormalities**: Due to defective synthesis of coagulation factors and decreased vitamin K absorption, all patients with liver disease should be presumed to have coagulation abnormality, until proven otherwise. Moreover, hepatic disease-associated coagulopathy can only be corrected by fresh-frozen plasma.
- **Cardiomyopathy**: In cirrhotic patients, the cardiac output is increased and is dependent upon above normal filling pressures and below normal systemic vascular resistance. So, these patients are poor tolerant of hypovolemia.
- **Renal functions**: The most severe expression of hepatic abnormalities is development of the hepatorenal syndrome. The hepatorenal syndrome is a functional renal defect in hepatic patient characterized by progressive oliguria hypernatremia, azotemia, intractable ascites, and a very high mortality rate.
- **Central nervous system manifestation**: Hepatic encephalopathy is characterized by alterations in mental status with fluctuating neurological signs and characteristic electroencephalographic changes (symmetric high-voltage, slow-wave activity). Precipitating factors include gastrointestinal bleeding, hypokalemic alkalosis (from vomiting or diuresis), infections, and worsening liver function. Encephalopathy should always be aggressively treated preoperatively by correcting precipitating factor. Sedatives should not be used in patients with encephalopathy.
- **Viral markers**: Elective surgery should be postponed in patients with acute hepatitis until its resolution, as indicated by normalization of liver tests. Presence of hepatitis B and C virus markers warrants extra precaution, to prevent their transmission to hospital staff and other patients.

Perioperative Considerations

Premedication

To minimize drug exposure, sedatives must be avoided in premedication.

Induction

Thiopentone or propofol for hemodynamically stable patient. For unstable patients, ketamine (or etomidate) is preferred. *Ramifentanil* is the most preferred opioid.

Maintenance

Anesthesia is maintained by air oxygen mixture along with a volatile agent. Desflurane is the preferred volatile agent. Cisatracurium is the muscle relaxant of choice for maintenance.

Monitoring

It depends upon patient's condition and surgical procedure. Unstable patients and/or lengthy procedures require invasive monitoring such as central venous pressure (CVP) and invasive blood pressure. These patients also require thromboelastography (monitoring of clot strength).

Perioperative Fluid

Glucose-containing fluids are preferred and lactated Ringer solution is avoided. Excessive crystalloids should be avoided. It is better to use colloids (preferably albumin) when excessive fluid is required.

Precautions

Following precautions are recommended in all cases with hepatic disease:
- **Avoid hypotension** as this can severely impair hepatic blood flow.
- **Avoid hyperventilation**: Hyperventilation can lead to alkalosis and can precipitate encephalopathy.
- **Maintain euglycemia**: Due to poor glycogen storage, and impaired gluconeogenesis, these patients are at risk for hypoglycemia.
- **Maintain urine output**: Any reduction in urine output or renal perfusion may precipitate hepatorenal syndrome.

Postoperative Care

Oxygen supplementation: Oxygen should be supplemented for 24 hours, as intrapulmonary shunting is increased after anesthesia.

BILIARY DISORDERS

Preoperative Considerations

These patients most commonly present for endoscopic retrograde cholangiopancreatography, and cholecystectomy. The cholecystectomy in these cases is usually performed laparoscopically, except in acalculous cholecystitis which usually occurs in critically ill patients and requires emergency operation.

Defective absorption of vitamin K (a fat soluble vitamin) in these patients may lead to vitamin K deficiency-associated coagulopathy. Vitamin K should be given parenterally which requires atleast 24 hour for effective response. Emergency surgery may necessitate administration of fresh frozen plasma.

Bile salts deposition on sinoatrial node may lead to bradycardia and other conduction abnormality, so electrocardiogram (ECG) is advised in all cases. High bilirubin increases the risk of postoperative renal failure also, so it is essential to maintain hydration.

Intraoperative Considerations

Biliary excreted drugs (vecuronium) show prolonged action and should be avoided. Agents dependent on renal elimination are preferable.

Monitoring

Routine laparoscopic cholecystectomy require only basic monitoring, i.e., ECG, noninvasive blood pressure, SpO_2. Patients with acalculous cholecystitis and those with severe cholangitis require invasive monitoring such as CVP and direct arterial blood pressure monitoring. Anesthetic management of laparoscopic surgeries has been discussed in detail in Chapter 37.

Postoperative Care

Same as that of patients with hepatocellular disease.

LAST-MINUTE REVISION

- All volatile agents reduce hepatic blood flow, maximum reduction is seen with halothane and least with desflurane.
- Agents of choice are volatile agent (desflurane); opioids (remifentanil); muscle relaxant (cisatracurium > atracurium).

REFERENCE

1. Carmichael FJ, Crawford MW, Khayyam N, Saldivia V. Effect of propofol infusion on splanchnic hemodynamics and liver oxygen consumption in the rat. A dose-response study. Anesthesiology. 1993;79(5):1051-60.

REVIEW QUESTIONS

1. Which of the following anesthetic agent increase hepatic blood flow?
   a. Halothane
   b. Propofol
   c. Thiopentone
   d. Morphine

2. In a patient of viral hepatitis which of the following agent should be avoided for anesthesia?
   a. Ketamine
   b. Halothane
   c. Propofol
   d. Etomidate

3. Volatile agent of choice in a patient with hepatic dysfunction:
   a. Halothane
   b. Isoflurane
   c. Enflurane
   d. Desflurane

4. Which of the following muscle relaxant is excreted through bile?
   a. Succinylcholine
   b. Vecuronium
   c. Atracurium
   d. Pancuronium

5. A patient suffered hepatitis after halothane administration now he is posted for laryngeal surgery. Which volatile agent is considered as safer for him?
   a. Isoflurane
   b. Desflurane
   c. Enflurane
   d. Sevoflurane

Note: Sevoflurane is a volatile agent of choice as it does not produce trifluoroacetic acid, the compound suppose to be associated with halothane hepatitis.

ANSWERS

1. b   2. b   3. d   4. b   5. d

CHAPTER 26

Anesthesia for Patients with Neuropsychiatric Disease

Anshul Jain, Keshav Goyal

INTRODUCTION

Patients with neuropsychiatric disease frequently present to the operating room for procedures unrelated to nervous system, e.g., an epileptic patient presenting for an incidental hernia surgery. Many of these patients are on medications which interact with anesthetics drugs, such patients need special care. In this chapter, we will discuss important neuropsychiatric disorders and their anesthetic considerations.

EPILEPSY

Epilepsy is characterized by recurrent, unprovoked seizures. Management of an epileptic patient posted for incidental surgery is based on following considerations:

Preoperative Considerations

Most anticonvulsants are hepatotoxic, so liver functions must be evaluated. Anticonvulsant therapy must be continued till the morning of surgery with usual doses and frequency, even in pregnant women.

Chronic anticonvulsant therapy induces hepatic enzymes; this increases the dose requirement of intravenous anesthetics and nondepolarizing neuromuscular blocking agents (NMBAs) and simultaneously increases the hepatotoxic potential of halothane.

KEY POINTS

Conditions where dose requirement of skeletal muscle relaxant increases:
- Burn
- Patient taking antiepileptics

Intraoperative Management

Anesthetic drugs with possible epileptogenic potential should be avoided, these include:
- **Induction agent**: Ketamine^Q and methohexital
- **Muscle relaxant**: Atracurium (due to its metabolite laudanosine)
- **Volatile agent**: Enflurane
- **Opioid**: Meperidine

Thiopentone^Q is the drug of choice for induction. Propofol^Q and etomidate^Q does not suppress epileptogenic foci, so they are the inducing agent of choice in patients posted for epileptic surgery.

CEREBROVASCULAR DISEASE

History of transient ischemic attacks (TIAs) or stroke signifies cerebrovascular disease. Cerebrovascular disease increases the risk of perioperative stroke. Risk is higher in patients undergoing neurologic and cardiovascular surgery. Following stroke elective procedures should be avoided for minimum of 6 weeks.

Preoperative Management

The type of stroke (thrombotic or hemorrhagic), presence of neurologic deficits and the extent of residual impairment should be determined and documented.

Most of these patients are on warfarin or antiplatelet therapy. Contrary to previous beliefs, low dose asprin and clopidogrel should be continued perioperatively.

Intraoperative Management

No single anesthetic technique is clearly superior to another. The goal of anesthetic management is to maintain blood pressure (BP) and glucose level close to their preoperative level. In general, any episode of severe hypotension or hypertension increases the risk of stroke, thrombotic or hemorrhagic, respectively.

DEGENERATIVE AND DEMYELINATING DISEASE

Parkinson's Disease

Parkinson's disease is characterized by bradykinesia, rigidity, postural instability and resting (pin-rolling) tremor. Treatment includes levodopa, anticholinergic agents, monoamine oxidase (MAO) inhibitors, amantadine (an antiviral drug) or a dopamine-receptor agonist.

Anesthetic Considerations

Antiparkinsonian drugs should be continued till the morning of surgery, as abrupt withdrawal of levodopa can worsen muscle rigidity and may interfere with ventilation. Phenothiazines and metoclopramide may exacerbate symptoms and should be avoided. Diphenhydramine is preferred for premedication and intraoperative sedation in patients with profound tremors.
- Chronic levodopa therapy depletes norepinephrine stores, which enhances the chances of orthostatic hypotension in these patients.
- Induction of general anesthesia in patients receiving long-term levodopa therapy can also produce hypotension or hypertension.
- Cardiac irritability readily leads to arrhythmias; so halothane, ketamine and local anesthetic solutions containing epinephrine are relatively contraindicated.
- Among muscle relaxants succinylcholine (SCh) can produce hyperkalemia, response to nondepolarizers remains normal.
- For treatment of hypotension direct-acting vasopressor are preferred.
- Therapeutic surgical intervention (thalamotomy or pallidotomy) are usually performed through awake craniotomy.

Alzheimer's Disease

Alzheimer's disease (AD), the most common neurodegenerative disease of geriatric patients, is characterized by progressive impairment of memory, judgment, decision-making and emotional liability. Treatment includes cholinesterase inhibitors which slow down the deterioration of mental status.

Anesthetic Considerations

Disorientation and noncooperation often complicates anesthetic management. Consent must be obtained from the legal guardian, if the patient is legally incompetent.

General anesthesia is usually preferred as these patients are not cooperative, which is the foremost requirement for regional anesthesia. Sedatives are avoided in premedication. Inhalation agents are preferred for induction of general anesthesia because of their rapid elimination. Glycopyrrolate, is the preferred anticholinergic as it does not cross blood-brain barrier.

Multiple Sclerosis

Multiple sclerosis is characterized by reversible demyelination primarily affecting patients between 20 years and 40 years of age, clinical manifestations include sensory disturbances (paresthesias), visual problems (optic neuritis and diplopia) and motor weakness.

Anesthetic Considerations

As stress of surgery and anesthesia might worsen the symptom, elective surgery should be avoided till patient improves completely. Spinal anesthesia can exacerbate the disease. Epidural and other regional techniques are safe. In general anesthesia, SCh is contraindicated because of the risk of hyperkalemia.

Importantly, irrespective of the technique, increases in body temperatures should be avoided, an increase of as little as 0.5°C may completely block conduction in the demyelinated fibers.

Guillain-Barré Syndrome

Guillain-Barré syndrome (GBS) is a relatively common disorder characterized by a sudden onset of ascending motor paralysis, areflexia and variable paresthesias.

Anesthetic considerations include respiratory complications, exaggerated hypotensive and hypertensive responses. In GBS, because of the reports which state the worsening of GBS after regional anesthesia, central neuraxial blocks are contraindicated. For general anesthesia, all drugs except SCh can be used.

PSYCHIATRIC DISORDERS

Depression

Depression, the most common psychiatric disorder, is distinguished from normal sadness and grief by the severity and duration of the mood disturbances.[1]

Anesthetic Considerations

Most of these patients are on antidepressant therapy in the form of tricyclic antidepressant (TCA), MAO inhibitors, etc. Antidepressant drugs are generally continued perioperatively. These drugs increase the requirement of anesthetic agents. TCA increase the response of both direct and indirect acting vasopressors and other sympathetic stimulants, so pancuronium, ketamine, meperidine and epinephrine containing local anesthetic solutions are avoided. Arrythmogenic potential of halothane is increased. For management of intraoperative hypotension, direct-acting vasopressor should be used in reduced doses.

The practice of discontinuing MAO inhibitors at least 2 weeks prior to elective surgery is controversial. Many authorities recommend their continuation. However, in patients receiving MAO inhibitors, opioids and halothane should be used cautiously as serious interactions have been reported. Most serious reactions are with meperidine,[Q] resulting in hyperthermia, seizures and coma. Rest protocols are similar to patients receiving TCA.

Mania

Mania is a mood disorder characterized by elation, hyperactivity and flight of ideas. Lithium, the most frequently used drug can produce diabetes insipidus, electrolyte disbalance.

Lithium prolong the duration of muscle relaxants, so neuromuscular function should be closely monitored. The other concern is the possibility of perioperative lithium toxicity. Sodium depletion can precipitate lithium toxicity. So, sodium-containing fluids should be administered and over diuresis has to be avoided.

Schizophrenia

Schizophrenia is one of the major psychotic disorder and is characterized by abnormal thought processes. If patient is on antipsychotic medication, drugs should be continued.

Many antipsychotics have sedative property, so dose of sedatives should be reduced. Ketamine is contraindicated in these patients, due to its vivid psychotic effects.

ANESTHESIA FOR ELECTROCONVULSIVE THERAPY

Electroconvulsive therapy (ECT) is indicated for treating severe depression or mania. The electric current produces a grand mal seizure consisting of a brief tonic phase followed by a more prolonged clonic phase.

Electroconvulsive therapy produces significant cardiovascular and central nervous system effects. Cardiovascular effects include initial bradycardia, and reduction in BP secondary to transiently increased parasympathetic activity. This is followed by sympathetic nervous system activation, resulting in tachycardia and hypertension lasting several minutes.

Anesthetic Management

Anesthesia for ECT must be brief. Atropine is the preferred anticholinergic which is administered 2 minutes before induction of anesthesia, so as to decrease salivation and bradycardia.

Methohexital[Q] (*induction agent of choice*) or Propofol (second preferred) is used to induce the patient. Succinylcholine (preferred due to its ultrashort action) is administered in doses of 0.3–0.5 mg/kg to attenuate the skeletal muscle contractions and to prevent bone fractures that can result from post-ECT seizure activity. Mivacurium is used in cases where SCh is contraindicated. Oxygen is supplemented till there is complete recovery.[2]

 LAST-MINUTE REVISION

- Epileptic drugs enhance the requirement of skeletal muscle relaxant.
- Lithium prolongs the duration of muscle relaxants.
- For ECT, methohexitone and thiopentone are the inducing agents of choice and SCh is the muscle relaxant of choice.

REFERENCES

1. Bains N, Abdijadid S. Major depressive disorder. [Updated 2022 Jun 1]. In: StatPearls [Internet]. Treasure Island (FL): StatPearls Publishing; 2022 Jan-. Available from: https://www.ncbi.nlm.nih.gov/books/NBK559078/
2. Reasoner J, Rondeau B. Anesthetic Considerations in electroconvulsive therapy. [Updated 2022 May 17]. In: StatPearls [Internet]. Treasure Island (FL): StatPearls Publishing; 2022 Jan-. Available from: https://www.ncbi.nlm.nih.gov/books/NBK576431/

REVIEW QUESTIONS

1. A. Assertion: Dose of nondepolarizing muscle relaxant is reduced in patients taking anticonvulsants.
   B. Reason: All anticonvulsants have got intrinsic property of relaxation, which potentiate nondepolarizing neuromuscular blocking:
   a. Both A and B are correct
   b. A is correct but B is wrong
   c. B is correct but A is wrong
   d. Both A and B are wrong
2. In electroconvulsive therapy which of the muscle relaxant is preferred?
   a. Atracurium
   b. Mivacurium
   c. Succinylcholine
   d. Pancuronium
3. A patient has been posted for hernia surgery. During preanesthetic check-up, it was found that he has got the history of epilepsy and last attack was 1 month back, presently he is taking phenytoin, regarding its anesthetic management which of the following statement is correct?
   a. Postpone the surgery for 2 months
   b. Ask him to take phenytoin even on the day of surgery
   c. Induce him with etomidate
   d. Dose requirement of vecuronium is reduced
4. Perioperative hyperthermia has got the most deleterious effect on:
   a. Parkinsonism
   b. Alzheimer disease
   c. Multiple sclerosis
   d. Guillain-Barré syndrome
5. Which of the following statement is correct regarding anesthetic management of patients with psychiatric disorders?
   a. Meperidine should be avoided in patients taking MAO inhibitors
   b. Duration of action of vecuronium is prolonged in patients taking lithium
   c. Ketamine should be avoided
   d. All of the above

ANSWERS

1. d   2. c   3. b   4. c   5. d

CHAPTER 27

Anesthesia for Patients with Musculoskeletal Disease

Keshav Goyal

Neuromuscular (NM) disorders though uncommon, challenge both perioperative management and intensive care because of their peculiar pathophysiology. Though rare one may encounter a patient with musculoskeletal disease for incidental and related surgery. Current chapter has been focused to the general anesthetic concepts and principles involved in the management of such patients.

MYASTHENIA GRAVIS

Myasthenia gravis (MG) the most important NM disorder is characterized by weakness and easy fatigability of skeletal muscle due to autoimmune destruction of postsynaptic acetylcholine receptors at the NM junction. About 10–15% cases of MG are associated with thymoma.

Patients with myasthenia may present for thymectomy or for unrelated surgical procedures. In all cases, patients should be assessed and treated accordingly preoperatively.

Preoperative Evaluation

These patients might have respiratory and oropharyngeal weakness which has to be assessed by pulmonary function test. Other autoimmune disorders (hypothyroidism, hyperthyroidism, rheumatoid arthritis) may be present, and should be ruled out.

Most of these patients are on anticholinesterase therapy. As a rule, patients must continue anticholinesterase medication even on the day of surgery.Q

These patients are very sensitive to respiratory depressants. Any drugs which can suppress ventilation should not be given preoperatively.

Patients with respiratory or bulbar involvement are at increased risk for pulmonary aspiration. So, aspiration prophylaxis should be undertaken in these cases.

Choice of Anesthesia

Whenever possible, regional anesthesia (peripheral or central neuraxial block) is preferred over general anesthesia.

Intraoperative Considerations

Induction

Propofol is a preferred intravenous agent; volatile induction can also be used. Deep anesthesia with a volatile agent alone may provide relaxation sufficient for tracheal intubation and surgical procedures. Succinylcholine can be used if needed but these patients need largerQ than normal doses because of the decreased number of functional acetylcholine receptors.

Maintenance

With the exception of muscle relaxant, standard maintenance (O_2 + N_2O + volatile agent) can be used. If essential then, a short acting nondepolarizing neuromuscular blockers (NDMB), like mivacuriumQ or cisatracuriumQ can be used. Long-acting nondepolarizers are strictly contraindicated.

Monitoring

Neuromuscular blockade should be monitored very closely along with routine monitoring. Interestingly NM monitoring with a peripheral nerve stimulator is not always reliable in MG patients. So, it is always better to avoid NDMB or if essential, use only small incremental doses.

Postoperative Care

Extubation should be performed only after ensuring full recovery. Postoperative mechanical ventilation is required in many cases.

LAMBERT–EATON MYASTHENIC SYNDROME

Lambert–Eaton myasthenic syndrome (LEMS) is a paraneoplastic syndrome characterized by proximal muscle weakness that typically begins in the lower extremities, but may involve upper limb, bulbar, and respiratory muscles. LEMS is usually associated with small cell carcinoma of the lung. Pathologically, LEMS is characterized by antibodies against voltage-gated calcium channels, this reduces the quantal release of acetylcholine at the motor end-plate. Thus, resulting in a presynaptic defect in NM transmission (in myasthenia syndrome defect is postsynaptic).

In these patients anticholinesterase are not much effective.

Anesthetic Considerations

Lambert–Eaton myasthenic syndrome patients are sensitive to both depolarizing and nondepolarizing muscle relaxants.^{Q} The response to other drugs used in anesthesia in usually normal.

Management protocol is same as that of myasthenia patient.

PERIODIC PARALYSIS (HYPERKALEMIC AND HYPOKALEMIC)

Both are genetically (autosomal dominant) transmitted disorders. Hyperkalemic periodic paralysis (HyperPP) is characterized by attacks of flaccid weakness associated with increased serum potassium. A potassium-rich meal or stressful situations may provoke the onset of paralysis.

In hypokalemic periodic paralysis, attacks are precipitated by a decrease in potassium levels in blood. The severity is usually greater hyperkalemic paralysis.

Anesthetic Considerations

Potassium, cholinesterase inhibitors, and depolarizing muscle relaxants aggravate paralysis in HyperPP patients. So, neostigmine and succinylcholine are contraindicated in HyperPP patients. Potassium-free maintenance fluids (e.g., DNS) are used.

Management of HypoPP patients should focus on avoiding events that produce hypokalemia.

MUSCULAR DYSTROPHIES

Duchenne's muscular dystrophy is the most common and most severe form of muscular dystrophy. Other major variants include Becker's, myotonic, limb-girdle dystrophies.

In Duchenne's muscular dystrophy, patients characteristically develop symmetric proximal muscle weakness and by age 12, most patients are confined to wheelchairs. Cardiac abnormalities are common.

Anesthetic Considerations

In patients of Duchenne and Becker's muscular dystrophy gastric emptying time is prolonged, which increases the risk for aspiration. So, aspiration prophylaxis should be taken in all cases.[1]

Preoperative premedication with sedatives or opioids is best avoided. Regional anesthesia is preferred wherever possible.

For general anesthesia total intravenous anesthesia^Q is preferred. Muscular dystrophies are associated with malignant hyperthermia, so all triggering agents are avoided. Sensitivity to NDMB is increased, so shorter-acting agents are used. Succinylcholine and volatile agents are contraindicated as they may precipitate cardiac arrest and malignant hyperthermia.

KEY POINTS

- Lambert-Eaton myasthenic syndrome versus myasthenia gravis
  - LEMS patients have depressed or absent reflexes, experience autonomic changes and characteristically have incremental rather than decremental responses (feature of myasthenia gravis) on repetitive nerve stimulation.
- Most common malignancy associated with LEMS: Small cell lung carcinoma.

Anesthetic Considerations in Myotonic Dystrophy

In myotonic dystrophy (most common muscular dystrophy in adults) succinylcholine is contraindicated[Q] as SCh can precipitate intense myotonic contractions; (trismus) making intubation and ventilation impossible. Other precipitating agents, include methohexital, etomidate, propofol, and neostigmine. Triggering factors for myotonic reactions are hypothermia, shivering, and mechanical or electrical stimulation. Treatment of myotonic reactions includes phenytoin (4–6 mg/kg/day) or quinine (0.3–1.5 g/day). It is better to use short-acting NDMB or avoid muscle relaxants.

Decreased ability to cough leading to the accumulation of oral secretions predisposes these patients to postoperative respiratory tract infections.

METABOLIC MYOPATHIES

Metabolic myopathies include glycogen storage disorders type I and type II. Glycogen storage disease type I is due to the defect in glucose-6-phosphatase, an enzyme that converts glucose 6-phosphate to glucose in the liver. Lysosomal acid alpha glucosidase is deficient in GSD type II.

Anesthetic Considerations

There is no special consideration in patients with GSD type I diseases except for the precaution to avoid lactate-containing solutions as these patients are not able to convert the lactic acid to glycogen.

GSD type II is more severe and these patients are always at risk for intraoperative cardiac failure. Succinylcholine is contraindicated because of its hyperkalemic potential. Halothane can precipitate cardiac arrest and should be avoided. Propofol by reducing afterload increases the risk of myocardial ischemia. Ketamine is preferred due to its ability to maintain SVR and contractility.

MALIGNANT HYPERTHERMIA

Malignant hyperthermia (MH) or malignant hyperpyrexia is a rare life-threatening condition that is usually triggered by exposure to certain drugs used for general anesthesia, specifically the volatile anesthetic agents and the NM blocking agent, succinylcholine. Exposure to the triggering agent can induce a drastic and uncontrolled increase in skeletal muscle which raises the body temperature and overwhelms the body's capacity to supply oxygen, removes carbon dioxide that eventually leads to circulatory collapse and death if not treated quickly.

Etiology

Malignant hyperthermia is inherited as an autosomal dominant disorder, for which there are at least six genetic loci, most prominently in the ryanodine receptor gene (RYR1). MH is associated with arthrogryposis multiplex, osteogenesis imperfecta,[Q] congenital ptosis and strabismus, kyphoscoliosis and Duchenne muscular dystrophy.

Pathophysiology

Malignant hyperthermia is a myopathy which remains subclinical until the patient is exposed to the triggering factors. On exposure to triggering factors there is acute loss of control over intracellular calcium. Normally immediately after muscle contraction Ca^{2+} is rapidly removed back from cytosol to bring down the concentration of

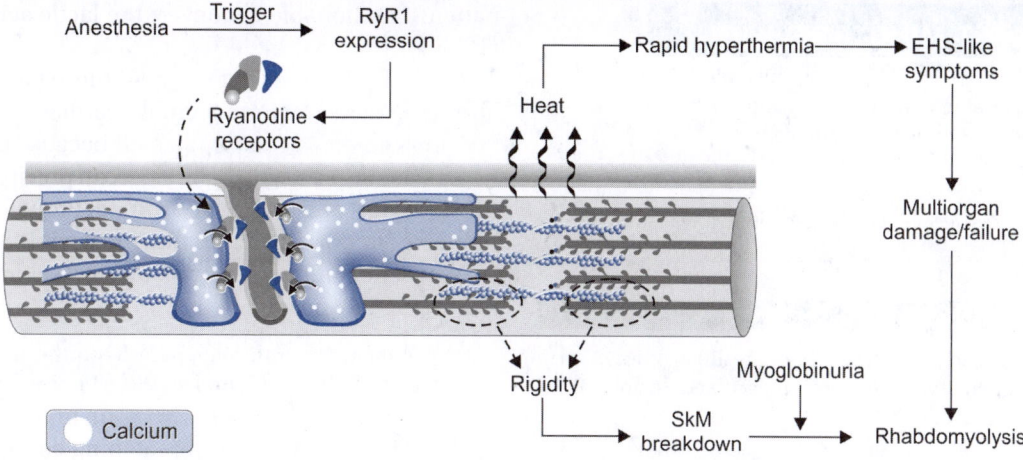

Fig. 27.1: Pathophysiology of heat production and rigidity in malignant hyperthermia.

intracellular calcium. As the cytosolic concentration of Ca^{2+} reaches below the threshold level, muscle relaxes. The rapid removal of Ca^{2+} is essential for normal muscle relaxation. In MH there is defect in RYR receptor, as a result of which intracellular Ca^{2+} remains high and muscle remains contracted. Further to maintain contraction energy is consumed and heat is produced, which increases body temperature **(Fig. 27.1)**.

Triggering Factors

- **Anesthetic drugs:** Halothane, enflurane, isoflurane, desflurane, sevoflurane. Desflurane and sevoflurane are less potent triggers. Nitrous oxide is also a weak trigger of MH.
- **Awake triggering:** Exercise, heat stroke, anoxia and excitement can trigger MH.

KEY POINTS

- **Fever:** AM temperature of >37.2° (98.9°F) or a PM temperature of >37.7°C (>99.9°F)
- **Hyperpyrexia:** A fever >41.5°C (>106.7°F)
- **Hyperthermia:** Uncontrolled increase in body temperature that exceeds the body ability to loose heat. Hyperthermia does not usually involve pyrogen.

Diagnosis

Perioperatively MH is defined by the rate of raise of temperature more than 1°C per 5 minutes after exposure to the agents which are known to trigger MH. Other features include muscle spasm, acidosis, hypercapnia.

Thyrotoxicosis and neuroleptic malignant syndromes are the most common differential diagnosis.

Intraoperative Management

- Withdraw volatile agent and ventilate patient with 100% oxygen.
- Dantrolene sodium[Q] is the drug of choice. Dantrolene reduces the calcium release from the sarcoplasmic reticulum. Dose is 1–2 mg/kg which may be increased up to 10 mg/kg.[2]
- Supportive measures like cold IV fluid, surface cooling.

Anesthesia in a Patient Susceptible to Malignant Hyperthermia

Regional anesthesia is preferred wherever possible. Total intravenous anesthesia using intravenous inducing agents, nondepolarizing muscle relaxants, opioid is safe alternative where regional anesthesia is not feasible.

LAST-MINUTE REVISION

Features common for all muscular disorders:
- **Contraindication**: Succinylcholine, halothane, long-acting nondepolarizers
- **Anesthetic agent of choice**:
  - *Volatile*: Isoflurane
  - *Intravenous*: Propofol
  - *Muscle relaxant*: Cisatacurium, mivacurium

REFERENCES

1. Lo Cascio CM, et al. Gastrointestinal dysfunction in patients with Duchenne muscular dystrophy. PLoS One. 2016;11: e016377.
2. Rosenberg H, et al. Malignant hyperthermia: a review. Orphanet J Rare Dis. 2015;10:93. doi: 10.1186/s13023-015-0310-1.

REVIEW QUESTIONS

1. Correct statement regarding anesthetic management of myasthenia gravis includes all, *except*:
   a. Dose of succinylcholine is enhanced
   b. Effect of nondepolarizing blockers is prolonged
   c. Chances of postoperative respiratory complications are high
   d. General anesthesia is preferred over regional anesthesia

2. Muscle relaxant that has to be avoided in myotonic dystrophy:
   a. Succinylcholine
   b. Mivacurium
   c. Doxacurium
   d. Atracurium

3. Agent causing malignant hyperthermia:
   a. Succinylcholine
   b. N_2O
   c. Ether
   d. Verapamil

4. Which anesthetic agent is contraindicated in a patient with family history of malignant hyperthermia?
   a. Propofol
   b. Succinylcholine
   c. Thiopentone
   d. Ether

5. Treatment of choice for a patient suspicious of having malignant hypothermia intraoperatively:
   a. Dantrolene
   b. Propofol
   c. Esmolol
   d. Halothane

ANSWERS

| 1. d | 2. a | 3. a | 4. b | 5. a |

CHAPTER 28

Anesthesia for Patients with Endocrinal Disease

Anshul Jain, Ashok Mittal

INTRODUCTION

Endocrinal disease dramatically affects the anesthetic management through multiple physiologic and pathologic changes. The common endocrine disorders (in order of decreasing prevalence) are diabetes, hypothyroidism, hyperthyroidism, Cushing's disease and pheochromocytoma. In current chapter we will discuss anesthetic management of patients with common endocrinal disorders posted for surgery.

DIABETES MELLITUS

It is characterized by impairment of carbohydrate and fat metabolism secondary to an absolute or relative deficiency of insulin or insulin responsiveness.

Diagnostic Criteria for Diabetes Mellitus (Adapted for American Diabetes Association)

- **Glycated hemoglobin (HbA1C) test:** It measures the percentage of blood sugar attached to hemoglobin. Doesn't require fasting, shows average blood sugar level for the past 2 to 3 months. HbA1C level of 6.5% or higher on two separate tests signifies diabetes. An A1C between 5.7% and 6.4% signifies prediabetes and below 5.7% is considered normal.
- **Random blood sugar test:** A blood sample will be taken at a random time irrespective of the last meal, a blood sugar level >200 mg/dL suggest diabetes.
- **Fasting blood sugar test (after 8 hour fasting):** A fasting blood sugar level >126 mg/dL on two separate test confirm diabetes. Level between 100–125 mg/dL (5.6–6.9 mmol/L) are diagnostic of prediabetes.
- **Oral glucose tolerance test:** After overnight fasting, first the fasting blood sugar level is measured. Then the patient is asked to have a sugary liquid, and blood sugar levels are tested regularly for the next two hours. A blood sugar level <140 mg/dL is normal. A reading of >200 mg/dL signifies diabetes and a reading between 140 and 199 mg/dL signifies prediabetes.

Preoperative Evaluation

The preoperative evaluation should emphasize the cardiovascular, renal, neurologic, and musculoskeletal systems **(Table 28.1)**. The presence of an autonomic neuropathy predisposes the patient to perioperative dysrhythmias, intraoperative hypotension, gastroparesis and hypoglycemia unawareness. Silent ischemia must be ruled out in patient with diabetic neuropathy **(Fig. 28.1)**.

Besides routine blood investigations, 12 lead electrocardiogram (ECG), chest X-ray, renal function tests are indicated in all cases.

Table 28.1: Complications of diabetes relevant to anesthesia.

Preoperative	Perioperative
Hypertension	Hypotension
Coronary artery disease	Bradycardia
Silent ischemia	Hyperglycemia
Joint immobility (difficult intubation)	Hypoglycemia (usually asymptomatic)
Effect of drugs	Myocardial ischemia (usually silent)
	Ketoacidosis
	Hyperglycemic hyperosmolar state

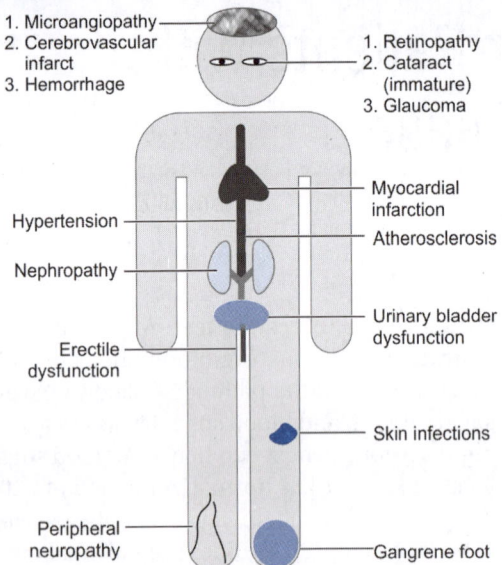

Fig. 28.1: Multisystem manifestation of diabetes.

"*Stiff joint syndrome (SJS)*" is a rare condition seen in long standing type 1 diabetes mellitus characterized by tight waxy skin and limited joint mobility or joint contractures. SJS initially affects the small joints of the digits and hands, involvement of the atlanto-occipital joint may prohibit proper extension of the neck making intubation difficult. Failure to approximate the palmar surfaces of the interphalangeal joints (*prayer sign*) is highly correlated with SJS.

> **KEY POINTS**
>
> **Why hyperglycemia is dangerous?**
> - It is associated with hyperosmolarity, infection, and poor wound healing. More importantly, it may worsen outcome following an episode of cerebral ischemia, acute myocardial infarction and compromise outcome following cardiac surgery.
> - Hyperosmolarity secondary to hyperglycemia leads to hyponatremia and its associated problems.

For patients on oral hypoglycemics, following protocol is followed:
- **Well-controlled type 2 diabetics posted for minor surgery:** Do not switch over to insulin, they can continue with their regular therapy.
- **Oral hypoglycemics**: Type 2 diabetes treatment has undergone major changes with the development of new drug classes. The perioperative management of these drugs depends upon the surgery, drug class **(Table 28.2)**.[2]
- Poorly controlled type 2 diabetics and all type 1 diabetics posted for minor surgery and all diabetics posted for major surgery need insulin.
- For major surgery, short duration crystalline insulin is preferred.

Blood sugar must be evaluated by bedside glucometers before anesthetizing the patient. It is wise to postpone, major elective surgery, if the plasma glucose is more than 270 mg/dL.[Q] If the serum glucose is >400 mg/dL, even minor surgery should be postponed.

Choice of Anesthesia

General anesthesia is usually preferred, except for minor surgeries which can be performed in low spinal block. In patients with autonomic and/or peripheral neuropathy spinal anesthesia is relatively contraindicated irrespective of type of surgery.

Anesthetic Management

The primary goal of perioperative management is to minimize hyperglycemia and avoid hypoglycemia. Due to delayed gastric emptying all diabetics must be considered full stomach.

In general anesthesia, all inducing agents except ketamine[Q] can be used. Ketamine by virtue of its sympathetic stimulating property raises blood sugar. Except historic volatile agents (trilene, ether, chloroform) all volatile agents can be used.

Both hypotension and hypertension may be seen perioperatively. Episodes of hypotension and bradycardia are usually unresponsive to atropine and respond only to adrenaline or isoprenaline.

Intraoperative Glycemic Control

There are several perioperative management regimens for diabetic patients. The most common method is to administer half of the total morning insulin dose in the form of intermediate-acting

Table 28.2: Perioperative management of oral hypoglycemics.

Class	Known mechanism of action	Generic name	Half-life	Day before ambulatory surgery	Minor or major surgery	Emergency surgery
Sulfonylurea	Stimulation of insulin secretion by inhibition of K-ATP channel, provoking calcium influx into the cell	Chlorpropamide Gliclazide Gliclazide MR Glimepiride Glyburide (glibenclamide)	36 h 10 h 16 h 5–9 h 10 h	Should be continued (attention to the time of surgery and fasting)	Stop the morning of the surgery and restart after food intake is resumed	Stop
Meglitinides	Stimulation of insulin secretion by inhibition of K-ATP channel, provoking calcium influx into the cell	Repaglinide	1 h	Should be continued (attention to the time of surgery and fasting)	Stop the morning of the surgery and restart after food intake is resumed	Stop
Biguanides	Inhibition of mitochondrial respiratory chain and activation of AMPK, reduction in hepatic gluconeogenesis and insulin resistance	Metformin Metformin XR	6–18 h 24 h	Should be continued (attention in case of contrast use and renal failure)	Restart after 24 h with stabilized renal	Stop
Thiazolidinediones	Enhanced insulin sensitivity by activation of PPAR γ	Pioglitazone Rosiglitazone	3–7 h 3–4 h	Should be continued	Should be continued	Stop
α glucosidase inhibitor	Inhibition of intestinal glucose absorption	Acarbose	2–4 h	Should be continued	Omit the dose if meal is skipped and restart after food intake is resumed	Stop
Dipeptidyl peptidase-4 inhibitors	Inhibition of GLP-1 degradation	Linagliptine Saxagliptine Sitagliptine Alogliptine	12 h 2.5 h 12 h 21 h	Should be continued	Should be continued	Stop
Sodium glucose cotransporter 2 inhibitors	Inhibition of renal glucose reabsorption, promoting glucosuria	Canaglifozin Dapagliflozin Empagliflozin Ertugliflozin	13 h 13 h 12 h 16 h	Should be continued	Stop the morning of the surgery and restart after food intake is resumed	Stop

(AMPK: 5' adenosine monophosphate-activated protein kinase; DDP4: dipeptidyl peptidase 4; GLP-1: glucagon-like peptide-1; K-ATP: potassium adenosine triphosphate; MR: modified release; PPAR: peroxisome proliferator-activated receptor; XR: extended release)

insulin provided blood sugar is ≥150 mg/dL. To decrease the risk of hypoglycemia, an infusion of 5% dextrose solution (1.5 mL/kg/hr) is started simultaneously. Supplemental dextrose can be administered if the patient becomes hypoglycemic (<100 mg/dL). Intraoperative hyperglycemia (>150–180 mg/dL) is treated with intravenous regular insulin according to a sliding scale.^{Q} According to which one unit of regular insulin given to an adult usually lowers plasma glucose by 25–30 mg/dL.

An alternative method is to administer regular insulin as a continuous infusion. The advantage is more precise control of insulin delivery. In this regimen 250 U of regular insulin can be added to 250 mL of normal saline and the infusion begun at 0.1 U/kg/hour. 20 mEq of KCl should be added to each liter of this fluid, as insulin causes an intracellular potassium shift. If blood sugar fluctuates, insulin infusion can be adjusted according to the following formula:

$$\text{Units per hour}^Q = \frac{\text{Plasma glucose (in mg/dL)}}{150}$$

Target for the intraoperative blood glucose level is 120–150 mg/dL for general surgery and 110–120 mg/dL for neurosurgery and cardiac surgery.

Monitoring

In addition to routine monitoring, plasma glucose level should be monitored frequently. In ECG monitoring, special attention should be paid to ST segment as diabetics are prone to silent ischemia, in fact silent myocardial ischemia is the most common cause of death in these patients.

Postoperative Care

ECG and glucose monitoring to be continued, supplemental oxygen may be administered.

THYROID DISORDERS

Thyroid gland secretes two hormones: triiodothyronine (T3) and thyroxine (T4). Although gland releases more T4 than T3, the later is more potent and less protein bound. Most T3 is formed peripherally through partial deiodination of T4.

Hypothyroidism

Hypothyroidism or myxedema is a relatively common disease affecting 0.5–0.8% of the adult population. In India also hypothyroidism is more common than hyperthyroidism. Clinical features suggestive of hypothyroidism include weight gain, cold intolerance, muscle fatigue, lethargy, constipation, hypoactive reflexes and depression. Diagnosis of primary hypothyroidism is confirmed by reduced levels of FT_4, FT_3 and an elevated TSH level.

Anesthetic Considerations

Preoperative

Severe hypothyroid patient should be rendered euthyroid prior to elective surgery. In patients with neck swelling indirect laryngoscopy, X-ray neck anteroposterior (AP) and lateral view should be advised to assess tracheal deviation and compression **(Figs. 28.2A and B)**. Under current practice CT scan is usually advised by ENT surgeon which supplant the use of X ray neck. One can estimate the exact tube size using the CT scan and also gets the information about the site of the narrowing, so as to place the tube distally to narrowing.

Choice of Anesthesia

Both regional and general anesthesia can be used. In regional anesthesia, intravascular volume should be maintained so as to prevent hypotension.

Premedication

- Avoid sedatives
- Administer aspiration prophylaxis (H_2 antagonists and metoclopramide)
- All patients should receive their usual dose of thyroid medication in the morning of surgery.

Intraoperative Management

- **Induction**: Hypothyroid patients are more susceptible to the hypotensive effect of anesthetic agents. *Ketamine because of its sympathetic stimulating property is induction*

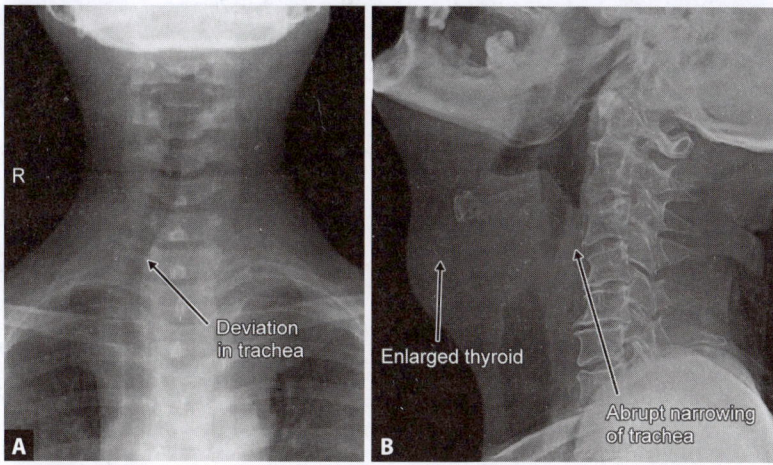

Figs. 28.2A and B: X-ray of neck: (A) anteroposterior view; (B) lateral view
Note: Tracheal deviation in AP view; tracheal compression in lateral view.

agent of choice.Q In patients with large goiter, awake fiberoptic-guided intubation is preferred.
- **Maintenance**: No specific recommendation. These patients are susceptible to cardiac depressant effects of volatile agents, so dose should be reduced.
- **Monitoring**: Besides routine monitoring, neuromuscular monitoring is indicated in all cases. CVP and invasive bold pressure (BP) monitoring are reserved for major surgery or patients with fluctuating thyroid function.

Postoperative Care

Recovery may be delayed in hypothyroid patients and patients should remain intubated until fully awake. For postoperative pain nonsteroidal anti-inflammatory drugs (NSAIDs) are preferred over opioids.

Hyperthyroidism

Patients with hyperthyroidism may come to OT for thyroid surgery, thymectomy, or more commonly for an incidental surgery.

Anesthetic Considerations
Preoperative

Elective surgery (including thyroid surgery) should be postponed till patient achieve euthyroid state. Preoperative preparation include normalization of thyroid function tests, with a goal to bring resting heart rate <85 beats/min. Antithyroid medications and beta-adrenergic antagonists are continued till the morning of surgery.

Premedication

- **Diazepam**: For preoperative sedation
- **Fentanyl**Q is the opioid of choice. Opioids producing sympathetic stimulation (*pentazocine, pethidine, butorphenol*) should be avoided.

> **KEY POINTS**
>
> **Problems of hypothyroidism relevant to anesthesia**
> - Swollen oral cavity, edematous vocal cords, or goitrous enlargement (airway compromise and difficult intubation).
> - Decreased gastric emptying (increased risk of regurgitation and aspiration).
> - Decreased cardiac output, stroke volume, heart rate, baroreceptor reflexes (increased risk of intraoperative hypotension and increased susceptibility to cardiac depressant anesthetic agents).
> - Reduced BMR (hypothermia occurs quickly and is difficult to treat).
> - Anemia, platelet and coagulation factor dysfunction (increased surgical bleeding).
> - Decreased neuromuscular excitability (increased potency and duration of neuromuscular blockers).
>
> (BMR: basal metabolic rate)

Choice of Anesthesia

Both regional and general anesthesia can be used. Nerve blocks are preferred wherever possible.

Intraoperative Management

- **Induction**: *Thiopental is the induction agent of choice as it possesses antithyroid property.* Ketamine, pancuronium, and other drugs that stimulate the sympathetic nervous system should be avoided because of the possibility of exaggerated elevations in BP and heart rate. Thyrotoxicosis is associated with myasthenia gravis, so neuromuscular blocking agent should be used cautiously. For managing intraoperative hypotension, a direct-acting vasopressor (phenylephrine) is preferred over indirect acting.
- **Monitoring**: Same as in hypothyroid patient.

Postoperative Management

There are several surgical complications which may be seen after thyroid surgery in postoperative period. Recurrent laryngeal nerve injury resulting in failure of one or both cords to move. Hematoma formation over surgical wound can cause severe airway obstruction secondary to tracheal collapse. Immediate opening of wound and sutures is the only treatment.

Unintentional removal or damage to blood supply of the parathyroid glands can cause acute hypocalcemia within 12–72 hours.

ADRENAL GLAND

Hypercortisolism (Cushing's Syndrome)

Cushing's syndrome can be due to excessive secretion of adrenocorticotropic hormone (ACTH) by pituitary (Cushing's disease) or excessive production of cortisol by abnormal adrenocortical tissues.

Anesthetic Considerations

The goal of anesthesia management is to prevent stress (including surgical stress) induced steroid release.

KEY POINTS

Thyroid storm
- The most severe problem in the perioperative period is thyroid storm, which is characterized by hyperpyrexia, tachycardia, altered consciousness and hypotension.
- Main differential diagnosis of thyroid storm is malignant hyperthermia (MH). Muscle rigidity, excessive hyperthermia, severe acidosis seen in MH are absent in thyroid storm.
- Treatment of thyroid storm includes maintenance of hydration, cooling, esmolol or IV propranolol for tachycardia, propylthiouracil orally or by nasogastric tube followed by sodium iodide and correction of any precipitating cause.

General anesthesia is preferred over regional anesthesia due to presence of vertebral body collapse, muscle weakness (even low spinal can compromise respiration).

Etomidate^Q is the inducing agent of choice as it transiently decreases the synthesis and release of cortisol by the adrenal cortex.

Adrenal Insufficiency

The most common cause of adrenal insufficiency (AI) is exogenous steroids. Steroids suppress pituitary adrenal axis and hence endogenous steroid secretion.

Management of Anesthesia

The goal is to ensure adequate steroid replacement therapy during the perioperative period. It is recommended to administer 100 mg of hydrocortisone phosphate every 8 hour beginning in the evening before or on the morning of surgery. There are no specific anesthetic agents and/or techniques for patients of adrenal insufficiency. Etomidate inhibits the synthesis of cortisol and is contraindicated.

PHEOCHROMOCYTOMA

Pheochromocytomas are catecholamine secreting tumors that arise from chromaffin cells of the sympathoadrenal system. Persistent or paroxysmal hypertension is the most frequent manifestation of the disease.

Anesthetic Considerations

Preoperative Preparation

Before surgery, medical treatment is advised to all patients with the goal of normotension, resolution of symptoms, elimination of ST-T changes and correction of arrhythmias. *Beta blocker phenoxybenzamine*^{Q} *is the drug of choice. Optimum duration of therapy is 2 weeks.*

Beta blockers are advised if there is tachycardia or other arrhythmias.

Note: A nonselective β-blocker should never be administered prior to α blockade as it may result in unopposed α-agonist, leading to vasoconstriction and hypertensive crises.

Intraoperative Management

The goal is to avoid any drug or maneuver that may potentiate catecholamine release.

Anesthetic drugs that appear safe include propofol, thiopental, etomidate, benzodiazepines, fentanyl, sufentanil, alfentanil, enflurane, isoflurane, nitrous oxide, vecuronium, and rocuronium. Drugs which should be avoided are atropine, pancuronium, succinylcholine, morphine, atracurium and halothane.

Sodium nitroprusside^Q *is the drug of choice for treating intraoperative hypertension.*

Hypotension following tumor vein ligation is a common occurrence. It is due to:
- Decrease in plasma catecholamines
- Residual effect of phenoxybenzamine
- Intraoperative fluid and blood loss.

To prevent this hypotension, it is recommended to administer fast fluid prior to tumor vein ligation. Lactated Ringer's solution or physiologic saline are the preferred fluids for this use.

Decrease in plasma catecholamines following resection increase insulin levels, this can produce hypoglycemia, so a dextrose-containing solution should be added after tumor resection.

Glucocorticoid therapy should be administered if bilateral adrenalectomy is performed.

Monitoring

Besides routine monitoring, arterial catheter, central venous pressure monitoring are indicated in all cases.

Postoperative Management

Hypotension is the most frequent cause of death in the immediate postoperative period. Large volumes of fluid are necessary to compensate sudden vasodilation after tumor resection. Patients usually remain in the intensive care unit for at least 24 hours.

LAST-MINUTE REVISION

- Ketamine is contraindicated in diabetics.
- **Insulin unit per hour is calculated as:** Plasma glucose/150
- Target for intraoperative blood glucose level is 120–150 mg/dL for general surgery and 110–120 mg/dL for neurosurgery.
- In hyperthyroid patient, thiopentone is drug of choice.
- In Cushing's syndrome, etomidate is drug of choice.

REFERENCES

1. Pippitt K, Li M, Gurgle HE. Diabetes mellitus: screening and diagnosis. Am Fam Physician. 2016;93(2):103-9. Erratum in: Am Fam Physician. 2016;94(7):533. PMID: 26926406.

2. Preiser JC, Provenzano B, Mongkolpun W, Halenarova K, Cnop M. Perioperative management of oral glucose-lowering drugs in the patient with type 2 diabetes. Anesthesiology. 2020; 133:430-38.

Unit V: Anesthesia and Associated Diseases

REVIEW QUESTIONS

1. Induction agent of choice in a hyperthyroid patient posted for thyroid surgery:
    a. Propofol
    b. Thiopentone
    c. Etomidate
    d. Ketamine

2. A patient aged 48 years had been posted for total hip replacement, He was a known diabetic, for which he was taking metformin, On the recommendation of medicine department he stopped metformin and insulin was started. On the day of surgery his blood glucose was 140 mg/dL in the morning. For surgery, combined spinal epidural (CSE) anesthesia was administered two hours after administration of CSE his blood sugar increased to 250 mg/dL. Which of the following statement is correct regarding his glycemic control?
    a. Start insulin at the rate of 1.25 IU/hour intravenously
    b. There is no need to take any action
    c. Administer metformin with a small sip of water
    d. Give 5 U bolus insulin followed by 2 IU/hour

3. A patient with hyperthyroidism, posted for thyroid surgery. Immediately after incision, his BP raises to 220/120 mm Hg. Differential diagnosis includes all, *except*:
    a. Thyroid storm
    b. Myxedemic coma
    c. Malignant hyperthemia
    d. Light plane of anesthesia

4. Agent of choice for controlling intraoperative hypertension in pheochromocytoma:
    a. Labetalol
    b. Sodium nitroprusside
    c. Nitroglycerine
    d. Esmolol

ANSWERS

1. b   2. a   3. b   4. b

CHAPTER 29

Anesthesia for Patients with Renal Disease

Anshul Jain

INTRODUCTION

The kidney is the principal organ involved in water conservation, electrolyte homeostasis and acid-base balance. Surgery and anesthesia can have important effects on renal function, this is particularly true in patients with pre-existing renal disease. Current chapter deals with the basic anesthetic considerations in a patient with renal disease posted for nonrenal surgery.

EFFECT OF ANESTHETIC AGENT ON RENAL PHYSIOLOGY

Volatile Agents

Methoxyflurane is associated with polyuric renal failure. Compound A, a product of sevoflurane is also toxic to kidney. So a fresh gas flow of at least 2 L/min is recommended with sevoflurane to prevent significant production of compound A.

Intravenous Agents

Propofol reduces glomerular filtration rate (GFR). Opioids and barbiturates have minimal effect on renal physiology when they are used alone. Whereas ketamine tends to preserve renal function during hemorrhagic hypovolemia.[1]

Direct Surgical Effects

There are certain surgical procedures that can significantly alter renal physiology. The pneumoperitoneum during laparoscopy can significantly reduce the renal perfusion. Other surgical procedures involving cross-clamping of the aorta or dissection near the renal arteries also reduce the renal perfusion.

EFFECT OF RENAL DISEASE ON ANESTHETIC AGENTS

Intravenous Agents

Patients with renal disease exhibit increased sensitivity to barbiturates during induction. Decreased protein binding in patients with hypoalbuminemia enhances the effects of etomidate and benzodiazepines.

The metabolites of morphine (morphine-6-glucuronide) and meperidine gets accumulated and prolong respiratory depression in some patients with renal failure.

The agents whose pharmacokinetics remains unaltered are propofol, ketamine, thiopentone, remifentanil, opioid agonist-antagonists (butorphanol, nalbuphine, and buprenorphine).

Inhalation Agents

Methoxyflurane, enflurane and sevoflurane (with <2 L/min gas flows) are considered undesirable in patients with renal disease because of their potential for fluoride accumulation. Desflurane[Q] is the volatile agent of choice in renal patients.

Muscle Relaxants

Succinylcholine[Q] is contraindicated when serum potassium is more than 5 mEq/L. Cisatracurium[Q] and atracurium are the relaxants of choice.[Q] Effect of vecuronium and rocuronium is prolonged. Pancuronium, pipecuronium, alcuronium and doxacurium are primarily dependent on renal excretion, so it is better to avoid these agents.

PREOPERATIVE CONSIDERATIONS

Preoperative evaluation of patients focuses on concomitant drug therapy and evaluation of systemic effects of renal failure, which includes:

Hematologic

Chronic renal failure (CRF) is associated with refractory anemia, i.e., this anemia is resistant to blood transfusion. Erythropoietin therapy can increase the hemoglobin level in these patients. Thrombocytopenia and other coagulopathies may be present which must be treated prior to elective surgery.

Cardiorespiratory

Pleural and pericardial effusion may be present. Hypertension, the most common systemic manifestation of CRF, should be treated appropriately.

Electrolytes

Renal failure is associated with hyperkalemia, hypernatremia, hypocalcemia, hypermagnesemia and acidosis. These abnormalities must be corrected prior to surgery.

Diabetes and liver diseases are commonly associated with renal disease, so they should be ruled out.

Preparation

Patients on hemodialysis should undergo dialysis during the 24 hours preceding elective surgery. It is recommended that the serum potassium should not exceed 5.5 mEq/L on the day of surgery. Antihypertensive drug therapy must be continued.

Premedication

Sedatives are avoided due to unexpectedly high sensitivity of these patients to central nervous system depressant drugs.

PERIOPERATIVE CONSIDERATIONS

Choice of Anesthesia

General anesthesia is usually preferred over regional anesthesia due to coexisting coagulopathies, anemia.

Induction

Any agent can be used in reduced dose; etomidate is preferred in hemodynamically unstable patients.

Nondepolarizing muscle relaxants are preferred over succinylcholine. Cisatracurium being the relaxant of choice.

Maintenance

Anesthesia is maintained by a short-acting opioid with isoflurane or desflurane (volatile agent of choice).

Fluid Therapy

- **5% dextrose**: Preferred fluid in non-diabetic patients undergoing minor surgery.
- Lactated Ringer's solution should be avoided in hyperkalemic patients as it contains potassium (4 mEq/L). Blood loss is replaced with packed red blood cells.

Monitoring

In addition to routine noninvasive monitoring, intra-arterial, central venous, and pulmonary artery pressure monitoring are often indicated in patients undergoing major procedures.

POSTOPERATIVE MANAGEMENT

Inadequate reversal is common and should be considered in anephric patients who show signs of skeletal muscle weakness in the postoperative period.

LAST-MINUTE REVISION

- **Nephrotoxic volatile anesthetic agent**: Methoxyflurane; sevoflurane.
- **Muscle relaxants contraindicated in renal failure**: Pipecuronium, pancuronium, doxacurium and gallamine.
- **Muscle relaxant of choice in renal failure**: Cisatracurium.
- **Fluid of choice**: 5% dextrose.

REFERENCE

1. Sahinovic MM, Struys MMRF, Absalom AR. Clinical pharmacokinetics and pharmacodynamics of propofol. Clin Pharmacokinet. 2018;57(12):1539-58.

REVIEW QUESTIONS

1. Muscle relaxant of choice for the patient of chronic renal failure posted for nephrolithotomy:
   a. Pancuronium
   b. Vecuronium
   c. Cisatracurium
   d. Atracurium

2. All of the following agents are nephrotoxic, *except*:
   a. Sevoflurane
   b. Methoxyflurane
   c. Pethidine
   d. Desflurane

3. Glomerular filtration rate is reduced by all anesthetic agents, *except*:
   a. Propofol
   b. Thiopentone
   c. Ketamine
   d. Etomidate

4. Opioid of choice for a patient with acute renal failure:
   a. Pethidine
   b. Morphine
   c. Butorphanol
   d. Cocaine

ANSWERS

1. c   2. d   3. c   4. c

CHAPTER 30

Anesthesia for Obese Patients

Sarvesh Kumar

INTRODUCTION

Obesity and its associated health concerns now represent major causes of morbidity and mortality. Previously obesity was considered a problem of developed countries, but now India ranks number one in the population of both obese and starved. In the current chapter, author will discuss basic principles of anesthetic management in an obese individual.

CLASSIFICATION

Most accepted classification of obesity is according to body mass index (BMI). BMI can be easily calculated by following formula:

$$BMI^Q = \frac{\text{Weight (in kg)}}{[\text{Height (in meter)}]^2}$$

Patient with BMI >40 are called as extreme obese (old-term morbid obese). Superobese is the newer term for patient with BMI > 50 **(Table 30.1)**.

Table 30.1: Categorization of obesity.

Classification	BMI (kg/m^2)
Underweight	<18.5
Normal weight	18.5–24.9
Over weight	25.0–29.9
Obese	
Class 1	30.0–34.9
Class 2	35.0–39.9
Class 3	40.0–49.9
Superobese	≥50

Obesity is associated with increased risk of many disease and leads to many deleterious effects. Obesity has got its maximum effects on respiratory system. Oxygen demand, CO_2 production, is increased because of increased tissue mass. Superimposed to this obesity reduce chest wall compliance, diaphragm movement, and lung volumes to the extent that person feels dyspnea in supine position **(Fig. 30.1)**.

Obesity Hypoventilation Syndrome (Pickwickian Syndrome)

A complication of extreme obesity, characterized by hypercapnia, cyanosis-induced polycythemia, right-sided heart failure, and somnolence. These patients are at higher risk for perioperative complications. Airway management might be difficult and postoperatively they may land in upper airway obstruction.

ANESTHETIC CONSIDERATIONS

Preoperative

Obese patients must be evaluated by an electrocardiogram (ECG), and pulmonary function tests in addition to routine evaluation to exclude hidden disease **(Table 30.2)**.

Intraoperative Considerations

Choice of Anesthesia

Obscured landmarks, difficult positioning, and extensive fat tissue make regional anesthesia very difficult. In addition to this it might be very difficult to intubate an obese person under

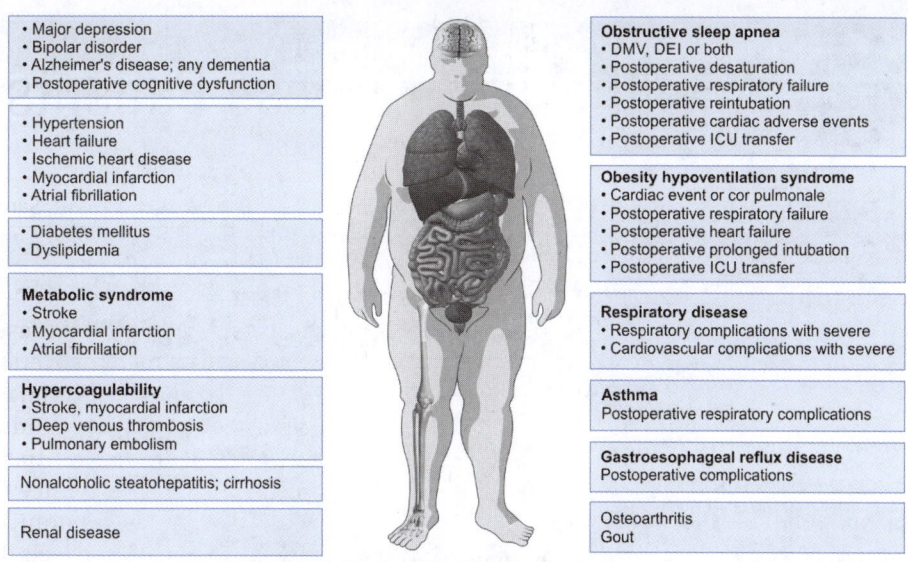

Fig. 30.1: Multisystem effect of obesity.

Table 30.2: Obesity: A multisystem problem.

Organ system	Associated disease and effects
Cardiovascular system	Hypertension, coronary artery disease, stroke, cardiac failure
Respiratory system	Obstructive sleep apnea, pulmonary hypertension, restrictive lung disease, reduced functional residual capacity, obesity hypoventilation syndrome (Pickwickian syndrome)
GIT	Hiatal hernia, gastroesophageal reflux, poor gastric emptying, and hyperacidic gastric fluid
Nervous system	Increased sensitivity to sedatives and anesthetic agents
Endocrinal system	Diabetes mellitus, metabolic syndrome (triad of obesity, hypertension, and type II diabetes)
Hepatobiliary system	Fatty liver, cholelithiasis

(GIT: gastrointestinal tract)

emergency situation, which may arise in regional anesthesia. So, *fully controlled general anesthesia is preferred mode of anesthesia in these patients.*

If airway appears to be difficult, awake fiberoptic guided intubation is strongly recommended. As breath sounds may be difficult to appreciate; successful endotracheal intubation is confirmed by detection CO_2 in expired air.

For short procedures regional anesthesia can be administered. It must be noted that obese patients require 20–25% less local anesthetic for epidural anesthesia **(Fig. 30.2)**.[1]

Anesthetic Drugs and Dosing

Obese patients show exaggerated response to opioids, propofol, and benzodiazepines. Short and rapid acting agents are preferred, thus propofol is induction agent of choice. In volatile agents desflurane (followed by sevoflurane) is agent of choice.

For fat-soluble drugs dose is calculated by actual body weight.

In contrast, for water-soluble drugs (rocuronium, propofol and remifentanil) dosing is based on ideal body weight to avoid overdosing.

ANESTHESIA FOR THE OBESE PATIENT: BMI >35 KG/M²

Preoperative Evaluation

S	Snoring: Do you snore loudly (louder than taking or heard through a closed door)?
T	Tired: Do you often feel tired fatigued or sleepy during the daytime?
O	Observed: Has anyone observed you stop breathing during your sleep?
P	Blood pressure: Do you have or are being treated for high blood pressure?
B	BMI: BMI >35 kg/m²
A	Age: Age >50
N	Neck: Neck circumference >40 cm (16 inches)
G	Gender: Male

Any of:
- Poor functional capacity
- Abnormal ECG
- Uncontrolled BP/IHD
- SpO_2 <94% on air
- If bicarb >28 OHS likely
- Previous DVT/PE
- stop-BANG >5

Yes →
Consider:
- Blood gases/sleep studies
- Preoperative CPAP
- Echocardiagram
- Cardiorespiratory referral

Need experienced anesthetic team
If major surgery consider HDU

No → May be suitable as day case surgery see below

Central obesity (waist >half height)
difficult airway/ventilation problems
more likely greater risk of CVS disease, thrombosis
↑ Risk of metabolic syndrome:
Central obesity plus hypertension
Dyslipidemia, insulin resistance

Most weight is:
Above the waist ←
Below the waist →

Peripheral obesity
(fat outside body cavity)
Less comorbidity

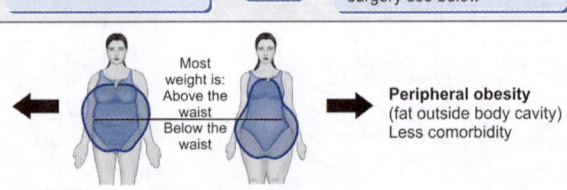

Apple body shape versus pear shape body

Intraoperative Management

Suggested equipment
- Suitable bed/trolley and operating table
- Gel padding, wide strapping, table extensions/arm boards
- Forearm cuff or large BP cuff
- Ramping device, step for anesthetist, difficult airway equipment, ventilator capable of PEEP and pressure modes. Hover mattress or equivalent
- Long spinal, regional and vascular needles
- Ultrasound machine.
- Depth of anesthesia and neuromuscular monitoring
- Enough staff to move patient

Ramping
Ear level with sternum. Reduces risk of difficult laryngoscopy, improves ventilation.

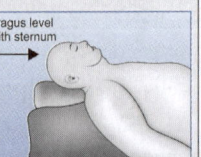

Tragus level with sternum

Anesthetic technique
- Consider premed antacid and analgesia, careful glucose control and DVT prophylaxis
- Self-position on operating table.
- Preoxygenate and intubate in ramped position +/– CPAP
- Minimize induction to ventilation interval to avoid desaturation. Commence maintenance anesthesia promptly
- Tracheal intubation is recommended.
- Avoid spontaneous ventilation. Use PEEP
- Use short-acting aents, e.g., desflurane or propofol infusion, short-acting opioids, multimodal analgesia PONV prophylaxis
- Ensure full NMB reversal
- Extubate and recover in head up position

Drug dosing—what weight to use?
Induction agents: Titrate to cardiac output—this equates to lean body weight in a fit patient.
Competitive muscle relaxants: use lean body weight.
Suxamethonium: Use total body weight
Neostigmine: Increase dose. Measure response
Opioids: Use lean body weight. Care with obstructive apnoea
TCI propofol: IBW plus 40% excess weight

If in doubt, titrate and monitor effect!

Lean body weight: This exceeds ideal body weight in the obese and plateaus = 100 kg for a man, = 70 kg for a woman.
Ideal body weight in Kg - Broca formula
Men: height in cm minus 100, Women: height in cm minus 105

Suggested dosing regimes for anesthetic drugs	
Lean Body Weight Up to Max: Males 100 kg, Females 70 kg	**Adjusted Body Weight** Ideal plus 40% excess
Propofol induction	Propofol Infusion
Thiopentone	Alfentanil
Fentanyl	Neostigmine (max 5 mg)
Rocuronium	Sugammadex (see package insert)
Atracurium	Antibiotics
Vecuronium	Low molecular weight heparin
Morphine	
Paracetamol	
Bupivacaine	
Lidocaine	

Postoperative Management

PACU discharge: Usual discharge criteria should be met. In addition, SpO_2 should be maintained at preoperative levels with minimal O_2 therapy, without evidence of hypoventilation.
OSA or obesity hypoventilation syndrome: Sit up. Avoid sedatives and postoperative opioids. Reinstate CPAP if using it preoperatively. Additional time in recovery is recommended, only discharge to the ward if free of apnoeas without stimulation. Patients untreated or intolerant of CPAP who require postoperative opioids are at risk of hypoventilation and require continuous oxygen saturation monitoring. Level 2 care is recommended. Effective CPAP reduces this risk to near normal.
Ward care: Escalation to Level 1, 2 or 3 care may be required based on patient comorbidity, the type of surgery undertaken and issues with hypoventilation discussed above. General ward care includes: multimodal analgesia, caution with long-acting opioids and sedatives, early mobilization and extended thromboprophylaxis.

Fig. 30.2: Summary guidelines: Perioperative management of an obese patient.

Positioning

Positioning is particularly important in obese patient as excessive pressure on weight-bearing points can lead to tissue necrosis. All pressure points must be carefully padded.

Postoperative Care

Supplemental oxygen should be provided to all. Semisitting position improve ventilation and oxygenation. Other common postoperative complications in obese patients include wound infection, deep venous thrombosis, and pulmonary embolism.

LAST-MINUTE REVISION

- **Technique of choice**: General anesthesia
- **Drug of choice**: Propofol, sevoflurane
- **Super obese**: BMI ≥50.

REFERENCE

1. Panni MK, Columb MO. Obese parturients have lower epidural local anaesthetic requirements for analgesia in labour. Br J Anaesth. 2006 Jan;96(1):106-10. doi: 10.1093/bja/aei284.

REVIEW QUESTIONS

1. Dose requirement of following anesthetics decrease in obese patient, *except*:
   a. Propofol
   b. Thiopentone
   c. Atracurium
   d. Rocuronium
2. "Morbid" obese is a term used for patients with body mass index:
   a. >20
   b. >30
   c. >40
   d. >50
3. True about anesthetic management of obese person includes all, *except*:
   a. Regional techniques are difficult
   b. Dose of many intravenous agent are reduced
   c. Intubation is difficult
   d. Proseal LMA cannot be used

ANSWERS

1. c   2. c   3. d

UNIT VI

Anesthesia Practice

Unit Outline

31. Anesthesia for Difficult Airway
32. Anesthesia for Ophthalmic Surgery
33. Anesthesia for Ear, Nose and Throat Surgery
34. Anesthesia for Orthopedic Surgery
35. Anesthesia for Genitourinary Surgery
36. Anesthesia for Laser Surgery
37. Anesthesia for Laparoscopy
38. Anesthesia for Neurosurgery
39. Anesthesia for Cardiothoracic Surgery
40. Geriatric Anesthesia
41. Obstetric Anesthesia
42. Pediatric Anesthesia
43. Anesthesia Outside Operating Room
44. Anesthesia for Day Care Surgery
45. Hypotensive Anesthesia
46. Anesthesia for Organ Donation

COMPETENCIES COVERED IN UNIT VI

Competency Number	Competency Name	Chapter Number
AS4.4	Observe and describe the principles and the steps/techniques in maintenance of vital organ functions in patients undergoing surgical procedures.	31–42
AS4.6	Observe and describe the principles and the steps/techniques involved in day care anesthesia.	44
AS4.7	Observe and describe the principles and the steps/techniques involved in anesthesia outside the operating room.	43

CHAPTER 31

Anesthesia for Difficult Airway

Anshul Jain, Apurva Abhinandan Mittal

INTRODUCTION

Difficult airway can be arbitrarily defined as the airway in which mask ventilation and/or endotracheal intubation is difficult. Difficult airway can be encountered clinically in two ways:
1. **Anticipated difficult airway**: When it is well known that patient airway pose problem during airway management, e.g., a patient with restricted mouth opening.
2. When difficulty is encountered after administration of anesthetic agents *(called as unanticipated difficult airway)*, e.g., patient with undiagnosed laryngeal tumor.

It can be understood very well, that second condition is more problematic and life-threatening, if proper management is delayed.

KEY POINTS

Conditions with difficult mask ventilation
- Obesity
- Lack of teeth
- Presence of beard
- History of snoring

ANESTHETIC MANAGEMENT

Anticipated Difficult Airway

There are many conditions, which make intubation and mask ventilation difficult (important ones are mentioned in **Table 31.1**).

In general, any condition that restricts mouth opening or limit neck movement or reduces or alters the diameter or curvature of larynx or trachea makes airway difficult.

Table 31.1: Conditions associated with difficult airway.

Reduced mouth opening	Restricted neck movements
• Submucosal fibrosis • Mandibular fracture • Temporomandibular joint ankylosis **Infections** • Submandibular abscess • Peritonsillar abscess • Epiglottitis **Congenital anomalies** • Pierre Robin syndrome • Treacher Collins syndrome • Laryngeal atresia • Craniofacial dysostosis	• Ankylosing spondylosis • Cervical spine injury **Anatomic variations** • Micrognathia • Prognathism • Large tongue • Arched palate • Prominent upper incisors **Other** • Obesity • Pregnancy • Malignant lesion of oropharynx and tongue

Management

In 2022 American Society of Anesthesiologists (ASA) revised the difficult airway management algorithm **(Fig. 31.1)**. The 2022 ASA difficult airway management guidelines forms the basis of difficult airway management.

As per 2022 difficult airway management guidelines awake intubation (usually under fiberoptic guidance) is the technique of choice for difficult airway management.

Other Options

- **Intubating laryngeal mask airway:** Specialized LMA through which endotracheal tube can be passed.
- **Retrograde intubation:** A catheter is passed transtracheally which is then brought out through mouth. Endotracheal tube is passed over that catheter.

UNANTICIPATED DIFFICULT INTUBATION

Unanticipated difficulty with direct laryngoscopy is a serious problem and an anesthesiologist must be skilled in at least one alternative technique of airway management otherwise patient may depart to heaven. Difficult airway society (DAS) algorithm is the standard guide for management of such conditions **(Fig. 31.2)**.

Cannot Intubate Cannot Ventilate Situation

This situation can be defined as one where ventilation with noninvasive techniques (e.g., mask) fails to maintain oxygenation and tracheal intubation proves impossible **(Table 31.2)**. In this situation, percutaneous airway via cricothyrotomy is the technique of choice **(Fig. 31.2)**.

AWAKE FIBEROPTIC INTUBATION

Awake fiberoptic intubation (AFOI) is a technique which allows a flexible oral or nasal route to provide a clear visualization of the vocal cords, and subsequent passage of an endotracheal tube into the trachea under direct vision **(Figs. 31.3A to E)**. AFOI is an essential skill in the management of a patient with a known difficult airway.

Indications for AFOI

- History of difficult airway or AFOI (suggested by previous anesthetic records)
- Previous difficulty in mask ventilation
- Anticipated difficult airway as found on preassessment, with other complicating factors such as contraindications to the use of succinylcholine.
- To avoid iatrogenic injury during laryngoscopy, e.g., unstable C-spine fracture.

Contraindications for AFOI

- Patient refusal or uncooperative patient
- Lack of airway skills
- Allergy to local anesthetic agents
- Infection/contamination of the upper airway—blood, friable tumor, open abscess
- Grossly distorted anatomy
- Fractured base of skull (contraindication to nasal route).

Preparations

- Ensure the familiarity with the fiberoptic scope, and review manufacturer's guidance on its use, including handling, channels and operation.
- Make sure the availability of all the appropriate resuscitation equipment. Plain lignocaine, xylometazoline or oxymetazoline nasal spray (or any other available topical vasoconstrictors) should be available.
- The patient should be fully monitored throughout the procedure (blood pressure, pulse oximetry, ECG). Ideally, capnography should be available.

Procedures

- Obtain intravenous access and administer glycopyrrolate (alternatively atropine) to minimize the airway secretions.
- Identify the patient's most patent nasal passage.
- Spray vasoconstrictor (oxymetazoline/xylometazoline) in the nasal mucosa.

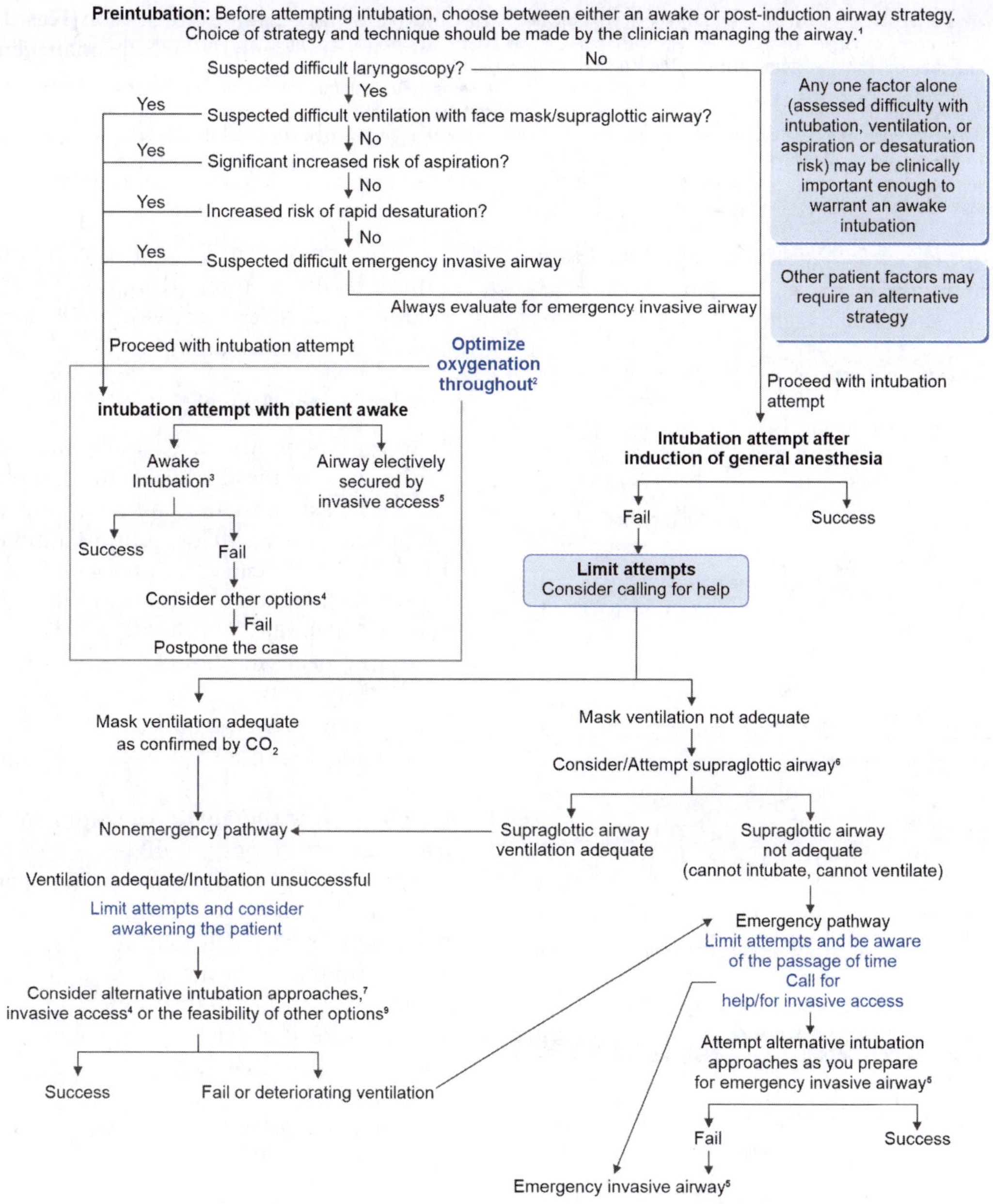

Chapter 31: Anesthesia for Difficult Airway

Preintubation: Before attempting intubation, choose between either an awake or post-induction airway strategy. Choice of strategy and technique should be made by the clinician managing the airway.[1]

- Suspected difficult laryngoscopy? → Yes
- Suspected difficult ventilation with face mask/supraglottic airway? → Yes / No
- Significant increased risk of aspiration? → Yes / No
- Increased risk of rapid desaturation? → Yes / No
- Suspected difficult emergency invasive airway → Yes

Always evaluate for emergency invasive airway

Any one factor alone (assessed difficulty with intubation, ventilation, or aspiration or desaturation risk) may be clinically important enough to warrant an awake intubation

Other patient factors may require an alternative strategy

Proceed with intubation attempt

Optimize oxygenation throughout[2]

Proceed with intubation attempt

Intubation attempt with patient awake
- Awake Intubation[3]
- Airway electively secured by invasive access[5]
  - Success
  - Fail → Consider other options[4] → Fail → Postpone the case

Intubation attempt after induction of general anesthesia
- Fail / Success
- Limit attempts / Consider calling for help

Mask ventilation adequate as confirmed by CO_2 ← → Mask ventilation not adequate

Consider/Attempt supraglottic airway[6]

- Nonemergency pathway ← Supraglottic airway ventilation adequate
- Supraglottic airway not adequate (cannot intubate, cannot ventilate)

Ventilation adequate/Intubation unsuccessful
Limit attempts and consider awakening the patient

Consider alternative intubation approaches,[7] invasive access[4] or the feasibility of other options[9]
- Success
- Fail or deteriorating ventilation

Emergency pathway
Limit attempts and be aware of the passage of time
Call for help/for invasive access

Attempt alternative intubation approaches as you prepare for emergency invasive airway[5]
- Fail → Emergency invasive airway[5]
- Success

Fig. 31.1: ASA difficult airway algorithm for adult patients.

1. The airway manager's choice of airway strategy and techniques should be based on their previous experience; available resources, including equipment, availability and competency of help; and the context in which airway management will occur.
2. Low- or high-flow nasal cannula, head elevated position throughout procedure. Noninvasive ventilation during preoxygenation.
3. Awake intubation techniques include flexible bronchoscope, videolaryngoscopy, direct laryngoscopy, combined techniques, and retrograde wire-aided intubation.
4. Other options include, but are not limited to, alternative awake technique, awake elective invasive airway, alternative anesthetic techniques, induction of anesthesia (if unstable or cannot be postponed) with preparations for emergency invasive airway, and postponing the case without attempting the above options.

5. Invasive airway techniques include surgical cricothyrotomy, needle cricothyrotomy with a pressure-regulated device, large-bore cannula cricothyrotomy, or surgical tracheostomy. Elective invasive airway techniques include the above and retrograde wire–guided intubation and percutaneous tracheostomy. Also consider rigid bronchoscopy and ECMO.
6. Consideration of size, design, positioning, and first versus second generation supraglottic airways may improve the ability to ventilate.
7. Alternative difficult intubation approaches include but are not limited to video-assisted laryngoscopy, alternative laryngoscope blades, combined techniques, intubating supraglottic airway (with or without flexible bronchoscopic guidance), flexible bronchoscopy, introducer, and lighted stylet or lightwand.
8. Adjuncts that may be employed during intubation attempts include tracheal tube introducers, rigid stylets, intubating stylets, or tube changers and external laryngeal manipulation.

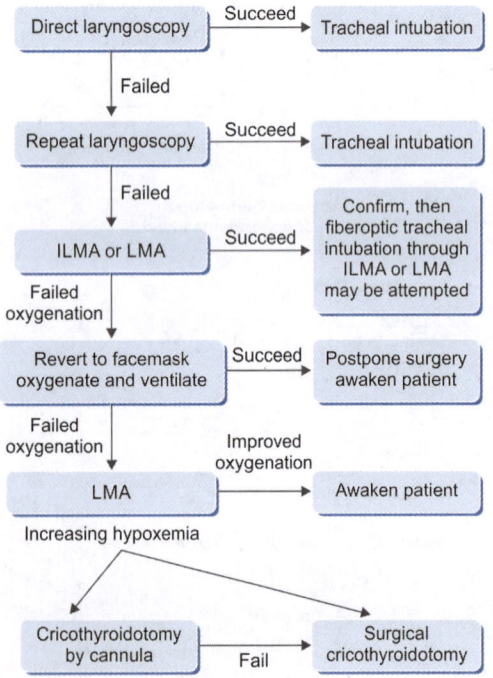

Fig. 31.2: Emergency difficult airway algorithm.
(ILMA: intubating laryngeal mask airway; LMA: laryngeal mask airway)

Table 31.2: Prerequisite for awake intubation.

Requirement	Achieved by
Anesthesia of oral cavity	Lignocaine spray or gargles
Abduction of vocal cords	Superior laryngeal nerve block
Anesthesia of larynx	Superior laryngeal nerve block
Anesthesia of trachea	Translaryngeal injection of local anesthetic by piercing cricothyroid membrane

- Administer oxygen 4L/min to the opposite nostril using a nasal cannula.
- *Communicate with patient, throughout the procedure. This will gain patient confidence and reduce the anxiety.*

- Position the patient in semi-recumbent or supine position, depending on operator's preference/patient convenience, for the endoscopy and intubation.

Anesthetizing the Airway

- **Nose and nasopharynx**: Insert the cotton swab (soaked in local anesthetic) into the nasal cavity (inferior nasal meatus) and posterior nasal space, leaving it *in situ* for around 3 minutes.
- **Tongue and oropharynx**: Spray 4 puffs of 10% lignocaine into the throat (over tonsillar pillars and back of throat).
- **Pharynx and larynx above cords**: Anesthetized by 1–4% lignocaine spray using a spatula or laryngoscope. Spray additional 4 puffs of 10% lignocaine into the nose and postnasal space.
- **Larynx below the cord**: Anesthetized by a transtracheal injection, of 3–5 mL of 1–4% lignocaine using a 21–23G needle. The patient is asked to exhale prior to the injection. Remove the needle immediately following injection, to prevent trauma of the airway when the patient coughs. The resultant inspiration and cough aids the spread of the local anesthetic within the tracheobronchial tree.
- *Make sure that the total administered dose of lignocaine should not exceed the recommended safe dose.*

Endoscopy and Intubation

- Load the endotracheal tube over the bronchoscope. Introduce the fiberscope through the nostril, into the lower nasal meatus (inferior, largest). Identify nasal septum medial, floor of nose superior, turbinate lateral.
- Beyond the nasal septum, enter the nasopharynx. Steer the fiberscope into the oropharynx, once

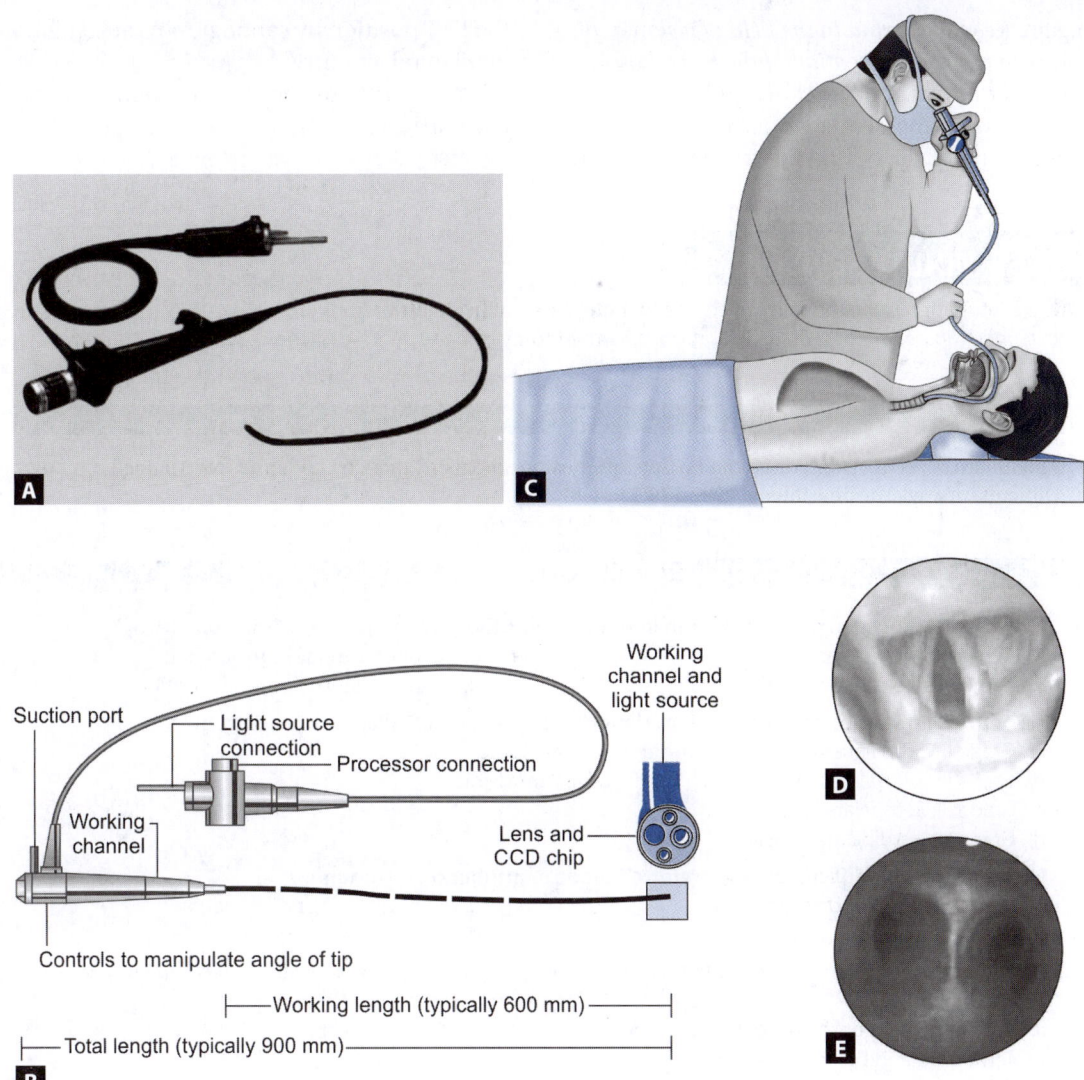

Figs. 31.3A to E: (A) Fiberoptic bronchoscopy instrument; (B) Fiberoptic bronchoscope parts; (C) Technique of insertion of bronchoscope; (D) View of larynx; (E) View showing tracheal bifurcation when bronchoscope is just above the level of carina.

in the oropharynx, one may see the epiglottis, the 1st landmark.
- Advance the fiberscope into the laryngeal opening. Advance it further until it enters the subglottic space, and identify the trachea, 2nd landmark. Few more spays of local anesthetic may be required which can be administered via bronchoscope. This again may cause the patient to cough.
- When cough subsides advance the fiberscope again into the trachea, identifying the carina, 3rd landmark.
- **Intubation:** Glide the loaded ETT, over the fiberscope. Advance the ETT with a gentle rotating motion through the nose, naso/oropharynx, pharynx and larynx. If any resistance is felt, do not force the tube, but withdraw slightly, rotate the ETT 90° anti-clockwise, and advance gently

again. *Keep the carina in the field of vision at all times to prevent dislocation of the bronchoscope out of the larynx into the esophagus.*
- Remove the fiberscope whilst visualizing, to ensure tip of the ETT is in the trachea. Confirm the ETT position by capnography, auscultation of bilateral air entry.
- After ensuring proper ETT placement *induce the patient using appropriate anesthetic agents.*

LAST-MINUTE REVISION

- Awake intubation is the modality of choice for anticipated difficult intubation.
- *In cannot intubate cannot ventilate* situation, cricothyrotomy is the technique of choice.

REFERENCE

1. Apfelbaum JL, et aL. 2022 American Society of Anesthesiologists Practice Guidelines for Management of the Difficult Airway. Anesthesiology. 2022;136(1):31-81.

REVIEW QUESTIONS

1. Which is the most dangerous situation in terms of anesthetic management of difficult airway?
   a. Can intubate can ventilate
   b. Cannot intubate can ventilate
   c. Can intubate cannot ventilate
   d. Cannot intubate cannot ventilate

2. All of the following correctly represent, clinical examination of Mallampati grading, *except*:
   a. Grade I: Soft palate, tip of uvula, faucial pillars are visible
   b. Grade II: Soft palate, base of uvula, faucial pillars are visible
   c. Grade III: Soft palate is visible
   d. Grade IV: Hard palate is visible

3. For a patient with difficult airway preferred mode of intubation is through:
   a. Rapid sequence induction
   b. Awake fiberoptic intubation
   c. Intubation through LMA
   d. Retrograde intubation

4. Retrograde intubation is a suitable technique for airway management in all of the following condition, *except*:
   a. Postburn neck contracture
   b. Cervical fracture
   c. Temporomandibular joint ankylosis
   d. Submucosal fibrosis

Note: Retrograde intubation requires transtracheal cannulation for passing catheter. As tracheal ring would be difficult to appreciate in neck contracture, it is not a suitable technique for this condition.

5. Pre-requisite for awake fiberoptic intubation includes all, *except*:
   a. Patient cooperation
   b. Adequate anesthesia of oral cavity
   c. Neck extension
   d. Antisialogogues

ANSWERS

1. d   2. b   3. b   4. a   5. c

CHAPTER 32

Anesthesia for Ophthalmic Surgery

Saurabh Nanda

INTRODUCTION

Due to increased life expectancy ocular surgeries are becoming very common. Cataract surgery is the most common ocular surgery. It is the most common surgery in elder age group. If we exclude traumatic conditions, patients undergoing ocular surgery belongs to extremes of age, i.e., either pediatric or geriatric. For proper anesthetic management one must know problems of these age groups along with basic ocular anatomy.

ANATOMY OF EYE

The eye is a sphere about 24 mm in diameter. The wall of the globe has three layers—the sclera, the uveal tract, and the retina.

The transparent cornea is the most anterior part of the sclera. Middle layer comprises of the uveal tract which has three structures—the choroid, the iris, and the ciliary body.

The innermost eye layer is the retina. Light stimulates retinal photoreceptors to produce neural signals that are carried to brain by optic nerve. There are no capillaries in the retina and oxygen is supplied by choroid layer.

Blood Supply

The ophthalmic artery, a branch of internal carotid artery provides most of the blood supply to the orbital structures. Venous drainage is *via*. superior and inferior ophthalmic veins which then drain directly into the cavernous sinus.

Nerve Supply

Eye is supplied by optic nerve (CN II) which carries the neural signals from the retina. The oculomotor, trochlear, and abducens control the extraocular muscles. Sensations of the lower lid are carried *via*. the maxillary nerve; whereas frontal branch of the ophthalmic nerve carries sensations of the upper lid.

The facial nerve provides motor innervation to the orbicularis muscle *via*. zygomatic branch.

OCULAR PHYSIOLOGY

Intraocular Pressure Dynamics

The eye can be considered a hollow sphere with a rigid wall. So, its content exert a pressure against its wall; this pressure called as the *intraocular pressure* (IOP, normal: 12–20 mm Hg) is very important for normal visual mechanics and ocular perfusion. The blood supply of eye depends on the intraocular perfusion pressure which in turn is equal to the difference between the mean arterial pressure and the IOP. Thus high IOP impairs the perfusion.

Coughing, straining, and vomiting are the most common factor that can increase IOP. This increase is transient and does not have any deleterious effect on normal eye. However, in an open eye, even this minor increase can result in loss of intraocular contents, and permanent vision loss.

Intravenous succinylcholine raises IOP by 6–12 mm Hg which lasts for 5–10 minutes. So, use of succinylcholine for induction in patients with open-globe injury is contraindicated.

Oculocardiac Reflex

Traction on the extraocular muscles or pressure on the globe causes bradycardia, atrioventricular block, ventricular ectopy, or asystole. It is especially seen with traction on the *medial rectus muscle*,[Q]

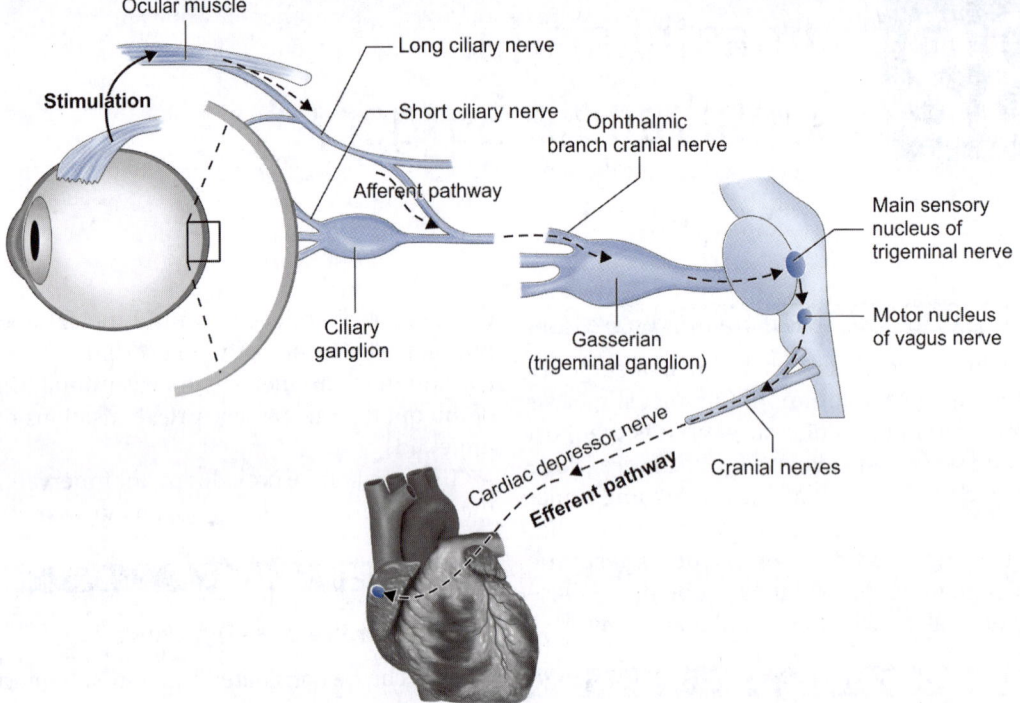

Fig. 32.1: Oculocardiac reflex pathway.

but can occur with stimulation of any of the orbital contents, including the periosteum **(Fig. 32.1)**.

The afferent limb of this reflex is formed by ophthalmic division of the trigeminal nerve which carries fibers to the sensory nucleus of the trigeminal near the fourth ventricle. The efferent limb is *via* the vagus nerve to the heart.

The reflex is more common under topical anesthesia and is exacerbated by hypercapnia or hypoxemia.

In the event of this reflex, surgeon must stop manipulation. If bradycardia is persisting or severe, intravenous atropine can be administered.

ANESTHETIC MANAGEMENT

Preoperative Evaluation

Cataract surgery is the most common surgery in the elderly. These are quick outpatient procedures that do not involve blood loss or much postoperative pain. So, one should not order irrelevant investigations.

Laboratory Studies

The American Heart Association classified ophthalmic procedures such as cataract extraction as low-risk procedures. For these procedures, laboratory evaluation is required only if patient have findings on physical examination.

Perioperative Management

Choice of Anesthesia

Regional anesthesia is preferred over general anesthesia, as it provides significant postoperative analgesia with less chance of nausea and vomiting.

Techniques of regional anesthesia include:
- **Facial nerve blocks**: A facial nerve block is done when complete akinesis of the eyelid is desired.
- **Retrobulbar block**: The retrobulbar block provides excellent akinesia and anesthesia of the eye.
  - A 3 cm, blunt Atkinson needle is recommended to reduce ocular perforation.

- *Complications include*: Retrobulbar hemorrhage *(most common)*; proptosis; subconjunctival ecchymosis; optic nerve damage and ocular perforation.
- Intravascular injection can occur despite a negative aspiration test. However, the total dose required is so small that even if the total dose is given intravenously, systemic effects would be unlikely.
- **Posterior peribulbar block**[Q]: Due to less chances of retrobulbar hemorrhage, posterior peribulbar anesthesia has become more popular. Currently the regional block of choice for ocular surgeries.[1]
  - *Advantages*:
    i. Less painful
    ii. Less chances of retrobulbar hemorrhage, globe perforation
    iii. Separate facial nerve blockade is not required
  - *Disadvantages*: Slower onset time (9-12 minutes) and incomplete akinesia.
- **Topical anesthesia:** Cataract surgery particularly phacoemulsion can be done under topical anesthesia alone. This avoids the potential complications associated with retrobulbar and peribulbar injections. In addition, patients have the most rapid visual rehabilitation, with improved vision almost immediately after the procedure.
  - *Disadvantages* include the potential for eye movement during surgery, increased patient anxiety, and discomfort from the microscope light.

General Anesthesia

The choice of general versus regional anesthesia depends upon the duration of the surgery, the relative risks and benefits of each technique for the patient, and patient preference. The goals of general anesthesia include a smooth intubation, stable IOP, avoidance of oculocardiac reflexes, a motionless field, and smooth emergence.

> **Note:** Nitrous oxide presents a special problem in some vitreoretinal procedures. In the technique called fluid gas exchange, the surgeon injects an intravitreal air bubble to tamponade the retina against the wall of the globe. Sulfur hexafluoride is a poorly soluble gas used to prolong the resorption of intravitreal air bubbles. Nitrous oxide if administered simultaneously, diffuses and causes bubble expansion, with the potential for dangerous increases in IOP. So, nitrous oxide must be shut off for 15 minutes before placing the sulfur hexafluoride bubble and should be avoided for 7–10 days thereafter.

The laryngeal mask airway can be used for ophthalmologic surgery and is associated with less coughing on emergence when compared with endotracheal intubation.

Anesthesia for Pediatric Ophthalmologic Procedures

Pediatric patient require anesthesia for procedures ranging from simple ophthalmic examination to complex squint surgery. Intramuscular ketamine sometimes can be a good choice if raised IOP is not hazardous.

The most common eye surgery in children is for squint and the main problem with this surgery is nausea and vomiting. Ondansetron is an effective antiemetic. Malignant hyperthermia and myotonic dystrophy also have been associated with strabismus. So, succinylcholine should be used cautiously.

LAST-MINUTE REVISION

- Regional technique of choice for ophthalmic surgery—posterior peribulbar block.
- **Drugs of choice:**
- **Anticholinergic:** Atropine is preferred over glycopyrrolate due to its better vagolytic activity.
- **Inducing agent:** Propofol (ketamine to be avoided)
- **Muscle relaxant:** Rocuronium (due to its rapid onset)
- **Volatile agent:** Sevoflurane

REFERENCE

1. Lodhi O, Tripathy K. Anesthesia for Eye Surgery. [Updated 2023 Jul 19]. In: StatPearls [Internet]. Treasure Island (FL): StatPearls Publishing; 2023 Jan-. Available from: https://www.ncbi.nlm.nih.gov/books/NBK572131/

REVIEW QUESTIONS

1. Muscle especially notorious for activation of oculocardiac reflex:
   a. Medial rectus
   b. Lateral rectus
   c. Superior oblique
   d. Inferior oblique
2. Most of the cataract surgeries are performed under which regional block:
   a. Trigeminal block
   b. Retrobulbar block
   c. Peribulbar block
   d. Facial nerve block

ANSWERS

1. a
2. c

CHAPTER 33

Anesthesia for Ear, Nose and Throat Surgery

Sachin Maheshwari

INTRODUCTION

Ear, nose and throat (ENT) surgery includes a variety of procedure varying in duration, severity and complexity. Nose and throat surgery pose special problem of "shared airway" as both anesthesiologist and surgeon work in same anatomical region. Current chapter deals with the basic principles of anesthesia for ear, nose or throat surgery.

EAR SURGERY

Anesthetic Management

Preoperative Assessment

In preoperative assessment, beside normal protocols specific attention must be paid to hypertension or other cardiovascular disease, which contraindicates or limits hypotensive anesthesia.

Choice of Anesthesia

External ear procedures can be performed very well under local anesthesia. Middle ear and inner easy procedures usually require general anesthesia.

Local Anesthesia

The sensory nerve supply of the ear comes from the "auriculotemporal nerve, greater auricular nerve" (*both of them can be blocked by infiltrating local anesthetic over anterior and posterior external meatal wall*), auricular branch of the vagus nerve and tympanic nerve (*blocked by topical infiltration of local anesthetic on the tympanic membrane*). Infiltration through an aural speculum blocks the auricular branch of the vagus.

General Anesthesia

Choice of drugs depends upon the patients, though propofol is usually a preferred induction agent due to its beneficial effect upon nausea and vomiting. Specific perioperative issues include:

- **Use of nitrous oxide**: Nitrous oxide due to its more solubility diffuses into air spaces within the body; diffusion into the middle ear cavity increases the pressure and may displace the graft of tympanoplasty. Reverse happens at the end of surgery, i.e., after discontinuation, rapid reabsorption of nitrous oxide can produce negative middle ear pressures, resulting in graft displacement. Thus in ear surgeries involving application of graft, nitrous oxide is best avoided and patient is ventilated with air oxygen mixture.
- **Patient position**: Rotation of the head and extension of the neck is necessary for most ear procedures; this position can compress internal and external jugular veins and the carotid artery. A lateral tilt of the operating table may improve surgical access without the need for extreme head and neck rotation.
- **Facial nerve monitoring**: Facial nerve monitoring is used to prevent and detect facial nerve injury during middle ear surgery. When the nerve is stimulated, there is contraction of muscles

> **KEY POINTS**
>
> Choice of anesthesia for ear procedures:
> - **External ear**: Local anesthesia
> - **Middle ear**: General anesthesia preferred
> - **Inner ear**: General anesthesia

supplied by facial nerve. Neuromuscular blockade hamper facial nerve monitoring by attenuating muscle contractions secondary to nerve stimulation. So at the time of facial monitoring neuromuscular blockade is reversed and anesthesia is maintained by short-acting opioid, most preferred one is remifentanil.

- **Antiemetics**: Middle ear and inner ear procedures are at higher risk for postoperative nausea and vomiting than general surgical procedures, so antiemetics should be administered prophylactically.
- **Recovery**: Smooth emergence and recovery are vital to prevent graft disruption. Laryngeal mask airway (LMA) may be put in place of endotracheal tubes prior to reversal as LMA provides smooth emergence. This technique of reversal is known as the *Bailey maneuver*.

NASAL SURGERY

Septal and sinus surgery are the most commonly performed nasal procedures; nowadays, they are usually performed endoscopically by the procedure called as functional endoscopic sinus surgery.

Preoperative Evaluation

These patients might have total nasal airway obstruction which may make face mask ventilation difficult, particularly when associated with other causes of difficult ventilation (e.g., obesity, maxillofacial deformities). Nasal polyps are often associated with allergic disorders such as asthma and cystic fibrosis. *Samter's triad*, the association of nonsteroidal anti-inflammatory drug (NSAID) sensitivity in patients with asthma and nasal polyps should be kept in mind.

Patient should be specifically assessed for obstructive sleep apnea, bleeding disorders.

Nasal Vasoconstrictors

Vasoconstrictors are commonly used to reduce bleeding from vascular nasal mucosa, epinephrine, and phenylephrine are commonly used vasoconstrictors.

Anesthetic Management

Choice of Anesthesia

Short procedures like septoplasty, turbinectomy, can be performed under local anesthesia provided patient is cooperative. General anesthesia is preferred for rest of the cases.

Local Anesthesia

Sensory supply of septum and lateral wall is derived from anterior ethmoidal nerve and sphenopalatine nerves. Both can be blocked simply by packing the nose with gauze soaked in local anesthetic.

General Anesthesia

Propofol remains the preferred inducing agent. Special considerations include:
- Reinforced or preformed right angle endotracheal tube are preferred over normal endotracheal tube due to their less susceptibility to kinking and furthermore these tubes do not hamper surgeons access.
- A throat pack around a tracheal tube is often used to prevent blood entering the oropharynx, and to reduce the entry of surgical debris in the laryngopharynx.
- Because of the proximity of the surgical field, patient's eyes must be padded to avoid a corneal abrasion.
- Extubation should be smooth, with minimum coughing or straining, as this will increase venous pressure and can cause bleeding.

INTRAORAL SURGERY

Tonsillectomy

Tonsillectomy and adenoidectomy are the most common throat procedure in pediatric age group. Both procedures involve sharing of airway, and possess a potential for blood contamination of the lower airway.

Both of these procedures are almost always performed under general anesthesia with nasal (preferred) or oral endotracheal intubation.

Preoperative Evaluation

Aims are to identify patients with loose teeth, bleeding disorders, anemia and active respiratory tract infection. Active respiratory tract infections increase the risk of bleeding and laryngospasm, so it is wise to postpone surgery for at least 4 weeks.

Intraoperative Management

The goals of anesthesia are to maintain a sufficient depth and prevent reflex-induced hypertensive responses. At the end of procedure, a careful inspection for blood should be performed.

Postoperative Care

A high-quality care is essential to identify problems in the immediate postoperative period. The child is placed in a left lateral or semiprone (tonsil position), position with slight head-down tilt and often a pillow is placed under the chest. This allows blood or secretions to drain out through mouth.

Postoperative analgesia can be provided with NSAIDs.

Laryngeal Procedures

Laryngeal and tracheal operations are unique as in that the anesthesiologist and the surgeon have to utilize the same anatomic field. Procedures range from minor vocal cord nodule excision to laryngectomy.

Preoperative Evaluation

Beside routine evaluation, anesthesiologist must assess the size, mobility and location of the lesion and its impact on airway management. Presence of stridor indicates a significantly narrowed airway, but the absence of stridor does not rule out narrowed airway. Supraglottic lesions, if mobile, can obstruct the airway and obscure the visualization of the laryngeal inlet.

Anesthetic Techniques

There is no ideal anesthetic technique for endoscopy procedures. Choice exists between two techniques. First one is "closed" system in which a cuffed tracheal tube is employed for protection of the lower airway, and second one is "open" system which uses either spontaneous ventilation and insufflation techniques or muscle paralysis with jet ventilation. Closed system provides better protection and control of airway while open system provides better surgical access.

LAST-MINUTE REVISION

- Nitrous oxide should better be avoided during middle ear surgery.
- In tonsillectomy, nasal intubation is preferred over oral intubation.
- When facial nerve is being monitored, neuromuscular blocking is contraindicated.

REVIEW QUESTIONS

1. Which of the following anesthetic agent should not be used in patient posted for tympanoplasty?
   a. Isoflurane
   b. Enflurane
   c. Nitrous oxide
   d. Thiopentone

2. Regarding anesthetic management of tonsillectomy, all statements are true, *except*:
   a. Nasal intubation is preferred over oral intubation
   b. Surgery is best performed when child has an acute attack of tonsilitis
   c. In immediate postoperative period, child is placed in semiprone position
   d. Propofol is the preferred inducing agent

ANSWERS

1. c   2. b

CHAPTER 34

Anesthesia for Orthopedic Surgery

Anshul Jain

INTRODUCTION

Orthopedic patients represent broad scope of problems, ranging from an elderly patient with multiple comorbid conditions to a young, trauma patient who has associated injuries.

Many orthopedic procedures are now performed as ambulatory surgery, and the anesthesiologist must take step by which patients can be discharged and their pain can be managed very well. Under current chapter we will discuss basic problems of anesthesia in orthopedic surgery and there solutions.

PREOPERATIVE EVALUATION

Routing testing is recommended as per the ASA categorization.[1] Any orthopedic patient could represent problem for anesthetist, but there are some group (geriatric, acute trauma) which are frequently associated with anesthetic problems, and they should be evaluated accordingly.

Choice of Anesthesia Technique

Wherever possible, regional anesthesia is the preferred choice. Advantages include:
- Less incidence of perioperative complications like deep vein thrombosis (DVT), pulmonary embolism (PE)
- Less intraoperative bleeding
- Better postoperative pain management
- In some orthopedic patients (ankylosing spondylitis) airway might be difficult, regional anesthesia avoids manipulation of the airway under such circumstances. But one should not think that general anesthesia is harmful or contraindicated in orthopedic surgery; final decision always depends upon patient condition and type of surgery.

PERIOPERATIVE COMPLICATIONS

Cardiac Complications

American Heart Association (AHA) classifies orthopedic surgery as intermediate-risk surgery. Older patients have an increased risk of perioperative myocardial morbidity and mortality after orthopedic surgery. β-blockers have shown to reduce risk of perioperative myocardial ischemia in high-risk patient.

Respiratory Complications

Orthopedic patient particularly elder ones are at risk. The hypoxia in these patients reflects respiratory changes caused by age, and embolization of bone marrow debris to the lungs. High spinal block can reduce tidal volume in elder patients by paralyzing abdominal muscles, so should be avoided.

Neurologic Complications

Delirium is the third most common complication seen in elderly patients after orthopedic surgery. Events that may trigger delirium include hypoxemia, hypotension, abnormal electrolytes, infection, sleep deprivation, pain, and administration of drugs like benzodiazepines, anticholinergics.

Incidence of delirium can be reduced by identifying and preventing risk factors, early mobilization, adequate pain control and maintenance of normal sleep cycles.

Fat Embolism Syndrome

Fat embolization is a well-known complication of skeletal trauma and surgery. Fat embolization and fat embolism syndrome (FES) are different. The embolization of fat occurs in all patients of pelvic or femoral fracture, but the incidence of FES is less than 1%. *It is more likely to occur in patients with multiple long bone and pelvic fractures. Femoral shaft fractures and tibial fracture carries highest risk of FES.* Age also seems to be a factor in the development of FES; young men with fractures are at increased risk.

The presentation of FES can be gradual, developing over 12–72 hours, or fulminant presenting as acute respiratory distress and cardiac arrest.

The pathophysiology of FES is not fully known, but most likely involves the embolization of fat and bone marrow debris into the lungs and other end organs where it obstructs the capillaries and triggers systemic inflammatory response.

Gurd suggested major and minor criteria for the diagnosis of FES. The presence of any one major finding plus four minor criteria and evidence of fat macroglobulinemia suggest diagnosis of FES **(Box 34.1)**.[2]

Petechial rash *(pathognomonic of FES)* are usually present on the conjunctiva, oral mucosa, and skin fold of the neck and axilla. *Respiratory signs* are common and chest X-ray shows bilateral alveolar infiltrates. *$ETCO_2$ begins to fall to an extent that it may become zero, if embolus is large. Central nervous system symptoms* range from drowsiness and confusion to obtundation and coma. MRI brain can reveal characteristic lesions of fat embolization.

Treatment

- Early resuscitation and stabilization.
- Oxygen therapy with a goal to keep SPO_2 more than 90%.
- If SPO_2 continues to remain below 85%, patient should be intubated and mechanically ventilated. Positive end-expiratory pressure may be valuable under such conditions.
- Heparin and ethanol once considered as essential components are now outdated, rather contraindicated due to problems of enhance bleeding with heparin and mental obtundation with ethanol.

Tourniquet-related Complications

In extremity surgery, tourniquets are often inflated to reduce the intraoperative bleeding, but they are associated with many complications **(Table 34.1)**.

> **KEY POINTS**
>
> **Safe tourniquet period:** Should never exceed 2 hours, for both upper and lower limb with pressure not exceeding 100 mm Hg above systolic or 250 mm Hg.

ANESTHETIC MANAGEMENT OF DIFFERENT PROCEDURES

Lower Extremity

Arthroscopy

Arthroscopic procedures of knee, hip, and ankle are usually performed as ambulatory procedure. Thus, the goal of anesthetic management is uncomplicated postoperative recovery with minimal pain.

BOX 34.1

Major criteria (at least one)
- Respiratory insufficiency (dyspnea)
- Cerebral involvement (confusion)
- Petechial rash

Minor criteria (at least four)
- Pyrexia
- Tachycardia
- Retinal changes
- Jaundice
- Renal changes

Laboratory features
- Fat microglobulinemia (required)
- Anemia
- Thrombocytopenia
- High erythrocyte sedimentation rate

Table 34.1: Tourniquet complications.

During inflation	Tourniquet period	During deflation	Post tourniquet
Hypertension due to increased circulating blood volume	Pain	Hypotension due to release of toxic metabolites like thromboxane	Neuropathy
	Acidosis secondary to ischemia	Hypercapnia release due to accumulated CO_2 in limb	
		Metabolic acidosis	

Deflation is the most dangerous period.

Choice of Anesthesia

Spinal anesthesia with pencil-point needles is the preferred anesthetic technique. Postoperative analgesia can be provided with intra-articular bupivacaine with or without morphine. Special mention is required for hip arthroscopy, a common outpatient procedure, which is performed in either supine or lateral position (operative side up). In positioning the patient, the anesthesiologist must ensure that the pudendal nerve is not compressed.

Hip Fractures

Hip fractures are common particularly in elderly and are associated with many perioperative complications like DVT, delirium, etc.

Early surgery (within 12 hours) results in lower pain scores, reduced perioperative complications, and thus reduces the duration of hospital stay.

Patients with hip fracture are often dehydrated and anemic because the fracture site can accommodate considerable extravasated blood. A normal intravascular blood volume must be restored before anesthesia and surgery.

Regional anesthesia results in better outcome compared with general anesthesia in these patients because of above-mentioned reasons. *Combined spinal-epidural anesthesia*[Q] is the anesthetic technique of choice where spinal anesthesia provides benefit of early onset and intense intraoperative analgesia, while epidural catheter provides extended analgesia for postoperative pain.

Pelvic Fractures

Pelvic fractures are usually associated with other injuries and can themselves result in fatal retroperitoneal bleeding. Hypotension and an increase in abdominal girth suggest intra-abdominal bleeding which require emergent exploratory surgery.

As iatrogenic sciatic nerve injury is the most frequent surgical complication (approximately 18%), many surgeons use *neuromuscular monitor* during the operation because of which neuromuscular blockers should be avoided. A combination of a general anesthesia with the placement of an epidural catheter for postoperative analgesia is the most appropriate anesthetic technique.

> ### ⚡ KEY POINTS
> **Safe tourniquet period:** Should never exceed 2 hours, for both a **spinal/epidural does not hamper neuromuscular monitoring, how?**
> Central neuraxial block acts at the level of spinal cord, and if a peripheral nerve is stimulated directly, there would be muscle contraction. In contrast, when neuromuscular blockers are administered, there would be no contraction. Upper and lower limb with pressure not exceeding 100 mm Hg above systolic or 250 mm Hg.

Hip and Knee Arthroplasty/Replacement

Total hip arthroplasty may be performed via an anterior or lateral approach. Most surgeons prefer the lateral posterior approach, in which the patient is placed in lateral decubitus position. *A combined spinal epidural anesthesia is the technique of choice.*Q

Blood loss during total hip arthroplasty can be significant, which can be reduced by providing hypotensive anesthesia. In addition to reduced blood loss, hypotensive anesthesia improves the cement prosthesis to bone fixation.

"Bone cement implantation syndrome," (BCIS) though rare but specific complication seen in total hip replacement, where prosthesis is fixed by bone cement (methyl methacrylate).

Bone cement implantation syndrome can result in intraoperative hypotension, hypoxia and cardiac arrest. Mechanisms for BCIS include embolization of bone marrow debris *(most likely)* secondary to pressurization of the femoral canal, toxic effects of circulating methyl methacrylate monomer, and the release of cytokines that promote microthrombus formation and pulmonary vasoconstriction. The hypotensive events should be treated with epinephrine. BCIS can be prevented by prophylactic high-pressure pulsatile lavage of the femoral canal and drilling a vent hole in the femur before prosthesis insertion.

Patients posted for total knee arthroplasty (TKA) are also managed by same principles. Here also, *central neuraxial blockade (spinal or epidural)* is the preferred technique.Q TKA patients have severe postoperative pain, which can be best managed by epidural analgesia.

Upper Extremity Surgeries

Surgery for the upper extremity, from the shoulder to the hand, can be performed successfully by blocking the brachial plexus at several points. Brachial block provide postoperative analgesia also.

Intravenous regional anesthesia can also be used for minor forearm and hand surgeries.

Spinal Surgeries

Spinal surgery includes procedures ranging from microdiscectomies for a herniated disk to complex reconstructive surgery for spinal deformities.

Most spinal surgeries require general anesthesia. In patients with pre-existing arthritic condition or other airway problems, awake fiberoptic intubation is the safest approach to general anesthesia. This is the standard technique in a patient with cervical instability too.

Intraoperative Considerations

Most important consideration for spinal surgery is positioning of patient as spinal surgery is usually performed in prone position, which is associated with many problems **(Table 34.2)**.

Complications

Postoperative neurologic deficit is the most feared complications of complex spinal reconstructive surgery. Somatosensory evoked potential, motor evoked potential and electromyogram should be monitored in complex surgeries to diagnose spinal cord damage intraoperatively.

Postoperative visual loss is another devastating complication of spinal surgery particularly after prone position. Causes include ischemic optic neuropathy *(most common)*, retinal artery or vein occlusion and cortical brain ischemia. To prevent this, systolic blood pressure must be kept above 90 mm Hg.

Table 34.2: Complications of the prone position.

Airway	Endotracheal tube kinking, dislodgment Upper airway edema
Neck	Hyperextension or hyperflexion Cervical rotation—compromised blood flow to brain
Eyes	Central retinal artery occlusion, supraorbital nerve compression, corneal abrasion
Upper extremity	Stretching of brachial plexus, ulnar nerve compression
Lower extremity	Occlusion of femoral vein, deep vein thrombosis, kinking of vascular grafts, peroneal nerve palsy (pressure lateral to fibula), lateral femoral cutaneous nerve palsy (pressure on iliac crest)

Postoperative Pain Management

For lumbar fusions, an epidural catheter placed at a level above the incision can be used for patient-controlled epidural analgesia. For surgeries involving multiple spinal levels, intrathecal morphine administered during surgery provides reliable postoperative pain control.

LAST-MINUTE REVISION

- **Maximum risk for fat embolism:** Upper femur and tibial fracture
- **Technique of choice for total hip replacement and knee replacement:** Combined spinal epidural
- **Technique of choice for upper limb orthopedic surgery:** Brachial block
- **Technique of choice for spine surgery:** General anesthesia

REFERENCES

1. Hasan O, Fahad S, Mustafa M, Hashmi P, Noordin S. Does more testing in routine preoperative evaluation benefit the orthopedic patient? Case control study from a resource-constrained setting. Ann Med Surg (Lond). 2021;66:102439.
2. Gurd AR. Fat embolism: An aid to diagnosis. J Bone Joint Surg Br. 1970; 52:32-737.

REVIEW QUESTIONS

1. Total hip replacement can be performed in all of the following anesthetic technique, *except*:
    a. Sciatic nerve block
    b. Epidural anesthesia
    c. Spinal anesthesia
    d. General anesthesia
2. A patient is being operated for shaft femur fracture, under SA, intraoperatively all of the following are major signs for the diagnosis of fat embolism syndrome, *except*:
    a. Respiratory insufficiency
    b. Irritability
    c. Tachycardia
    d. Petechiae

ANSWERS

1. a 2. c

CHAPTER 35

Anesthesia for Genitourinary Surgery

Anshul Jain

INTRODUCTION

Urological procedures account for 10–20% of operative procedures. Many of these patients have coexisting medical illnesses, particularly renal dysfunction. Current chapter deals with the perioperative management of common genitourinary surgeries.

ANESTHETIC CONSIDERATIONS

For proper regional technique, one must know the neural innervation of genitourinary organs **(Table 35.1)**.

Cystoscopy

Cystoscopy is the most commonly performed urological procedure. Choice of anesthesia depends on the age of the patient and indication for the procedure. General anesthesia is necessary for children and is preferred in short diagnostic studies of male patient. Topical anesthesia in the form of viscous lignocaine with or without sedation is sufficient for diagnostic studies in women, because of their short urethra. Spinal anesthesia is preferred in therapeutic cystoscopies expected to last more than 30 minutes.

Regional anesthesia, however, does not abolish the *obturator reflex* (*external rotation and adduction of the thigh secondary to stimulation of the obturator nerve by electrocautery current through the lateral bladder wall*). The reflex (muscle contraction) can only be reliably blocked by neuromuscular blockers during general anesthesia.

Transurethral Resection of the Prostate

Transurethral resection of the prostate (TURP), the surgical procedure of choice for benign prostatic hyperplasia (BPH), is performed by inserting a resectoscope through the urethra and resecting prostatic tissue with an electrically powered cutting-coagulating metal loop. As BPH is the problem of older age group, problems of geriatric age group must be considered in all patients.

Choice of Anesthesia

Spinal anesthesia is the anesthetic technique of choice for TURP.[Q] It has got following advantages over general anesthesia:
- Mental status of the patient can be monitored intraoperatively, which aids in early recognition of complications like TURP syndrome and transient blindness.
- Decreases the incidence of deep vein thrombosis.
- Less intraoperative blood loss.
- Signs and symptoms of bladder perforation (restlessness, diaphoresis, nausea, abdominal pain, dyspnea, shoulder pain and hiccups) can be recognized early in a conscious patient under spinal anesthesia.
- Better control of postoperative pain.

Table 35.1: Pain conduction of the genitourinary system.

Organ	Spinal levels of pain conduction
Kidney	T10–L1
Ureter	T10–L2
Bladder	T11–L2 (dome), S2–4 (neck)
Prostate	T11–L2, S2–4
Penis	S2–4
Scrotum	S2–4
Testes	T10–L1

In spinal anesthesia, a T10^Q level is sufficient in most cases. Sensory levels above T9 are undesirable because pain caused by perforation of the prostatic capsule (capsular sign) would be missed if capsule gets perforated.

Intraoperative Management

Transurethral resection of the prostate requires continuous irrigation to wash tissue debris and blood. An irrigation solution for TURP should be isotonic, electrically inert, nontoxic, transparent, easy to sterilize and inexpensive. Unfortunately, such a solution does not exist. Commonly used solutions are glycine: 1.2 and 1.5%, mannitol: 3–5%, glucose: 2.5–4%, sorbitol: 3.5%, Cytal (a mixture of sorbitol 2.7%, and mannitol 0.54%). All these solutions are slightly hypotonic.

TURP can be associated with a number of serious complications viz:

TURP Syndrome

When large amount of irrigation fluid (usually >2 liters) is absorbed, a constellation of symptoms and signs appears, commonly referred to as the TURP syndrome. Absorption depends on the duration of the resection, as well as the height (pressure) of the irrigation fluid. On an average, 20 mL/min^Q of the irrigating fluid is absorbed.

Manifestations of TURP are primarily those of circulatory fluid overload, water intoxication, and occasionally toxicity from the solute in the irrigating fluid. The hypotonicity of these fluids can lead to acute hyponatremia and hypo-osmolality, which produces serious neurological manifestations. Earliest symptom is perioral numbness.^{Q}

KEY POINTS

Why isotonic normal saline cannot be used as TURP irrigant fluid?
Normal saline in solution exists in ionized form as Na$^+$ and Cl$^-$; both of them are good conductors of electric current. Thus electric current of cautery can disperse and damage the normal tissue.

Treatment of TURP syndrome depends on early recognition and severity of the symptoms. Most patients can be managed with fluid restriction and a loop diuretic, so as to excrete absorbed water. Seizure activity (if occurs) can be terminated by small doses of midazolam. Hypertonic saline solution is indicated only in cases not responding to fluid restriction.

Glycine Toxicity

In case of glycine irrigant, marked hyperglycinemia has been reported. Absorption of glycine may result in central nervous system toxicity as a result of oxidative biotransformation of glycine to ammonia. Glycine has also been implicated in the myocardial depression, hemodynamic changes and transient blindness.[1]

Bladder Perforation

Cutting loop or knife electrode can perforate bladder. Most perforations are extraperitoneal, and in a conscious patient, they result in pain in the periumbilical or suprapubic regions. Sweating, abdominal rigidity, nausea, vomiting and hypotension are other signs.

Hypothermia

Irrigation fluid, if cold, may lead to hypothermia and can cause shivering.

Bleeding and Coagulopathy

A hypertrophied prostate is highly vascular, and operative bleeding can be significant. Average blood loss is 2–5 mL/min of resection time.

Transient bacteremia and septicemia are other complications.

Monitoring

In addition to routine monitoring, mental status in the awake patient is the best monitor for detection of early signs of the TURP syndrome and bladder perforation. A decrease in arterial oxygen saturation is an early sign of fluid overload.

Radical Prostatectomy

Radical prostatectomy is indicated in prostate cancer. The most common intraoperative problem is hemorrhage and massive blood loss requiring blood transfusion. Blood loss is less in continuous epidural anesthesia.

Renal Transplantation

Renal transplantation, the most common visceral organ transplant is indicated in end-stage renal disease. Most renal transplant candidates are on long-term dialysis and have associated systemic problems secondary to renal disease.

Perioperative Considerations

Optimization of the patient's medical condition with dialysis is mandatory. Current organ preservation techniques allow ample time (24–48 hours) for preoperative dialysis of cadaveric recipients. The recipient's serum potassium concentration should be below 5.5 mEq/L and existing coagulopathies should be corrected.

Although both spinal and epidural anesthesia have been successfully employed, most transplants are done under general anesthesia. Among volatile agents, except enflurane and sevoflurane all can be used desflurane is agent of choice. Cisatracurium (atracurium and rocuronium as second choice) is the muscle relaxant of choice.[Q]

LAST-MINUTE REVISION

- **Cystoscopy**: Performed as daycare surgery mostly under general anesthesia through laryngeal mask airway.
- **TURP**: Spinal anesthesia is preferred technique, TURP syndrome is the main complication, which occurs mainly due to fluid overload.

REFERENCE

1. Demirel I, Ozer AB, Bayar MK, Erhan OL. TURP syndrome and severe hyponatremia under general anaesthesia. BMJ Case Rep. 2012;2012:bcr-2012-006899. doi: 10.1136/bcr-2012-006899.

REVIEW QUESTIONS

1. Anesthetic technique of choice for TURP:
   a. General anesthesia
   b. Spinal anesthesia
   c. Caudal block
   d. Epidural block

2. In a patient posted for renal transplantation, which of the following agent should not be used for anesthetic management?
   a. Atracurium
   b. Isoflurane
   c. Methoxyflurane
   d. Propofol

3. Early feature of TURP syndrome includes all, *except*:
   a. Perineal pain
   b. Tachycardia
   c. Perioral tingling
   d. Breathlessness

4. All of the following are being used as irrigant in TURP, *except*:
   a. Sorbitol
   b. Urea
   c. Cytal
   d. Distilled water

ANSWERS

1. b   2. c   3. a   4. d

CHAPTER 36

Anesthesia for Laser Surgery

Sarvesh Singh

INTRODUCTION

The word *laser* is a short form for *light amplification* by *stimulated emission* of *radiation*. Presently, lasers are an accepted and often preferred member of the surgical armamentarium. Anesthesia management is guided by the site and as such based on general principles. But one must know the basic hazards associated with laser surgery which are of utmost importance for the perioperative management.

LASER HAZARDS

The hazards associated with laser use can be divided into four major categories:

A. Atmospheric Contamination: Laser Plume

Laser vaporization of tissue produces smoke and fine particulates that might get inhaled and deposited in the alveoli. Odor of this smoke can produce tearing, and nausea in sensitive persons.

Laser smoke may also be mutagenic, teratogenic, and a vector for viral infection. *Maximum smoke is produced by carbon dioxide (CO_2) lasers.*[Q]

B. Tissue and Vessel Perforation

Misdirected laser energy can lead to perforation of viscera or a large blood vessel. This perforation and bleeding may not occur until edema and necrosis reach to its maximum, thus may evident only after several days postoperatively.

C. Embolism

Venous gas embolism might be seen in Nd:YAG laser system particularly during hysteroscopic surgery and resection of laryngeal or tracheal tumor.

D. Energy Transfer to an Inappropriate Location

If laser control trigger is pressed at the wrong time or site, then it can deliver laser energy to sites at which surgical ablation was not desired viz:

Eye

Carbon dioxide laser can produce serious corneal injury, whereas argon, potassium-titanyl-phosphate (KTP): Nd:YAG, or ruby lasers may burn the retina. So, eyelid of nonoperated eyes should be taped closed and then covered with an opaque metal shield. Operating room personnel must wear safety goggles or lenses specific for the laser being used.

Endotracheal Tube

One of the most severe complications of laser during airway surgery is endotracheal (ET) tube fire. Chances are high, if ET tube is in proximity to surgical site.

Fires results when laser beam *(either direct or reflected)* strikes particles of tissue blown from the surgical site. Leak or unrecognized deflation of the tube cuff permits oxygen-enriched gas to enter the operative site and increase the risk of fire.

Strategies to Prevent Airway Fire

To reduce the incidence of airway fire two strategies are used:
1. **Reduction in the flammability of the ET tube:** Modern polyvinyl chloride (PVC) tubes are very sensitive to CO_2 laser and produce toxic

combustion products. Silicone tubes are the most resistant to ignition, but they generate white silica ash, which can produce silicosis.
- *Protection of the endotracheal tube*: Wrapping tubes with metalized foil tape reduce laser dissipation and thus combustion. Aluminum and copper foils are commonly used. *The Merocel Laser Guard is a Food and Drug Administration (FDA)-approved metal foil for this purpose.*
- *Metal endotracheal tubes*: Specialized laser tubes include laser Flex tube (an airtight stainless steel spiral tube) for CO_2 and KTP laser, Bivona tube (*aluminum spiral tube with an outer covering of silicone*) for pulsed CO_2 lasers. These tubes are slightly bulky and may abrade tracheal mucosa.
- If specialized laser tubes are not available, then red rubber tube is the preferred ET tube for laser surgery.

2. **Respiratory gas mixture:** Combustion is more likely when excessive oxygen is present. Reduction in FiO_2 to less than 0.40 reduces fire chances. N_2O also favors combustion, so air-oxygen or oxygen-helium mixture (better) is preferred.

Airway Fire Protocol

If an airway fire or explosion occurs, then surgeons and the anesthesiologists must act quickly in a coordinated fashion:
- Remove the source as quickly as possible.
- Stop ventilation (so as to prevent the entry of smoke in lower airways).
- Disconnect the breathing circuit from the anesthesia.
- Direct laryngoscopy and rigid (Venturi-ventilating) bronchoscopy to survey damage and to remove debris.
- If the fire was of the "interior blowtorch" type, gentle bronchial lavage may be indicated.
- If any airway damage is apparent, then patient should be reintubated.
- If the damage is severe, then a low tracheostomy may be indicated.

LAST-MINUTE REVISION

- Carbon dioxide laser produces maximum smoke surgery.
- If specialized laser tubes are not available, then red rubber tube is the preferred ET tube for laser surgery.

REVIEW QUESTIONS

1. Which of the following is not included into the strategies to reduce the airway fire in laser surgery?
   a. Ventilation with 100% oxygen
   b. Intubation with metallic ET tube
   c. Use of saline for inflation of ET tube cuff
   d. Use of jet ventilation for ventilating the patient

2. A patient is being operated for vocal nodule excision through laser, In the midway of surgery, there is flaming from the ET tube. All of the following represent management strategies, *except*:
   a. Disconnect the breathing circuit
   b. Stop ventilating the patient
   c. Stop all anesthetic agents and start ventilating with 100% oxygen
   d. Stop surgery

ANSWERS

1. a   2. c

CHAPTER 37

Anesthesia for Laparoscopy

Anshul Jain, Chris L Lemos

INTRODUCTION

The provision of better equipment and optics, along with enhanced medical knowledge, has allowed the development of endoscopy for diagnostic and operative procedures. Since the introduction of the first laparoscopic cholecystectomy procedure, laparoscopy has expanded both in scope and volume. Laparoscopy provides benefits of improved and more rapid recovery, reduced postoperative fatigue and less postoperative pain. Stress response is much less after laparoscopic surgery when compared with open surgery. These overall translates to early discharge, early return of activity and decreased economic burden.

Though laparoscopy has got multiple benefits over open procedures, it also poses some risks which must be weighed against benefits.

In laparoscopic surgery, pneumoperitoneum is created to provide the working space for laparoscope (Figs. 37.1A and B). The pneumoperitoneum along with the positioning required for laparoscopy, induce pathophysiologic changes that complicates anesthetic management.

PHYSIOLOGICAL AND PATHOLOGICAL CONSEQUENCES OF PNEUMOPERITONEUM

Pneumoperitoneum is most commonly created by intraperitoneal insufflation of carbon dioxide (CO_2). Veress needle is introduced through abdominal wall into the peritoneal cavity, through this needle CO_2 flows into peritoneal cavity. As peritoneal cavity expands various ports are inserted. It should be noted that insufflated CO_2 is being absorbed continuously into the systemic

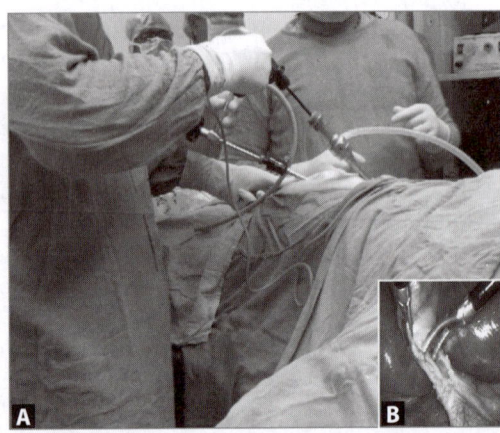

Figs. 37.1A and B: (A) Laparoscope in situ (Note the abdominal distension); (B) Image taken, during laparoscopic cholecystectomy.

circulation, so it is necessary to provide continuous flow of CO_2 to maintain static intra-abdominal pressure (IAP). The increased IAP secondary to pneumoperitoneum results in ventilatory and respiratory changes and can produce four principal respiratory complications, viz:

- CO_2 subcutaneous emphysema
- Pneumothorax
- Endobronchial intubation
- Gas embolism

As peritoneal cavity expands, diaphragm is pushed up (results in basal atelectasis) which reduces thoracopulmonary compliance and decreases functional residual capacity which can lead to raised peak and mean airway pressures. Both of these factors increase physiological dead space. These changes are more marked, if IAP is above 14 mm Hg.

Carbon dioxide absorbed from peritoneum increases the partial pressure of arterial CO_2

($PaCO_2$). Usually, the $PaCO_2$ progressively increases to reach a plateau 15–30 minutes after the beginning of CO_2 insufflation. Any significant increase in $PaCO_2$ after this period requires a search for some other causes, independent to CO_2 insufflation, such as CO_2 subcutaneous emphysema.

Subcutaneous Emphysema

Subcutaneous emphysema can develop as a complication of accidental extraperitoneal insufflation or as side effect of certain laparoscopic surgical procedures that require intentional extraperitoneal insufflation, e.g., inguinal hernia repair.

Under these circumstances, both $PaCO_2$, and end-tidal carbon dioxide concentration ($ETCO_2$) increases which does not respond to adjustment of ventilation.

If subcutaneous emphysema is suspected, then laparoscopy must be temporarily interrupted to allow CO_2 elimination and can be resumed after correction of hypercapnia.

> ### KEY POINTS
> **Why CO_2 preferred for pneumoperitoneum over O_2 and N_2?**
> - More soluble than O_2 and N_2 so is absorbed/eliminated more quickly.
> - In case of intravenous insufflation, margin of safety is much higher for CO_2 than N_2 and O_2.
> - Lethal dose of embolized CO_2 is five times greater from O_2.
> - Does not support combustion.

Pneumothorax, Pneumomediastinum and Pneumopericardium

Creation of a pneumoperitoneum can produce pneumomediastinum, unilateral or bilateral pneumothorax, and more seriously pneumopericardium. This can be due to opening of embryonic channels of communication between the peritoneal cavity and the pleural and pericardial sacs, secondary to increased intraperitoneal pressure.

Pneumothorax may also develop secondary to alveolar rupture or pleural tears.

Spontaneous CO_2 pneumothorax usually resolves spontaneously within 30–60 minutes. Positive end-expiratory pressure (PEEP) application enhances the rate of resolution. However, if the pneumothorax is secondary to rupture of pre-existing bullae, thoracocentesis is mandatory and PEEP application is contraindicated.

Endobronchial Intubation

Pneumoperitoneum displaces diaphragm cephalad, this may results in cephalad movement of the carina potentially leading to an endobronchial intubation. Chances further increase in head-down position.

Gas Embolism

Although rare, gas embolism is the most feared and dangerous complication of laparoscopy.[Q] Direct needle or trocar placement into a vessel can result in intravascular injection of gas, or it may occur as a consequence of gas insufflation into an abdominal organ. This complication develops principally during the creation of pneumoperitoneum, and is more common in patients with previous abdominal surgery. The rapid injection of gas under high pressure produces a "gas lock" in the vena cava and right atrium; thereby completely obstructing the venous return. Subsequently, there is fall in cardiac output or even circulatory collapse. Physical signs such as tachycardia, cardiac arrhythmias, hypotension, alteration in heart tones (i.e., mill-wheel murmur), cyanosis, immediately after initiation of peritoneal insufflation suggest gas embolism. Sudden decrease in $ETCO_2$ approaching toward zero is highly suggestive of gas embolism.

Carbon dioxide is more soluble in blood and rapidly eliminated, thus increases the margin of safety in case of intravenous injection of CO_2. This is one of the reason because of which CO_2 is preferred for pneumoperitoneum.

Treatment

- Immediate cessation of CO_2 insufflation.
- The patient is placed in steep head-down and left lateral decubitus (Durant's) position.
- All anesthetic agents are discontinued and patient is ventilated with 100% O_2. Hyperventilation increases CO_2 excretion.
- If these simple measures are not effective, then a central venous or pulmonary artery catheter can be introduced for aspiration of the gas. Cardiopulmonary resuscitation must be initiated, if necessary.
- Hyperbaric oxygen treatment should be strongly considered, if cerebral gas embolism is suspected.

Hemodynamic Problems

Hemodynamic changes of laparoscopy result from the combined effects of pneumoperitoneum, patient position, anesthesia and hypercapnia secondary to the absorbed CO_2 (**Fig. 37.2**).

Urine output, renal plasma flow and glomerular filtration rate decrease to less than 50% of baseline values.

Contrary to previous belief splanchnic blood flow does not decrease. This is due to the direct vasodilating effect of CO_2 on splanchnic circulation which counteracts the mechanical effect of increased IAP.

Lower limb venous stasis (more pronounced in head-up position) increases the risk of thromboembolic complications.

The reduction in venous return and cardiac output can be attenuated by increasing circulating volume prior to the pneumoperitoneum.

Gastrointestinal Problems

Aspiration of Gastric Contents

Patients undergoing laparoscopy are at risk for acid aspiration syndrome due to increased IAP.

Nausea and Vomiting

One of the main complaints of laparoscopy is postoperative nausea and vomiting (PONV). Perioperative opioids increase the incidence of PONV, whereas propofol anesthesia markedly reduces it.

Neurologic Problems

Rise in intracranial pressure maybe seen due to multiple factors like head low position, increased partial pressure of CO_2 and elevated SVR which can result in decrease in cerebral perfusion pressure.

Problems Related to Patient Positioning

Patient positioning depends on the site of surgery; head-down tilt is used for pelvic and lower abdominal surgery, whereas the head-up position is preferred for upper abdominal surgeries, e.g., cholecystectomy.

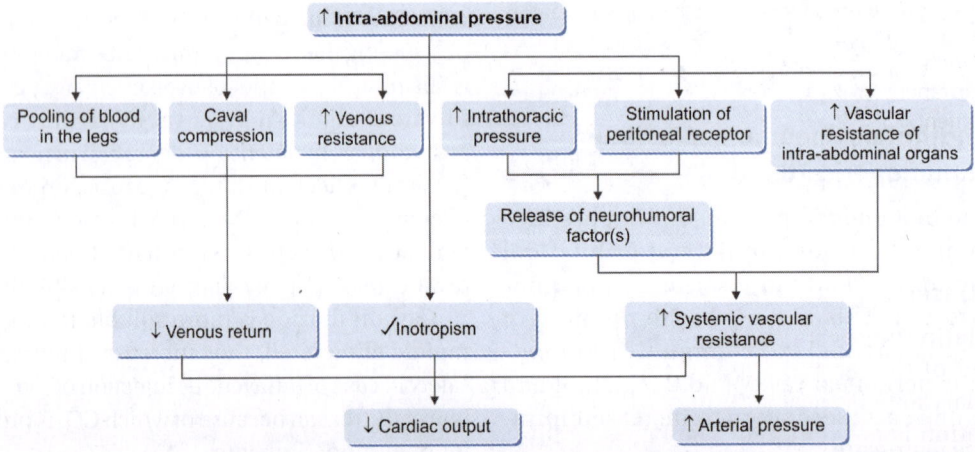

Fig. 37.2: Hemodynamic effects of pneumoperitoneum.

Physiologic effects and problems secondary to patient position include:
- *Cardiovascular effects*: Head-down position increase central venous pressure (CVP), intracranial pressure and intraocular pressure.
- Conversely with the head-up position (adopted in cholecystectomy), there is reduction in cardiac output and mean arterial pressure secondary to reduced venous return. This decrease is accentuated by hemodynamic changes induced by pneumoperitoneum.
- *Respiratory changes*: Head-down position reduce the functional residual capacity, total lung volume and the pulmonary compliance. These changes are more marked in obese, elderly and debilitated patients. The head-up position is usually favorable to respiration and tends to counter the respiratory effect of pneumoperitoneum.
- *Nerve injury*: Nerve compression is a potential complication in head-down position.

Postoperative Pain

Both intensity and duration of postoperative pain are much lower after laparoscopic surgery. Nature of pain also varies, in open surgery parietal pain is much more while in laparoscopic visceral pain is high. Postlaparoscopy shoulder-tip pain resulting from diaphragmatic irritation[Q] due to CO_2 is particularly problematic in postoperative period.

KEY POINTS
Techniques to prevent postlaparoscopy shoulder tip pain: Intraperitoneal saline infusion and pulmonary recruitment.

ALTERNATIVES TO CO_2 PNEUMOPERITONEUM

Inert Gases

Insufflation of inert gas (e.g., helium, argon) instead of CO_2 avoids the increase in $PaCO_2$ secondary to peritoneal absorption. Thus, hyperventilation is not required. The hemodynamic changes produced by pneumoperitoneum using inert gas are similar to those observed with CO_2. But, the low blood solubility of the inert gases increases the mortality risk of gas embolism.

Gasless Laparoscopy

In gasless laparoscopy, the peritoneal cavity is expanded using abdominal wall lift obtained with a fan retractor. This avoids the hemodynamic and respiratory repercussions of increased IAP and the consequences of the use of CO_2. Elderly and patients with compromised cardiopulmonary reserve can be considered for gasless laparoscopy.

ANESTHETIC MANAGEMENT

Preoperative Evaluation and Premedication

Proper preoperative evaluation is necessary, to determine the tolerability of pneumoperitoneum. Patients with severe congestive heart failure and terminal valvular insufficiency are more prone to develop cardiac complications than patients with ischemic cardiac disease.

Premedication depends on the duration of the laparoscopy. Preoperative nonsteroidal anti-inflammatory drugs reduce postoperative pain and opiate requirements. Benzodiazepines tend to reduce hemodynamic responses of pneumoperitoneum.

Anesthetic Techniques

General, local and regional anesthesias have all been used successfully and safely for laparoscopy.

General Anesthesia

General anesthesia with endotracheal intubation and controlled ventilation is certainly the safest and most commonly used technique for inpatients and for long laparoscopic procedures.

During pneumoperitoneum, controlled ventilation must be adjusted to maintain end tidal CO_2 pressure ($pETCO_2$), between 35 and 40 mm Hg. To achieve, ventilation has to be increased by 15–20%. *Increase in respiratory rate rather than tidal volume* is preferable; this avoids alveolar overinflation and reduces the risk of pneumothorax.

Second generation supraglottic airway devices can be used as an alternative to endotracheal intubation. It allows controlled ventilation and accurate monitoring of pETCO$_2$ with reduced chances of postoperative sore throat.[Q] The ProSeal™ LMA guarantees an airway seal up to 30 cm H$_2$O and is preferred over LMA Classic™.

Local and Regional Anesthesia

Regional anesthesia, including epidural and spinal techniques, combined with the head-down position can be used for short gynecological laparoscopic procedures.[1]

Choice of drugs: Use of nitrous oxide is associated with increased bowel distension. It can increase size of CO$_2$ bubbles and potentiate risk for gas embolism and can also support combustion, hence it is recommended to avoid using N20 in laparoscopic procedures. Also increases risk of PONV.

Analgesia: Local anesthetic blocks such as transverse abdominis plane block can be used for analgesia which can help reduce opioid consumption as a part of multimodal approach with paracetamol and NSAIDs.

Propofol is the preferred inducing agent, among volatile agents sevoflurane, desflurane, isoflurane can be used safely.

Intraoperative Care

Patient Positioning and Monitoring

Patients must be positioned with great care. All pressure points must be padded to prevent nerve and pressure injuries.

Induction and release of the pneumoperitoneum must be smooth and progressive. IAP should be kept as low as possible to reduce hemodynamic and respiratory changes, and in no case allowed to exceed 20 mm Hg.

Liberal perioperative intravenous fluid therapy decreases hemodynamic changes from pneumoperitoneum and PONV and improves postoperative recovery.

Monitoring

Irrespective of type of laparoscopy, noninvasive blood pressure, heart rate, electrocardiography, capnometry, and pulse oximetry must be continuously monitored. Invasive hemodynamic monitoring (CVP, arterial blood pressure) may be required in patients with cardiac diseases.

Recovery and Postoperative Care

Hemodynamic monitoring should be continued in the early postoperative period as hemodynamic changes outlast the release of the pneumoperitoneum. Patients undergoing laparoscopic surgery are at higher risk for PONV, hence prevention and treatment are very important.

LAPAROSCOPY IN CHILDREN AND DURING PREGNANCY

The most common nonobstetric surgical problems during pregnancy are appendicitis and cholecystitis, and they are amenable to laparoscopic surgery. Laparoscopy during pregnancy increases the risk of miscarriage or premature labor. Another concern is the risk of damaging the gravid uterus which can be avoided by alternative entry sites for the Veress needle and trocars. For safe laparoscopy in pregnant patients, recommendations are:

- Preoperative discussion with obstetric team.
- Consider use of rapid sequence induction for pregnancy >12 weeks.
- Compression stockings use for DVT prophylaxis.
- The operation should be done before the 23rd week of pregnancy.
- Fetal monitoring may be performed using transvaginal ultrasonography.
- Mechanical ventilation must be adjusted to maintain a physiologic maternal alkalosis.
- Gasless laparoscopy is an alternative to avoid the potential side effects of CO$_2$ pneumoperitoneum.

In children, laparoscopy is frequently performed for appendectomy. CO_2 pneumoperitoneum induces the same hemodynamic changes as in adults. Further, pediatric patients are more prone for the deleterious effect of increased IAP.

In pediatric patients, $pETCO_2$ may sometimes overestimate $PaCO_2$.

Principles of anesthetic management are same as that in adults.

LAST-MINUTE REVISION

- In pneumoperitoneum, IAP should be kept below 14 mm Hg.
- Serious complications of pneumoperitoneum are pneumothorax, air embolism, pneumopericardium and arrhythmias.
- Postlaparoscopy shoulder tip pain is due to CO_2 induced diaphragmatic irritation.
- General anesthesia is the preferred choice. Drugs that should be avoided are ketamine and pancuronium.

REFERENCE

1. Bajwa SJ, Kulshrestha A. Anaesthesia for laparoscopic surgery: General vs regional anaesthesia. J Minim Access Surg. 2016;12(1):4-9. doi: 10.4103/0972-9941.169952. PMID: 26917912; PMCID:PMC4746973.

REVIEW QUESTIONS

1. For laparoscopic cholecystectomy, patient is placed in which position:
   a. Supine
   b. Trendelenburg position
   c. Reverse Trendelenburg position with right side up
   d. Trendelenburg position with right side up

2. Gas used for creating pneumoperitoneum in laparoscopy:
   a. O_2
   b. CO_2
   c. N_2O
   d. N_2

3. A patient posted for laparoscopic cholecystectomy has been induced with propofol and rocuronium. Patient was alright till the insertion of Veress needle, immediately after CO_2 insufflation, patient become pulseless and his $ETCO_2$ drops to 3 mm Hg, what could not be the probable cause:
   a. Gas embolism
   b. Pneumothorax
   c. Cardiac arrest
   d. Ventricular fibrillation

ANSWERS

1. a
2. c
3. b

CHAPTER 38

Anesthesia for Neurosurgery

Keshav Goyal

INTRODUCTION

Historically, advice of neurosurgery in patients, is like their ticket to some other world and data also proves this. Till 1980s, any neurosurgery lasting >5 hours had >50% mortality. If we move to present statistics, mortality is <2%. This improved outcome of modern neurosurgery is the result of better anesthetic management, better imaging techniques, further it is not wrong to say that improved neuroanesthesia is the outcome of better understanding of neurophysiology and pharmacology. Current chapter covers important aspects of cerebral physiology and pharmacology in relation to anesthesia and anesthetic management of common neurosurgical procedure.

CEREBRAL PHYSIOLOGY AND PHARMACOLOGY

Cerebral Metabolism

Brain is responsible for 20% of total oxygen consumption. *Average cerebral metabolism rate ($CMRO_2$), expressed in terms of cerebral oxygen consumption rate is 3–3.8 mL/100 g/minute or 50 mL/minute.* $CMRO_2$ is highest in gray matter of cerebral cortex. *Because of relatively high oxygen consumption, as little as 10 seconds interruption of cerebral perfusion can produce unconsciousness. If blood flow is not established within minutes (maximum 8 minutes) irreversible neuronal injury occurs.* Hippocampus and cerebellum are most sensitive to hypoxic injury.

Glucose is the principal source of energy for neurons and acute hypoglycemia is equally as devastating as hypoxia. In brain, more than 90% of glucose is metabolized aerobically *(reason behind paradoxical exacerbation of hypoxic brain injury in hyperglycemia).*

Under hypoxic conditions, glucose is metabolized anaerobically with production of lactic acid which further exacerbates acidosis and neuronal injury creating a vicious cycle. Because of this reason, glucose-containing fluids should be avoided in neurosurgery.

Cerebral Blood Flow

Average cerebral blood flow (CBF) is 50 mL/100 g/minute^Q (80 mL/100 g/minute in gray matter while 20 mL/100 g/minute in white matter).

Regulation of Cerebral Blood Flow

- **Cerebral perfusion pressure**: Cerebral perfusion pressure (CPP) is the difference between mean arterial pressure (MAP) and intracranial pressure (ICP) or cerebral venous pressure (whichever is higher). Since ICP is normally <10 mm Hg, CPP usually parallels MAP. Normally CPP varies between 80 and 100 mm Hg, and a CPP <25 mm Hg results in irreversible brain damage.
- **Autoregulation**: Brain has got the best autoregulatory power in the body which maintains CBF at a relatively constant level between MAP of 60–160 mm Hg. Beyond these, limit cerebral perfusion become, pressure dependent. In chronic hypertensives cerebral autoregulation curve shift to right, means they can well tolerate high blood pressure while during episodes of hypotension CBF declines rapidly.

- **Other factors:**
  - *CO_2 content of blood*: CBF is directly proportional to $PaCO_2$. Hypercapnia increases CBF, while hypocapnia decreases blood flow. This is due to change in CSF pH. CBF does not depend much on arterial oxygen tension and only marked hypoxemia increases CBF.
  - *Temperature*: Hyperthermia increase CBF, while hypothermia decreases it.

Intracranial Pressure

Intracranial pressure by convention means supratentorial CSF pressure measured in lateral ventricles and is normally <10 mm Hg.

Cranial vault is a rigid structure with a fixed total volume. Contents of cranium include brain tissue (80%), blood (12%) and CSF (8%). Raise in the volume of any component of vault must be accompanied by equivalent decrease in another component otherwise ICP will increase. These contents exert a continuous lateral pressure against noncompliant bony cranium. In general, ICP should be maintained at <20 mm Hg and CPP should be maintained at >60 mm Hg.

> **Why increased intracranial pressure is dangerous?**
> Increased ICP tends to decrease CPP and can lead to brain herniation. Decreased CPP and neuronal damage produce cerebral edema, which further increase ICP thus creating a vicious cycle.

Diagnosis of Increased Intracranial Pressure

Early symptoms of elevated ICP include drowsiness and a diminished level of consciousness.[Q] Headache; vomiting; blurred vision; mental change; somnolence are other common symptoms of increased ICP.[1]

> **KEY POINTS**
> - **Cushing reflex:** Hypertension and bradycardia in association with raised ICT.
> - All volatile agents increase ICP by increasing cerebral blood flow.

Signs include hypertension, bradycardia and papilledema.

Computed tomography (CT) shows midline shift (> 0.5 cm), obliteration of basal cistern, loss of sulci, ventricular effacement.

Effect of Anesthetic Agents on Brain Physiology (Table 38.1)

Inhalational Agents

All volatile agents reduce cerebral metabolic rate; maximum reduction is seen with isoflurane while halothane has least effect. All volatile anesthetics dilate cerebral blood vessels and impair autoregulation, halothane has the greatest effect. The increased blood flow coupled with decreased cerebral metabolic rate produce a state of enhanced perfusion, called as luxury perfusion.[Q] However, it

Table 38.1: Comparative effects of anesthetic agents on cerebral physiology.

Agent	CMR	CBF	CSF (Production/Absorption)	ICP
Halothane	↓↓	↑↑↑	↓ / ↓	↑↑
Isoflurane	↓↓↓	↑	± / ↑	↑
Nitrous oxide	↓	↑	± / ±	↑
Barbiturates	↓↓↓↓	↓↓↓	± / ↑	↓↓↓
Etomidate	↓↓↓	↓↓	± / ↑	↓↓
Propofol	↓↓↓	↓↓↓	effect not properly studied	↓↓
Benzodiazepines	↓↓	↓	± / ↑	↓
Ketamine	±	↑↑	± / ↓	↑↑
Opioids	±	±	± / ↑	±

± little or no change
(CMR: cerebral metabolic rate; CBF: cerebral blood flow; CSF: cerebrospinal fluid; ICP: intracranial pressure)

should be clear that volatile agents do not increase blood flow in ischemic areas, thus in cases with focal ischemia blood is redistributed away from ischemic area to normal areas *(circulatory steal phenomenon)*. Volatile agents have no effect on CO_2 response and hypocapnia can blunt or reverse the volatile agent induced increase in blood flow.

Enflurane increases CSF production while halothane decreases CSF absorption, so both of them tend to increase CSF volume.

Summarizing the above discussion, *halothane has got most deleterious effect while isoflurane has maximum beneficial effects and is the volatile agent of choice*[Q] *in neurosurgery.*[2]

Intravenous Agents

Except ketamine, all intravenous agents reduce CMR and CBF. Cerebral autoregulation and CO_2 responsiveness remain normal with all agents.

Thiopentone, because of the following properties is induction agents of choice in neuroanesthesia:
- Hypnosis
- Reduce ICP (by reducing CBF and enhancing CSF absorption)
- Anticonvulsant

Proportionally, there is higher reduction in $CMRO_2$ than CBF, so metabolic supply exceeds demand. It is important to mention that barbiturates reduce CBF only in normal areas. As a result, there is redistribution of blood from normal to focal ischemic areas. *This phenomenon is called as Robin Hood or reverse steal phenomenon.*[Q] Due to these properties barbiturate prophylaxis is effective in preventing brain injury during focal ischemia *(but not during global ischemia)*.

Propofol and etomidate also reduce CMR, CBF and ICP. Propofol is the second induction agent of choice (where thiopentone is contraindicated).

Ketamine[Q] is the only intravenous agent that dilates cerebral vasculature, increase CBF, and CMR. Ketamine impede CSF absorption and increase ICP, so is contraindicated in neuroanesthesia **(Table 38.1)**.

Among neuromuscular blocking agents, *succinylcholine (SCh) and histamine-releasing nondepolarizers (tubocurarine, atracurium, metocurine, mivacurium) increase ICP.*[Q] With SCh, this increase is minimal and short-lived, so SCh is still intubating muscles relaxant of choice in emergency neurosurgery particularly where airway is difficult: Rocuronium is preferred over vecuronium as the intubation relaxant of choice in elective neurosurgery **(Table 38.1)**.

ANESTHETIC MANAGEMENT

Principles for Safe Anesthesia Management

- Maintenance of normal intracranial temperature (ICT) **(Table 38.2)**
- To protect brain against ischemic injury **(Fig. 38.1)**
- Avoidance of position-related problems
- Proper management of associated problem (if any).

Maintenance of ICP carries highest priority

Table 38.2: Measures to reduce intracranial pressure.

Compartment	Volume control measures
Brain tissue (neurons, glia, tumor)	Surgical removal
Extracellular and intracellular fluid (cerebral edema)	Diuretics (mannitol, hypertonic saline), steroids principally in tumors
Cerebrospinal fluid	Drainage
Arterial blood	Hypocapnia-induced vasoconstriction, barbiturates
Venous blood	Improve venous drainage by head-up position

Management of Increased Intracranial Pressure (Flowchart 38.1)

As mentioned earlier, in conditions with increased ICT, cerebral perfusion pressure reduces markedly. Thus, in order to bring CPP toward normal, it is very essential to reduce ICP. This can only be achieved by reduction in one or more compartment of brain,

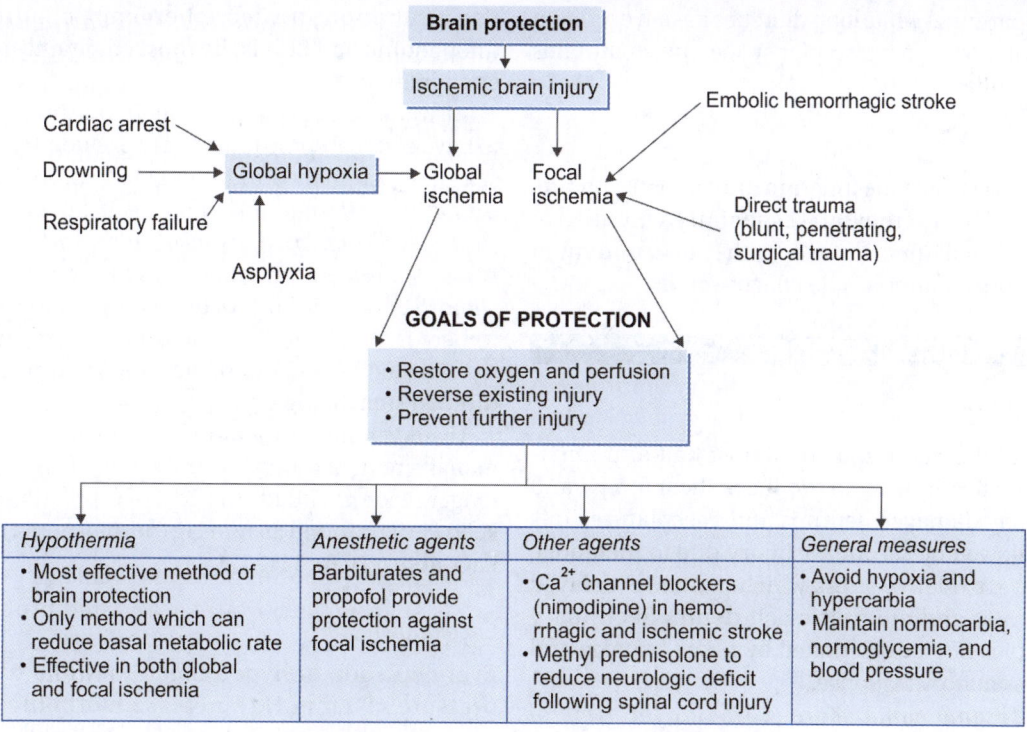

Fig. 38.1: Protection against ischemic brain injury.

i.e., brain tissue, CSF, blood, intracellular and extracellular fluids **(Table 38.2)**.

International Societies of Neurosurgery recommends, stepwise management starting from positional therapy to decompressive craniectomy (removal of part of cranium) **(Flowchart 38.1)**.

A special note is required for diuretics and steroid in conditions with increased ICT.

Diuretics

Diuretics mainly reduce the extracellular fluid compartment of brain. Though both osmotic and loop diuretics can be used for this purpose; *osmotic diuretics (mannitol, hypertonic saline) are the preferred one*. Due to hyperosmotic nature mannitol withdraw fluid from extravascular space; however, it is effective only when some degree of blood-brain integrity is preserved. If blood-brain barrier is disrupted (intraparenchymal hemorrhage) mannitol extravasates and can increase edema. Administration of furosamide

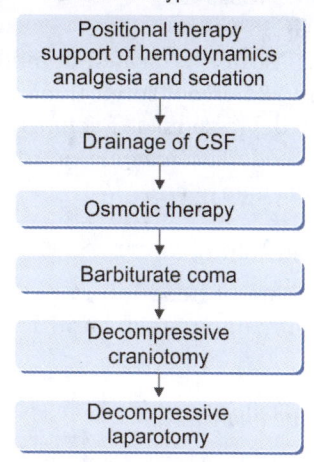

Flowchart 38.1: Stepwise management of intracranial hypertension.

(CSF: cerebrospinal fluid)

along with osmotic diuretics is based on the rationale that osmotic diuretics draw water from extracellular compartment, to intravascular compartment while loop diuretics hasten excretion of water from intravascular space, thus maintains the gradient.

Steroids

Steroids reduce the inflammation and membrane permeability, they are especially valuable in intracranial tumor,[Q] however, they take minimum 24 hours for appreciable effect.

SPECIFIC CONDITIONS

Head Injury

Head injury accounts for almost half of trauma-related death. Trauma produces shear forces, and directly damages neurons and vasculature. This is followed by secondary injury due to metabolic failure, oxidative stress which produces delayed necrotic and apoptotic cell death. Secondary injury is often exacerbated by tissue hypoxia and inflammatory response.

Glasgow coma score (GCS) at the time of admission, it the most important prognostic factor.[Q] Based on GCS head injury can be:
- **Mild: GCS score**: 13–15
- **Moderate**: GCS: 9–12
- **Severe**: GCS ≤ 8.[Q]

Urgent CT scan is indicated in moderate and severe injury. Emergent surgical management is indicated for depressed skull fractures, evacuation of epidural, subdural hematoma, and debridement of penetrating injury.

Preoperative Management

Anesthetic care of head injury patient begins in emergency department and follows ABC algorithm.

Airway and Breathing (A, B)

Hypoxemia mostly coexists with head injury. In patient with normal breathing effort and reflexes, oxygen supplementation with mask is enough. Patients with obvious hypoventilation, absent gag reflex or GCS < 8, requires endotracheal intubation. For intubation in such emergency condition thiopentone and SCh is the most commonly used combination.

All traumatic head injury patients are presumed to have cervical spine injury until excluded (by CT scan) and supposed to be full stomach. So, *oral intubation with manual inline head stabilization (to avoid movement at cervical spine) and cricoid pressure (Sellick maneuver) is the technique of choice.*[Q] Blind nasal intubation is contraindicated, if there is suspicion of basal skull fracture which is suggested by CSF rhinorrhea, hemotympanum, raccoon sign, battle sign.

Hyperventilation therapy, long a mainstay in the management of traumatic brain injury (TBI), is no longer recommended. The goal of ventilation is to keep $PaCO_2$ around 35 mm Hg (normocapnia) and PaO_2 above 70 mm Hg.

Circulation (C)

Every episode of hypotension (systolic blood pressure <90 mm Hg) increase morbidity and mortality in traumatic brain injury. Active bleeding must be controlled and hypotension must be corrected. Current goal is to maintain euvolemic state (normovolemia) for which crystalloid fluids are preferred over vasopressor, later should be used only when fluids alone are not sufficient. *Hypertonic or normal saline is the preferred fluid while glucose-containing fluids are contraindicated*[Q] (for the reason mentioned above). In cases of significant bleeding, transfusion may be started in order to keep hematocrit <30%.

An intraventricular catheter can be inserted to monitor ICP. The goal is to maintain CPP >60 mm Hg and ICP <20 mm Hg.

Diagnostic studies: After maintaining ABC; CT and CT angiography (if needed) can be performed to know the exact pathology.

Intraoperative Management

- Follow steps as per **Flowchart 38.1** and **Box 38.1**.
- If patients is already intubated anesthesia can be maintained on $N_2O : O_2$ + isoflurane

BOX 38.1

Intraoperative management for head injury (common for all patients).
- Establish airway, breathing and circulation
- Maintain systolic BP >90 mm Hg
- Ventilate to maintain $PaCO_2$ around 35 mm Hg
- Provide supplemental O_2 to keep PaO_2 >70 mm Hg or SpO_2 >94%
- Keep Hct 30–33%
- Maintain serum sodium at 140–145 unless patient has ICP elevations
- Maintain normothermia
- Ensure good head and neck alignment
- Start anticonvulsant therapy for the first 7 days after injury; phenytoin is the agent of choice
- Reduce unnecessary noxious stimuli
- Manage raised ICT in stepwise manner

(ICT: intracranial temperature; ICP: intracranial pressure; Hct: hematocrit)

+ rocuronium/vecuronium. *Nitrous oxide should be avoided when there is suspicion of pneumocephalus.* Under such conditions, air is used instead of N_2O, as N_2O expands the closed air spaces.
- For unintubated patients, protocol of emergency airway management is followed.
- Intraoperative hypertension should be managed by deepening anesthesia and β-blocker.
- Vasodilator should be avoided until dura is opened. Disseminated intravascular coagulation and neurogenic pulmonary edema can complicate head injury intraoperatively and are managed accordingly.

KEY POINTS

Brain senses pain but brain parenchyma itself is not sensitive to pain.

The decision to extubate at the end of surgery depends upon patient hemodynamic status, surgical procedure, associated injury and preoperative status.

Note: It must be mentioned that brain parenchyma itself is not sensitive to pain and it is only scalp and dura which has pain fibers, so neurosurgery patients requires analgesia sufficient enough to tolerate endotracheal tube.

Monitoring

In addition to routine monitoring; ICP, urine output, arterial blood pressure, CVP should be monitored in all patients.

Postoperative Care

Diabetes insipidus, stress gastric ulcers, and convulsive attacks are the common complications of TBI in postoperative period.

INTRACRANIAL MASS LESIONS

Intracranial mass lesion can be neoplastic, infectious (abscess) or vascular (hematoma, AV malformation). Regardless of the cause intracranial mass lesion produces symptoms related to mass effect, location and increased ICT.

Preoperative Evaluation

Goal is to find the intensity of intracranial hypertension. All patients should be assessed for neurologic deficit, which if present must be documented. Current medication of patient should be reviewed with special reference to steroids, diuretics *(may cause electrolytic abnormalities)* and anticonvulsant.

Anesthetic Management

In patients with intracranial hypertension premedication is avoided. Anesthetic agents of choice are thiopentone, rocuronium, isoflurane. *Succinylcholine is best avoided in elective situation, when there is raised ICT, and in patients with paralytic abnormalities (produce severe hyperkalemia).*

Anesthesia is maintained with O_2: N_2O/air with isoflurane. Hyperventilation is no longer recommended (correctly speaking contraindicated).[3]

Goal is to maintain normocarbia and avoidance of hypoxia. Hypercapnia ($ETCO_2$ >40 mm Hg) must be avoided as above 40 mm Hg, each mm Hg raise in $PaCO_2$ would increase CBF by 20–30 mL and hence, increase ICT markedly. Invasive monitoring (CVP, arterial blood pressure) is indicated in complex procedures only.

Intravenous Fluids

Normal saline, Ringer lactate *(some books have mentioned RL is contraindicated, this is wrong)* are the preferred fluid for intraoperative fluid therapy. *Glucose containing fluids are contraindicated.*[Q]

Postoperative Management

Anticonvulsant must be continued. Hypoxia and hypercarbia must be avoided.

Patients who are undergoing craniotomy through subfrontal approach may exhibit delayed emergence, lethargy in immediate postoperative period. This phenomenon is called *frontal lobey and should be managed accordingly.*[Q]

POSTERIOR FOSSA PROCEDURES (CRANIOTOMY IN SITTING POSITION)

Posterior fossa procedures present unique problems related to obstructive hydrocephalus, possible injury to brainstem, surgical position (sitting position) pneumocephalus and above all, these procedures carry highest risk of venous air embolism (VAE).

Problem of Posterior Fossa Surgery

Obstructive Hydrocephalus

Infratentorial tumor can obstruct CSF flow which leads to severe intracranial hypertension. Such cases often require ventriculostomy before anesthesia, so as to reduce ICP.

Positioning (Fig. 38.2)

Posterior fossa procedures are most commonly performed in sitting position. This position is associated with many problems including maximum chances of VAE.

Important problems of sitting position are:
- **Pneumocephalus**: In sitting position, air may enter in subarachnoid space. This pneumocephalus can compress brain after dural closure and delays recovery from anesthesia along with other deleterious effects.
- **Hemodynamic instability**: In sitting position, there are increased chances of hypotension and cardiovascular instability.
- **Quadriplegia**: Neck flexion is sitting position can stretch or compress the cervical spinal cord which may lead to quadriplegia. Risk is high in patient with pre-existing cervical pathology.
- **Brainstem stimulation**: Surgical instruments by irritating, medulla and extracranial portion of 5th cranial nerve, produce cardiovascular instability.

Venous Air Embolism

Venous air embolism (VAE) can occur in any surgery, whenever venous pressure in the surgical area is subatmospheric.

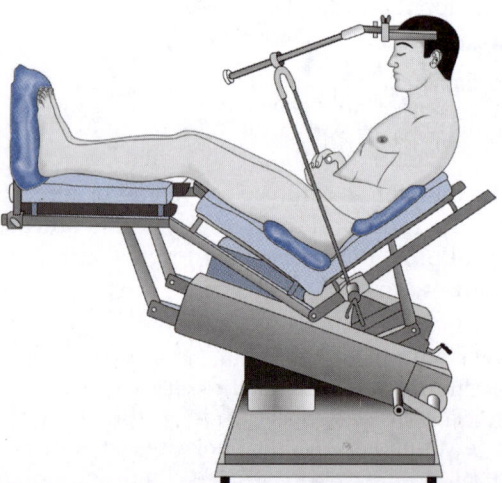

Fig. 38.2: Sitting position for posterior fossa procedure.

If any valveless vein gets open in such area, then it will suck air. Incidence of VAE is maximum in sitting position.

Pathophysiology

Air enters through vein and reaches right atrium (RA); from RA air can go to pulmonary circulation via right ventricle or left atrium *(if foramen ovale is patent)*; from left atrium it may go to systemic circulation *(paradoxical embolism)* and can block end arteries.

In pulmonary circulation, fate depends upon the amount of air, small air bubbles diffuses through alveoli and are not problematic. When air amount or bubble size exceeds pulmonary clearance, they get lodged in pulmonary artery and blocks circulation which increase right ventricular afterload, when air amount is very large, it produces gas lock at right ventricle outflow and can lead to acute right ventricular failure.

Diagnosis

Clinical signs are often absent in small embolism. If air amount is very large, signs are hypertension, tachycardia, cyanosis and mill wheel murmur. Decreased $ETCO_2$ and arterial saturation are usually the initial signs. *When air amount is very large, $ETCO_2$ suddenly drops to zero (no diffusion across alveoli) and $PaCO_2$ raise.* Most sensitive test for VAE is transesophageal echo (detect 0.02 mL) followed by precordial Doppler (detect 0.25 mL of air).

Prevention of Venous Air Embolism

Continuous irrigation of wound by normal saline, which creates a water barrier between subatmospheric venous pressure and air.

Management of an Acute Air Embolism

- **Prevent further air entry**
  - Ask surgeon to pack surgical field
  - Compress jugular veins
  - Place the patient in head-down position
- **Reduce intravascular air**
  - Aspirate right atrial catheter
  - Discontinue N_2O ventilate patient with 100% O_2
  - Administer inotropes
  - Chest compression, if needed.

Note: N_2O by virtue of its high diffusion capacity, readily diffuses into closed cavity, thereby increase the size of pneumocephalus and VAE. So, N_2O is contraindicated in sitting craniotomies.

INTRACRANIAL ANEURYSMS AND ARTERIOVENOUS MALFORMATION

Anesthetic management is based on the same protocols of brain protection.

In intracranial aneurysm, there is associated vasospasm, so hyperventilation *(which exaggerates vasospasm)* should be avoided. *Contrary to this in AV malformation, hypoventilation might be required to improve surgical visualization of affected vessel.*[Q]

SEIZURE SURGERY

Seizure surgery (resection of anteromedial temporal lobe or *amygdalohippocampectomy*) is indicated in patients with refractory epilepsy.

Preoperative Evaluation

All patients should undergo Wada test and functionally to localize the hemisphere that controls speech.

All patients should be informed regarding the operative procedure and requirement of awareness during surgery. *Anticonvulsive drugs should be stopped or reduced* as they will interfere with the localization of seizure foci.

In premedication, agents with anticonvulsant effect (benzodiazepines) are contraindicated.

Intraoperative Management

The objective of seizure surgery is specific selection of seizure foci, which is accomplished through intraoperative stimulation of cortex and checking, whether it is producing seizure. So, any medication with anticonvulsant property is avoided. The goal of anesthetic management is light level of anesthesia; combination of choice is *propofol*

+ *ramifentanyl/fentanyl with laryngeal mask airway.*[Q] Scalp is anesthetized by local infiltration, addition of dexmedetomidine improves analgesia and sedation.

After opening the dura, cortical surface is stimulated so as to find exact seizure foci. If no seizure activity is observed, provocative measures can be employed. Methohexital and etomidate are used as provocative drugs. During stimulation seizure can be very severe and under such circumstances, propofol can be used as an anticonvulsant. In postoperative period, anticonvulsant drug should be continued and then withdrawn gradually.

AWAKE CRANIOTOMY

Awake craniotomies are frequently being used in neurosurgical centers for the excision of epileptic foci and eloquent brain areas surgery.

Conscious sedation in addition to a scalp block is the commonly used anesthetic technique, which allows for the titration of the level of sedation and analgesia according to surgical events, leading to quick recovery. As obstructive apnea leading to hypoventilation is a risk, a plan for securing the airway rapidly if need arises must be part of the anesthetic management. Dexmedetomidine is used in some centers as it is not associated with respiratory depression. The use of an asleep-awake-asleep technique with a laryngeal mask airway (LMA) is an alternative technique used in many centers. Routine monitoring as for a craniotomy should be used. This includes a urinary catheter if the procedure is expected to be prolonged. Patient's feeling of claustrophobia.

TRANSSPHENOIDAL SURGERY

Transsphenoidal surgery is usually done for pituitary adenoma. Anesthesia is challenging as it takes into considerations of endocrine abnormalities associated with the disease process. Transnasal transsphenoidal (TTNS) excision has benefits in terms of recovery and reduced mortality.

Pituitary tumors are more commonly associated with acromegaly, gigantism and Cushing disease. These patients have also associated diabetes mellitus, hypertension and obstructive sleep apnea. They also have airway abnormalities owing to presence of acromegaly.

Intraoperative anesthesia management is based on size of tumor and associated comorbidities, and physiological disturbances. Dexmedetomidine and remifentanil are newer and excellent drugs used for maintenance of hemodynamic stability. Postoperative management includes strict monitoring, and looking for complications such as diabetes insipidus and CSF leak.

Anesthesia management includes perioperative hemodynamic stability, maintenance of normal intracranial pressure, smooth surgical conditions such as lax brain, maintenance of adequate cerebral blood flow, rapid recovery, and emergence at completion of surgery.

Glucocorticoids are supplemented in patients with hypopituitarism on evening before surgery with 100 mg hydrocortisone, and is repeated just before or at the beginning of surgery and third dose is given in evening after the operation.

KEY POINTS

Wada Test
- The test is usually performed prior to ablative surgery for epilepsy and sometimes prior to tumor resection. The aim is to determine which side of the brain is responsible for certain vital cognitive functions, namely speech and memory.
- A barbiturate (which is usually sodium amobarbital) is introduced into the internal carotid artery of left side then on right side. The purpose is to anesthetize one hemisphere at a time.

Chapter 38: Anesthesia for Neurosurgery

 LAST-MINUTE REVISION

Drug of choice:
- **Induction agent for elective neurosurgery:** Thiopentone
- **Volatile agent of choice:** Isoflurane
- All volatile agents increase ICT
- Ketamine is the intravenous inducing agent that increases CBF, $CMRO_2$ and ICP.

REFERENCES

1. Pinto VL, Tadi P, Adeyinka A. Increased Intracranial Pressure. [Updated 2022 Aug 1]. In: StatPearls [Internet]. Treasure Island (FL): StatPearls Publishing; 2022 Jan-. Available from: https://www.ncbi.nlm.nih.gov/books/NBK482119/
2. Kitano H, Kirsch JR, Hurn PD, Murphy SJ. Inhalational anesthetics as neuroprotectants or chemical preconditioning agents in ischemic brain. J Cereb Blood Flow Metab. 2007;27(6):1108-28. doi: 10.1038/sj.jcbfm.9600410. Epub 2006 Oct 18. PMID: 17047683; PMCID: PMC2266688.
3. Zhang Z, Guo Q, Wang E. Hyperventilation in neurological patients: from physiology to outcome evidence. Curr Opin Anaesthesiol. 2019;32(5):568-73. doi: 10.1097/ACO.0000000000000764. PMID: 31211719; PMCID: PMC6735527.

REVIEW QUESTIONS

1. A patient sustained road traffic accident and has got multiple fractures in long bones, mandible, ribs, on admission his GC score is 11, after 2 hours of admission his GC score becomes 8 and emergency intubation was planned. Under such circumstances, intubating relaxant of choice is:
   a. Rocuronium
   b. Succinylcholine
   c. Thiopentone
   d. Atracurium
2. Which of the following agents exhibit Robin Hood phenomenon?
   a. Etomidate
   b. Propofol
   c. Thiopentone
   d. Ketamine
3. Least suitable volatile agent for neurosurgery:
   a. Halothane
   b. Propofol
   c. Isoflurane
   d. Sevoflurane
4. Intubation with manual inline stabilization is performed in:
   a. Lumbar spine injury
   b. Thoracic spine injury
   c. Chest trauma
   d. Head injury
5. Sitting position craniotomy is associated with enhanced risk of following complications, *except*:
   a. Venous air embolism
   b. Facial nerve palsy
   c. Pneumocephalus
   d. Quadriplegia

ANSWERS

| 1. a | 2. c | 3. a | 4. d | 5. b |

CHAPTER 39

Anesthesia for Cardiothoracic Surgery

Reena, Anshul Jain

INTRODUCTION

Due to improvement in surgical and anesthetic techniques more and more patient are being operated for cardiac problems. Anesthesia for cardiovascular surgery requires a thorough understanding of circulatory physiology, pharmacology, and pathophysiology as surgical manipulations often have a profound impact on circulatory function.

Before considering anesthetic management of cardiothoracic surgery it is essential to know about cardiopulmonary bypass (CPB).

CARDIOPULMONARY BYPASS

Cardiopulmonary bypass is a technique that diverts venous blood away from the heart, adds oxygen, removes CO_2, and returns the blood to a large artery (usually the aorta) thus bypassing heart and lung.

In CPB (**Fig. 39.1**), an extracorporeal circuit is placed in series with the systemic circulation which provides both artificial ventilation and perfusion. For proper surgical access surgeon requires cardiac stand still, this is achieved by injecting cardioplegic solution in the heart (a chemical solution which arrests myocardial electrical and mechanical activity).

Cardiopulmonary bypass operation requires a perfusionist—a highly specialized technician who manages CPB pump. Optimal results with CPB require close cooperation and communication between the surgeon, anesthesiologist and perfusionist.

Circuit

The CPB machine has five basic components:
1. **Venous reservoir**: Reservoir receives unoxygenated blood from the patient via one or two venous cannulas in the right atrium or the superior and inferior vena cava. Blood flows to the reservoir by gravity drainage.
2. **Oxygenator**: Blood from the bottom of the venous reservoir goes to the oxygenator. Modern CPB machines have membrane-type oxygenator in which there is a very thin, gas-permeable silicone membrane. This blood-gas interface allows blood to equilibrate with the gas mixture (primarily oxygen).
3. **Heat exchanger**: Blood from the oxygenator enters the heat exchanger. The blood is then either cooled or warmed; heat transfer occurs by conduction. As blood temperature rises, gas solubility decreases so a filter is built into the unit to catch any bubbles that may form during rewarming.
4. **Main pump**: Modern CPB machines use either an electrically driven double-arm roller (positive displacement) or a centrifugal pump to propel blood through the CPB circuit.
    - Centrifugal pumps are nonocclusive, less traumatic to blood than roller pumps. Unlike roller pumps, which are placed after the oxygenator; centrifugal pumps normally lie between the venous reservoir and the oxygenator. Both pumps produce a continuous nonpulsatile flow.
    - Pulsatile blood flow is possible with some roller pumps by varying the rate of rotation of the roller heads. Pulsatile flow besides being

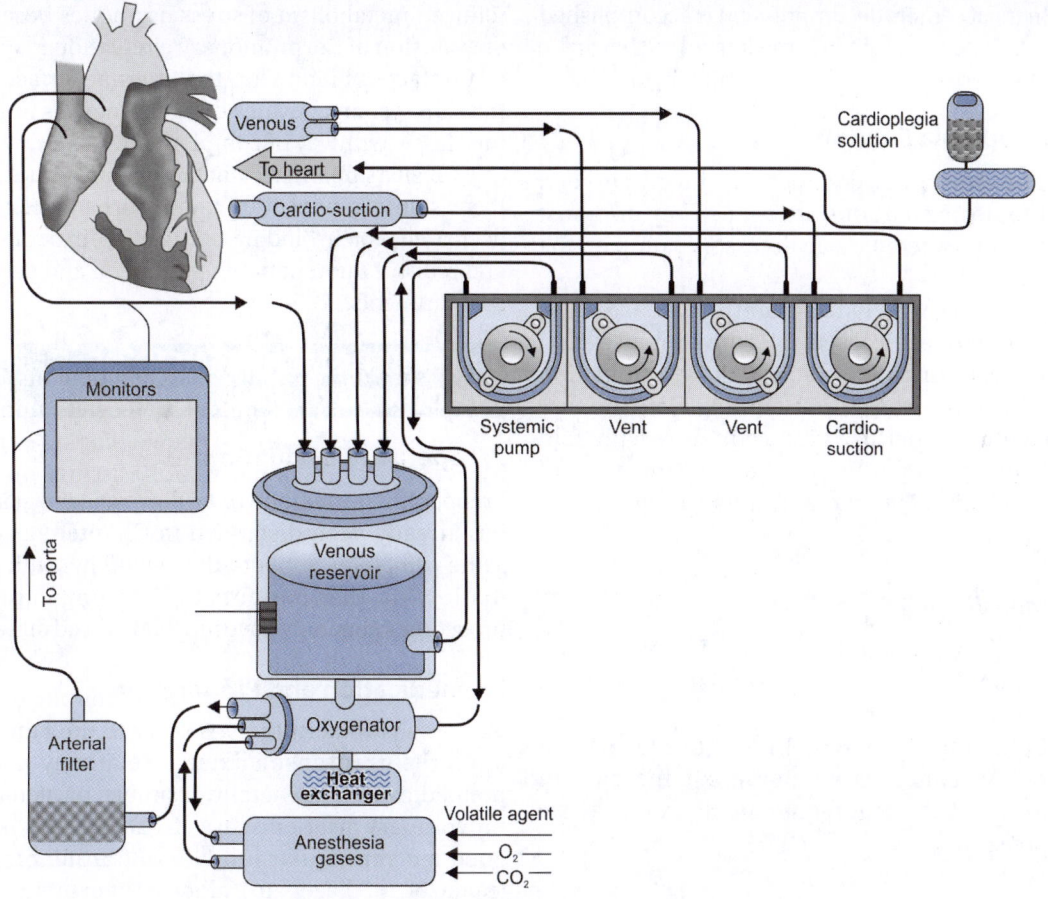

Fig. 39.1: Generic cardiopulmonary bypass circuit.

physiological, improves tissue perfusion, enhances oxygen extraction, attenuates the release of stress hormones, and results in lower systemic vascular resistances (SVRs) during CPB.

5. **Arterial filter**: Particulate matter (e.g., thrombi, fat globules) commonly enters in CPB circuit. To prevent this an in-line, arterial filter is mandatory.

Once filtered, the propelled blood returns to the patient, usually via cannula placed in the ascending aorta. A normally functioning aortic valve prevents blood from entering the left ventricle.

Accessory Pumps and Devices

Cardiotomy Suction

The cardiotomy suction pump aspirates blood from the surgical field during CPB and returns it to the main pump reservoir.

Left Ventricular Vent

Blood flowing from the bronchial arteries and thebesian vessels (or as a result of aortic regurgitation) distends the left ventricle. Distension of left ventricle compromises myocardial preservation and thus requires decompression.

In most centers decompression is accomplished by a catheter inserted into the left ventricle via the right superior pulmonary vein and left atrium.

Cardioplegia Solution

To prevent cardiac contractions during surgery, cardioplegic solutions are used. They are most often administered via an accessory pump on the CPB machine.

The most widely used method of arresting myocardial electrical activity is the administration of potassium-rich crystalloid. Following initiation of CPB, and aortic cross-clamping, the coronary circulation is perfused intermittently with cold cardioplegic solution. As the concentration of cardioplegic solution raises, the heart gets arrest in diastole.

Composition

Although there is wide variability in the composition of cardioplegic solution. Essential constituents include:
- Potassium (<40 mEq/L)—higher levels can be associated with a paradoxic increase in myocardial energy requirements and excessive potassium loads.
- Sodium (<140 mEq/L).
- Calcium (0.7–1.2 mmol/L) to maintain cellular integrity.
- Magnesium (1.5–15 mmol/L) to control excessive intracellular influxes of calcium.
- A buffer most commonly bicarbonate is necessary to prevent excessive build-up of acid metabolites.
- Other components like mannitol, procaine, lidocaine or glucocorticoids (for their membrane stabilizing effect). Energy substrates are provided as glucose, glutamate or aspartate.

Physiological and Pharmacological Effects of Cardiopulmonary Bypass

Cardiopulmonary bypass is associated with a marked increase in stress hormones and systemic inflammatory response. This is partially due to reduced metabolism of stress hormones because of exclusion of the pulmonary circulation.

Contact of blood with the internal surfaces of the CPB system activates both alternate as well as the classic pathway of complement.

CPB alters pharmacokinetics of many drugs via: Increase in volume of distribution with hemodilution, decreased protein binding, and changes in perfusion and redistribution between peripheral and central compartments.

ANESTHETIC MANAGEMENT OF CARDIAC SURGERY IN ADULTS

Preoperative Evaluation

Preoperative evaluation of cardiovascular diseases has already been discussed in Chapter 22. The same principles apply to these patients with the distinction that patients undergoing cardiac procedures generally have more advanced disease.

Premedication and Preparation

The term cardiac surgery is scary to the patients and creates intense anxiety. Relatively heavy premedication is generally desirable, particularly for coronary artery disease (CAD) patients with good left ventricular function. Benzodiazepine (midazolam; diazepam), alone or in combination with an opioid (usually morphine) are commonly used for this purpose. The dose of a benzodiazepine should generally be halved when the drug is combined with an opioid.

In cardiac surgery, ideally two large-bore (16-gauge or larger) intravenous catheters should be placed. One of which should be in a large central vein. Blood must be readily available if needed.

Intraoperative Management

Anesthetic techniques for cardiac surgery range from primarily volatile inhalation anesthesia, to total intravenous anesthesia, and combined neuraxial blockade with light general anesthesia. Except ketamine all drugs can be used in CAD patients. Drug of choice in valvular surgery is same as for patients undergoing noncardiac surgery.

Among volatile agents sevoflurane and desflurane are the agent of choice.[Q] Isoflurane is the second choice. Propofol or etomidate are most commonly used intravenous agents for induction. Nitrous oxide (N_2O) is usually avoided because of its tendency to expand any intravascular air bubbles that may form during CPB.

Rocuronium and vecuronium are the preferred muscle relaxants. Succinylcholine is reserved only for endotracheal intubation in difficult airway patient.

Monitoring

In addition to all basic monitoring NIBP, ECG, invasive BP monitoring and CVP monitoring is indicated in all cases. Arterial cannulation and central venous cannulation is generally performed prior to induction of anesthesia, as the induction period represents a time of major hemodynamic stress.

Routine use of a pulmonary artery catheter is controversial. In general, it is reserved for patients with compromised ventricular function (ejection fraction <40–50%) or pulmonary hypertension and in those undergoing complicated procedures.

It must be noted that pulmonary artery catheters often migrate distally during CPB and may spontaneously wedge without balloon inflation. Inflation of the balloon under these conditions can rupture a pulmonary artery and may produce lethal pulmonary hemorrhage.

Blood gases, hematocrit, serum potassium, ionized calcium, and glucose measurements should be performed at least once intraoperatively.

Transesophageal Echocardiography

Transesophageal echocardiography (TEE) is extremely beneficial in detecting cardiac function during surgery. TEE can detect regional and global ventricular abnormalities, chamber dimensions, valvular anatomy, and the presence of intracardiac air. The two most commonly used views are the four-chamber view and the transgastric (short-axis) view.

Transcranial Doppler

Transcranial Doppler (TCD) is useful in detecting cerebral emboli noninvasively, and can be used whenever available.

Intraoperative Course

Prebypass Period

Anesthetic course in prebypass period is frequently associated with hypotension, followed by periods of intense stimulation that can produce tachycardia (skin incision, sternotomy and sternal retraction, opening the pericardium). The anesthetic depth should be adjusted appropriately in anticipation.

Accentuated vagal responses may be seen during sternal retraction or opening of the pericardium resulting in marked bradycardia and hypotension.

Anticoagulation

Anticoagulation must be established prophylactically prior to CPB so as to prevent acute disseminated intravascular coagulation and formation of clots in the CPB pump. Heparin is the preferred anticoagulant for this purpose.

Bypass Period

At the onset of CPB, arterial pressure dips abruptly. Levels of 30–40 mm Hg are not unusual. However, persistent and excessive decreases (<30 mm Hg) must prompt a search for unrecognized aortic dissection or pump malfunction.[1]

Ventilation

Ventilation of the lungs should be continued until the heart stops ejecting blood. If ventilation is discontinued prematurely, pulmonary blood flow acts as a right-to-left shunt that can promote hypoxemia.

Ventilation is resumed at the conclusion of CPB when the heart begins to eject blood.

Cerebral Protection

Neurological complications are of major concern following CPB. Intracardiac (valvular) procedures, elder patients, and patients with pre-existing cerebrovascular disease are at high risk. In most of the cases air or atherosclerotic embolism is the responsible factor. Epiaortic echocardiography is the most sensitive and specific technique to detect embolization.[2]

Termination of Cardiopulmonary Bypass

Discontinuation of bypass is accomplished serially through following steps:
- **Rewarming**: Rewarming must be gradual as rapid rewarming often results in large temperature gradients between well-perfused organs and peripheral vasoconstricted tissues.
- Complete evacuation of air
- Removal of the aortic cross-clamp
- Reinstitution of lung ventilation.

Accepted guidelines for separation from CPB include the following:
- The core body temperature more than or equal to 37°C.
- Stable rhythm (preferably sinus) with heart rate around 80–100 beats/minute.

If both criteria are satisfied CPB should be discontinued gradually by progressively clamping the venous return line (tubing). As the beating heart fills, ventricular ejection resumes. Pump flow is then gradually reduced.

Few patients fail to emerge from CPB. In such cases, CPB is reinstituted while inotropic therapy is initiated. Intra-aortic balloon pump (IABP) is initiated before another attempt is made to wean the patient. The efficacy of IABP depends on proper timing of inflation and deflation of the balloon. The balloon is ideally inflated just after the dicrotic notch to augment diastolic blood pressure and coronary flow. Early inflation can increase afterload and exacerbate aortic regurgitation, whereas late inflation reduces diastolic augmentation.

Postbypass Period

After ensuring proper hemostasis, bypass cannulas are removed, anticoagulation is reversed, and the chest is closed. Most patients require additional blood volume after termination of bypass. A final hematocrit of 25–30% is well tolerable.

Reversal of Anticoagulation

Once bypass is terminated heparin activity is reversed with protamine.

Postoperative Period

Most patients remain on mechanical ventilation for 2–12 hours postoperatively. Sedation may be accomplished by small doses of morphine or propofol infusion. In first few postoperative hours patient should be intensively monitored for excessive postoperative bleeding. Chest tube drainage more than or equal to 250–300 mL/hour (10 mL/kg/hour) is considered significant and often requires surgical re-exploration.

OFF-PUMP CORONARY ARTERY BYPASS SURGERY

Advanced epicardial stabilizing devices, such as the octopus, has allowed coronary artery bypass grafting without the use of CPB. These suction based retractors, lift the anastomotic site rather than compress it down, and results in greater hemodynamic stability. Such type of bypass operations are known as off-pump coronary artery bypass (OPCAB).

Off-pump coronary artery bypass was initially developed for one- or two-vessel bypass grafting on patients with good left ventricular function, but its better results have allowed it to be used routinely for multigraft surgery, redo operations, and patients with compromised left ventricular function.

Off-pump coronary artery bypass reduces bleeding and CPB-related complications. But, the incidence of postoperative neurological complications remains same.

ANESTHESIA FOR THORACIC SURGERY

Thoracic surgery presents a unique set of physiological problems for the anesthesiologist that includes physiological derangements caused by opening the chest (open pneumothorax), placing the patient with one side down (lateral decubitus position), and the frequent requirement for one-lung ventilation.

In addition to tuberculosis and suppurative pneumonitis common indications for thoracic surgery includes lung and esophageal malignancies, chest trauma and mediastinal tumors.

PHYSIOLOGICAL CONSIDERATIONS

Lateral Position

Most thoracic operations require lateral position **(Fig. 39.2)**. This position significantly alters the normal pulmonary ventilation or perfusion relationships in an anesthetized individual. Due to gravity perfusion is higher in the dependent (lower) lung, whereas ventilation progressively favors the less perfused upper lung. The resulting ventilation perfusion mismatch markedly increases the risk of hypoxemia. This is in contrast to an unanesthetized awake individual where in lateral position both ventilation and perfusion are higher in dependent lung **(Fig. 39.3)**.

The Open Pneumothorax

The lungs are normally kept expanded by a negative pleural pressure. When one side of the chest is opened, the negative pleural pressure is lost and the elastic recoil of the lung on that side tends to collapse it. Spontaneous ventilation with an open pneumothorax in the lateral position results in paradoxical respirations and mediastinal shift. Controlled positive-pressure ventilation is essential to overcome this effect.

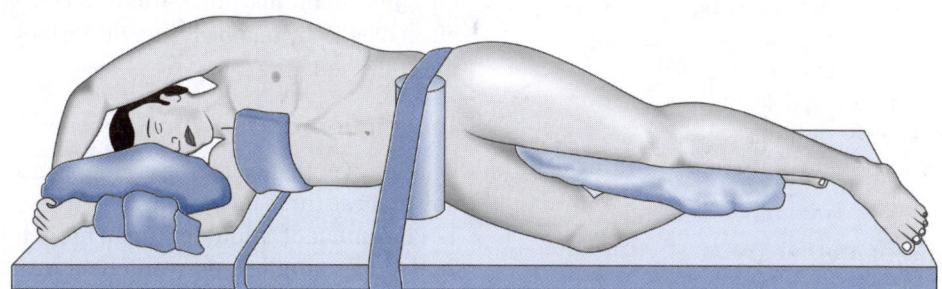

Fig. 39.2: Lateral decubitus position for lateral thoracotomy (Note the position of pads between lower limbs).

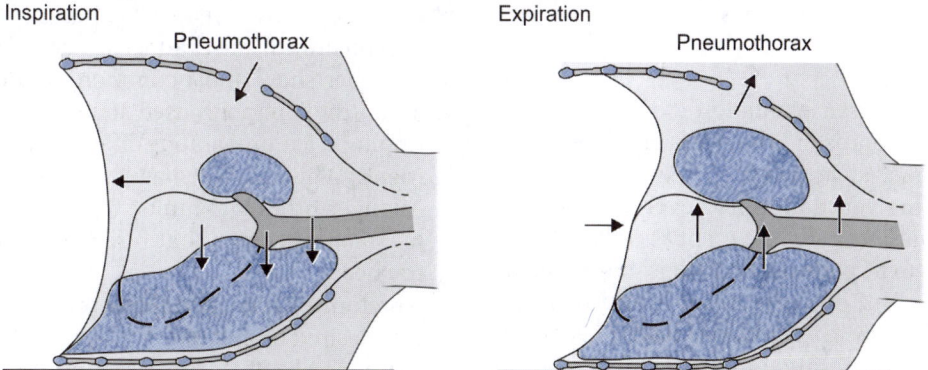

Fig. 39.3: Physiological effect on ventilation in lateral position after thoracotomy
Note: Pendulum-like movement of gases (pendelluft phenomenon)

Spontaneous ventilation in a patient with an open pneumothorax also results in to-and-fro gas flow between the dependent and nondependent lung (pendelluft phenomenon).^{Q} During inspiration, the pneumothorax increases, and gas flows from the upper lung across the carina to the dependent lung. During expiration, the gas flow reverses and moves from the dependent to the upper lung **(Fig. 39.3)**.

One-Lung Ventilation

For facilitating surgical procedures, intentional collapse of the lung on the operative side is indicated in many cases:

Indications for One-Lung Ventilation

Patient-related

- Confine infection to one lung
- Confine bleeding to one lung
- Separate ventilation to each lung
- Bronchopleural fistula
- Tracheobronchial disruption
- Large lung cyst or bulla
- Severe hypoxemia due to unilateral lung disease.

Procedure-related

- Repair of thoracic aortic aneurysm
- Lung resection
- Pneumonectomy
- Lobectomy
- Segmental resection
- Thoracoscopy
- Esophageal surgery
- Single-lung transplantation
- Anterior approach to the thoracic spine
- Bronchoalveolar lavage.

One-lung ventilation however greatly complicates anesthetic management as collapsed lung continues to be perfused and but is not ventilated. The mixing of unoxygenated blood from the collapsed lung with oxygenated blood of dependent lung widens the alveolar-to-arterial oxygen gradient (PA-aO$_2$) and often results in hypoxemia.

Fortunately, lung has got the defense mechanism called hypoxic pulmonary vasoconstriction (HPV)^Q which produces vasoconstriction in nonventilated areas, thus tends to reduce perfusion in nonventilated areas. Factors which inhibit HPV, tends to increase the right-to-left shunting and must be avoided in one-lung ventilation. These factors include:

- Too high or too low pulmonary artery pressures
- Hypocapnia
- High or very low-mixed venous PO$_2$
- Drugs such as nitroglycerin, nitroprusside, alpha adrenergic agonists (including dobutamine and salbutamol) and calcium channel blockers
- Pulmonary infection
- Inhalational anesthetics

Factors that decrease blood flow to the ventilated lung are equally detrimental as they counteract the effect of HPV by relatively increasing blood flow to the collapsed lung.

Techniques for One-Lung Ventilation

One-lung ventilation can be accomplished through any of these three techniques:

1. Placement of a double-lumen bronchial tube
2. Use of a single-lumen tracheal tube in conjunction with a bronchial blocker or
3. A single-lumen bronchial tube.

Double-lumen tubes (DLT) **(Figs. 39.4A to D)** are most commonly used as they are relatively easy to place, can be used to ventilate either single or both lungs, and provide the channel for suction of either lung. Robertshaw (most common), Carlen's and White are the commonly used double lumen tubes.

Common features among different types of DLT (Carlen's; White; Robertshaw) are:

- A longer bronchial lumen and another shorter tracheal lumen that remains in the lower trachea.
- A preformed curve that allows preferential entry into desired bronchus
- A bronchial cuff
- A tracheal cuff.

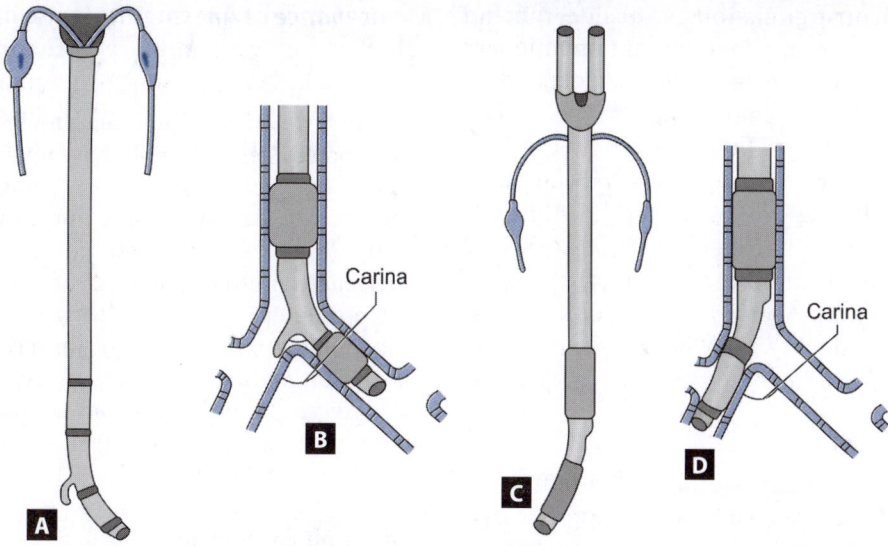

Figs. 39.4A to D: Carlen's and Robertshaw tube: (A) Carlens tube; (B) Placement at the carina; (C) Right Robertshaw tube; (D) Placement at the carina.

Carlen tube and White tube are bronchus specific (Carlen for right bronchus and White for left) both possess carinal hook. Robertshaw tube lack bronchial hook and can be used for both lungs. Carinal hook can produce injury which makes Robertshaw tube a preferred choice. Ventilation can be delivered to only one of the two lungs by either the bronchial or tracheal lumen with both cuffs inflated; opening the port of the appropriate lumen allows the one lung to collapse.

Complications of Double-Lumen Tubes

Double-lumen tube is associated with many complications. Major ones are:
- Trauma to airway
- Tube malplacement or occlusion, which can lead to hypoxemia
- Tracheobronchial rupture resulting from over-inflation of the bronchial cuff
- Inadvertent suturing of the tube to bronchus during surgery.

ANESTHETIC MANAGEMENT OF LUNG RESECTION

Lung resection is indicated for the treatment of lung tumors, necrotizing pneumonitis, and rarely for bronchiectasis.

Preoperative Considerations

Most important is to determine feasibility of resection. Although the decision of pneumonectomy is clinical, it is important to establish that patient can tolerate this loss of lung mass postoperatively. The most commonly used criterion for operability is a predicted postoperative forced expiratory volume at 1 second (FEV1) >800 mL.

If FEV1 is <800 mL, the ability of the remaining pulmonary vasculature to tolerate total blood flow has to be tested, in which the main pulmonary artery on the diseased side is occluded with a balloon catheter; if the mean pulmonary artery pressure exceeds 40 mm Hg or the PaO_2 decreases to <45 mm Hg, the patient is not a candidate for pneumonectomy.

After ensuring feasibility, beside routine investigations, comprehensive cardiopulmonary function test are indicated in all cases.

Patients with malignancy should be evaluated for paraneoplastic syndromes also.

Preoperative chest radiographs and computed tomography (CT) and magnetic resonance imaging (MRI) scans should be reviewed carefully. Tracheal or bronchial deviation can complicate tracheal intubation and proper positioning of bronchial tubes. The location of any bullous cysts or abscesses should be noted.

Premedication

Sedatives are usually avoided in patients with moderate to severe respiratory compromise. As oropharyngeal secretions can obscure visualization through fiberoptic bronchoscope, anticholinergics are administered routinely to reduce these secretions.

Intraoperative Management

Induction

Intravenous induction is preferred in most cases, selection of an induction agent is based on the patient's preoperative status.

Tracheal intubation is achieved with succinylcholine or a nondepolarizing agent.

Controlled positive-pressure ventilation prevents atelectasis, paradoxical breathing, and mediastinal shift; it also allows control of the operative field to facilitate the surgery.

Positioning

Following confirmation of correct tracheal or bronchial tube position, and application of all monitoring, patient is positioned for surgery. Most lung resections are performed via posterior thoracotomy with the patient in the lateral decubitus position **(Fig. 39.2)**. Pillows should be placed between the arms and legs, and an axillary roll is positioned just beneath the dependent axilla to avoid injury to the brachial plexus.

Maintenance of Anesthesia

In most cases anesthesia is maintained by the combination of a potent volatile agent (halothane, sevoflurane or desflurane) and an opioid. Halogenated agents generally have minimal effects on HPV in doses <1 MAC.

Nitrous oxide is generally not used because it limits high FiO_2 and exacerbate pulmonary hypertension in some patients.

The greatest risk of one-lung ventilation is hypoxemia. So, the period of time of one-lung ventilation should be kept to a minimum and 100% oxygen should be used for ventilation. If peak airway pressures rise excessively (>30 cm H_2O), tidal volume may be reduced to 6–8 mL/kg and the ventilatory rate may be increased to maintain the same minute ventilation.

Other measures to improve oxygenation are:
- Periodic inflation of the collapsed lung with oxygen.
- Continuous positive airway pressure (CPAP) (5–10 cm H_2O) to the collapsed lung; perhaps the most effective measure but unfortunately compromises the surgical exposure.

When a patient undergoing one-lung ventilation develops hypoxia, apply first step is to apply CPAP[Q] to the collapsed lung, and then, if the patient is still hypoxic, positive end-expiratory pressure (PEEP) to the ventilated lung. If hypoxemia persists, collapsed lung should be immediately expanded and position of the bronchial tube (or bronchial blocker) should be rechecked.

Postoperative Management

Early extubation is preferred in most cases, to decrease the risk of pulmonary barotrauma [particularly "blowout" (rupture) of the bronchial suture line] and pulmonary infection. If ventilation is essential DLT should be replaced with a regular single-lumen tube.

Postoperative hemorrhage is a rare but serious complication and is associated with high mortality. Signs of hemorrhage include increased chest tube drainage (>200 mL/hour), hypotension, tachycardia, and a falling hematocrit.

Postoperative Analgesia

Adequate analgesia is the foremost component of thoracic surgery as any pain tends to restrict respiratory movement and reduces tidal volume.

Techniques for postoperative analgesia after thoracic surgery include intercostal or paravertebral nerve blocks; thoracic epidural; cryoanalgesia and intravenous opioids. Among all, thoracic epidural is the best.^Q

Anesthesia for Thoracoscopic Surgery

Thoracoscopy is being used for lung biopsy, segmental and lobar resections, pleurodesis, esophageal procedures, and even pericardiectomy. Most procedures are performed through three or more small incisions in the chest with the patient in the lateral decubitus position.

Anesthetic management is similar to that for open procedures (above) except that one-lung ventilation is preferred in all cases.

LAST-MINUTE REVISION

- On pump CABG requires CPB, whereas off pump CABG is accomplished by specialized suction based retractors.
- Off pump bypass surgery is more physiological.
- In bypass period, blood flow is nonpulsatile, so end organs are vulnerable for ischemic damage.
- Thoracic surgery:
  - Most lung surgery require one lung ventilation, which can be accomplished through DLT or bronchial blockers
  - Carlen's and Robertshaw are the important DLTs.
  - Continuous positive airway pressure to the collapsed lung is the most effective measure to treat perioperative hypoxemias but it compromises the surgical exposure.
  - Postoperative analgesia is must after thoracic surgery, thoracic epidural is the most preferred technique for postoperative analgesia.

REFERENCES

1. Miao Q, et al. Target blood pressure management during cardiopulmonary bypass improves lactate levels after cardiac surgery: a randomized controlled trial. BMC Anesthesiol. 2021;21(1):309. doi: 10.1186/s12871-021-01537-w. PMID: 34879822; PMCID: PMC8653567.

2. Sarkar M, Prabhu V. Basics of cardiopulmonary bypass. Indian J Anaesth. 2017;61(9):760-7. doi: 10.4103/ija.IJA_379_17. PMID: 28970635; PMCID: PMC5613602.

REVIEW QUESTIONS

1. **Preferred technique of postoperative analgesia after lung resection:**
   a. Cryoanalgesia
   b. Thoracic epidural
   c. Intercostal block
   d. Intravenous morphine

2. **In all of the following surgeries double-lumen endotracheal tube is used, *except*:**
   a. Thoracoscopic resection of pleura
   b. Resection of upper lobe of left lung
   c. Congenital diaphragmatic hernia
   d. Lung transplantation

3. **Induction agent of choice for an ischemic heart disease patient posted for coronary artery bypass graft (CABG). Whose ejection fraction is 48%.**
   a. Propofol
   b. Thiopentone
   c. Etomidate
   d. Morphine

   Morphine is preferred over etomidate as it provides analgesia too.

4. Robertshaw endotracheal tube differs from Carlen's tube in which respect:
   a. Robertshaw has single lumen whereas Carlen has double-lumen
   b. Carlen's tube possess hook which is absent in Robertshaw
   c. Carlen's tube can be used for unilateral left lung ventilation whereas Robertshaw cannot be
   d. Carlen is for left lung while Robertshaw is for right lung

5. True statement regarding off-pump coronary artery bypass (OPCAB) grafting includes all, *except*:
   a. Uses low doses of cardioplegic solution
   b. Cardiac bypass is not required
   c. Bleeding is less
   d. Postoperative recovery is fast

ANSWERS

1. b   2. c   3. d   4. b   5. a

CHAPTER 40
Geriatric Anesthesia

Anshul Jain

INTRODUCTION

Aging alters many normal process of human being than not only includes drug metabolism but physiological responses as well. Current chapter deals with the basic anesthetic considerations in the elder patients.

PHYSIOLOGICAL CHANGES WITH AGING

Aging is characterized by declining end-organ reserve, increasing imbalance of homeostatic mechanisms, with high prevalence of pathologic changes, viz (**Fig. 40.1**):

Nervous System

Most elder patients have memory impairment. Structurally, cerebral atrophy occurs with aging in a selective and differential manner. Changes in autonomic system with aging include a decreased response to β-receptor stimulation and an increase in sympathetic nervous system activity. Thus, elder patient are not able to increase their heart rates in response to stress and are susceptible for acute cardiac failure.

Neuraxial changes include a reduction in the volume of the epidural space, increased permeability of the dura, and decreased volume of cerebrospinal fluid. In peripheral nerves, inter-Schwann cell distance is decreased, so is conduction velocity.[Q] These changes render geriatric patient more sensitive to neuraxial and peripheral nerve block (**Fig. 40.1**).

Cardiovascular System

The aging process is associated with decreased myocyte number, left ventricular wall thickening, and decreased left ventricular compliance. Functionally, these changes translate to decreased contractility, increased myocardial stiffness and decreased β-adrenergic sensitivity.

In vessels, there is atherosclerosis which results in reduced elasticity and caliber, this translates to elevated mean arterial pressure and increased pulse pressure.

During surgery, these patients are poor tolerant of both fluid loss and fluid overload. Both of them may manifest as acute cardiac failure and/or pulmonary edema.

Respiratory System

With aging there is loss of elastic recoil, decreased surfactant, both contribute to an increase in lung compliance. Due to loss of elasticity, small airways collapse early on expiration (*or closing capacity encroaches functional residual capacity*) and does not take part in air exchange. There also is a progressive loss of alveolar surface area. The functional results of these pulmonary changes are increased anatomic dead space, decreased diffusing capacity, and increased closing capacity all leading to impaired gas exchange.

In younger individuals, closing capacity is below functional residual capacity, by sixth decade, closing capacity becomes equal to functional residual capacity in the upright position. When closing capacity surpasses functional residual capacity, ventilation-perfusion mismatch occurs and there is impaired oxygenation of blood even with normal alveolar oxygen tension.

Under anesthesia, this effect becomes evident by the fact that preoxygenation will not raise the arterial oxygen tension to the extent as it rises in younger patients.

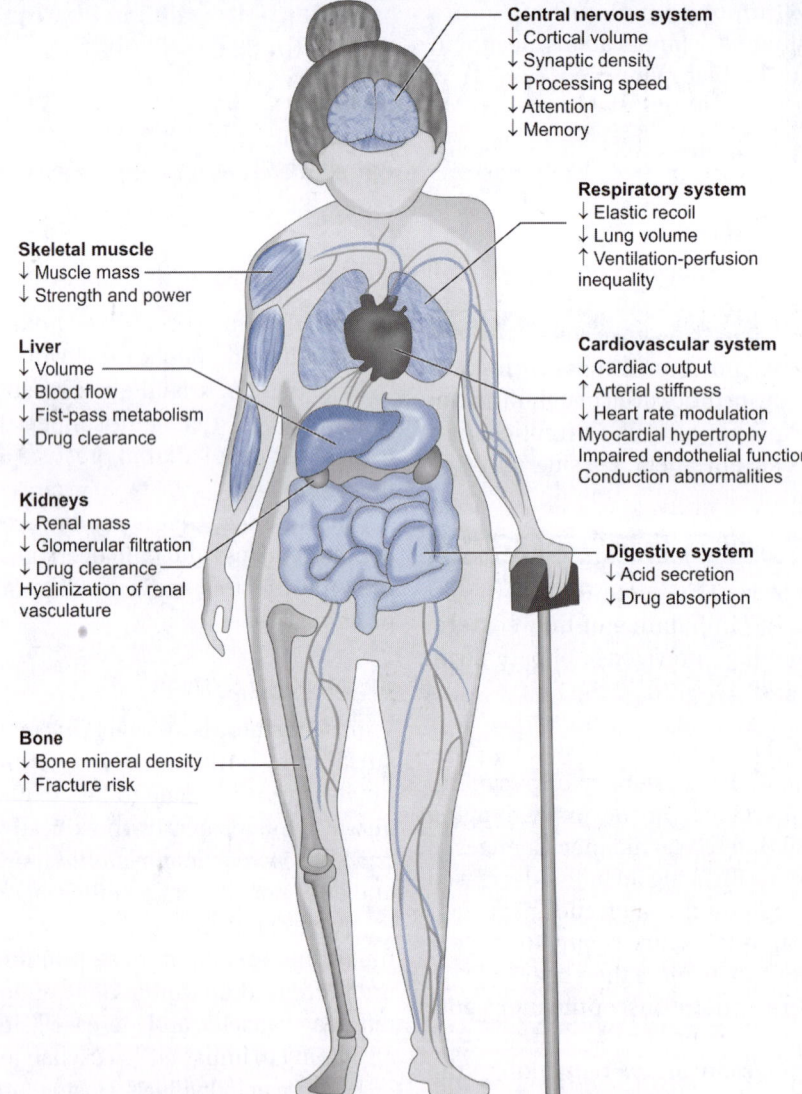

Fig. 40.1: Aging related changes in various organ system.

Urinary System

There is a progressive decline in creatinine clearance with age, yet with normal aging, serum creatinine remains relatively unchanged. This is due to the fact that muscle mass also decreases with aging. Thus it is not wrong to say that serum creatinine is a poor predictor of renal function in elderly patients.^Q

Additional Problems

In addition to previous mentioned changes and disease, there are some other problems which increase the perioperative risk in adult patient.

These include:
- Nutritional problems
- Depression

- **Immobility**: Immobile patient have more chances of pulmonary complications, deep vein thrombosis and cardiac failure.
- Hypothermia.

ANESTHETIC MANAGEMENT

Preoperative Evaluation

Geriatric patient should always be assessed for all those diseases which are common in elderly patient. Cardiovascular disease and diabetes are particularly prominent followed by lung disease especially chronic obstructive pulmonary disease.

Another important aspect is assessment of functional reserve and frailty.

Frailty

Frailty refers to a loss of physiologic reserve. The components of the frailty syndrome include decreased mobility, muscle weakness, poor exercise tolerance, unstable balance and body related factors *(weight loss, malnutrition and muscle wasting)*. Frail patients are more likely to develop disability.

Choice (Regional versus General Anesthesia)

In psychologically stable persons, regional anesthesia is preferred over general anesthesia provided patient is cooperative.

Elder patient exhibits exaggerated response to most general anesthetic. This gross change in pharmacology of drugs is due to alteration in:
- **Plasma protein binding**: With aging the albumin level decreases while that of α-1 acid glycoprotein increases. As a result, free fraction of drugs bound to albumin increases and shows exaggerated responses.
- **Body content**: Aging is associated with decrease in lean body mass, an increase in body fat, and a decrease in total body water.
- **Drug metabolism**: It might be grossly altered due to decreased hepatic and renal clearance.
- **Pharmacodynamics**: Elder patients are more sensitive to anesthetic agents, and further drug effect is often prolonged.

Important Alteration in Pharmacology of Anesthetic Drugs

Inhaled Anesthetics

The minimum alveolar concentration decreases approximately 6% per decade after fifth decade.

Intravenous Anesthetics

There is no change in brain sensitivity to thiopental with age. However, due to decrease in the initial distribution volume of the drug, the dose of thiopental decreases with age. Sensitivity of propofol increases in elders; in addition, clearance of propofol is reduced.

Opiates

Morphine clearance is decreased and its metabolite morphine-6-glucuronide[Q] tends to get accumulated.

Potency of sufentanil, alfentanil and fentanyl increase by two times due to increased brain sensitivity.

Muscle Relaxants

Duration may be prolonged due to altered liver or renal metabolism. Pharmacokinetics of atracurium[Q] is little and cisatracurium[Q] is not altered by age.

Postoperative Considerations

Common problems in the postanesthesia care unit are:

Postoperative Pain

An important problem in geriatric patients is pain assessment. A greater problem occurs in patients with cognitive impairment. Verbal pain scales are superior to nonverbal methods in elderly patients.

Postoperative Delirium

Postoperative delirium *(characterized by acute onset of variable and fluctuating changes in level of consciousness accompanied by a range of other mental symptoms)* is seen in 10% elderly patients after major elective surgery, incidence is higher after cardiac surgery and hip fracture repair.[1]

Management of delirium includes recognition and treatment of any predisposing or precipitating factor and correction of metabolic and electrolyte disorders.

 LAST-MINUTE REVISION

- **Inducing agent of choice in geriatric patient:** Thiopentone > Propofol
- **Muscle relaxant of choice in geriatric patient:** Cisatracurium
- **Volatile agent of choice in geriatric patient:** Sevoflurane.

REFERENCE

1. Marcantonio ER. Postoperative delirium: a 76-year-old woman with delirium following surgery. JAMA. 2012;308(1):73-81. doi: 10.1001/jama.2012.6857. PMID: 22669559; PMCID: PMC3604975.

REVIEW QUESTIONS

1. All of the following are true regarding anesthetic management of supracondylar fracture of humerus in an 80-year-old woman, *except*:
   a. Dose of midazolam is reduced
   b. Dose of propofol has to be increased
   c. Brachial plexus block can be used, if patient is cooperative
   d. Laryngeal mask airway is preferred over endotracheal intubation
2. Muscle relaxant of choice in a 90-year-old posted for cholecystectomy:
   a. Rocuronium
   b. Vecuronium
   c. Atracurium
   d. Cisatracurium

ANSWERS

1. b
2. d

CHAPTER 41

Obstetric Anesthesia

Anshul Jain, Reena

INTRODUCTION

Obstetric cases represent one of the most commonly encountered patient groups. Most of these patients come for cesarean section. Proper management of these patients demands knowledge of physiological changes that pregnancy produces in body and their anesthetic implications.

PHYSIOLOGICAL CHANGES IN PREGNANCY AND THEIR ANESTHETIC IMPLICATIONS (FIG. 41.1)

Cardiovascular System (Table 41.1)

Cardiac output increases fifth week onwards and reaches to its maximum at approximately 32 weeks. The increased stroke volume and raised heart rate, both contribute to increased cardiac output.

Despite increased cardiac output, arterial blood pressure remains unaffected. This is due to reduction in peripheral vascular resistance.^Q

Gravid uterus compresses inferior vena cava (IVC), to compensate this, collateral routes of venous return develop, via paravertebral veins to the azygos vein. In the third trimester as uterine size is very big, IVC compression is profound, and can cause significantly reduced cardiac output, particularly in supine position and gets relieved when women assume left lateral position. Some parturients, at term develop severe hypotension while assuming the supine position.

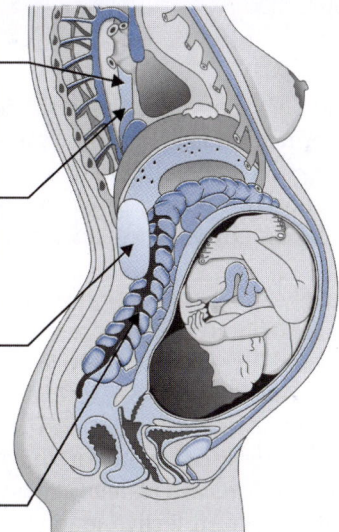

Impact of pregnant physiology

Cardiac
- Increased heart rate
- Increased renal and uterine blood flow
- Increase in total body water, blood volume and capillary hydrostatic pressure
  - Clinically this could necessitate higher initial and maintenance dose of hydrophilic drugs to obtain therapeutic plasma levels
- Reduced serum albumin protein concentration
  - Increase in unbound active drug

Respiratory
- Increased vascularity and edema of upper respiratory mucosa
  - Inhaled medications may be more readily absorbed by pregnant patients

Renal
- Dilation of urinary collecting system and urinary stasis
  - Predisposes pregnant women to UTIs
- Increased renal blood flow and glomerular filtration rate
  - Increase renal clearance and elimination rates and reduce drug half-lives
- Sodium and water retention leading to volume expansion
  - Reduction in serum concentrations of hydrophilic drugs

Gastrointestinal
- Delayed gastric emptying and prolonged small bowel transit time
  - Alter bioavailability of oral drugs
- Increase in gastric pH and reduced gastrointestinal motility
  - Reduce or delay absorption of drug

Fig. 41.1: Anatomical, physiological and changes in pregnancy.

Table 41.1: Cardiovascular changes in pregnancy.

Parameter	Change
Heart rate	Increased by 20–30%
Stroke volume	Increased by 20–50%
Cardiac output	Increased by 30–50%
Central venous pressure	Unchanged
Pulmonary capillary wedge pressure	Unchanged
Systemic vascular resistance	Decreased by 20%
Systemic blood pressure	Slight decrease in second trimester, then rises
Pulmonary vascular resistance	Decreased
Pulmonary artery pressure	Decreased

This phenomenon known as supine hypotension syndrome, is due to the compression of both aorta and IVC.

Anesthetic Implications

- Due to hyperdynamic circulation, parturients are prone for congestive heart failure (CHF).
- Anesthetic drugs that produce vasodilation; and central neuraxial blockade may exacerbate the impact of aortocaval compression. So, as a precaution, in the operating room, a small pillow or "wedge" should be placed under right buttock, which provides left uterine displacement of 15–20°.

Hematologic System

Maternal blood volume begins to increase early in pregnancy and by term, plasma volume increases by up to 45% whereas red cell volume increases by 30%. This differential increase produces a state of anemia called as "physiological anemia of pregnancy".

If coagulation is taken into account pregnancy is a state of hypercoagulability. All factors except II and XI (reduced) are increased[Q] **(Table 41.2)**. There is marked increase in fibrinogen level. The platelet count mostly remains unchanged, and gets reduced slightly in the third trimester. But, this is usually accompanied by increased platelet activity.

Hypercoagulable state is a protective adaptation to reduce the bleeding that occurs at the time of delivery. This, however, makes obstetrics patients prone for thromboembolism, which remains a leading cause of maternal mortality.

Table 41.2: Coagulation factors in pregnancy.

Factor	Change
Factor II	Unchanged
VII	Increased
VIII, IX, X, XII	Increased
XI	Reduced
Fibrinogen	Increased
Platelets	Stable

Respiratory System (Table 41.3)

Due to bulky uterus all lung capacity except tidal volume gets reduced. The most significant change in maternal lung dynamics is a reduction of functional residual capacity (FRC), which at term may decrease by as much as 20% of prepregnancy values. Minute ventilation increases by 45%, primarily due to increase in tidal volume as the respiratory rate remains unchanged.

Table 41.3: Respiratory changes in pregnancy.

Parameter	Change
Respiratory rate	Unchanged
Tidal volume	Increased
Minute ventilation	Increased
Work of breathing	Increased
Functional residual capacity	Decreased
Closing capacity	Unchanged

Anesthetic Implications

- Because of reduced FRC and increased oxygen (O_2) consumption parturients desaturate at a much faster rate when compared with non-pregnant women.
- Due to increased minute ventilation, inhalational induction is faster.
- Preoxygenation for 5 minutes reduces the rate of desaturation. In an acute emergency setting, four deep breaths with 100% O_2 are considered sufficient.

Other changes include capillary engorgement and edema of orotracheal mucosa which may result in a difficult intubation with increased chances of trauma. Due to this, a relatively smaller endotracheal tube (size 6–7.0) is preferred.[Q]

Most of the respiratory changes in pregnancy are due to progesterone. Progesterone sensitizes the respiratory center to carbon dioxide and is responsible for increase in ventilation.

Gastrointestinal System

Changes in gastrointestinal function is a topic that continues to be controversial. Progesterone by relaxing smooth muscle impairs esophageal and intestinal motility during pregnancy.

Interestingly pregnancy (in contrary to previous thinking) enhances gastric emptying. But, the residual volume of stomach increases which increases the chances of pulmonary aspiration (Mendelson syndrome). The pain of labor, however, may delay gastric emptying and promote emesis. These changes are due to the effects of placental gastrin.

KEY POINTS

Mendelson syndrome
Chemical pneumonitis caused by aspiration during anesthesia especially during pregnancy. Aspirated contents may include gastric juice, blood, bile, water, undigested food. Risk is higher, if residual gastric volume is >25 mL and gastric pH <2.5.

Anesthetic Implications

- The patients should always be considered as full stomach.
- Endotracheal intubation is preferred over laryngeal mask airway (LMA) for airway protection, if general anesthesia (GA) is required.

Renal System

Progesterone and increased cardiac output induce following changes in renal system:
- Increased glomerular filtration rate (GFR) and renal plasma flow
- Increased creatinine and uric acid clearance, which reduces the normal value of creatinine and urea.

Hence, marginally elevated blood urea nitrogen and creatinine levels usually indicate severe renal impairment in parturients.

Central Nervous System

Pregnant women exhibit increased sensitivity to both regional and general anesthetics. The minimum alveolar concentration (MAC) value of volatile anesthetics is reduced. The exact mechanism of the decreased anesthetic requirements remains unclear. Both progesterone and increased endogenous opioids seem to play role.

As pregnancy advances, epidural veins get engorged (due to compression of IVC). As the volume of spinal canal is constant, engorged veins reduce the size of subarachnoid space and epidural space. So, drug injected in subarachnoid space may spread high and consequently produce higher block.

Anesthetic Implications

- Dose requirement of local anesthetics is reduced.
- Chances of epidural venous puncture are increased.
- Chances of high spinal are increased.
- To achieve same level of block, pregnant females require 30% less dose in comparison to nonpregnant female.

PLACENTAL TRANSFER OF ANESTHETIC DRUGS

Many medications administered to a pregnant woman cross the placenta, and affect the fetus. Drugs cross the placenta by three main processes:
1. Simple diffusion
2. Active transport
3. Pinocytosis.

The extent of transfer depends on, molecular weight, protein binding, degree of lipid solubility, maternal drug concentration, and maternal and fetal pH. Larger molecules and highly ionized substances with poor lipid solubility (e.g., nondepolarizing muscle relaxants) have limited transfer.

Once a drug crosses the placenta, fetal pH and protein binding affect drug disposition. The liver is the first fetal organ exposed to transfer drug. Hepatic drug uptake in the fetus may protect the fetus from the deleterious effects of certain drugs on the fetal nervous system.

Placental transfer[Q] of anesthetic drugs is one of the reason because of which regional anesthesia is preferred over GA in parturients.

EVALUATION OF THE FETUS

Fetal well-being is of major importance to both the obstetrician and anesthesiologist and should be addressed in the preanesthetic evaluation of the parturient.

Fetal well-being can be assessed by fetal heart rate (FHR) monitoring. The normal FHR varies between 120 and 160 beats/minute with a variability of 5–25 beats/minute. Reduced variability suggests quiescent phases (corresponding to "sleep"), effect of drugs, fetal hypoxia and acidosis.

Fetal pulse oximetry is a recent addition to the tools available to monitor the fetus. A probe is inserted through the cervix and placed between the fetal cheek and uterine wall. This technology allows early detection of acidosis, when used in combination with continuous FHR monitoring.

ROLE OF INTRAUTERINE RESUSCITATION

Intrauterine resuscitation (IUR) refers to the attempts or measures targeted to improve oxygenation of fetus.

Commonly adopted measures include left lateral knee-chest positioning, O_2 supplementation, rapid infusion of crystalloid solution, and discontinuation of oxytocin infusion.

ANESTHESIA FOR SPONTANEOUS VAGINAL DELIVERY (LABOR ANALGESIA)

Before proceeding to various analgesic options available to the parturient, it is important to understand the mechanisms and pain pathways of labor.

During the *first stage of labor*, pain impulses arise primarily from the uterus. Uterine contractions result in myometrial ischemia, which leads to release of bradykinin, histamine and serotonin.

In addition, there is stretching and distension of the lower uterine segment and cervix. Patients describe this pain as dull and poorly localized. *The pain is in the distribution of T10, T11, T12 and L1 spinal segments.*[Q]

In second stage of labor, pain due to stretching of the perineum predominates and is in the distribution of the S2, S3 and S4 levels **(Fig. 41.2)**.[Q]

Techniques for Labor Analgesia

Psychoprophylaxis

Probably the oldest method. It includes education program, breathing techniques, and relaxation techniques of voluntary muscles. Indeed, even the presence of close relative or husband during labor has a positive effect on outcomes, including the duration of labor.

Transcutaneous Electrical Nerve Stimulation (TENS)

It provides analgesia by nociceptive inhibition at a presynaptic level in the dorsal horn.[Q] TENS also enhances release of endorphins and dynorphins centrally.

Systemic Medication

Opioids are the most commonly used analgesics in laboring women. All opioids, however, cross

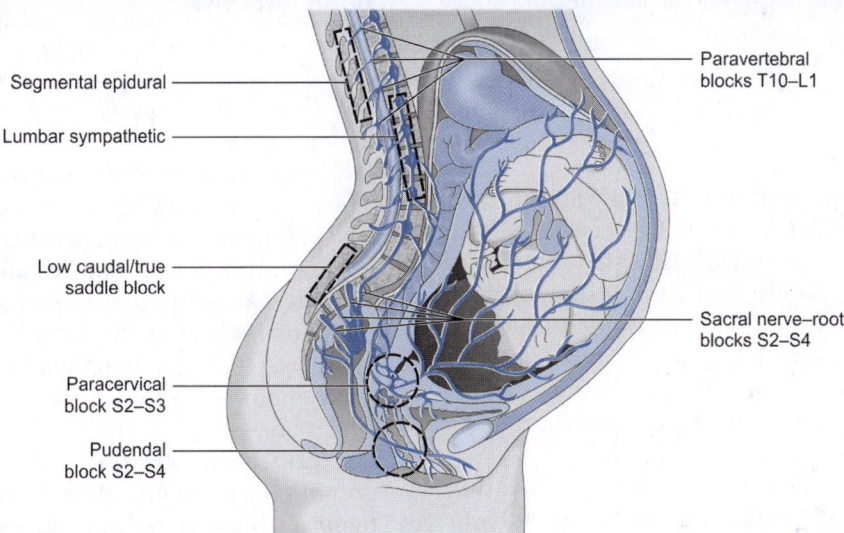

Fig. 41.2: Nerve pathways transmitting labor pain and the available nerve blocks that can be used to block them.

placental circulation freely and may cause respiratory depression in the newborn. Sedative-tranquilizers and ketamine are other systemic drugs. Pethidine is still the most commonly utilized systemic opioid for labor pain as it can be easily administered by midwives. Remifentanyl is being preferred over pethidine (whenever available) due to its faster onset and shorter duration.

Inhaled Analgesia

Inhaled analgesia should not be confused with inhaled anesthesia that produces unconsciousness and loss of protective laryngeal reflexes. Inhaled analgesia provides a limited amount of pain relief, which usually remains insufficient for most mothers. It however has a place as an adjunct to neuraxial techniques or in parturient where regional anesthesia is not possible. Entonox (50:50 N_2O/O_2 mixtures) has been used for many years as both a sole analgesic and an adjuvant for labor. Recent studies suggest sevoflurane as an effective labor analgesic. An inspired concentration of 0.8% appears to be acceptable and effective for labor analgesia.

Regional Analgesia

Regional analgesic techniques are the most effective and most commonly adopted means of providing labor analgesia[Q] that too with minimal depressant effects on the mother and fetus.

The most commonly performed regional techniques for labor are epidural, spinal and combined spinal-epidural blocks.[Q] These blocks always require anesthetist. Less frequently used paracervical, pudendal blocks, and local perineal infiltration techniques can be performed by the obstetrician. Each technique has its own merits and demerits. Proper patient evaluation and preparation is mandatory before administering blocks.

REGIONAL TECHNIQUES FOR LABOR ANALGESIA

Patient Evaluation and Preparation

Before administration of a regional block it is important to assess the patient. Assessment involves a focused medical and obstetric history, clinical examination, and evaluation of the airway.

Epidural Analgesia

Lumbar epidural analgesia is a safe and effective technique for labor analgesia. It is versatile and may be extended to provide anesthesia for operative delivery. *Low concentration of local anesthetic (LA) or opioid combinations is administered to provide a continuous T10-L1 sensory block during the first stage of labor.*[Q] In second stage, further supplementation may be required to achieve a sacral block.

Principle lies behind the fact that low concentration (0.0625% for bupivacaine; 0.1% for ropivacaine) of LA produces only sensory block without appreciable motor block.

The benefits of epidural analgesia include effective pain relief without appreciable motor block, reduction in maternal catecholamines, and versatility to achieve surgical anesthesia. *Absolute contraindications* to neuraxial analgesia include patient refusal, overt maternal coagulopathy, frank infection at the injection site, and maternal hemodynamic instability. Other high-risk conditions, such as fixed cardiac output states (critical aortic stenosis), must be considered on a case-by-case basis.

Choice of Drugs

Ropivacaine is the local anesthetic of choice followed by bupivacaine **(Table 41.4)**. This is because of the differential blockade of ropivacaine, which results in dense sensory blockade with relative preservation of motor activity.[1]

Epidural Test Dose

This is a controversial issue whether a test dose is indicated in labor epidural or not. The commonly followed practice is to avoid test dose because of the following reasons:[2]

- **For intravenous detection**: Routinely, lignocaine with epinephrine is used for test dose. Epinephrine is not sensitive enough in pregnancy to detect intravascular injection. As maternal heart rate variability because of the pain of uterine contractions interferes with heart rate response to epinephrine. Further intravenous epinephrine has got deleterious effects on uterine blood flow.
- **For intrathecal injection**: In labor, epidural drug is injected via epidural catheter. Of course there are chances (rather chances are more in pregnant woman) of accidental subarachnoid migration of epidural catheter, and one must be thinking why test dose is avoided. Here the answer! *Normally,* if lignocaine (of test dose) is injected in subarachnoid space it will result in profound motor blockade, means failure to proceed into normal labor or failure of labor analgesia. Moreover in ultra-dilute concentrations *(as used in labor epidural)* subarachnoid injections do not pose a serious threat.
- The best way of prevention is to administer drug only after catheter aspiration, administration should be at a slow rate with continuous

> **KEY POINTS**
> **Labor analgesia**
> - Continuous lumbar epidural is the technique of choice.
> - Pethidine is the preferred opioid.

Table 41.4: Suggested dosages for continuous epidural labor analgesia.

Drug	Initial injection	Continuous infusion
Bupivacaine	10–15 mL of a 0.125% solution	0.0625–0.125% solution at 8–15 mL/hour
Ropivacaine	10–15 mL of a 0.1–0.2% solution	0.05–0.2% solution at 8–15 mL/hour
Fentanyl	50–100 µg in a 10 mL volume	1–4 µg/mL

monitoring of maternal conscious state and electrocardiogram (ECG). If patient remains comfortable with active limb movements, proper epidural catheter placement is ensured.

Spinal Analgesia

A single-shot intrathecal injection of diluted LA or opioid provides effective and rapid onset of labor analgesia particularly when patient is distressed in pain. The problems are of short duration and postdural puncture headache (PDPH).

Combined Spinal-Epidural Analgesia

Combined spinal-epidural (CSE) analgesia is the most recent addition to labor analgesia. This technique provides the advantages of both early onset and prolongs analgesia, through the use of an epidural catheter. Moreover if operative delivery is required, analgesia can be deepened to anesthesia. The commonly used drugs are bupivacaine (0.0625%) and ropivacaine. In such concentration even intrathecal injection are devoid of motor blockade.

The CSE technique has also made ambulation possible for many women. Because of the minimal motor block with this technique, it has been termed "the walking epidural".[2]

Paracervical and Pudendal Blocks

The paracervical block is an alternative technique for labor analgesia in which neuraxial block is contraindicated. It is a relatively simple block to perform, provides pain relief for the first stage of labor, and does not adversely affect the progress of labor. The block is mostly performed by obstetricians.

The pudendal nerve block provides satisfactory analgesia for vaginal delivery and forceps delivery, but it is not useful for labor analgesia.

ANESTHESIA FOR CESAREAN SECTION

The cesarean birth rate is increasing day by day. Increased use of the procedure has been attributed to the liberalization of indications for fetal "distress" as well as elective repeat cesarean sections.

Choice of Anesthesia

This depends on the indications for the surgery, the degree of urgency, maternal status, and desires of the patient. Let us see the merits and demerits of each anesthetic technique for cesarean delivery.

Spinal Anesthesia

As a general rule single-shot spinal anesthesia is the anesthetic technique of choice[Q] until there are contraindications.

Advantages

- Rapid onset and provides a dense sensory and motor block.
- Require very less amount of LA (2–3 mL), so risk of LA toxicity is very low and there is only a minimal transfer of drug to the fetus.
- Decreased risk of failed intubation.
- Decreased risk of aspiration of gastric contents.
- Less neonatal exposure to potentially depressant general anesthetic drugs.
- Mother remains awake and enjoys the birthing experience.
- Blood loss is less under regional anesthesia for cesarean delivery.

Disadvantages

- Short duration of anesthesia (2–3 hours)
- Higher incidence of hypotension
- Higher incidence of PDPH

Choice of Drug

Hyperbaric 0.5% bupivacaine is the most commonly used agent,[Q] it provides blocks which last up to 1.5–2 hours in most cases.[Q] Drug dose should not exceed 3 mL (2.5 mL is sufficient for most cases).

The quality of the spinal anesthesia can be improved by the addition of fentanyl or sufentanil.

Note: In pregnant women enlarged epidural veins, reduce the volume of subarachnoid space, as a result given volume of LA spreads to a higher level when compared with nonpregnant state. Therefore to prevent high spinal anesthesia, the dose of LA has to be reduced by 30–40%.

Epidural Anesthesia

In epidural anesthesia, duration can be extended with top-ups and postoperative pain can also be controlled. So, for a potentially prolonged cesarean section a combined spinal and epidural technique with catheter is a better choice.

In addition, women with indwelling epidural catheters which were inserted for labor analgesia, who now require cesarean section usually receive the additional LA through those catheters, i.e., by converting epidural analgesia into anesthesia.

Disadvantage of epidural anesthesia includes delayed onset, variable effect, technically difficult procedure, require large dose of local anesthesia, increased chances of intravascular injection. To reduce the risk of intrathecal or intravascular injection following measures are taken:
- Catheter must be aspirated before use and an appropriate test dose is administered. Even in patients with catheter *in situ* (as for labor analgesia), there are chances of catheter migration, so test dose must be administered prior to full dose.
- Local anesthetic should be administered in fractionated doses, i.e., inject 2 mL, wait for 30 seconds again inject 2 mL so on.
- Safer drugs (e.g., chloroprocaine and lidocaine) or the newer amide LAs (e.g., ropivacaine and levobupivacaine) should be used preferably.

> **Note:** It looks bit confusing that test dose is not indicated in patients posted for labor epidural while indicated in epidural anesthesia for cesarean delivery. Answer lies in the fact that concentration used for labor analgesia is very low (which is relatively nontoxic) and the motive is to produce sensory block only, whereas in epidural anesthesia concentration is high and the goal is to block both sensory and motor fibers.

Combined Spinal-Epidural Technique

The CSE provides rapid onset of dense surgical anesthesia while allowing the ability to prolong the block with an epidural catheter. Postoperative pain can also be controlled. However the technique is difficult, time consuming and if epidural catheter fails block cannot be prolonged.

Complications of Spinal and Epidural Anesthesia

- **Hypotension**: Hypotension[Q] (systolic blood pressure <100 mm Hg or a fall exceeding 20% of the baseline readings) is the most common complication of central neuraxial block and is seen most commonly after spinal anesthesia.[Q] The incidence and severity of hypotension depends on the level of the block, the position of the parturient and hydration status. Prophylactic measures that decrease the risk of hypotension include intravenous administration of fluids, avoidance of aortocaval compression (by left uterine displacement). If recognized and treated promptly, transient maternal hypotension has no ill effect. Intravenous ephedrine[Q] or phenylephrine[Q] *(preferred but costly)* are the drugs of choice.[Q]
- **Accidental dural puncture**: A problematic complication of epidural placement is accidental puncture of the dura ("wet tap"). This complication can lead to the development of PDPH in up to 70% of cases.
- **Postdural puncture headache**: *Both chances and severity of PDPH are increased in pregnant women.*[Q] PDPH has the typical features of a postural headache that is worsened by standing or straining and relieved by lying down.
  - Generally, PDPH is initially treated conservatively with increased intake of both oral and intravenous water. Drugs that have been used to treat PDPH include caffeine, vasopressin, theophylline, sumatriptan, and adrenocorticotropic hormone (ACTH). If the symptoms are severe enough to limit a mother's activity or if evidence of cranial nerve involvement is noted, an epidural blood patch *(most effective treatment)* should be considered.[Q]
- **Total spinal block**: A total spinal block is a rare and life-threatening complication that occurs after excessive cephalic spread of the LA. This is usually seen as result of inadvertent intrathecal spread of epidural medication after unintentional dural puncture or catheter

migration but rarely it may follow single-shot spinal anesthesia.
- **Backache**: Incidence of postpartum backache increases after epidural block.

General Anesthesia

With improved regional anesthesia indications of GA for cesarean delivery have dramatically declined. Currently, it is indicated mainly for the management of emergency situations, like maternal hemorrhage, overt coagulopathy, life-threatening fetal compromise, or if patient refuses regional anesthesia.

General anesthesia provides advantages of immediate onset, better control of the hemodynamics. However, over all GA has got 16 times higher risk of mortality in cesarean section than regional anesthesia. Potential problems associated with GA in pregnant women include failed intubation, pulmonary aspiration of gastric contents, neonatal depression and maternal awareness.

For safe administration of GA in pregnant women, following steps are followed:
- **Aspiration prophylaxis**: Administer a nonparticulate antacid. Additional agents like metoclopramide or an H_2-blocker should also be administered in patients at high-risk for aspiration.
- **Prepare patient and yourself**: Apply routine monitors, (ECG, pulse oximetry and capnography). Ensure availability of emergency drugs, equipments for difficult intubation.
- **Patient position**: Position the patient in a manner to achieve left uterine displacement and optimal airway position.
- **Preoxygenation**: Preferably preoxygenate the patient with 100% of O_2 for 3–5 minutes. In cases of dire emergency four vital capacity breaths with high flow 100% O_2 are optimal.Q
- **Induction**: After the drapes are applied and the surgeon is ready, initiate rapid-sequence induction with thiopental, 4.0–5.0 mg/kg, and succinylcholine, 1.0–1.5 mg/kg. Apply cricoid pressure and continue until correct position of the endotracheal tube is verified and the cuff is inflated. In hypotensive patients, ketamine, 1.0–1.5 mg/kg, can be substituted for thiopental.
- **Maintenance**: Oxygen/N_2O mixture (50:50) with a volatile anesthetic, and a nondepolarizer muscle relaxant. Goal is to maintain normocarbia. After delivery, increase N_2O to 70%, and an opioid and/or benzodiazepine can be administered. Add oxytocin to intravenous fluids to facilitate uterine contraction.

> **Note:** Volatile anesthetics have to be used only in low concentrations as they relax myometrium and increase chances of postpartum hemorrhage (PPH). Isoflurane is the preferred volatile agent in cesarean section.

- **Extubation**: Endotracheal tube is removed only when the patient is awake, and is following commands.

SPECIFIC CONDITIONS

Pre-eclampsia and Eclampsia

Pre-eclampsia [pregnancy-induced hypertension (PIH)] complicates around 8% of pregnancies. PIH is usually defined as a systolic blood pressure >140 mm Hg or diastolic pressure >90 mm Hg, or, alternatively, as a consistent increase in systolic or diastolic pressure by 30 mm Hg and 15 mm Hg, respectively, above the patient's normal baseline. Clinically, it is characterized by the triad of hypertension, proteinuria and edema.Q When seizures occur in the presence of above triad, syndrome is termed eclampsia.Q

On the basis of severity, pre-eclampsia may be classified as mild or severe **(Table 41.5)**.

Treatment includes bed rest, sedation, antihypertensive drugs (labetalol, hydralazine, methyldopa 250–500 mg orally), and magnesium sulfate, if convulsions are there. Esmolol has potentially adverse fetal effects, so it should not be used. Calcium channel blockers are also avoided because of their tocolytic action and potentiation of magnesium-induced circulatory depression.

The HELLP syndrome is a term used for PIH associated with hemolysis, elevated liver enzymes, and a low platelet count.

Table 41.5: Grading of pre-eclampsia.

	Mild	Severe
Systolic BP	<160 mm Hg	>160 mm Hg
Diastolic BP	<110 mm Hg	>110 mm Hg
Urinary protein	<5 g/24 hours	>5 g/24 hours
Urine output	>500 mL/24 hours	<500 mL/24 hours
Headache	No	Yes
Visual disturbances	No	Yes
Epigastric pain	No	Yes
Abdominal pain	No	Yes
Pulmonary edema	No	Yes
Cyanosis	No	Yes
HELLP syndrome	No	Yes
Platelet count	>100,000/mm³	<100,000/mm³

(BP: blood pressure)

Anesthetic Management

Patients with mild PIH require nothing more than a little extra care during anesthesia and standard anesthetic techniques can be used. After spinal and epidural anesthesia there is an accentuated fall in arterial blood pressure in these patients.

Patients with severe disease, require stabilization prior to anesthesia. Hypertension should be controlled and hypovolemia needs to be corrected before anesthesia. *In the absence of coagulopathy, continuous epidural anesthesia is the anesthetic technique of choice.* A central venous line may be used to guide perioperative fluid replacement. Hypotension must be treated with small doses of ephedrine (5 mg/IV).

As magnesium potentiates muscle relaxants, doses of nondepolarizing muscle relaxants have to be reduced in patients receiving magnesium therapy.

In active eclampsia, rapid sequence induction using thiopentone and succinylcholine is the anesthetic technique of choice.

Antepartum Hemorrhage

Antepartum hemorrhage is one of the most severe morbidities complicating obstetric anesthesia. Causes in decreasing order are placenta previa, abruptio placentae and uterine rupture.

Placenta Previa

In this condition, placenta either overlies or encroaches the cervical os. An anterior lying placenta previa increases the risk of excessive bleeding during cesarean section. Placenta previa usually presents as painless vaginal bleeding. In fact, all pregnant females with vaginal bleeding are assumed to have placenta previa until proven otherwise.

Abruptio Placentae

In this condition, there is premature separation of a normal placenta, oozed blood gets collected into the basal layers of the decidua. Expansion of the hematoma progressively extends the separation. The blood occasionally may extend into the myometrium (Couvelaire uterus). Patients usually experience painful vaginal bleeding with uterine contraction and tenderness.

Severe abruptio placentae can lead to intrauterine fetal death, coagulopathy which may progress to disseminated intravascular coagulation (DIC). Severe abruption is a life-threatening emergency that necessitates an emergency cesarean section under GA.

Uterine Rupture

Relatively uncommon but can occur as a result of, dehiscence of a previous uterine surgery scar; intrauterine manipulations or use of forceps (iatrogenic) or spontaneous rupture following prolonged labor. Uterine rupture can present as continuous abdominal pain, hypotension, frank hemorrhage, fetal distress, loss of uterine tone.

Treatment includes volume resuscitation and immediate laparotomy under GA. Ligation of the internal iliac (hypogastric) arteries with or without hysterectomy might be required to control bleeding.

Management of Anesthesia

In all cases (except mild placenta previa), emergency cesarean is required and GA is the anesthetic technique of choice.^Q Massive blood transfusion, including replacement of coagulation factors and platelets, may be necessary in abruption and uterine rupture.

ANESTHESIA FOR NONOBSTETRIC SURGERY DURING PREGNANCY

It is estimated that approximately 2% of pregnant women undergo nonobstetric surgeries in pregnancy. Most of them are emergency procedures, appendectomy being most common followed by cholecystectomy and adnexal surgery.

Principles of anesthetic management are:
- A rapid preoperative assessment that must include airway evaluation.
- Aspiration prophylaxis *(H_2 antagonist and a nonparticulate antacid just prior to induction of anesthesia)* should be administered to all pregnant patients beyond 14 weeks' gestation.
- Choice of anesthesia depends upon surgery and patient condition. Regional anesthesia is preferred over general anesthesia usually.
- If GA is necessary, a rapid-sequence technique after preoxygenation for at least four vital breaths should be used.
- Maternal $PaCO_2$ should be maintained in the normal range for pregnancy (30 mm Hg) as maternal hyperventilation reduces placental blood flow.
- In addition to maternal monitoring, fetus should be monitored wherever possible.

BASIC LIFE SUPPORT IN PREGNANCY

In any unconscious pregnant patient, continuous cricoid pressure should be applied during positive-pressure ventilation to minimize the risk of regurgitation.

As the diaphragm and abdominal contents are elevated by the gravid uterus, chest compressions should be performed at the site slightly higher than usual, i.e., slightly above the midpoint of the sternum. Rate and depth of compression remains same as in nonpregnant female.

ANESTHESIA FOR MANUAL REMOVAL OF PLACENTA

Retained placenta is one of the important causes of PPH. Manual removal of placenta is an emergency procedure to control PPH secondary to retained placenta. Under such circumstances GA with volatile agent is procedure of choice. Among available volatile agents desflurane is the agent of choice, as it provides intense uterine relaxation, which lasts only for a brief period.

LAST-MINUTE REVISION

- For labor analgesia, epidural analgesia is considered as best.
- For cesarean section, spinal analgesia is preferred.
- **Walking epidural**: Combined spinal + epidural anesthesia for the purpose of labor analgesia.
- In PIH continuous epidural anesthesia is the technique of choice, provided coagulopathy has been ruled out.
- Labor epidural is the only epidural where test dose is not given.
- For manual removal of placenta desflurane is the agent of choice (previously halothane was the agent of choice).

REFERENCES

1. Jain A, Mittal A, Sharma S, Deep A. Comparative evaluation of intrathecal dexmedetomidine and fentanyl as an adjuvant for combined spinal-epidural analgesia for labor. Anesth Essays Res. 2022;16:197-202.
2. Massoth C, Wenk M. Epidural test dose in obstetric patients: should we still use it? Curr Opin Anaesthesiol. 2019;32(3):263-7.

Unit VI: Anesthesia Practice

REVIEW QUESTIONS

1. **Assertion:** Ropivacaine is the drug of choice in labor epidural
   Reason: Ropivacaine is cheaper than bupivacaine
   a. Both assertion and reason are correct
   b. Assertion is correct but reason is wrong
   c. Assertion is wrong but reason is correct
   d. Both assertion and reason are wrong

2. All of the following statements are correct in reference to cardiovascular changes during pregnancy, *except*:
   a. There is increase in heart rate
   b. There is an increase in cardiac output
   c. There is increase in blood pressure
   d. There is increase in stroke volume

3. All of the following anesthetic techniques can be used to abolish pain of labor, *except*:
   a. Spinal analgesia
   b. Epidural anesthesia
   c. Paracervical block
   d. Pudendal nerve block

4. Local anesthetic of choice for labor epidural:
   a. Ropivacaine
   b. Bupivacaine
   c. Lignocaine
   d. Procaine

5. True statement regarding epidural block in a pregnant women includes all, *except*:
   a. Local anesthetic dose is reduced
   b. Chances of accidental dural puncture are high
   c. Chances of intravascular injection are low
   d. Onset time is less

6. Drugs of choice for controlling BP in a PIH patient in perioperative period:
   a. Hydralazine
   b. Labetalol
   c. Nitroglycerine
   d. Na Nitroprusside

7. Mendelson syndrome is secondary to:
   a. Gastric aspiration in perioperative period
   b. Trauma in chest
   c. Pneumonia
   d. Postspinal lung atelectasis

ANSWERS

1. b	2. c	3. d	4. a	5. c	6. b
7. a					

CHAPTER 42

Pediatric Anesthesia

Anshul Jain, Reena

INTRODUCTION

Pediatric patients should not be considered as small adults, because they have physiological and anatomical differences from adults.

Safe anesthetic management in pediatric patients requires detailed knowledge of their physiological, anatomical and pharmacological characteristics.

ANATOMICAL AND PHYSIOLOGICAL DIFFERENCES

Airway (Figs. 42.1A and B)

Pediatric (especially infant) airway management introduced is difficult because of the following reasons:

- Tongue is relatively large, which increases the risk of airway obstruction and simultaneously makes laryngoscopy difficult.
- Larynx is anterior and higher (more cephalic), it lies at the level of C4 in comparison to adults where it lies at the level of C6. Due to this straight blade is preferred over curved blade for laryngoscopy.
- Epiglottis is shaped differently, it is short, stubby, omega-shaped, and is angled over the laryngeal inlet; control with the laryngoscope blade is therefore more difficult.
- Vocal cords are angled, so a blindly passed endotracheal tube may get lodged in anterior commissure.
- Infant larynx is funnel-shaped and the narrowest part is at the level of cricoid cartilage (subglottis). So an endotracheal tube that easily passes through the vocal cord may not be able to pass easily through subglottic area.
- Due to this reason, uncuffed endotracheal tube is preferred over cuffed endotracheal tube till 6 years of age, as inflation of cuff can compress subglottic area and may lead to postoperative croup, tracheal edema. To prevent this, tube should be loose enough to allow some air leak, if airway pressure rose above 30 cm H_2O.
- Too undersize tube should also be avoided as this would increase the chances of aspiration.
- Recently introduced microcuff tube, allows more uniform distribution of cuff pressure thereby reducing the chances of edema and simultaneously provide protection against aspiration. However, they are very expensive.
- Infant head is proportionately large in comparison to adults, due to this intubation is better in neutral or slight flexed position (in adults atlanto-occipital extension is required).
- Trachea of infants divides into right and left bronchus at an angle of 55° on both sides (this angle remains equal up to 3 years). Thus, in children up to 3 years endotracheal tube may pass into right or left bronchus with equal risks (*in adults tube usually passes into right bronchus*).

> **KEY POINTS**
>
> Classically, it is taught that in adult, glottis is the narrowest part of the airway; but recent autopsy data had shown subglottis to be the narrowest part in adults too. However, the proportional narrowing is much less because of which endotracheal tubes pass subglottic area easily.

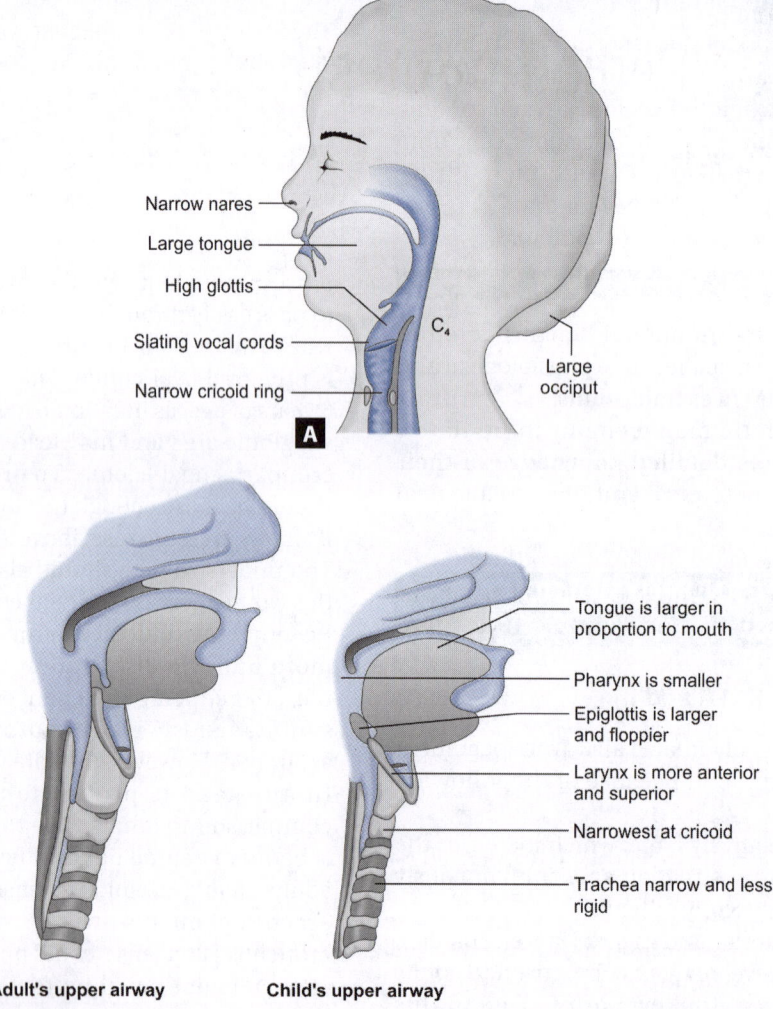

Figs. 42.1A and B: (A) Distinct characteristics of pediatric airway; (B) Adult vs. pediatric upper airway.

Respiratory System

Several anatomic differences make respiration less efficient in infants:
- Infants have less alveoli and their alveolar diameter is also less, both factors increase airway resistance (alveoli increases in number and size till 8 years of age).
- Compliance of both lung and chest is high, so there is functional airway closure in each breath or it can be said that work of breathing is much higher in infants.
- In diaphragm and intercostal muscles, type I fibers are less which contributes to easy fatigability of respiratory muscles. So, in infant ventilation should always be assisted.

Note: This enhanced work of breathing is not the negative aspect for infant as this increased work provides stimulus for the proper growth of respiratory muscles.

Cardiovascular System

- Though functional closure of ductus arteriosus, foramen ovale, ductus venosus occurs at birth in response to increased blood oxygen content. True mechanical closure does not occur until 3 weeks of age. Before 3 weeks, there is flip-flop circulation, i.e., any event that decreases oxygen content or increases pulmonary artery pressure can reopen these shunts and revert to fetal circulation.
- Due to low compliance and poor development of left ventricle, stroke volume is fixed and therefore, cardiac output is heart rate dependent.
- Vasoconstriction response is poorly developed, so infants are poor tolerant of intravascular fluid depletion and hemorrhage.
- Infant cardiac calcium stores are very low, that is why they are more susceptible to myocardial depressant action of inhalational agents.

Hepatorenal System

Neonates are obligate sodium loser, and are always at risk for hyponatremia, so sodium rich fluids should be infused for fluid maintenance. Further ability to handle salt and water load is also impaired up to 2 years as complete maturation of kidneys occurs only after 2 years of age. Half-life of renally excreted drugs is also prolonged.

Infant liver is immature and phase II metabolism (conjugation) is impaired, though phase I metabolism is adequate. Plasma albumin is low, so the action of albumin bound drugs is enhanced.

Gastrointestinal System

Neonates have high incidence of gastroesophageal reflux as they have poor ability to coordinate swallowing with respiration.

Thermoregulation

Pediatric patients are vulnerable to hypothermia because:
- They have a large surface area per kilogram of weight; skin is thin.
- The ability to generate heat is poor.
- The ability to conserve heat is also less.

The major mechanism of heat production in neonates is nonshivering thermogenesis by metabolism of brown fat; that too is reduced under anesthesia. Cold stress increases oxygen consumption and can cause metabolic acidosis.

The best way to prevent hypothermia in pediatric patient is by keeping operating theater temperature around 28°C. *Hot air blankets are the most efficient method for warming children.*

Metabolic Differences

Due to low glycogen storage, children (especially neonates) are very prone for hypoglycemia. So fasting should be as minimum as possible and always be accompanied by intravenous (IV) administration of glucose-containing fluids.

Central Nervous System

The blood-brain barrier is poorly developed and myelinization is also incomplete, so neonates are sensitive to almost all anesthetic agents. However, for unexplained reason, minimum alveolar concentration (MAC) value of volatile anesthetic is highest in infants of 3–6 months of age.

Neuromuscular Function

Neuromuscular (NM) functions are immature until 2 months of age, this makes neonates ultrasensitive to nondepolarizers.

Further, due to presence of extrajunctional receptors and undiagnosed myopathies succinylcholine should better be avoided in pediatric age group.

PHARMACOLOGICAL DIFFERENCE

Inhaled Anesthetic

High cardiac index and rapid respiration result in rapid induction and rapid recovery from volatile anesthetic.

Nonvolatile Anesthetics

Due to larger central volume and greater clearance, induction dose of most nonvolatile anesthetics is higher in infants. In neonates, dose requirement of thiopentone is reduced due to low fat stores.

Sedative Analgesics

Midazolam is the only benzodiazepine approved by US Food and Drug Administration (US-FDA)for use in neonates. Remifentanil[Q] is the safest opioid in pediatric patients.

Muscles Relaxant

Due to their higher extracellular fluid volume, dose of succinylcholine (SCh) is increased in infant. Incidence of cardiac arrest (after SCh) is also higher in pediatric patient, so atropine must be administered before succinylcholine.

Among nondepolarizers, cisatracurium[Q] and atracurium are the preferred agents, especially in neonates, as their liver functions are poorly developed. Rocuronium has emerged as the relaxant of choice[Q] for intubation in pediatric patients.

ANESTHETIC CONSIDERATIONS

Preoperative Evaluation

- The goal is to reduce the anxiety of parents and child.
- Upper respiratory tract infection (URI) must be ruled out in every pediatric patient. Children with URI are at increased risk for laryngospasm, bronchospasm, postintubation croup, atelectasis and episodes of desaturation. The risk is more in endotracheal intubation when compared with supraglottic devices like LMA. It is always wise to defer elective surgery in a child with active URI for 6 weeks.
- Fasting period should be minimum and should always be accompanied by IV fluids **(Table 42.1)**.

Premedication

- It is wise to avoid sedatives in infants up to 6 month or if the child is very sick.

Table 42.1: Preoperative fasting.[1]

Age	Fasting time (hours)	
	Milk and solid	Liquid
< 6 months	4	2
>6 months <36 months	6	3
> 36 months	8	3

- Oral midazolam is the most commonly administered sedative agents in pediatric patients.
- Atropine should be administered in neonates if succinylcholine is supposed to be used.

Induction

In pediatric patients, following techniques can be used for induction:
- **Inhalational induction**: Induction method of choice. Sevoflurane[Q] and halothane are the volatile agents of choice for induction.
- **Intravenous induction**: Most reliable and rapid method of induction; the only prerequisite is presence of patent IV line. Intravenous induction is specifically indicated in patients with full stomach; sick patient. Ketamine and thiopentone are the most commonly used inducing agents.
- **Intramuscular (IM) induction**: Ketamine (5 mg/kg) IM can be used as inducting agent, the disadvantages include delayed onset and painful injection.

Laryngoscopy and Tracheal Intubation

Straight laryngoscope blade is preferred in infants; in older children, curved blade can be used.

Uncuffed endotracheal tubes are preferred up to the age of 6 years for the reasons mentioned previously. Tube size (diameter) can be calculated by following formula:

$4 + Age/4$ = Tube diameter (or size)

For neonate, 3.5 mm tube is appropriate, and for preterm child 3.0 mm tube is sufficient.

Monitoring

Essential monitoring for pediatric patient include:
- Noninvasive blood pressure monitoring

- Precordial stethoscopy
- $ETCO_2$
- Temperature monitoring

Regional Anesthesia

Caudal block and brachial block are the most common regional techniques in pediatric patients. Both brachial and caudal blocks are performed under light general anesthesia in pediatric patients.

Postoperative Care

Two common postoperative problems in pediatric patients are:
1. **Laryngospasm**: Postoperative laryngospasm usually occurs when child is extubated in light planes of anesthesia. To prevent this complication extubation is done when child is either awake (opening the eyes) or in deep plane. Treatment of laryngospasm includes positive pressure ventilation, intravenous lidocaine. Succinylcholine is indicated for refractory cases.
2. **Postintubation croup**: This occurs due to glottis or tracheal edema. Intravenous dexamethasone prevents edema formation while nebulized epinephrine in normal saline is the effective treatment for croup.

Postoperative Pain Management

It is difficult to assess postoperative pain in pediatric age group, particularly in infants as they are unable to speak. Management is however very crucial, as pain can hamper their physical and mental development. Example: if an infant has injury over right hand then he will restrict its movement which will lead to reduced growth of that limb. Among various techniques available, caudal block is the preferred technique for postoperative pain management after abdominal and perineal surgeries.

Commonly used drugs for postoperative pain management in pediatric patients are:
- Acetaminophen (drug of choice in infants)
- Fentanyl
- Ketorolac

ANESTHETIC MANAGEMENT OF SPECIFIC DISORDERS

Tracheoesophageal Fistula

Tracheoesophageal fistula (TOF) is characterized by abnormal connection between trachea and esophagus.

There are five types of TOF out of which most common in type IIIB (upper end of esophagus is blind and there is fistula between lower end of esophagus and trachea). Clinically, it is diagnosed by inability to pass suction catheter into the stomach.

Tracheoesophageal fistula may be associated with other anomalies of VACTER (vertebral defect, anal atresia, cardiac anomalies, TOF, esophageal atresia, radial dysplasia) syndrome which must be ruled out.

> **KEY POINTS**
>
> Conditions where positive pressure bag mask ventilation is contraindicated:
> - Tracheoesophageal fistula
> - Congenital diaphragmatic hernia
> - Full stomach

Preoperative Management

Stop feeding, place a suction catheter in esophagus and infant is placed prone so as to drain saliva.

If the infant has pneumonia then, treatment should be initiated and surgery should be postponed till pneumonia resolve.

Anesthetic Management

Positive pressure ventilation is avoided prior to intubation, as air may enter in stomach which leads to gastric distension, and subsequently vomiting and aspiration.

Due to dehydration and malnutrition, intubation can easily be performed without muscle relaxant.

The most crucial part of management is correct endotracheal tube position. Ideally, the tip of tube should lie between the fistula and carina.

Congenital Diaphragmatic Hernia

In this abnormality, abdominal viscus herniates through a defect in diaphragm (most commonly through foramen of Bochdalek on left side).

Hallmarks of diaphragmatic herniation include respiratory distress, scaphoid abdomen and evidence of bowel in the thorax by radiography. Depending on the timing of herniation, there is variable degree of pulmonary hypoplasia and pulmonary hypertension (early the herniation more would be pulmonary hypoplasia).

Anesthetic Management

Anesthetic management is based on following principles:
- High pressure bag and mask ventilation (produces over distension of stomach) is strictly contraindicated.
- The neonate is preoxygenated and intubated awake, without the aid of muscle relaxants.
- Anesthesia is maintained on air oxygen mixture with a volatile agent. Nitrous oxide is not used as it can cause bowel distension.
- For positive pressure ventilation, peak inspiratory airway pressure should be kept below 20 cm H_2O, peak pressure above this level can produce pneumothorax in contralateral lung.

Hypertrophic Pyloric Stenosis

In this condition there is gastric outlet obstruction which results in recurrent vomiting. Characteristic abnormality is hypokalemia, hypochloremic metabolic alkalosis with paradoxical aciduria.

Anesthetic management includes awake endotracheal intubation followed by low-dose rocuronium. Rapid sequence induction is an alternative technique.

LAST-MINUTE REVISION

- Infant larynx is funnel-shaped with subglottis as the narrowest part.
- Trachea of infant divides at equal angle, so tube can go to either bronchus with equal frequency.
- **Drug of choice**:
  - *Volatile*: Sevoflurane
  - *Intravenous*: Ketamine, thiopentone
  - *Muscle relaxant*: Rocuronium for intubation

REFERENCE

1. Frykholm P, et al. Preoperative fasting in children: review of existing guidelines and recent developments. Br J Anaesth. 2018;120(3):469-74.

REVIEW QUESTIONS

1. Airway of an infant differs from airway of an adult in all of the following respects, *except*:
   a. Larynx is more anterior
   b. Vocal cords are angled
   c. Right sided principal bronchus is in straighter course in relation to trachea
   d. Larynx is funnel-shaped

2. Preferred volatile agent in pediatric patient:
   a. Sevoflurane
   b. Halothane
   c. Desflurane
   d. Isoflurane

3. An infant of 11 months is being operated for intussusception, what would be the preferred technique for postoperative pain relief?
   a. Caudal block
   b. Spinal anesthesia
   c. Intravenous morphine
   d. Intravenous pentazocine

Chapter 42: Pediatric Anesthesia

4. Following are used for treatment of postoperative nausea and vomiting after squint surgery in children, *except*:
   a. Ketamine
   b. Ondansetron
   c. Promethazine
   d. Dexamethasone
5. In a child with intestinal obstruction and deranged liver function test, the anesthetic of choice is:
   a. Enflurane
   b. Isoflurane
   c. Halothane
   d. Sevoflurane
6. The most appropriate circuit for ventilating a spontaneously breathing infant during anesthesia is:
   a. Mapleson A or Magill circuit
   b. Mapleson C or Waters to-and-fro canister
   c. Jackson-Rees modification of Ayre's T-piece
   d. Bain circuit

ANSWERS

1. c   2. a   3. a   4. a   5. d   6. c

CHAPTER 43

Anesthesia Outside Operating Room

Anshul Jain

INTRODUCTION

Nonoperating room anesthesia (NORA) refers to administration of sedation/anesthesia outside the operating room to patients undergoing painful or uncomfortable procedures. Common procedures include MRI, diagnostic/therapeutic interventions, pediatric cardiac catheterization, psychiatric treatment, and dentistry. Anesthesiologists are frequently asked to provide NORA in these remote locations. Current chapter deals with the basic principles and techniques of anesthesia outside operating room.

Challenges and Risks

Beside the risk related to the disease condition, unique challenges with NORA include those related to the procedure, and environment.[1] The anesthesiologist must ensure the availability of monitoring devices resuscitation equipment. Inadequately trained or insufficient staff, and unavailable medication or equipment in emergency situations places both patients and anesthesiologists at risk. Accordingly, the American Society of Anesthesiology (ASA) has provided minimal guidelines for anesthesia in the nonoperating room to improve the quality of patient care **(Box 43.1)**. Complications from NORA range from mild difficulties like anxiety to serious one including cardiac arrest. One should communicate with the treating team and team where procedure is being performed.

BOX 43.1

Guidelines for nonoperating room anesthesia

Location related
- Reliable source of oxygen
- Adequate and reliable source of suction
- Adequate and reliable system for scavenging waste anesthetic gases
- Self-inflating hand resuscitator bag capable of administering >90% oxygen
- Adequate anesthesia drugs, supplies, and equipment for the intended anesthesia care
- Adequate monitoring equipment
- Sufficient electrical outlets to satisfy anesthesia machine and monitoring equipment requirements

Provision for adequate illumination
- The patient, anesthesia machine, and monitoring equipment
- Battery-powered illumination other than a laryngoscope immediately available

Sufficient space
- Accommodate necessary equipment and personnel
- Allow expeditious access to the patient, anesthesia machine, and monitoring equipment

Immediate availability of an emergency cart
- Defibrillator, emergency drugs, and other equipment to provide cardiopulmonary resuscitation

Staff
- Trained anesthesiologist
- Adequate staff trained to support the anesthesiologist

Appropriate postanesthetic management
- Adequate number of trained staff
- Appropriate equipment available to safely transport the patient to a postanesthesia care unit

Applicability

NORA can be performed not only to the general population undergoing diagnostic procedures but also to patients who are too ill to be considered for surgery. It is recommended that the anesthesiologist who delivers deep sedation or anesthesia should be trained in airway rescue and management. While performing NORA, the anesthesiologist must ensure that participating staff are adequately trained to assist in anesthesia as well as cardiopulmonary resuscitation.

Procedures and Techniques

Neuroradiology Procedures

Diagnostic and interventional radiology procedures like embolization of cerebral aneurysms and vascular malformation are performed in DSA suite. These procedures are not typically painful, but general anesthesia is preferred for better outcomes in the event of an unexpected complication during the procedure. It is important for the anesthesiologist to communicate with the radiologist or the neuro-interventionist regarding not only routine procedures but also disasters.

Cardiac Catheterization Procedures

Usually performed in sedation which is administered by cardiologist, many a times anesthesiologist may be called for the same. Although there is no ideal anesthetic technique for cardiac catheterization laboratories, it is important for the anesthesiologist to minimize the effects of anesthetics on the cardiovascular system.

Repair of atrial septal defects or ventricular septal defects require general anesthesia with endotracheal intubation and transesophageal echocardiography. Pediatric cardiac procedures differ from those performed in adults due to the type of disease and structure of the abnormal heart.

Gastrointestinal Endoscopy

It is the most commonly performed NORA procedure. Potential risks include hemodynamic instability due to limited cardiovascular reserve in the elderly population, dehydration resulting from bowel preparation, and vagal responses due to distention of the gastrointestinal tract. Patients are at risk of aspiration due to gastric bleeding or consumption of large amounts of bowel preparation agents, while access to the airway may be compromised due to prone positioning, dark rooms, or endoscopy itself, which blocks the airway.

Diagnostic Imaging Procedures

The magnetic resonance imaging (MRI) environment is different from other remote locations providing anesthesia. It possesses strong static and dynamic magnetic fields, high-frequency electromagnetic waves, and a pulsed magnetic field. All anesthesiologists are educated on the unique environment of the MRI suite and screened for the presence of ferromagnetic materials, foreign materials, or implanted devices. Patients should be specifically screened for insertion of foreign materials (eyeliner tattoos, metallic intraocular fragments, piercings), or implanted items (aneurysm clips, prosthetic heart valves, or coronary stents). MRI is contraindicated in patients with implanted electronic devices such as pacemakers, cardioversion defibrillators, or nerve stimulators. MRI suite demands specialized MRI compatible anesthesia machines and monitoring devices.

All anesthetic plans should be individualized with principles of daycare surgery. Its always wise for proper airway control and its very difficult to manage the airway once the patient is inside MRI gantry.

Monitoring should adhere to the ASA guideline "Standards for Basic Anesthesia Monitoring", and anesthetic equipment and drugs consistent with those in the OR should be available.

Lighting is also a problem in MRI suites and its difficult to visually interpret the patient condition.

Complications Regarding Patient Management

Respiratory Complications

The most common complication of NORA claims is inadequate oxygenation/ventilation. In most of the cases this is preventable with better monitoring, such as pulse oximetry and capnography.

Hypothermia

Hypothermia occurs frequently in areas heavily air-conditioned to avoid equipment overheating. Pediatric patients are vulnerable to hypothermia when exposed for prolonged periods, which may cause dangerous side effects. Methods of reducing hypothermia include warming blankets with surface heating, administering heated fluids, and pre-emptive warming in volunteers. Hypothermia must be managed seriously as, mild hypothermia is known to increase surgical blood loss and also reduce the drug metabolism.

Aspiration

Though rare it's a serious complication. So, preprocedure fasting should be followed in a fashion similar to preoperative fasting. However, prolonged fasting can cause dehydration and hypocalcemia in children, so fluid therapy should be performed according to the guidelines. Clear fluids are allowed 2 hours before induction, whereas solids regarded as a meals are withheld for at least 8 hours.

Postoperative Nausea and Vomiting

Postoperative nausea and vomiting (PONV) is one of the primary causes of unplanned hospitalization, and is easily recognizable and preventable.

Postoperative Care

Postoperative or postsedation care similar to that after general anesthesia must be provided in a standardized manner. Preventable adverse respiratory events occur during the recovery or postoperative periods, so strict surveillance is necessary until full recovery.

REFERENCE

1. Metzner J, Domino KB. Risks of anesthesia or sedation outside the operating room: the role of the anesthesia care provider. Curr Opin. Anaesthesiol. 2010;23:523-31.

REVIEW QUESTIONS

1. Anesthesia in MRI suite differs from anesthesia in operation theater, via all of the following respects, *except*:
    a. In MRI light is very low which may preclude the cyanosis
    b. In MRI steel laryngoscope blades could not be used
    c. In MRI intravenous anesthetic agents do not work
    d. In MRI specialized MRI compatible monitors are required
2. MRI compatible anesthesia machine are made up of:
    a. Aluminum
    b. Pure steel
    c. Silver
    d. Titanium
3. In MRI suite, which of the following cannot be used?
    a. Steel laryngoscopic blade
    b. Regional anesthesia
    c. Electrocardiogram ECG monitoring
    d. Neuromuscular monitoring

ANSWERS

1. c   2. a   3. a

CHAPTER 44
Anesthesia for Daycare Surgery

Akashdeep, Anshul Jain

INTRODUCTION

Ambulatory surgery is a planned nonemergency surgical episode where—(1) the patient requires less than 24 hours in hospital stay (daycare anesthesia); (2) patient can carry out his normal activities (ambulant) after anesthesia (ambulatory anesthesia). This is also *called outpatient anesthesia.*[Q]

Top priorities for successful daycare surgery are: alertness, ambulation, analgesia, alimentation, i.e., nutrition (four "A").

Patients Suitable for Daycare Surgery

- Normal term infants more than 6 weeks of age.[Q]
- American Society of Anesthesia (ASA) I or II and medically stable ASA grade III patients.
- Preferably literate patient which can follow discharge instruction.
- Place of residence should be close to hospital (can reach hospital within 1 hour).

ANESTHETIC MANAGEMENT

Preoperative Evaluation

Stabilize coexisting diseases (e.g., hypertension, diabetes), encourage exercise program and smoking cessation.

Premedication

In premedication agents with shorter duration are preferred over long acting drugs. Use appropriate prophylactic therapies to prevent postoperative complications (e.g., nausea, vomiting, pain and ileus).

> **KEY POINTS**
> Four most commonly performed daycare procedures:
> - Cataract surgery
> - Endoscopic retrograde cholangiopancreatography
> - Hernia surgery
> - Arthroscopy

Choice of Anesthesia

The choice of anesthetic technique depends on both surgical and patient factors. For many ambulatory procedures, general anesthesia remains the most popular technique. Regional anesthesia via peripheral nerve blocks, wound infiltration, and/or instillation that does not preclude early ambulation is the preferred choice wherever feasible. With central neuraxial blockade (spinal and epidural anesthesia) prolong immobility is the limiting factor.

Intraoperative Management

There is no specific protocol for daycare surgery. Overall anesthetic technique depends upon the surgical procedure. *Nasogastric tubes, surgical drains, and invasive monitoring should be avoided.*[Q]

Agents of Choice

- **Premedication**: *Midazolam*[Q] is the agent of choice due to its shorter duration.
- **Analgesics**: Remifentanil[Q] is opioid of choice, among NSAIDs selective COX-2 inhibitors *(oral-rofecoxib, celecoxib, valdecoxib parental-parecoxib)* should be used.
- **Inducing agents**: Propofol[Q] is the intravenous agent of choice while desflurane[Q] and sevoflurane[Q] are volatile agents of choice.

- **Muscle relaxants**: As succinylcholine is associated with postanesthesia myalgias, it should be avoided.[Q] Rocuronium[Q] is the intubating relaxant of choice. All intermediate acting nondepolarizers (cisatracurium, atracurium) can be used for maintenance.
- **Muscle relaxation**: Laryngeal mask airway (LMA) is preferred over endotracheal tube for airway management.

Postoperative Period

Ensure adequate pain control in the postoperative period preferably by nonopioid analgesics.

Allow patients who meet discharge criteria to be fast-tracked (i.e., *discharged earlier from recovery units*). Encourage early ambulation and resumption of normal activities of daily living.

Modified Aldrete score is used to assess fitness of patient for transfer from postanesthesia care unit to postoperative ward.

Fast Tracking

Fast tracking after ambulatory surgery is accomplished by taking the patient directly from the operating room to the day-surgery step-down unit[Q] (i.e., bypassing the postanesthesia care unit) or simply discharging the patient home from the postanesthesia care unit.

LAST-MINUTE REVISION

Agent of choice:
- **Intravenous induction:** Propofol
- **Inhalational induction:** Desflurane and sevoflurane
- **Opioid:** Remifentanil
- **Airway device:** Laryngeal mask airway

REFERENCE

1. Watkins AC, White PF. Fast-tracking after ambulatory surgery. J Perianesth Nurs. 2001;16(6):379-87.

REVIEW QUESTIONS

1. Volatile agent of choice for daycare surgery:
   a. Ether
   b. Isoflurane
   c. Sevoflurane
   d. Enflurane
2. Intravenous induction agent of choice for daycare surgery:
   a. Etomidate
   b. Ketamine
   c. Propofol
   d. Thiopentone
3. Aldrete score is used in reference to:
   a. Transfer of patient from postanesthesia room to postoperative ward
   b. As an alternative to ASA classification
   c. Grading of hypovolemia
   d. Assessment of airway

ANSWERS

1. c   2. c   3. a

CHAPTER 45

Hypotensive Anesthesia

Anshul Jain

INTRODUCTION

There are some procedures which demands hypotension to reduce perioperative bleeding and improve visualization. Example includes vascular surgery. Current chapter deals with the basic principles of inducing hypotension in an anesthetized individual.

Healthy young individuals can tolerate mean arterial pressures as low as 50–60 mm Hg without complications. On the other hand, chronically hypertensive patients with altered cerebral autoregulation can tolerate only 30% reduction to their baseline value.

So, following guidelines are used in this context:

> Reduce blood pressure (BP) up to 60 mm Hg (mean arterial pressure) or 80 mm Hg (systolic blood pressure) or 30% of base line whichever is higher.[1]

Example: In a patient with BP of 150/90 mm Hg systolic BP is lowered only up to 105 (150–0.3 × 150) mm Hg; whereas in patient with BP of 100/70 safe systolic BP is 80 mm Hg.

Indications

- Hypotensive anesthesia is used in following surgeries:
  - *Neurosurgery*: Cerebral aneurysm repair, brain tumor resection
  - *Cardiac surgery*: Aortic aneurysm repair, coarctation of aorta
  - *Oncosurgery*: Radical cystectomy, pheochromocytoma, resection of any vascular tumor.
- When blood is not available or if patient denies transfusion (Jehovah's witness).
- Any other surgery in which huge blood loss is being anticipated.

Contraindications

- Severe anemia or hypovolemia
- Atherosclerotic cardiovascular disease
- Renal or hepatic insufficiency
- Cerebrovascular disease
- Uncontrolled glaucoma

METHODS FOR INDUCING HYPOTENSION

Nonpharmacological

- **Proper positioning**: Elevation of the surgical site selectively reduces the BP at the surgical wound and reduces bleeding.
- **Positive-pressure ventilation**: Intermittent positive pressure ventilation (IPPV) with positive end-expiratory pressure (PEEP) application reduces venous return, cardiac output, and mean arterial pressure, thereby reduces both systolic and diastolic BP.

Pharmacological

Out of many drugs nitroglycerin and sodium nitroprusside (SNP) are the most commonly used pharmacological agent while isoflurane[Q] is the most commonly used volatile agent for inducing hypotension.

Clinical Considerations (Table 45.1)

Overall nitroglycerin and SNP infusion are the most frequently used drugs to induce hypotension.

Maximum recommended safe dose of SNP is 1.5 mg/kg. Main limitation of SNP is cyanide toxicity. Cyanide toxicity is suggested by development of acute resistance[Q] to its hypotensive effects

Table 45.1: Comparative evaluation of commonly used hypotensive agent for hypotensive anesthesia.

Organ effects	Nitroprusside	Nitroglycerin	Hydralazine	Trimethaphan	Adenosine
Heart rate	↑	↑	↑↑↑	↑	↑
Preload	↓↓	↓↓↓	0	↓↓	0
Afterload	↓↓↓	↓↓	↓↓↓	↓↓	↓↓
Cerebral blood flow	↑↑	↑↑	↑↑	0	↑↑
Onset	1 min	1 min	5–10 min	3 min	<1 min
Duration	5 min	5 min	2–4 hr	10 min	1 min
Metabolism	Blood and kidney	Blood and liver	Liver	Blood	Blood and liver
Dose					
Bolus	50–100 µg	50–100 µg	5–20 mg	NA	6–12 mg
Infusion (µg/kg/min)	0.5–10	0.5–10	0.25–1.5	10–100	60–120

(tachyphylaxis), and increase in venous oxygen content due to nonutilization of oxygen at cellular level^Q (histotoxic-hypoxia).

Nitroglycerin is the preferred agent in patients with cardiorespiratory disease as it decreases myocardial oxygen demand and increases supply, moreover it relaxes both pulmonary vasculature and bronchial smooth muscle.

Hydralazine^Q is the agent of choice for renal patients as renal blood flow is usually maintained or increased **(Table 45.1)**.

OTHER TECHNIQUES TO REDUCE INTRAOPERATIVE BLEEDING

- Elevation of surgical site as mentioned above.
- Use of tourniquet.
- Use of vasoconstrictors, e.g., adrenaline. Reduces cutaneous bleeding only and overuse can increase BP which then lead to increased bleeding.
- **Decreased surgical time:** Bleeding is proportional to surgical time, so complex procedures must be handled by experience surgeon.

LAST-MINUTE REVISION

- Sodium nitroprusside is the most common agent used to produce controlled hypotension. Main side effect is cyanide toxicity.
- Hydralazine is the only hypotensive agent which increases renal blood flow.

REFERENCE

1. Barak M, Yoav L, Abu el-Naaj I. Hypotensive anesthesia versus normotensive anesthesia during major maxillofacial surgery: a review of the literature. ScientificWorldJournal. 2015;2015:480728. doi: 10.1155/2015/480728. Epub 2015 Feb 23.

Chapter 45: Hypotensive Anesthesia

REVIEW QUESTION

1. A patient with renal artery stenosis is posted for craniotomy for excision of astrocytoma, surgeon wants hypotensive anesthesia which agent can be used for providing hypotension in perianesthetic period:
   a. Nitroglycerin
   b. Adenosine
   c. Hydralazine
   d. Nitroprusside

ANSWER

1. c

CHAPTER 46

Anesthesia for Organ Donation

Ghansham Biyani, Rajasekhar Metta, Tanvi M Meshram

INTRODUCTION

The goal of organ transplantation is to replace the function of a vital organ when its function is irreversibly lost due to acute or chronic illness or trauma. This process involves retrieving organ from a person who is living or deceased (the organ donor) and transplanting it into another person with an end stage organ failure (the recipient) **(Fig. 46.1)**. World organ donation day is observed on 13th of August with the aim to spread the awareness on organ donation.[1] So far, many of the organs and tissues have been successfully transplanted, but the concept of brain transplantation still remains in its infancy.[2-4]

TYPES OF ORGAN DONATION

Organs can be retrieved from either living or deceased donors **(Fig. 46.2)**. Organ donation from living donors can be from related family members or from unrelated donors (allogenic donors). Organ donors who were once considered as not ideal due

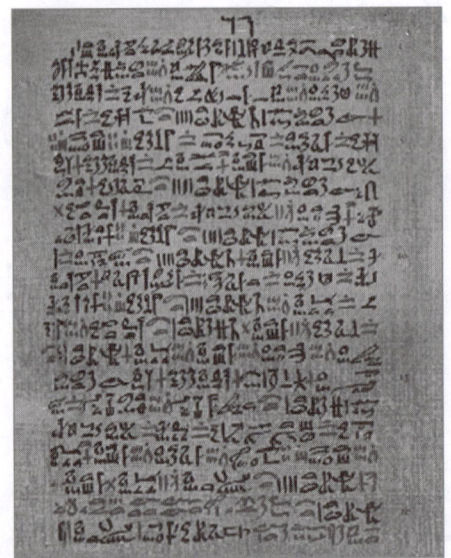

Fig. 46.1: Mention of skin grafting in Ebers Papyrus, Circa 1550 BC.
(*Image source*: Ebers Papyrus, University Library, University of Leipzig, Germany, https://commons.wikimedia.org, public domain)

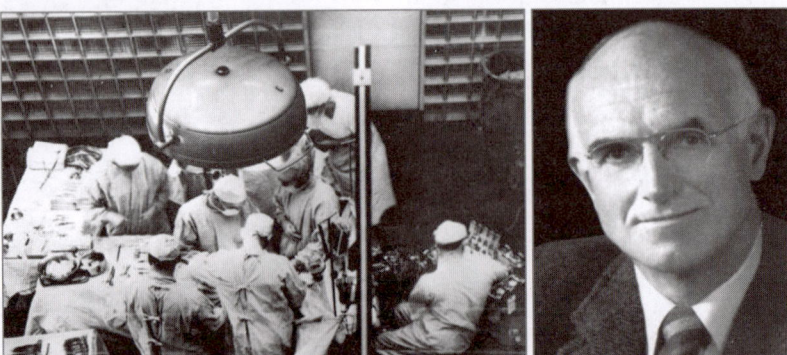

Fig. 46.2: Dr Joseph E Murray is credited for performing the first successful organ transplant in 1954, at Peter Bent Brigham Hospital in Boston.
(*Image source*: Brigham and Women's Hospital Photo https://web.stanford.edu/dept/HPST/transplant/html/history.html & Nobel Foundation Archive, www.nobelprize.org).

Chapter 46: Anesthesia for Organ Donation

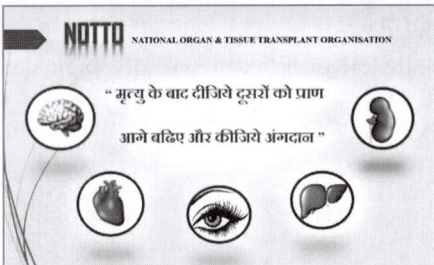

Fig. 46.3: Theme of National Organ and Tissue Transplant Organisation (NOTTO).
(*Image source*: www.mygov.in).

to coexisting medical conditions like age, diabetes and hypertension are now usually accepted.

Deceased donors include donation after circulatory death (DCD) and donation after brain death (DBD). Cardiorespiratory death is diagnosed after 5 minutes of observed continuous asystole. Brainstem death occurs after neurological damage when the brainstem has been irreversibly damaged, but the heart is still functioning and breathing is assisted using ventilator.[5]

In the United States majority of organs for transplantation come from DBD patients, while in India live related organ donation is most common. Underutilization of organs from DBD donors is the major reason for organ crisis in India. This needs a collective effort from the government, nongovernment organizations, and healthcare sector to spread the awareness **(Fig. 46.3)**, so that people dying because of end-organ failure can get an opportunity to live 2nd life. The forms for becoming voluntary organ donor are available at https://notto.gov.in/download-forms.htm.

CONTRAINDICATIONS TO ORGAN DONATION

Contraindications to organ donation is shown in **Box 46.1**.[6]

Warm and Cold Ischemic Times

Warm and cold ischemic times are shown in **Table 46.1**.[7]

ORGAN PRESERVATION

Interruption in perfusion to the vital organs (ischemic period) results in metabolic and pathological

BOX 46.1

Contraindications to organ donation
- Active cancer in the last 3 years excluding non-melanoma skin cancer and primary brain tumor
- Hematological malignancies like myeloma, lymphoma, leukemia
- Untreated systemic infection
- Prion disease transmissible spongiform encephalopathies
- Acquired immunodeficiency syndrome (AIDS)

Table 46.1: Warm and cold ischemic times.

The 'donor warm ischemia time'	It is defined as the interval from asystole or withdrawal of life support to the initiation of cold organ preservation
The 'cold ischemia time'	It refers to the interval between starting cold perfusion of the organs in the donor's body after the circulation has ceased or from keeping the organ in ice cold box to the removal of organ from the cold storage box
The 'recipient warm ischemia time'	It is defined as the interval from removal of the organ from cold storage until the restoration of normal reperfusion of transplanted graft in recipient's body

changes leading to intense inflammatory response and cellular injury. To minimize the effect of ischemia on the tissues and organs and to improve the graft function after transplantation, various protective measures are followed which includes storage of organs in preservative solutions and at very low temperature (4° Celsius). Various organ preservative solutions are available among which University of Winconsin (UW) and Histidine–Tryptophan-Ketoglutarate (HTK) solutions are most popular. These days organ specific solutions are also available. The accepted 'cold ischemic time' is 4 hours for lungs, 6 hours for heart, 12 hours for liver, and 24 hours for kidneys.[8]

PATHOLOGICAL CHANGES AFTER CIRCULATORY DEATH

The Maastricht classification of DCD is shown in **Table 46.2**. Expected DCD occur after planned withdrawal of life-sustaining ventilator support, whereas unexpected death refers to a donor who had an unanticipated cardiac arrest without successful resuscitation. Hence, in majority of DCD patients, there is a gradual decline in the vital parameters for a variable time frame before asystole occurs. This time period varies from few minutes to several hours. Therefore, organs retrieved from DCD patients are often subjected to variable degree of 'warm ischemia' during the dying process.

Table 46.2: Maastricht classification of donation after circulatory death (DCD) patients.

Classification	Description
I	Patients who are dead on arrival at the hospital
II	Unsuccessfully resuscitated patients
III	Patients in whom cardiac arrest is imminent
IV	Cardiac arrest in neurologic-dead donors
V	Unexpected arrest in the intensive care unit

Understandably, most extreme ischemia occurs in the time interval between the beginning of asystole to the onset of cold organ perfusion, but most of the vital organs are exposed to a longer period of ischemia in the period before asystole. Hence, a better measure of ischemic injury, often called as 'functional warm ischemia time' begins when the patient's systolic blood pressure falls below 50 mm Hg, or the oxygen saturation falls below 70%, or both. As a result, transplant-related outcome parameters for DCD differ compared with their DBD counterparts in terms of primary graft failure, graft rejection, delayed graft function, and other ischemic complications.[7]

PATHOLOGICAL CHANGES AFTER BRAIN DEATH

Neurologic death results in profound effects at the molecular levels of various organ systems, the understanding of which is essential in the management of DBD donors in ICU and in operation theaters (OT). If left untreated, it can result in autonomic, metabolic, and endocrine derangements causing organ deterioration and

BOX 46.2

Physiological goals in donation after brain death (DBD) patients
- PaO_2 >100 mm Hg, $PaCO_2$: 35–45 mm Hg, and pH 7.35–7.45
- SpO_2 >95% with lowest possible FiO_2 (ideally <0.4)
- Lung protective mechanical ventilation: Tidal volume of 6–8 mL/kg of ideal body weight, optimal positive end expiratory pressure, recruitment maneuvers, plateau pressure: <30 cm H_2O
- Heart rate: Sinus rhythm and rate between 60 and 100 beats/min
- SBP >100 mm Hg, MAP >60 mm Hg, CVP: 5–10 mm Hg, left ventricular ejection fraction >45%, cardiac index: >2.4 L/min/m² of body surface area
- Hemoglobin: >100 g/L (10 g)
- Blood glucose: 80–180 mg/dL
- Serum sodium: <155 mEq/L
- Core temperature: > 36°C
- Urine output: >1 mL/kg/hr (ideally 100 mL/hr)

thereby making DBD patients unsuitable for organ donation.[9] The various physiological goals of management are stated in **Box 46.2** (*see* chapter on 'Brain Death').

ANESTHETIC MANAGEMENT OF ORGAN DONORS IN OPERATION THEATER

The goal of anesthetic management is to maintain the cardiovascular function, oxygenation, acid-base balance, electrolyte levels, blood glucose, and temperature within the normal physiological range to optimize the quality of transplantable tissue or organ. Preanesthetic preparation should include preparing vasoactive and inotropic drug infusions, assuring availability of resuscitation drugs and equipment, cross matched blood, and discussing heparin dose with surgical team. Supportive measures started in the ICU should be continued in the intraoperative period.

Donor is placed in supine position with arms tucked by the sides. A forced-air warmer and fluid warming (hotline) should be used to maintain core temperature above 36°C. Even in the setting of brain death, both autonomic and motor spinal reflexes remain intact. Though the donor will have no pain perception, reflex sympathetic responses like tachycardia, hypertension, and movements of the neck, trunk, limbs can occur to surgical incision. These can be inhibited by the use of opioids, volatile anesthetics, and vasodilators. Muscle relaxants are used to optimize surgical conditions during organ procurement. Hence, drugs are administered to attenuate the physiological responses and not for providing anesthesia. Intravascular fluids and vasoactive drugs are used to maintain hemodynamics and to replace any lost blood. The calculated dose of heparin is given several minutes before the cross-clamping of aorta.[8]

Surgical exposure is obtained via a midline laparotomy incision extended by sternotomy. A cannula is placed in the aorta to perfuse the organs with the cold preservative solution and ice is applied to the surgical field to protect the organs. The organs are removed with their vascular supply after isolation in order of their susceptibility to ischemia, with the lungs first and the kidneys in the last. Prior to lung procurement, positive pressure breaths are administered to inflate them. Following this, the ventilator and monitors are turned off and organs are retrieved in the following order: lungs, heart, liver, small bowel, pancreas, and kidneys.[10]

CRIME AND LAWS RELATED TO ORGAN DONATION

Shortage in the supply of donor organs has led to illegal and unethical transplant practices especially in developing countries like India. Poor people consent to donate their organs due to economic issues, poverty, unemployment, and lack of stringent laws. For instance, 'Gurgaon kidney scandal' is one racket notoriously known for its illegal kidney sales from poor victims of Uttar Pradesh to recipients from across the globe.[11] Many such scandals across the country remain unearthed. Such incidents will only make the commoner question about the altruistic nature of organ donation.

Transplantation of Human Organs Act (THOA) was constituted in 1994 to regulate organ donation and for preventing commercial dealings of human organs in India. It was amended in 2011 and renamed as Transplantation of Human Organs and Tissues Act (THOTA), 1994.[12] National Organ Transplant Programme (NOTP) was initiated by Government of India to carry out the activities of the THOTA. The National Organ and Tissue Transplant Organisation (NOTTO) operates as an apex center for organ donation, and coordinates all the activities and networking for the procurement and distribution of organs and tissues within the country. The key points of THOTA and NOTTO are summarized in **Boxes 46.3 and 46.4** respectively.

BOX 46.3

Key points of Transplantation of Human Organs and Tissues Act (THOTA)
- Recognition of brain death as a legal death in India.
- Regulation of hospitals to conduct organ donation. Hospitals and tissue banks should be registered under the act to carry out organ donations. It is mandatory for such hospitals to have a transplant coordinator and a brain death declaration board.
- Prohibition of removal of organs for purposes other than therapeutic purpose, and to appoint authorities to prevent violation of the regulations.
- Punishment for removal of organs without authority, and for the illegal and commercial trading of the organs.
- Act has made provision of greater caution in case of minors and foreign nationals and prohibition of organ donation from mentally challenged persons.

BOX 46.4

Key points of National Organ and Tissue Transplant Organisation (NOTTO)
- To establish and maintain a national registry for human organs and tissues removal and storage.
- To maintain a national registry for organ transplant.
- To promote deceased organ and tissue donation.
- To train required manpower.
- To protect vulnerable poor from organ trafficking.
- To monitor organ and tissue transplant services and bring about policy and programme corrections/changes whenever needed.

Unit VI: Anesthesia Practice

LAST-MINUTE REVISION

- Live related organ donation (allogenic donors) is most common in India. Underutilization of organs from potential DBD patients is the major reason for organ crisis in India.
- The interruption of blood supply during the ischemic period in DCD patients and neurologic damage in DBD patients has profound effect at molecular and tissue level.
- The resulting metabolic derangement, inflammatory response, and cellular injury if left untreated, can result in organ impairment making them unsuitable for transplantation.
- The goals of anesthetic management are to maintain the cardiovascular function, oxygenation, acid-base balance, electrolyte levels, blood glucose, and temperature within the normal physiological range to minimize the untoward effects.

REFERENCES

1. Ranganath TS. Organ donation. RGUHS National Journal of Public Health 2016.
2. Gkasdaris G, Birbilis T. First Human Head Transplantation: Surgically Challenging, Ethically Controversial and Historically Tempting – an Experimental Endeavor or a Scientific Landmark?. Maedica (Bucur) 2019; 14(1): 5-11.
3. Nordham KD, Ninokawa S. The history of organ transplantation. Proc (Bayl Univ Med Cent). 2021; 35(1):124-8.
4. Singh V. Sushruta: The father of surgery. Natl J MaxillofacSurg. 2017; 8(1):1-3.
5. Van Zanden JE, Jager NM, Daha MR, Erasmus ME, Leuvenink HGD, Seelen MA. Complement Therapeutics in the Multi-Organ Donor: Do or Don't? Frontiers in Immunology. 2019;10: 329.
6. Westphal GA, Garcia VD, de Souza RL, Franke CA, Vieira KD, Birckholz VR, et al. Guidelines for the assessment and acceptance of potential brain-dead organ donors. Rev Bras Ter Intensiva. 2016; 28(3):220-55.
7. Manara AR, Murphy PG, O'Callaghan G. Donation after circulatory death. Br J Anaesth, 2012; 108: 21.
8. Brown MB, Abramowicz AE, Panzica PJ, Weber G. Anesthetic Considerations of Organ Procurement After Brain and Cardiac Death: A Narrative Review. Cureus. 2023;15(6):e40629. doi: 10.7759/cureus.40629. PMID: 37476138; PMCID: PMC10355135.
9. Pandit RA, Zirpe KG, Gurav SK, Kulkarni AP, Karnath S, Govil D, et al. Management of potential organ donor: Indian Society of Critical Care Medicine: Position statement. Indian J Crit Care Med. 2017; 21: 303-16.
10. Corbett S, Trainor D, Gaffney A. Perioperative management of the organ donor after diagnosis of death using neurological criteria. BJA Educ. 2021;21(5): 194-200.
11. Kidney racket busted in Gurgaon. The Times of India. 2008.
12. The Transplantation of Human Organs and Tissues Act, 1994.

REVIEW QUESTIONS

1. Which of the following is not a part of physiological goals in donation after brain death (DBD) patient?
    a. Hb of 10 g/dL
    b. Heart rate of 100 beats/min
    c. Blood sugar of 100 mg/dL
    d. MAP of 100 mm Hg
2. A donor has been brought to theater for multiorgan retrieval. As part of perioperative management, which of the following is true?
    a. Avoid neuromuscular blocking agent since the donor is deceased
    b. Inhalational agents can be used to mitigate sympathetic responses to surgery
    c. Opioid medications are of no use as the patient is not having any perception of pain
    d. Cold IV fluids must be administered to suppress the organ metabolism

3. Which of the following is a contraindication to organ transplantation?
   a. Untreated systemic infection
   b. HIV infection
   c. Patient whose core body temperature is below 34°C
   d. Patients on anticancer drugs
4. Donation after brain death means:
   a. Patient's cerebral activity is irreversibly lost
   b. Patient's cardiac activity is irreversibly lost
   c. Patient's brainstem function is irreversibly lost
   d. Patient's motor function is irreversibly lost
5. The recipient warm ischemia time is defined as:
   a. Interval between removal of the organ from cold storage until the restoration of normal reperfusion
   b. Interval from asystole or withdrawal of life support to the initiation of cold organ preservation
   c. Interval between keeping the organs in ice cold box to the removal of organ from the cold storage box
   d. None of the above

ANSWERS

1. d   2. b   3. a   4. c   5. a

UNIT VII

Pain Management

Unit Outline

47. Basic Concepts of Pain
48. Postoperative Pain Management
49. Chronic Pain and Palliation

COMPETENCIES COVERED IN UNIT VII

Competency Number	Competency Name	Chapter Number
AS8.1	Describe the anatomical correlates and physiologic principles of pain.	47
AS8.2	Elicit and determine the level, quality and quantity of pain and its tolerance in patient or surrogate.	47
AS8.3	Describe the pharmacology and use of drugs in the management of pain.	48
AS8.4	Describe the principles of pain management in palliative care.	49
AS8.5	Describe the principles of pain management in the terminally ill.	49

CHAPTER 47

Basic Concepts of Pain

Anshul Jain, Manish Kumar Singh

INTRODUCTION

The International Association for Study of Pain defines *pain as an unpleasant sensory and emotional experience associated with actual or potential tissue damage or described in terms of such damage.*

Thus, pain is a sensory and emotional experience. The emotional component is variable from person to person and in the same person from time to time. Fear, anxiety and sleeplessness are the factors which worsen the pain experience. Current chapter deals with the pain transmission, types and the methods to estimate pain.

TRANSMISSION OF PAIN

The peripheral bare nerve ending possess pain receptor called as nociceptor.[Q] Mechanical, thermal, electrical or chemical stimulation of the nociceptor generates electrical impulse in the peripheral nerves. *These impulses are then transmitted up through A-δ[Q] and C fibers to the dorsal horn of the spinal cord.* In the dorsal horn cells, the impulses get modified before onward transmission to the thalamus and the cerebral cortex where the pain is appreciated **(Fig. 47.1)**.

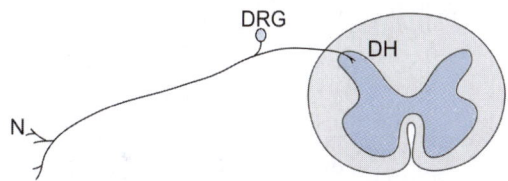

Fig. 47.1: Diagrammatic representation of the pain pathway from the nociceptor to the dorsal horn of the spinal cord.

(N: nociceptor; DRG: dorsal root ganglion; DH: dorsal horn of the spinal cord)

THEORIES OF PAIN

Till now many theories had been proposed for pain transmission out of them *"gate control theory"* (proposed by Melzack and Wall in 1965) is most popular. According to gate control theory, small (nociceptive) and large (touch, pressure) nerve fibers carry information from the site of injury to two destinations in the dorsal horn of the spinal cord: the *"inhibitory"* cells and the *"transmission"* or *"projection"* cells **(Fig. 47.2)**. Signals from both thin and large diameter fibers excite the

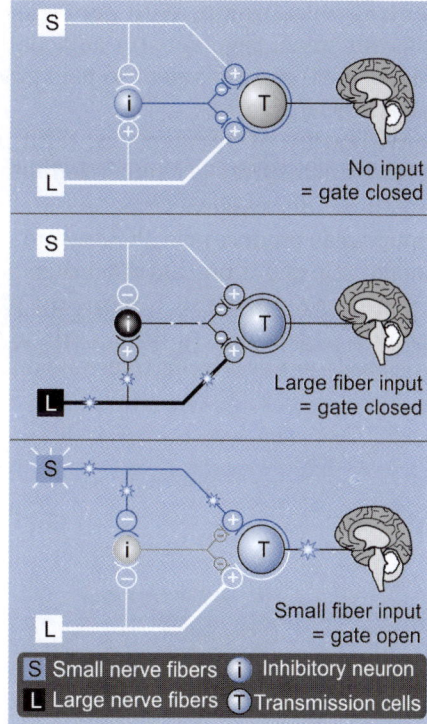

Fig. 47.2: Gate control theory of pain.

transmission cells, and when these signals exceed a critical level, impulse is further propagated to brain.

Inhibitory cells inhibit activation of the transmission cells **(Fig. 47.2)**. Thus, *transmission cells are the gate of pain, and inhibitory cells can close this gate.*

The thin fibers *impede* the inhibitory cells (tending to keep the gate open) while the large diameter fibers *excite* the inhibitory cells (tending to close the gate). This theory explains the fact that rubbing injury site decreases pain intensity, as rubbing excites large fibers which tend to close the gate **(Fig. 47.2)**.

It must be noted that even without additional injury the severity and area of pain increases initially, the reasons for this include:
- **Recruitment of nociceptor**: "Silent" or "sleepy" nociceptors that do not respond to noxious stimuli normally, gets activated in the inflamed tissues and same degree of peripheral stimulus generates more number of electrical impulses.
- **Central recruitment**: With persisting pain, adjacent spinal segments (or adjacent supra spinal areas) gets recruited, so pain gradually spreads to larger areas.
- **Sensitization of nociceptors**: With period of time nociceptors get sensitized and their threshold decreases. Thus, even a minor stimulus can produce pain. Prostaglandins have a major role in this process of sensitization.
- **Central sensitization ("wind-up phenomenon")**: The dorsal horn cells also get sensitized there by favoring transmission of pain impulses to higher centers. This is termed as "wind-up" phenomenon. N-methyl D-aspartate is the main neurotransmitter involved in the "wind- up" mechanism.

CLASSIFICATION OF PAIN (FIG. 47.3)

Broadly pain is of two types:
1. **Nociceptive pain**: Any pain caused primarily by stimulation of the nociceptor is said to be nociceptive pain. It is further subdivided to somatic and visceral pain, depending on site of origin.
2. **Neuropathic pain**: If pain is caused by impulse generation within the pathway proximal to the nociceptor (this could be in the nerve, the spinal cord or the brain), it is called *neuropathic* pain.

Neuropathic pain can be of three subtypes:
1. **Neural injury:** Pain is due to anatomical abnormality in peripheral nerves, or in the central pain pathway (e.g., pain in the upper limb secondary to the tumor-infiltrating the brachial plexus).

   The characteristic features of this pain are:
   - Shooting, stabbing, pricking, aching or burning nature
   - It has a neural or dermatomal distribution.
   - Often associated with abnormal sensation in the area of pain, e.g., allodynia, hyperalgesia.
2. **Nerve compression**: Pain occurs when some external structure compresses neural structure for example a nerve root compression in prolapsed intervertebral disk.

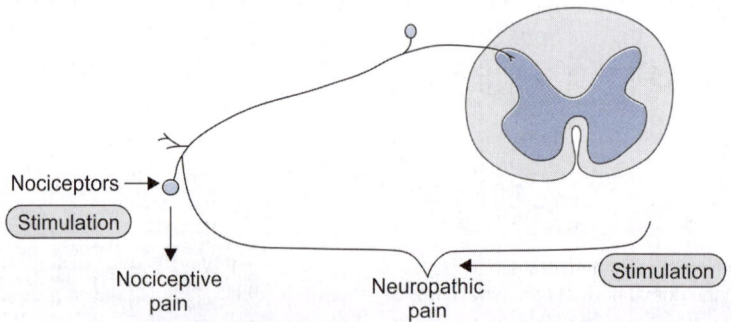

Fig. 47.3: Classification of pain according to etiology.

3. **Complex regional pain syndrome**: This includes reflex sympathetic dystrophy [*Complex Regional Pain Syndrome* (CRPS) *Type I*] and causalgia (CRPS type II). In CRPS there is associated edema, cutaneous blood flow changes and/or abnormal sudomotor activity which are absent in other neuropathic pain.

EVALUATION OF PAIN

One of the biggest problems in assessing pain is its subjectivity. So far many scales and scores have been devised to assess pain. But only McGill's questionnaire and visual analog scale (VAS) are popular.

Visual Analog Scale Score

It is the most commonly adopted method to assess acute pain (e.g., postoperative pain). VAS contains digits from 1 to 10. The person is asked to compare the severity of current pain with the worst pain he has ever faced in life. That severe pain is rated as 10 on VAS, whereas the current intensity is taken as VAS score. If patient says he is having most severe pain he had ever experienced then the VAS score is 10. In follow-up patient is asked to score pain by comparing his pretreatment pain **(Fig. 47.4)**.

> **KEY POINTS**
>
> Three most painful chronic pain syndromes:
> 1. Causalgia
> 2. Cluster headache
> 3. Trigeminal neuralgia

McGill's Pain Questionnaire

This scale assesses pain in a *multimodal way*.[Q] It measures the sensory, affective, evaluative and other aspects of pain. The questionnaire contains about 20 questions. 1 to 10 represents sensory aspects of pain, 11 to 15 represent affective aspect of pain, 16 represents evaluative aspect of pain, 17 to 20 represent other miscellaneous aspects of pain. Each question has 2 to 5 preformed answers, patient has to choose the most appropriate answer for him. The sum of all points, i.e., total value is called as pain rating index. Because of its multidimensional approach McGill's pain questionnaire evaluates many aspects of pain. However, evaluation is time-consuming, so it is used mainly in chronic pain.

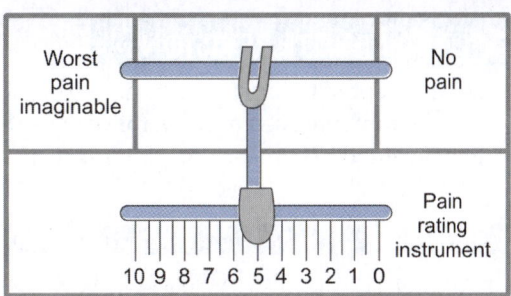

Fig. 47.4: Visual analog scales.

Evaluation of Pain in Neonate and Children

Pediatric age group patients may not be able to express pain with suitable words and it is much more difficult in preverbal age group. Pain in neonates is mostly assessed in an indirect way such as observing physiological changes or behavioral responses.[1]

Physiological changes include increased heart rate, respiratory rate, blood pressure and excessive palmar sweating.

Behavioral changes include changes in facial expression (eyebrow bulge, eye squeeze, nasolabial furrow, open lips, vertical or horizontal stretching of mouth, lip purse), body movement and type of cry. The neonate often show diffuse body movements to noxious painful stimuli.

In preschool age group *Smiley scale* and *Children's Hospital of Eastern Ontario Pain Scales (CHEOPS)* are used. The CHEOPS[Q] is a behavioral scale for evaluating postoperative pain in young children. It can be used to monitor the effectiveness of treatment also. CHEOP scale particularly suites in children between 1 year and 4 years of age. CHEOP scale uses crying, facial expression, verbal expression, touch position, body position and leg position for assessing pain. The *Oucher scale, color analog scale, Poker chip tool, ladder scale, and linear analog scale* are other methods for assessing pain in this age group.

Unit VII: Pain Management

LAST-MINUTE REVISION

- **Most accepted theory for pain:** Gate control theory
- **Most commonly used method for pain evaluation in adult:** VAS score
- **Pain evaluation in preschool children:** CHEOP scale

REFERENCE

1. Maxwell LG, Malavolta CP, Fraga MV. Assessment of pain in the neonate. Clin Perinatol. 2013;40(3):457-69.

REVIEW QUESTIONS

1. For monitoring severity of pain, most commonly adopted method is:
   a. Visual analogue scale
   b. Mc Gill's questionnaire
   c. Smile scale
   d. CHEOP scales
2. A Children Hospital of Eastern Ontario Pain Scale (CHEOPS) for rating postoperative pain in children includes all, except:
   a. Cry
   b. Touch
   c. Torso
   d. Oxygen saturation
3. Visual analog scale score of 10 signifies:
   a. Patient is totally pain free
   b. Patient has very severe pain
   c. Patient has mild pain
   d. Patient has moderate pain

ANSWERS

1. a   2. d   3. b

CHAPTER 48

Postoperative Pain Management

Anshul Jain, Manish Kumar Singh

INTRODUCTION

Pain after surgery can adversely affect both physical and physiological functions (e.g., postsurgical chest pain may inhibit the coughing, which is necessary to clear out pulmonary secretions). Postoperative pain can prolong recovery, increase the duration of hospital stay thereby increasing healthcare cost. Current chapter deals with drugs and other techniques for managing postoperative pain.

ASSESSMENT OF PAIN

Visual analog scale (VAS) is one of the most widely accepted methods to evaluate pain in the perioperative period. Patients with VAS score more than 3 require treatment. Assessment of pain should be repeated at regular intervals and the affectivity of treatment can be assessed by reduction in VAS scores.

METHODS OF POSTOPERATIVE PAIN MANAGEMENT

Broadly, postoperative pain management can be divided into pharmacological and nonpharmacological methods **(Fig. 48.1)**. The choice is guided by the ladder devised by World Health Organization (WHO) **(Fig. 48.2)**.

Pharmacological Methods

Systemic Analgesics

- **Nonsteroidal anti-inflammatory drugs (NSAIDs)**: NSAIDs play a major role in postoperative pain management. They are devoid of sedation but possess limitations of delayed onset, gastrointestinal (GI) irritation, etc. The combination of opioid and NSAID is ideal for treatment of severe postoperative pain.
- **Acetaminophen**: Though a commonly used analgesic and antipyretic, its low potency makes it less useful in perioperative periods. But its safety profile makes paracetamol[Q] the preferred postoperative analgesic for infants.
- **Opioids**: Moderate-to-severe pain which does not respond to nonopioids requires addition of opioids to pain medication regimens. Opioids possess the side effects of respiratory depression, drowsiness, euphoria, nausea, vomiting and constipation.

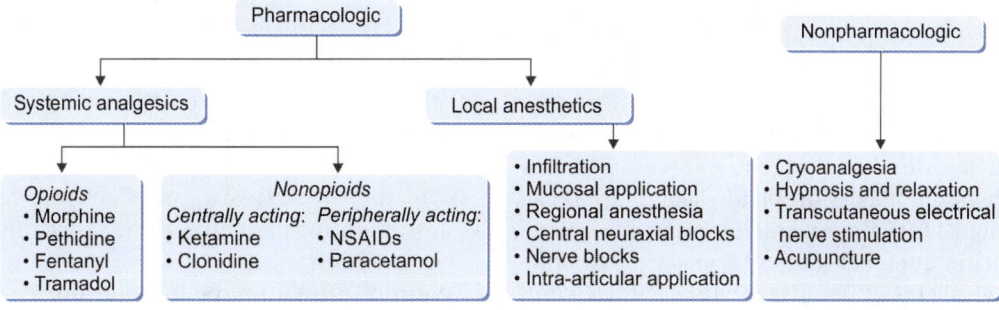

Fig. 48.1: Techniques for postoperative pain control.
(NSAIDs: nonsteroidal anti-inflammatory drugs)

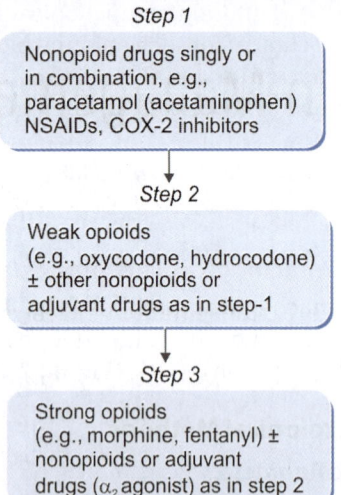

Fig. 48.2: Adaptation of the World Health Organization (WHO) analgesic ladder to control postoperative pain in patients undergoing ambulatory surgery.

(NSAIDs: nonsteroidal anti-inflammatory drugs; COX: cyclo-oxygenase)

- Morphine and pethidine are usually used to relieve moderate pain whereas, fentanyl and remifentanil are the drug of choice to relieve severe pain.^{Q} The common practice is to administer one bolus of fentanyl and maintenance with morphine. Morphine is the opioid of choice for patient control analgesia (PCA) too.^{Q} In PCA there is continuous infusion of an opioid; patient can administer additional bolus doses through a digital button. There is a lockout interval^Q which prevents overdose, i.e., if patient presses button again for additional bolus in lockout interval, drug would not be released by PCA pump. The purpose is to have placebo effect.
- **Ketamine**: It is the only intravenous-inducing agent which possesses significant analgesic effects. Favorably its analgesic concentration is much lower than that required for anesthesia. When combined with opioids, ketamine reduces opioid consumption and improves analgesia.
  - Limitation of ketamine is its vivid psychological effects, because of which it is used only in very severe pain not responding to opioids or when opioids cannot be used.
- **Dextromethorphan**: It is an N-methyl-d-aspartate (NMDA) antagonist analgesic that has got opioid sparing effect thereby reducing the opioid related side effects.
- **Clonidine**: A well-known antihypertensive but only recently introduced in anesthetic practice. Clonidine acts by stimulating presynaptic α-2 receptors and inhibits norepinephrine release from central and peripheral adrenergic neurons. Clonidine improves the duration and quality of postoperative analgesia when administered either epidurally/intrathecally or intravenously.
- **Dexmedetomidine**: Another selective α-2 adrenergic receptor agonist dexmedetomidine has sedative, analgesic, and antisympathetic effects, and is now widely used as an adjuvant in general anesthesia, spinal canal anesthesia, nerve block anesthesia, topical anesthesia, and postoperative analgesia.[1]
- **Flumazenil**: A benzodiazepine antagonist, which potentiates effects of opioids, and thus reduce opioids requirement.
- **Naloxone:** An opioid antagonist, which can effectively reduce opioid related adverse effects, and paradoxically improve analgesia.

Route of Administration

Drug should be administered using the least invasive route. Thus out of different routes (e.g., oral, parenteral, transmucosal, transdermal, and sublingual) oral route remained the mainstay for postoperative pain control. Parenteral route is reserved for patients in whom oral feed are withheld or if drug cannot be administered orally.

Local Anesthetics

Local anesthetics (LA) are widely employed for postoperative analgesia. LA can be used as:
- **Topical anesthesia**: Lignocaine gel application over the surgical site can effectively relieve postoperative pain after minor surgeries like circumcision.
- **Wound infiltration or instillation**: This can provide excellent postoperative analgesia facilitating a rapid and smooth recovery.

- **Continuous wound infusion**: Through pump driven continuous wound infusion one can provide sustained pain relief which aids in early ambulation.
- **Regional anesthesia**: Common blocks for postoperative pain control are the interscalene block for shoulder surgery and the femoral nerve block for anterior cruciate ligament reconstruction. These blocks are technically easy and provide excellent postoperative pain relief.
- Central neuraxial block (subarachnoid or epidural block) when feasible, provides better postoperative analgesia with lower incidence of side effects. Epidural analgesia including caudal analgesia is preferred central neuraxial blockade (CNB) for postoperative analgesia as the duration of analgesia can be extended by use of catheter technique. Caudal block is particularly preferred in children undergoing lower abdominal, perineal and lower extremity procedures. It is the most widely used local anesthetic technique for postoperative pain control in pediatric patients.^Q Further regional blocks are not associated with nausea and vomiting.
    - Addition of opioids or other adjuvants can improve the quality and duration of analgesia of CNB. Patient control epidural analgesia (PCEA) is a technique in which a patient controlled infusion pump is used through which a continuous infusion of LA in low concentration and additive (if any) is administered. If patient feels pain he can administer bolus doses through a digital button of infusion pump. Ropivacaine is the LA of choice^Q for such epidural blocks.
- **Intra-articular local anesthesia**: LA (20 mL bupivacaine of 0.25%) when given intra-articularly in arthroscopic knee procedures, can provide good analgesia and reduce postoperative opioid consumption.

Nonpharmacological Techniques

Acupuncture, transcutaneous electrical nerve stimulation (TENS) and continuous flow cold therapy are nonpharmacological modalities for postoperative control of pain.

Acupuncture, produce counter-irritation induced analgesia and can reduce postoperative analgesic requirement. Although, used rarely acupuncture and TENS are safe and effective in controlling postoperative pain.

Multimodal Analgesic Approach

It is the technique of combining multiple modalities of pain relief to provide more effective analgesia with lower incidence of adverse effects. This approach also prevents development of tolerance to individual medications. Multimodal analgesia^Q encompasses the combination of different classes of pain medications and different routes of administration. Examples include intravenous tramadol with rectal suppository of diclofenac. A multimodal approach is superior to any modality alone. WHO has also recommended a ladder approach for management of postoperative pain in patients undergoing ambulatory surgery **(Fig. 48.2)**.

LAST-MINUTE REVISION

- VAS score is the most widely adopted method to evaluate postoperative pain.
- PCA is the patient controlled analgesic infusion pump in which there is continuous infusion of an analgesic (most commonly morphine) and patient can himself inject the additional bolus.

REFERENCE

1. Tang C, Xia Z. Dexmedetomidine in perioperative acute pain management: a non-opioid adjuvant analgesic. J Pain Res. 2017;10:1899-1904. doi: 10.2147/JPR.S139387.

Unit VII: Pain Management

REVIEW QUESTIONS

1. **VAS score is used to measure:**
   a. Sleep
   b. Sedation
   c. Pain intensity
   d. Depth of anesthesia
2. **The purpose of lockout interval in PCEA device is to:**
   a. Lock the device so it cannot be misused by patient
   b. Prevent overdosing of analgesic
   c. To prevent underdosing of analgesic
   d. All of the above

ANSWERS

1. c
2. b

CHAPTER 49

Chronic Pain and Palliation

Anshul Jain, Manish Kumar Singh

INTRODUCTION

Chronic pain is defined as pain which persists beyond the period of natural course of initial insult. Arbitrarily a pain persisting at least a month beyond the usual course of an acute disease/insult is said to be chronic. It also includes pain which recurs after pain-free intervals of months or years.

ASSESSMENT AND MANAGEMENT

McGill's pain questionnaire^Q is the best tool to assess chronic pain because of its more subjective nature. It should also be kept in mind that chronic pain usually is not totally curable. The goals of chronic pain management include more comfort (as "pain-free" is often not possible) better physical functioning, lesser distress and to provide other positive outcomes. To accomplish these goals, chronic pain often is best managed by "multimodality" approach that includes a combination of following therapies:
- Drug therapies
- Psychological therapies
- Rehabilitative therapies
- Neurostimulatory therapies
- Surgical therapies
- Lifestyle changes (exercise)
- Alternative medicine therapies (acupuncture).

MANAGEMENT ACCORDING TO PAIN TYPES

Diabetic Neuropathy

It is the most common^Q neuropathic pain encountered in clinical practice. Management includes:

- Proper glycemic control
- Avoidance of possible neurotoxins (alcohol, smoking) and increase intake of vitamins (especially vitamin B_{12})
- Effective drugs are tricyclic antidepressants (*amitriptyline, desipramine, nortriptyline, imipramine*), selective serotonin reuptake inhibitors (duloxetine), anticonvulsants (gabapentin, pregabalin, carbamazepine, lamotrigine). Duloxetine and pregabalin are the newer agent approved by US Food and Drug Administration (US-FDA) for pain associated with diabetic neuropathy.

Trigeminal Neuralgia

It is due to the pathology of 5th cranial nerve, most often maxillary division. Management includes:
- **Drugs**: Carbamazepine is the drug of choice. Second choice drugs are phenytoin, baclofen, clonazepam.
- **Neuroablation**: Radiofrequency thermo-coagulation of trigeminal ganglion is the treatment of choice.^Q Gasserian ganglion block (associated with many complications), the preferred block for trigeminal neuralgia few decades back has become obsolete now.
- **Surgery**: Microvascular decompression is the surgical technique of choice in younger patients.

Postherpetic Neuralgia

- **Drugs**: *Gabapentin is the drug of choice.*^Q Pregabalin, amitriptyline hydrochloride, fluphenazine are other effective drugs.
- Lidocaine patches, intercostal nerve blocks provide short-term relief in very severe pain.

- Role of transcutaneous electrical nerve stimulation (TENS) is controversial, but it tends to improve the analgesic effects of gabapentin.

Phantom Pain

Phantom pain means pain in the amputated part. This occurs after limb amputation mainly, but has also been reported after mastectomy (as pain in removed breast). Pre-emptive analgesia, i.e., analgesia before pain occurs is the best preventive treatment; which can be accomplished through thoracic or lumbar epidural, nerve blocks. In established cases treatment includes gabapentin, nerve blocks, TENS, cordotomy.

Scar Pain

Scar pain can occur after any operation, but most commonly follow thoracotomy and mastectomy.

Most often it is due to neuroma formation where nerves have regenerated in abnormal manner.

Treatment

Treatment is by blocking the nerve supplying that area or local infiltration of neuroma itself. If this is unsuccessful cryoanalgesia may be helpful.

Complex Regional Pain Syndrome

Complex regional pain syndrome (CRPS) is a syndrome of pain and sudomotor (or vascular) instability. It is of two types, *viz.* CRPS Type I (reflex sympathetic dystrophy) which includes Raynaud's phenomenon, erythromelalgia, Sudeck's dystrophy, etc., and CRPS Type II which includes causalgia. In CRPS type I, there is no history of nerve injury while causalgia follows nerve injury. Both conditions are characterized by hyperalgesia, allodynia, changes in skin blood flow and edema.

Treatment

- Intravenous regional sympathetic blockade (chemical sympathectomy) using guanethidine and prilocaine.
- **Sympathetic blocks**: For upper limb CRPS stellate ganglion block is used, while lumbar sympathetic block is used for lower limb CRPS. If block gives good result, surgical sympathectomy can also be planned.

Low Backache

Low backache is the single most common problem for which an individual visits pain clinic. Before taking any step, surgical causes must be ruled out.

Treatment

- Analgesics
- Physiotherapy including hydrotherapy and exercises
- Injection of local anesthetics and steroids in facet joint (sacroiliac)
- Epidural steroids, this is particularly effective in disk prolapse pain
- Transcutaneous electrical nerve stimulation and acupuncture as an adjuvant.

Cancer Pain

In advance cancer, pain is the most prominent symptom. Cancer pain is typical as it possess both nociceptive and neuropathic component. Cancer pain often requires multimodal approach, World Health Organization (WHO) has advised three step ladder for cancer pain. NSAIDs should be the first drug, if pain does not responds weak opioids can be added, if pain is still unresponsive strong opioids can be used **(Fig. 49.1)**.

Neuraxial opioids can be used for intractable pain of gynecological malignancies. Regional

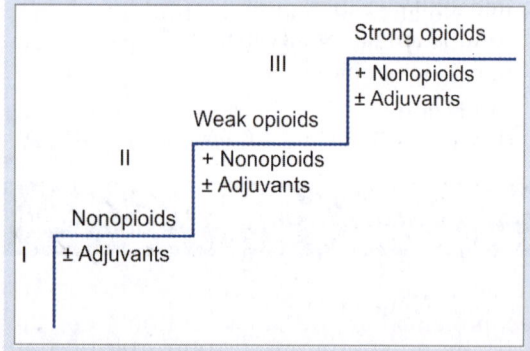

Fig. 49.1: World Health Organization (WHO) ladder for cancer pain management.

blocks like celiac plexus blocks can be used for gastrointestinal malignancy.

COMBINING PAIN MANAGEMENT WITH PALLIATIVE CARE

Palliative care is defined by WHO as "the active total care of patients whose disease is not responsive to curative treatment." Goal of palliative care is achievement of the best possible quality of life for patients and their families. Palliative care extends, if necessary, to support in bereavement.

Principles of Palliative Care

- Provides relief from pain and other distressing symptoms.
- Affirms life and regards dying as a normal process.
- Intends neither to hasten or postpone death.
- Integrates the psychological and spiritual aspects of patient care.
- Offers a support system to help patients live as actively as possible until death.
- Offers a support system to help the family cope during the patient's illness and in their own bereavement.
- Uses a team approach to address the needs of patients and their families, including bereavement counseling, if indicated.
- Will enhance quality of life, and may also positively influence the course of illness.

Thus the aim of treatment is to improve quality of life. No attempt is made to prolong life by a few hours or days at the expense of significant reduction in the quality of life.

Practically, palliative care is to allow patients what he wants, fulfill his wishes that do not possess a significant negative impact on the survival.

Example: In breathlessness due to terminal advanced malignancy, artificial ventilation or isolation of the patient in an ICU is not recommended, rather a familiar environment, correction of correctable causes like pleural effusion or bronchospasm. Oxygen is administered only if it relieves the symptom. Oral morphine may actually improve the situation by decreasing the sensation of breathlessness.

Similarly, in an intestinal obstruction due to advanced tumor, despite of inserting a nasogastric tube,[Q] corticosteroids (which help by decreasing peritumor edema) and large doses of prokinetic agents are used.

PAIN MANAGEMENT IN TERMINALLY ILL

Pain and discomfort at the end of life are frequently under-recognized and under treated. With the advent of modalities that help prolong life, there is a constant risk of prolonging suffering. Pain is the most common symptom associated with terminal diseases worldwide, namely cancer, heart failure, chronic obstructive pulmonary disease (COPD), and lung cancer.

Saunders conceptualized the concept of "total pain" in evaluating and managing pain in the dying. Total pain encompasses four components: Noxious stimuli, emotional discomfort, interpersonal conflicts, and the nonacceptance of one's own death. To alleviate the discomfort of the dying, all four components need to be addressed.

Evaluation

The evaluation of pain at the end of life follows the general pattern of pain assessment aimed at the site of pain, the onset of pain, character, radiation of pain, exacerbating, and relieving factors. Verbal description of the quality of pain is an important marker of the origin of pain. Somatic pain can be described as aching, whereas visceral pain may be described as cramping. Similarly, neuropathic pain may be burning or shooting in character. An evaluation of the intensity and duration of pain in the last 24 hours helps the caregiver quantify and manage pain. The cornerstone of efficient pain management includes round-the-clock assessment and repeated evaluations, especially following intervention.

Management

Cancer pain ladder devised by the World Health Organization (WHO) is the best guide for selecting pharmacological agents in managing pain. Nonsteroidal anti-inflammatory drugs (NSAIDs) are the most commonly used initial pharmacological agents for pain. Opioid analgesics are considered the gold standard of pain management at the end of life, providing the greatest pain relief.

Palliative nerve blocks: Carries important position, nerve blocks like celiac ganglion block for pancreatic cancer. Palliative nerve blocks provide superior pain relief and needs to be assessed in every patient wherever feasible.

Nonpharmacological Management

This includes measures aimed at avoiding pain triggers and psychosocial assistance in managing the end of life. Proper head positioning and neck support can avoid spasms of the neck, artificial tears and lubricants can help avoid painful keratitis. The use of gel foam pads on the skin-appliance interface can help avoid ulceration, for example, nasal bridge gel pads for noninvasive ventilation. Oral care and proper hydration can avoid painful ulcerations and dental decay. Frequent repositioning and offloading the dependent areas of the body can help avoid decubitus ulcers. In case of skin breaks, nonbulky, nonstinging chemical dressings can be used to avoid pain.[1]

LAST-MINUTE REVISION

- McGill's pain questionnaire is the evaluation method of choice for evaluation of chronic pain.
- **Treatment of choice**:
  - *Hepatic neuralgia*: Gabapentin
  - *Trigeminal neuralgia*: Radiofrequency thermocoagulation
  - *Complex regional pain syndrome*: Sympathetic blocks

REFERENCE

1. Sinha A, Deshwal H, Vashisht R. End of Life Evaluation And Management of Pain. [Updated 2022 Apr 4]. In: StatPearls [Internet]. Treasure Island (FL): StatPearls Publishing; 2022 Jan-. Available from: https://www.ncbi.nlm.nih.gov/books/NBK568753/

REVIEW QUESTIONS

1. Treatment of choice for trigeminal neuralgia:
   a. Gasserian ganglion block
   b. Radiofrequency coagulation of Gasserian ganglion
   c. Gasserian ganglionectomy
   d. Trigeminal neurectomy

2. Treatment of choice for postherpetic neuralgia:
   a. Gabapentin
   b. Lignocaine patch
   c. Paracetamol
   d. Diclofenac patch

3. Complex regional pain syndrome II is best treated by:
   a. Nerve blocks
   b. Lumbar sympathectomy
   c. IV Propofol
   d. Ketamine sniffs

ANSWERS

1. b   2. a   3. b

SECTION 2 CRITICAL CARE

UNIT VIII

Practice and Management in ICU

Unit Outline

50. Organization and Management of ICU
51. Oxygen Therapy Devices
52. Principles of Mechanical Ventilation
53. Clinical Management in ICU
54. Cardiopulmonary Resuscitation
55. Acid–base and Electrolyte Imbalance
56. Nutritional Support in Intensive Care Unit
57. Brain Death
58. Ethics related to Anesthesia and Critical Care Practice

COMPETENCIES COVERED IN UNIT VIII

Competency Number	Competency Name	Chapter Number
AS7.1	Visit, enumerate and describe the functions of an Intensive Care Unit.	50
AS7.2	Enumerate and describe the criteria for admission and discharge of a patient to an ICU.	50
AS7.3	Observe and describe the management of an unconscious patient.	53
AS7.4	Observe and describe the basic setup process of a ventilator.	52
AS7.5	Observe and describe the principles of monitoring in an ICU.	53
AS1.3	Enumerate and describe the principle of ethics as it relates to Anaesthesiology.	58
AS2.1	Enumerate the indications, describe the steps and demonstrate in a simulated environment, Basic Life Support in adults, children and neonates.	54
AS2.2	Enumerate the indications, describe the steps and demonstrate in a simulated environment, Advanced Life Support in adults and children.	54

CHAPTER 50

Organization and Management of ICU

Advaith A Chetan, Manu Varma MK

INTRODUCTION

Practice of critical care medicine originated in 1940s when intensive support was provided to polio patient. In the past two decades critical care medicine has emerged as a separate specialty. Successful management in critical care unit requires proper organization, coordination, cooperation and functioning of different specialties for the benefit of patients.

Intensive care, a term synonymously used for critical care, is a specialty which is multidisciplinary in nature and is dedicated to comprehensive management of patients to prevent or treat life threatening organ dysfunctions. It is a system of care delivered by skilled team from various professions. Critical care practitioners play a pivotal role in the organization of the intensive care unit (ICU).

Definition of ICU

An ICU is a specially staffed and equipped, separate, and self-contained area of a hospital dedicated to the management and monitoring of patients with life-threatening conditions. It provides special expertise and the facilities for the support of vital functions and uses the skills of medical, nursing, and other personnel experienced in the management of these problems.[1]

Classification of ICU

ICU could be classified depend upon cohort of patients (like postoperative, pediatric, burn ICU, etc.), or depend upon available care for severity of illness (Level of ICU).[1]

- **Level 0**: Patients whose needs can be met through normal ward care in an acute hospital.
- **Level 1 (Primary)**: Patients at risk of their condition deteriorating, or those recently relocated from higher levels of care, whose needs can be met on an acute ward with additional advice and support from the critical care team.
- **Level 2 (Secondary)**: Patients requiring more detailed observation or intervention including support for a single failing organ system or postoperative care or those 'stepping down' from Level 3 care.
- **Level 3 (Tertiary)**: Patients requiring advanced respiratory support alone, or basic respiratory support together with support of at least two organ systems. This level includes all complex patients requiring support for multiorgan failure.

OPEN VERSUS CLOSED UNITS

- **Open ICU**: ICU in which variety of physicians admit their patients and continue to act as the primary physician.
- **Closed ICU**: ICU in which both admission and clinical management are in the hands of intensivist (trained clinicians in Critical Care Medicine). Results of closed ICU are considered far better than open ICU.

ICU OPERATIONS

The aim of this chapter is to describe the optimal conditions to operate an effective, efficient, safe and patient-centered ICU with a goal of providing healing environment. A design based on functional requirements would enhance satisfaction of patients, staff and visitors.

Physical Space

- **Patient care zone:** This zone should not only serve for patient care but also be beneficial for visiting relatives. The patients need to be considered are privacy, prevention of cross infection and tolerant physical environment. Single rooms with glass walls, closed doors with provision for day light would be an ideal setup to meet the above set of goals. The ceiling should be painted with soft colors. The medical equipment is kept off the floor by the ceiling services. The ceiling services also allow the flexibility of the patient's bed. There should optimal clear space around the bed. This space should be at-least 4 feet at the head and foot and at-least 6 feet one each side. This space will be utilized for the bedside services like X-ray, and other patient care services. The medical gas, vacuum, data and electrical outlets need to be accessible as appropriately from all sides of the bed. In case of multibed ICU, each space should be at least 20 meter-square, excluding the service and walking areas. Supply of essential consumables and disposal of waste from the patient care zone should be adequately spaced. A negative pressure for airborne diseases and a positive pressure room (with separate air handling units) for immunosuppressant patients are recommended. Availability of soap, water and alcohol dispensers will increase the adherence of hand hygiene practices.[2] Alcohol dispensers are to be placed at entry or exit of the patient care with easy accessibility and reminding of the staff for the use of it.
- **Clinical support zone:** The nursing station provides space to accommodate monitoring and necessary staff functions. In a modular design each station should be capable of most of functions. The surface should be spaced for seating, charting, shelving, storing, overhead and task lighting.
- **Unit support zone:** This includes the office space, conference space, staff lounge with restrooms. Adequate space should be provided for these areas for smoother functioning of these units. Special rooms should be designated for the family counseling, pastoral care, social services and family support as per the local needs.
- **Family support zone:** Respite area to be designed for the comfort of the patient. A large space, with cafeteria and internet facilities. A private space with beds and washroom facilities to help relatives from far off places is advisable. Signage, with patient room number and orientation for visiting hours make relatives more comfortable.

Monitoring and Support Technology

Each monitoring unit includes the analysis, display of electrocardiogram, at least three fluid pressures and oxygenation, and preferably in both analog and digital formats. The alarms and settings should indicate critical values by both audible and visual means. The monitors should be located to permit easy access, viewing with minimal interruption to observe monitored status of each patient at a glance.[3] The space and electrical facilities should be designed accordingly.

Interiors

It is well known that physical environments have impact physiological, psychological, and social behaviors of human.

- **Ventilation**: Patient comfort is the criteria for temperature and air-conditioning. Appropriate filters are applied for air conditioning and recirculation of air. Air quality and safety are maintained by having at least a total of six air exchanges per hour. . The exhaust from toilets should be at least 75 cubic feet per minute capacity.[3]
- **Temperature**: The unit should have user controlled temperature settings. The physician, and in some cases the patient, should be able to decide the ambient temperature in the given clinical condition and set temperature accordingly.
- **Lighting**: Patients should be exposed to natural sunlight. General illumination with adjustable lighting levels, with minimal glare and indirect

lighting is preferred. Artificial lights with some high intensity sources for clinical procedure. These light sources should be designed to prevent burns. The total illumination should be targeted to less than 30 foot candles. Separate lighting should be placed in ceiling just above the patient for emergencies and should illuminate 150 foot candles and shadow free light.

- **Noise control**: Alarms, pumps, monitors, telephones, etc., will add to the noise overload in ICU. The challenge is to modulation of this sound to alert the medical staff but to be less noxious to the listener. The recommended noise levels in these areas are 45 dB(A) in day hours and 20 dB(A) in night hours.[3] Commonly the noise levels in the hospital will be around 50–70 dB(A), hence ceilings, floors and walls should be constructed with the materials that absorb sound. The symmetric positioning of the doorways and windows are avoided to reduce transmission.
- **Electricity supply**: Continuous supply of electricity is expected in ICU for constant functioning of the equipment. Grounded 110-volt electrical outlets with 30 amp circuit breakers should be provided for each bed. Voltage stabilizers (to attenuate voltage surges), automatic switch to backup supplies (to bridge power cuts) are crucial parts or electrical supply to ICU,[4] we provide guidance on some basic structural requirements, focusing on organization, staffing, and infrastructure. We suggest a closed-format ICU. The electrical outlets should be approximately thirty-six inches above the floor, or if at sides and foot of bed should be placed close to the floor to avoid tripping over electric cords.
- **Water supply**: Water supply is crucial for infection control, cleaning and dialysis and hence should be from a certified supplier. Hand washing units should be deep and wide and engineered with elbow or foot or automatic operators.[3]
- **Oxygen supply**: The common methods of oxygen supply are concentrators, cylinders, and piped oxygen systems. Concentrators absorb nitrogen from atmospheric air and supply up to 90% of oxygen. It is dependent on continuous power supply and require regular technical power maintenance. The centralized systems comprise one or more of liquid oxygen tank, oxygen concentrator, or large oxygen cylinders. These systems should have adequate backup plans for oxygen supply, power, and technical defects.[4] Two oxygen outlets, one compressed air outlet per bed is required. Audible, visible pressure alarms, manual shutoff valves should be located for each outlet at each patient area for better maintenance of the oxygen supply.
- **Floors and walls**: The door system should be wide and flexible to provide enough room for rapid transport of the patients. The surfaces should avoid the laminates, water traps, crevices, joints, fissures. The flooring should be made of resilient, smooth surface and extend into the wall to form a smooth junction. All the surfaces should be designed from the materials with infection control as the main objective.
- **Unit Décor**: Providing pleasant surroundings with help of appropriate color schemes, pictures and art works may decrease the incidence of delirium and stress in patients and families. Most often the bedridden patients would see the ceiling, hence careful design of ceiling will have additional impact on the patients well-being.[2]
- **Furniture**: The beds should be specially designed for the critically ill patients, preferably remote-controlled unit for easy positioning of the patient. Each patient should have access to chair (preferably a recliner chair) with an additional chair for the visitor. The bed space should be provided with containers for appropriate waste disposal.[2]
- **Gas supply**: Each bed space should be equipped with two oxygen outlets, one air outlet and one vacuum outlet. These connections should occur by a keyed plug to prevent accidental interchanging of gases. Manual shut-off valves are identified for immediate interruption of gases in case of emergency like fire, pressure or repair.[3]

Clinical Support Spaces

All the work areas in the ICU should be provided with space for storage and review of policy, manuals, formularies, telephone lists, computers, telephones and other resources as required by the users.

- **Storage area**: The storage areas for the consumables and reusables should be identified and designed. These areas should be planned to keep the area clear for smooth transport of patients and care providers. The areas should have the process for easy retrieval of the equipment and consumables. The charging points with grounded electric outlets should be provided sufficient to permit recharging of battery-operated items.[3]
- **Equipment specific storage**: It is recommended that each ICU should be equipped with point of care facilities for arterial blood gases, blood glucose measurements, lactate measurements and ultrasonography. There should be a designated area for the use and maintenance of these equipment.[4]
- **Other area**: Some of the point of care facilities can be made available to ICUs. This includes and not limited to ABGs, blood sugar analyzer prothrombin time. A pneumatic system for the transport of samples can decrease the transit time of the sample to the laboratories. The radiology units with portable X-rays and viewer boxes/digital access should be made available in every unit.
- **Clean and dirty utility room**: The contaminated room should have separate ventilation, exhaustion storage area and puncture proof materials for sharp penetrating medical wastes. The room should be equipped with drain, washing device for sanitizing the bedpans. The medical waste room should be designed in accordance with medical waste instructions.[5]
- **Procedure room**: If required a well-designed, spacious room with appropriate monitors, equipment, and safety considerations can be provided in a space adjacent to the ICU. The supplies should be adequate for smooth performance of the procedure without leaving the room.[3]

Human Resources

ICU involves multidisciplinary and team-based approach. Each personnel in the team should have undergone specialty training in ICU, as accredited by the universities or the professional organizations of the country. In India, Critical Care Medicine is now considered as superspecialty requiring three years of training in institutions recognized by National Medical Council (NMC). Similar programmes are recognized for master's degrees for nursing and allied health sciences. In addition, certification can be obtained in subspecialties like neurointensive care, echocardiography, etc. Also each unit should be appointed with team of pharmacists, physiotherapists, nutritionists, social workers, speech therapists, occupation therapists, psychologists, healthcare scientists, security personnel and support staff.

- **Critical care services**:[1] The daytime doctor-to-patient ratio must not normally exceed 1:12. This ratio is complex and needs to be cognizant of the seniority and competency of junior staff, the reason for admission and the number and complexity of emergency admissions and patient characteristics. The night-time ratio cannot be defined. All critical care units must have immediate 24/7 on-site access to a doctor with advanced airway skills. There must be a designated Clinical Director and/or a Lead Consultant for Intensive Care Medicine. Rotas for consultants and resident staff must be cognizant of fatigue and the risk of burnout. The patients must have a registered nurse/patient ratio of a minimum of 1:2 to deliver direct care.
- **Infection control practices**: The ICUs are built in accordance with national and international recommendations for best hospital infection control practices. Each hospital should develop individual policies and practices for infection control. The policies should have recommendations for the following:[4]
    - Rapid access and adequate access to personal protective equipment.
    - Sterility and use of masks, gowns, caps and drapes for invasive procedures.

- Hand hygiene and moments of hand washing practices.
- Easy accessibility for hand wash and hand hygiene.
- Alcohol-based solution is available after each contact with patient and surroundings.

AUDITS, RESEARCH EDUCATION AND QUALITY IMPROVEMENT

A regular change for improvization based on latest evidence is the constant in ICU. Documentation of patient records, adverse events, and performance indicators as per national and international records should be the routine in any given ICU. Each unit should develop bundle cares, protocols and checklists as applicable to the respective patient population. The unit should regularly be a part of national/international bench marking process.[4]

Challenges and Limitations

The ultimate objective of ICU design and operation is most likely compromised by cost, size details and competing interests.

CONCLUSION

The organization of the intensive care department has been changed over the past decades resulting in better patient outcome and reduction of cost. Besides future improvements of organizational structures within the ICU, the focus should also be on implementation of and compliance with proven beneficial organizational structures.

LAST-MINUTE REVISION

- APACHE II, and SAPS II scores are the most commonly used scoring system in ICU
- *Shock associated with increased cardiac output*: Septic shock, neurogenic shock
- *Type I respiratory failure*: Oxygenation failure
- *Type II respiratory failure*: Ventilation failure
- *Type III respiratory failure*: Perioperative respiratory failure.

REFERENCES

1. Guidelines for the Provision of Intensive Care Services | The Faculty of Intensive Care Medicine [Internet]. [cited 2022 Sep 1]. Available from: https://www.ficm.ac.uk/standardssafetyguidelinesstandards/guidelines-for-the-provision-of-intensive-care-services.
2. Thompson DR, Hamilton DK, Cadenhead CD, Swoboda SM, Schwindel SM, Anderson DC, et al. Guidelines for intensive care unit design. Critical Care Medicine 2012;40(5):1586-600.
3. Guidelines for intensive care unit design. Guidelines/Practice Parameters Committee of the American College of Critical Care Medicine, Society of Critical Care Medicine. Crit Care Med. 1995;23(3):582-8.
4. Papali A, Adhikari NKJ, Diaz JV, Dondorp AM, Dünser MW, Jacob ST, et al. Infrastructure and organization of adult intensive care units in resource-limited settings. In: Dondorp AM, Dünser MW, Schultz MJ (Eds). Sepsis Management in Resource-limited Settings [Internet]. Cham: Springer International Publishing; 2019. p. 31–68. Available from: https://doi.org/10.1007/978-3-030-03143-5_3.
5. Katirci Y, Şafak T, Aydemir S. A Review of Design Features of Intensive Care Unit in General Terms. Eurasian J Crit Care. 2019;1(2):51–8.

REVIEW QUESTIONS

1. The most common complication in ICU is:
   a. DVT
   b. Pneumonia
   c. UTI
   d. Delirium

2. Type III respiratory failure may occur after:
   a. Pneumothorax
   b. Basal atelectasis of right lung
   c. Pneumonia
   d. Pulmonary edema
3. A 62-year-old patient is admitted with signs of shock BP: 92/64 mm of Hg; heart rate 128/min; temperature 96.2°F. On echocardiography, his cardiac output was found to be increased. Pulmonary artery blood gas analysis shows increased oxygen tension. The most probable etiology in this patient is:
   a. Sepsis
   b. Hypovolemia
   c. Cardiac failure
   d. Cerebrovascular accident CVA.
4. Type I shock can be caused by all of the following except:
   a. Hypovolemia
   b. Trauma
   c. Cardiac tamponade
   d. Sepsis
5. True about type II, respiratory failure includes:
   a. $PaCO_2$ remains low
   b. Obstructive sleep apnea is one of the causes
   c. There is hyperventilation
   d. PaO_2 is high

ANSWERS

1. c
2. b
3. a
4. d
5. b

CHAPTER 51

Oxygen Therapy Devices

Sagarika Panda

Oxygen (O_2) is one of the most common therapies in critical care medicine. In the current pandemic of COVID-19 world realized the importance of oxygen therapy and now focus is shifting towards equipment/devices through which oxygen can be administered to the patient without wasting. Current chapter deals with the brief introduction of oxygen therapy and the devices used to administer oxygen.

HISTORICAL PERSPECTIVE

Oxygen was discovered by Carl Wilhelm Scheele in 1772; and it was first described by Joseph Priestley in 1775 in his work where he referred O_2 as 'dephlogisticated air'. In 1778 French chemist Antoine-Laurent Lavoisier described its role in respiration and named it as *oxygène*.

INDICATIONS OF OXYGEN USE

- For treatment of hypoxemia due to alveolar hypoventilation and ventilation/perfusion abnormalities.
- For improving oxygen supply to tissues, in situations with increase oxygen demand (sepsis)
- To decrease the work of breathing.
- During preoxygenation and maintenance of anesthesia.

Hypoxemia is defined as abnormally low O_2 tension in the arterial blood, and hypoxia is the failure of tissue oxygenation. Tissue hypoxia occurs when O_2 supply to the tissue is inadequate to meet the metabolic demands. Hypoxia can be classified into four major types, i.e., hypoxic hypoxia, anemic hypoxia, circulatory hypoxia and histotoxic hypoxia (**Table 51.1**).

Table 51.1: Types of hypoxia.

Type	Definition with example
Hypoxic hypoxia	Caused by low arterial oxygen tension (PaO_2) • High altitude • Hypoventilation • Ventilation-perfusion mismatch
Anemic hypoxia	Caused by decreased oxygen content (CaO_2) • Anemia • Blood loss • Carbon monoxide poisoning • Methemoglobinemia
Circulatory hypoxia	Caused by decreased perfusion • Decreased cardiac output
Histotoxic hypoxia	Caused by impairment of tissues to utilize oxygen • Cyanide poisoning • Shifting of O_2-Hb dissociation curve

The amount of O_2 delivered to the tissue depends on cardiac output and arterial oxygen content through the following equations (**Box 51.1**):

BOX 51.1

Calculation of arterial oxygen content and delivery
Arterial oxygen content (CaO_2) = [1.34 × (Hb) x SaO_2] and (0.003 × PaO_2)
Hb = hemoglobin (g/dL)
1.34 = O_2-carrying capacity of hemoglobin
SaO_2 = arterial oxygen saturation
PaO_2 = arterial partial pressure of O_2 (mm Hg)
0.0031 = solubility coefficient of O_2 in plasma
Calculation of oxygen delivery (DO_2) = CaO_2 × CO
CO = cardiac output

OXYGEN DELIVERY DEVICES

Oxygen delivery devices can be classified by number of methods, which includes:
- Fixed versus variable performance (based on performance)
- Low versus high gas flow (based on design)
- Patient-dependent versus patient-independent.

The variable performance systems are considered as 'patient-dependent' as they are based on the patient's ventilatory pattern including respiratory rate (RR) and minute ventilation as shown in **Table 51.2**. But fixed performance devices delivered a predetermined inspired oxygen concentration (FiO_2), hence considered as 'patient-independent' system.

Tables 51.3 and 51.4 show the classification of oxygen therapy devices according to the total gas flow and patient dependency, respectively. Low-flow system delivered O_2 from 1 L/minute to maximum of 15 L/min.

Table 51.2: Factors determining delivered FiO_2 in variable devices.

Broad category	Factors
Equipment related factors	Size of the O_2 reservoir
	O_2 flow rate
	Fitting of the mask (mask seal)
Patient related factors (patient's ventilatory pattern)	Peak inspiratory flow
	Tidal volume
	Respiratory rate
	Minute ventilation

Importance of Peak Inspiratory Flow

The point when fresh gas flow became less than the peak inspiratory flow of the patient and unable to meet the patient's demand, there will be entrainment of room air and dilution of FiO_2

Table 51.3: Classification of oxygen therapy devices according to the total gas flow.

	Type of devices	Delivered FiO_2	Advantages	Disadvantages
Low-flow	Nasal prongs	24–40%	• Comfortable • Ease of use • Able to eat and speak • Humidification not required	• Dryness, irritation and bleeding from nasal mucosa with high flow • Unpredictable FiO_2 • Maximum FiO_2 0.4
	Nasopharyngeal catheter	24–40%	Used in pediatric population	• Nasal and pharyngeal trauma due to improper insertion • Unpredictable FiO_2 • Need frequent clearing of catheter to prevent occlusion of holes
	Simple face mask	40–60%	Easy to apply	• Unpredictable FiO_2 • Rebreathing of CO_2 at low-flow <5 L/min
	Partial rebreathing mask	40–70%	• Easy to set up • Oxygen conservation capacity useful during transportation	• Variable FiO_2 • Significant rebreathing when oxygen flow is inadequate
	Nonrebreathing mask	70–90%	• Easy to use • Provides higher FiO_2	• Variable FiO_2 • Requires humidification

Contd...

Contd...

Type of devices		Delivered FiO$_2$	Advantages	Disadvantages
High flow	Venturi mask	24–60%	Useful in COPD patients where accurate titration of FiO$_2$ is needed to reduce the dead space ventilation	
	High-flow nasal cannula	21–100%	• Predictable FiO$_2$ • Decreased work of breathing • Better tolerated	Oxygen is not humidified at low-flow, dry nose, dry throat, and nasal pain
	Noninvasive ventilation	21–100%	Predictable FiO$_2$	• Excessive drying of nasal mucosa • Risk of self-inflicted lung injury

Table 51.4: Classification of oxygen therapy devices according to patient dependency.

Variable	Standard nasal cannula, simple face masks, partial rebreathing mask, nonrebreathing mask
Fixed	Venturi face masks, HFNC, NIV, invasive mechanical ventilation

of the fresh gas. In a tachypnoeic patient, when respiratory rate is increased the inspiratory time (Ti) became less. To deliver the same tidal volume (TV) the peak inspiratory flow becomes high (Flow=TV/Ti) and when it exceeds the fresh gas flow, entrainment of room air occurs. So, the FiO$_2$ of fresh gas will be diluted by the entrained air. Therefore, in order to deliver a predictable FiO$_2$ the fresh gas flow should exceed peak inspiratory flow of the patient.

LOW-FLOW DEVICES

Nasal Cannula

It is a low-flow variable performance device without a reservoir. It is a thin tube fixed behind the ear with two soft prongs inserted into the nostril (**Fig. 51.1**). It is used in mild to moderate hypoxemia. Oxygen is delivered through the cannula at a flow rate of 1–5 L/min to the nasopharynx which acts

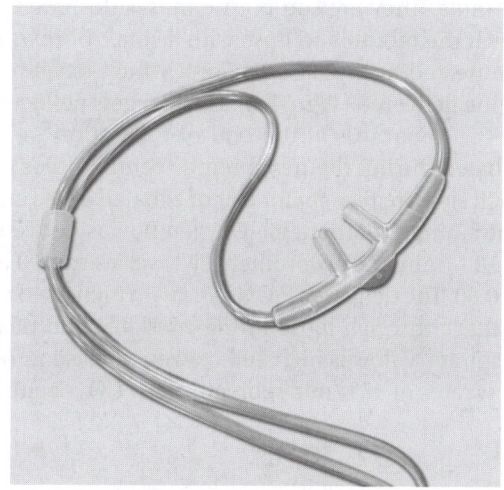

Fig. 51.1: Nasal cannula.

as an anatomical reservoir of approximately 50 mL which is one-third of normal anatomic dead space. Each 1 L/min of oxygen increases FiO$_2$ by 4% for patients with normal ventilatory pattern. So, FiO$_2$ achieved through this device is from 0.24 to 0.40. But the delivered FiO$_2$ greatly varies and depends on the patient's ventilatory pattern, respiratory rate, peak inspiratory flow and volume of the nasopharynx. Disadvantages are: Could not use in respiratory distress, and in cases of edematous nasal mucosa.

Nasopharyngeal Catheter

It is a low-flow variable performance device without reservoir. Catheters of variable size varying from 8–14 FG are available. The depth of insertion is equal to the distance between ala nasi to tragus. Oxygen delivers to the oropharynx which acts as an anatomic reservoir. The catheter should be changed daily and alternated between each nares every 8–12 hours. The disadvantage is that chances of catheter occlusion.

Simple Face Mask

It is a low-flow variable performance device with small reservoir of approximately 100–250 mL and provides higher FiO_2 than that of nasal cannula. They are soft plastic masks designed to cover the mouth and nose with a small-bore tube connected at the base through which oxygen is being delivered (**Fig. 51.2**). Oxygen gets collected in the apparatus at the end of expiration to be inhaled during the next breath. Vented holes on each side are present for exit of exhaled gases and entrainment of room air. Oxygen flow is between 5–10 L/min and accordingly FiO_2 varies from 0.35 to 0.60. The delivered FiO_2 is lost with increased air leakage through loose fitting-masks, when peak inspiratory flow is high and oxygen flow is low. At flow rates of <5 L/min rebreathing of CO_2 occur at the start of inspiration because exhaled air is not adequately flushed from the face mask.[1]

Partial Rebreathing Mask

This is a low-flow variable performance device with reservoir of 1000 mL. During inspiration the reservoir bag should not be fully deflated as it may lead to decreased FiO_2 because of entrainment of room air. Oxygen flows directly into the reservoir bag and to maintain the bag at least one-third to one-half full during inspiration. At exhalation the reservoir receives fresh oxygen and exhaled gas of volume equal to the anatomic dead space. Hence, during the next breath, the exhaled gas is inhaled along with fresh gas, accounting for the name partial rebreather. The rebreathing capacity potentially conserves oxygen use. It provides FiO_2 of 0.4 to 0.7 with a flow rate of 6-10 L/min. Minimum fresh gas flow must be 6 L/min to keep the bag inflated during the entire ventilatory cycle to minimize CO_2 rebreathing and ensure the delivery of highest FiO_2.

Nonrebreathing Mask

It is similar to partial rebreathing mask with the exception of having the presence of three unidirectional valves (**Fig. 51.3**). One valve

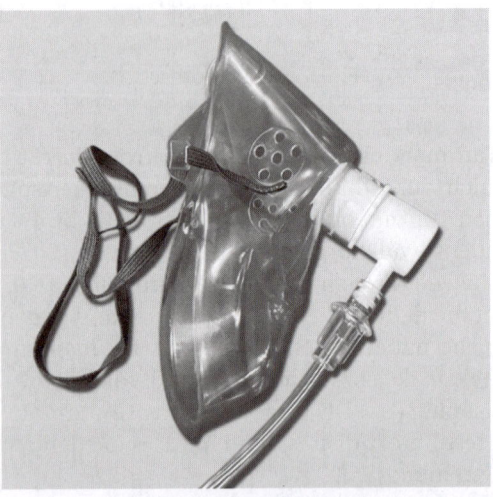

Fig. 51.2: Simple face mask.

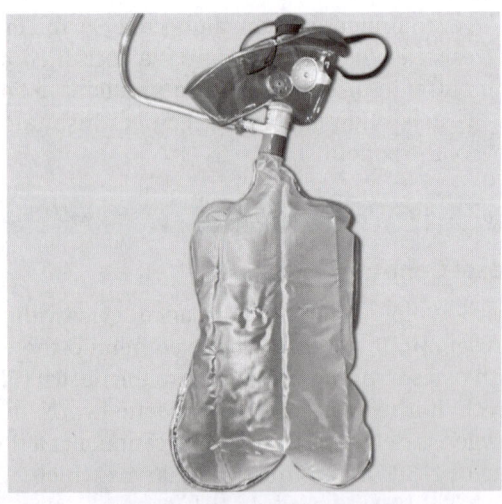

Fig. 51.3: Nonrebreathing mask.

present on each side of the mask minimizes the entrainment of atmospheric air and allows the exit of the exhaled gas. The third valve is situated between the mask and reservoir bag to prevent mixing of exhaled gasses with fresh oxygen. However, entrainment of atmospheric air is possible if there is leak between the mask and the face. At a flow rate of 12–15 L/min it delivers FiO_2 of 0.75 to 0.90.

HIGH-FLOW DEVICES

Venturi Mask

It is a high flow, fixed performance device where FiO_2 does not vary with respiratory pattern (**Fig. 51.4**). Oxygen is passed through narrow tubing under pressure to reach the jet orifice which is attached to the mask. The Venturi principle is based on the Bernoulli Effect which states that the sum of kinetic energy (flow velocity) and the potential energy (pressure) in any system is constant. When a fluid flows through areas of narrow diameters, there is increase in velocity and hence increases in kinetic energy and so the pressure is reduced. Venturi principle uses this phenomenon and when oxygen is passed through the small jet orifice, which is present in venturi mask, a low pressure is created and room air is entrained into the mask through the entrainment port located near to jet (**Fig. 51.5**).[2]

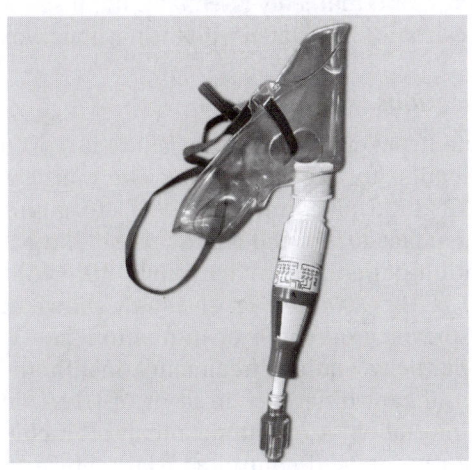

Fig. 51.4: Venturi mask.

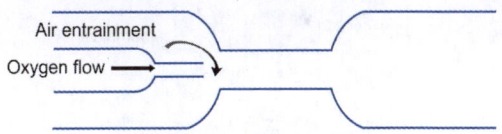

Fig. 51.5: Venturi principle.

Table 51.5: Venturi devices.

Oxygen flow rate (L/min)	Air entrainment (L/min)	Total flow	Delivered FiO_2
2	51	53	0.24
4	41	45	0.28
6	41	47	0.31
8	37	45	0.35
10	32	42	0.40
15	15	30	0.60

The size of the entrainment ports determines the FiO_2 and oxygen flow rate determines the total delivered flow through following formula.
Total gas flow is the sum of the oxygen flow and the amount of air entrained
Entrained air flow = O_2 flow from wall × (1 – FIO_2)/FiO_2 – 0.2
The masks are available in two varieties:
1. Color coded with fixed FiO_2 model with a given flow (**Table 51.5**)
2. Variable FiO_2 model with graded adjustment of the air entrainment port.

Advantages

It is useful in COPD patients when increase in dead space ventilation FiO_2 occurs. As it delivers high flow with no particulate water, it prevents precipitation of bronchospasm and hence it is beneficial in asthmatics.

High-flow Nasal Cannulas

It has been developed to provide humidified high-flow oxygen up to 60 L/min. It consists of a flow generator, active heated humidifier, single-limb heated circuit and nasal cannula (**Fig. 51.6**).
Air-oxygen blender with flow meter is the most popular flow generator, which enables stable

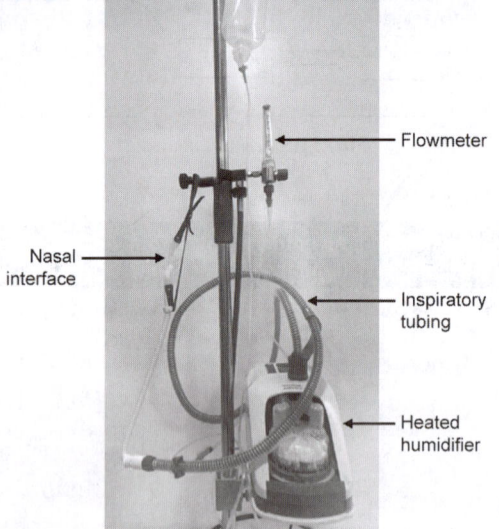

Fig. 51.6: High-flow nasal cannula.

delivery of both FiO_2 and gas flow. It achieves escalation of FiO_2 from 21 to 100% irrespective of flow rates.

Humidification is done by a heated humidification system, where blended gas is passed through a bundle of narrow tubes. It is adequate until flow exceeds 60 L/min. But when HFNC flow is less than the inspiratory flow of the patient and entrainment of ambient air happens, humidification gets affected.

Inspiratory Limb

Heated-wire circuits are incorporated into the inspiratory limbs to minimize condensation and for delivery of adequately humidified gas.

Interface

HFNC uses a slender nasal cannula whose internal diameter and nasal prong bore are narrow, and this results in high flow through the nasal prongs.

Physiological Effects

- **Decrease dead space ventilation:** The high flow rate delivers large volumes of air which exceeds the patient's physiological ventilation hence, displaces excess CO_2 with excess O_2 and leads to reduced respiratory rates and improved work of breathing. The increased alveolar oxygen thus generated creates a greater oxygen diffusion gradient and potentially improves oxygenation. Studies had shown that patients with a baseline high $PaCO_2$ had greatest improvement in work of breathing.[3] Thus patient HFNC is useful both in hypoxemic and hypercapnic respiratory failure.
- **Improvement in ventilation/perfusion ratio**: The heated and humidified gas helps in improving mucociliary function and thereby facilitates clearance of secretion and decreases the risk of atelectasis, and improves the oxygenation.
- **Positive end-expiratory pressure (PEEP) effect**: High-flow creates a PEEP to the lower airways that acts as a splinting force to prevent alveolar airways from collapsing during expiration and also allows for improved alveolar recruitment. But these effects are maximum only when patients keep their mouths closed. 1 cm H_2O of PEEP is generated for every 10 L/min of flow delivered with closed mouth breathing.
- Because the delivered flow is higher than the spontaneous inspiratory demand, it delivers higher and more predictable FiO_2.
- It decrease the work of breathing by providing flow rates that match the patient's inspiratory flow, and markedly attenuates the inspiratory resistance associated with the nasopharynx.

Indications

Acute hypoxemic respiratory failure is a primary indication for HFNC therapy. The multicenter FLORALI trial compared HFNC to standard oxygen face masks and NIV on rate of intubation in adult patients with tachypnea (RR > 25) and PaO_2/FiO_2 <300 mm Hg. The study showed that the primary outcome of intubation rate were similar between three treatment arms. There was a significant difference in favor of HFNC in 90 day mortality.[4] A recent meta-analysis including nine randomized controlled trials showed that HFNC was associated with lower intubation rate when compared to conventional oxygen therapy (RR 0.85, 95% CI 0.74–0.99), but there was no difference in mortality in the two groups (RR 0.94, 95% CI 0.67–1.31).[5]

HFNC also found to be comparable to NIV with respect to intubation rate in hypercapnic respiratory failure (OR 0.92, 95% CI: 0.45-1.88) as shown by PL and colleagues in a systematic review and meta-analysis.[6]

During HFNC therapy, it is desirable to assess the HFNC failure and not to delay intubation. The ROX index defined as the ratio of SpO_2/FiO_2 to RR is a simple noninvasive tool, used as a predictor for the need of intubation in patients receiving HFNC therapy.

Apart from hypoxemic and hypercapnic respiratory failure, it is also indicated during preoxygenation, bronchoscopy and post-operative respiratory failure. It has also been used in all populations such as neonates, children and adults.

NONINVASIVE VENTILATION

Noninvasive ventilation (NIV) refers to the delivery of mechanical ventilatory support through an artificial interface without the need for an invasive airway. Compared to invasive mechanical ventilation NIV is better tolerated hence requirement of sedation is less. NIV also allows talking and eating during intermittent break periods.

Physiological Effects

- Decreases work of breathing and improve gas exchange by alveolar recruitment and improving lung compliance
- By increasing closing capacity it increases the functional residual capacity and oxygenation
- Increased intrathoracic pressure has beneficial effects on left ventricular function
  - Decreases left ventricular transmural pressure, so decreases the afterload
  - Decreases the preload by decreasing the venous return
- Increased positive end-expiratory pressure decreases work of breathing
- Increased expiratory air flow and minute ventilation improve CO_2 clearance, hence hypercapnia.

Indication

Noninvasive ventilation is used both for hypercapnic and hypoxemic respiratory failure.[7] Strong recommendations are acute exacerbation of chronic obstructive pulmonary disease (COPD), weaning of COPD and cardiogenic pulmonary edema (**Table 51.6**). Other indications of NIV are obstructive sleep apnea, postoperative respiratory failure, post-traumatic respiratory failure, respiratory failure in immunosuppressed states and patients with do not intubate status.

Table 51.6: Indications of noninvasive mechanical ventilation.

Strong recommendation	• Acute respiratory failure due to COPD exacerbation • Weaning of COPD patients from mechanical ventilation • Acute respiratory failure due to cardiogenic pulmonary edema
Conditional recommendation	• Immunocompromised patients with ARF • Patients with postoperative ARF • Chest trauma patients with ARF

Contraindication

Absolute contraindication of NIV is respiratory arrest or immediate need of intubation. Relative contraindications are listed in **Box 51.2**.

BOX 51.2

Relative contraindications of NIV
- Hemodynamic instability
- Altered sensorium
- Uncooperative patient
- Inability to protect airway
- Excessive secretion
- Poor cough reflex
- Facial deformities

Table 51.7: Advantages and disadvantages of various NIV interfaces.

Mask	Advantages	Disadvantages
Nasal mask	• Less claustrophobic • Less dead space • Less risk of aspiration • Ability to eat and speak	• Trauma over nasal bridge • Nasal congestion • Mouth leak
Full face mask	Better tightness and less air leak	• Increased claustrophobic • Increased risk of aspiration • Increased dead space • Facial skin irritation • Ulceration over nasal bridge
Helmet	• Increase patient comfort • Less resistance to gas flow • Ability to talk • Better tightness	• Increased claustrophobic • Increased dead space

Equipment

Masks

Different types of masks include nasal mask, nasal pillow, face mask, total face mask and helmets (**Table 51.7**).

Breathing Circuit

It is available as single circuit or double circuit. Double circuit has disadvantages of larger weight; however, more accurate monitoring of ventilation is possible. Single circuit is simple in use and of low weight.

Setup and Initiation of NIV

After selecting the ventilator and interface, the procedure must be explained to the patient before initiating ventilation (**Box 51.3**). The efficacy and result of therapy largely depends on patient cooperation, hence repeated explanation should be done as the process continues. Ventilation begins with low IPAP and EPAP which includes IPAP of 8–10 cm H_2O and EPAP of 4–5 cm H_2O.

Monitoring

Close monitoring of patients with NIV is important because failure has been established

> **BOX 51.3**
>
> **Steps for Initiation of NIV**
> 1. Explaining the technique to the patient
> 2. Place the patient in an upright position
> 3. Select appropriate size and type of interface
> 4. Attach the mask and tighten the straps
> 5. Setting the IPAP at 8 cm H_2O and EPAP 5 cm H_2O
> 6. Turn on the ventilator
> 7. Monitor oxygen saturation and titrate the FiO_2 to target SpO_2 >90%
> 8. Titrate IPAP and EPAP to achieve adequate tidal volume, patient comfort and ventilator synchrony
> 9. Consider humidification
> 10. Monitor respiratory rate, heart rate, blood pressure, SpO_2 and minute ventilation
> 11. Obtain arterial blood gas within one hour

as an independent risk factor for mortality. HACOR (heart rate, acidosis, consciousness, oxygenation, and RR) is a validated score used as a predictor of NIV failure in patients with acute hypoxemic respiratory failure. A HACOR score > 5 after 1 hour of NIV predict patients with a >80% risk of NIV failure.

Chapter 51: Oxygen Therapy Devices

 LAST-MINUTE REVISION

- **HFNC (High-flow nasal cannula):** HFNC delivers warm, humidified oxygen at a high flow rate, providing better oxygenation and comfort. It is often used for patients who need a higher level of oxygen support but do not necessarily require mechanical ventilation.
- **NIV (Non-invasive ventilation):** NIV helps patients breathe by providing pressurized air through a mask. It is commonly used for people with conditions, such as sleep apnea or respiratory failure, as it assists with breathing without the need for invasive procedures, such as intubation.
- **Venturi mask:** A Venturi mask is designed to deliver a precise amount of oxygen. It mixes oxygen with room air, creating high-flow enriched oxygen air. This is useful for patients who require a specific and controlled concentration of oxygen.

REFERENCES

1. Bateman NT, Leach RM. ABC of oxygen. Acute oxygen therapy. BMJ. 1998;317(7161):798-801.
2. Adcock CJ, Dawson JS. The Venturi mask: more than moulded plastic. Br J Hosp Med (Lond). 2007;68:M28-9.
3. Mauri T, Turrini C, Eronia N, Grasselli G, Volta CA, Bellani G, et al. Physiologic effects of high-flow nasal cannula in acute hypoxemic respiratory failure. Am J Respir Crit Care Med. 2017;195(9):1207-15.
4. Frat J-P, Thille AW, Mercat A, Girault C, Ragot S, Perbet S. High-flow oxygen through nasal cannula in acute hypoxemic respiratory failure. N Engl J Med. 2015;372:2185-96.
5. Rochwerg B, Granton D, Wang DX, Helviz Y, Einav S, Frat JP, et al. High flow nasal cannula compared with conventional oxygen therapy for acute hypoxemic respiratory failure: a systematic review and meta-analysis. Intensive Care Med. 2019 ;45(5):563-72.
6. Huang Y, Lei W, Zhang W, Huang JA. High-Flow nasal cannula in hypercapnic respiratory failure: a systematic review and meta-analysis. Can Respir J. 2020;2020:7406457.
7. Rochwerg B, Brochard L, Elliott MW, Hess D, Hill NS, Nava S, et al. Official ERS/ATS clinical practice guidelines: noninvasive ventilation for acute respiratory failure. Eur Respir J. 2017;50(2):1602426.

REVIEW QUESTIONS

1. The highest percentage of inspired oxygen is delivered by:
   a. Nasal cannulae
   b. Simple oxygen face mask
   c. Venturi mask
   d. Non-rebreathing mask
2. High flow oxygen therapy devices includes all, *except*:
   a. Venturi mask
   b. HFNC
   c. NIV
   d. Nasal prongs

ANSWERS

1. d   2. d

CHAPTER 52

Principles of Mechanical Ventilation

Gautham Raju, Anshul Jain

INTRODUCTION

A *medical ventilator* (**Fig. 52.1**) can be defined as a *machine designed to mechanically move breathable air into the lungs and satisfy gas exchange needs of the body*. Ventilators perform the aforementioned function through application of positive pressure, moving the gases into the respiratory system in conformance with specific volume, pressure and time patterns.

In its simplest form, a ventilator system consists of the following:
- A compressible air reservoir or turbine and energy to drive the system
- Air and oxygen supply
- A control system to regulate the timing and size of breaths, and monitor performance of device and the patient condition
- A stable patient interface including invasive airway devices (or noninvasive) and circuits.

Ventilators are chiefly used in intensive care unit (ICU), emergency room (as standalone units), during administration of anesthesia (as a component of an anesthesia machine) and even homecare settings for supporting respiratory function in chronic respiratory ailments (e.g., chronic obstructive pulmonary disease, obstructive sleep apnea, etc.).

Physics and Physiology of Mechanical Ventilation

Ventilator function is based on the equations of motion for the respiratory system, while delivering pressure, volume and flow to the patient.[1]

In mechanical ventilation positive pressure is applied, via interface (like artificial airway), which generates an inward flow of gases *(directed from the ventilator to the patients)*, ventilator serves as the energy source by substituting the muscles of diaphragm and chest wall. Expiration is passive, driven by the recoil of lungs and chest wall. Under these circumstances pressure applied at the airway includes the positive pressure generated by ventilator (P_{vent}) plus the negative pressure generated by respiratory muscles (P_{mus})
The equation is as follows:

$$P_{mus} + P_{vent} = P_{res} + P_{el}$$

P_{res} = Resistive pressure which a function of airway resistance = (Flow × Airway resistance)
P_{el} = Elastic recoil pressure which is a function of lung elastance = (Volume × Elastance).
Hence $P_{mus} + P_{vent}$ = (Flow × Resistance) + (Volume × Elastance)

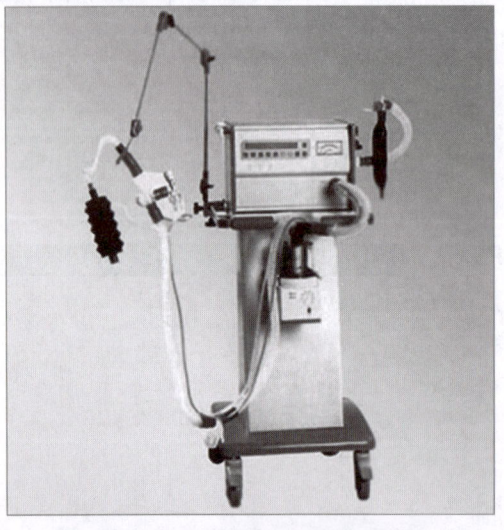

Fig. 52.1: An image of a medical ventilator.

In the expiratory phase, as pressure gradient is generated by the passive recoil of the chest and lung, ventilator circuit vents the expired gases to the atmosphere.

During spontaneous breathing, respiratory muscles *(mainly diaphragm)* generate a negative pressure (P_{mus}) that produce inspiratory flow and volume against the airway resistance and elastic lung tissue respectively and P_{vent} is 0. Thus, in spontaneous breathing pressure relationship can be described as: $P_{mus} = P_{res} + P_{el}$

Total and Partial Ventilator Support

Based on the relative contribution of patient's muscle work and ventilation, ventilation can be described as totally or partially ventilator controlled.

In total mechanical ventilation, P_{mus} is abolished by sedation and muscle relaxants, ventilator provides whole work of breathing.

In partial ventilation, ventilator provides a fixed amount of support thereby reducing patient P_{mus}. Here ventilator delivers a preset tidal volume/inspiratory flow in response to patient's inspiratory effort.

Indication of Mechanical Ventilation

Primary indication for initiation of mechanical ventilation is respiratory failure, which could have either clinical, mechanics or arterial blood gases-based criteria **(Table 52.1)**. There are two common types of respiratory failure:[2]

Table 52.1: Respiratory criteria for ventilatory support.

- Respiratory rate >35/minute or <8/minute
- Vital capacity <15 mL/kg
- Tidal volume <5 mL/kg
- Blood gas analysis:
  - PaO_2 <50 mm Hg on room air or <60 mm Hg at FiO_2 >0.5
  - pH <7.25
  - $PaCO_2$ >50 mm Hg
  - PaO_2/FiO_2 <250 mm Hg
  - $Pa(A-a)O_2$ gradient >350 mm Hg on 100% O_2

(FiO_2: an inspired oxygen fraction; PaO_2: partial pressure of oxygen; $PaCO_2$: partial pressure of carbon dioxide; $P(A-a)O_2$: alveolar-arterial oxygen gradient)

Hypoxemic Respiratory Failure (Type I or Oxygenation Failure)

It is defined by the PaO_2 <60 mm Hg with normal or subnormal $PaCO_2$. Here the gas exchange is impaired at the level of alveolo-capillary membrane. It could be due to ventilation perfusion mismatch and shunt. Example: cardiogenic or noncardiogenic pulmonary edema, severe pneumonia, acute respiratory distress syndrome (ARDS).

Hypercarbic Respiratory Failure (Type II or Ventilatory Failure)

It is characterized by arterial $PaCO_2$ > 50 mm of Hg and an arterial pH <7.30 with or without hypoxemia. Underlying factor is reduced alveolar ventilation and resultant failure to remove carbon dioxide. Alveolar ventilation can be inadequate due to failure of the respiratory pump or inability to overcome increased airway resistance in disease states, e.g., asthma, chronic obstructive airway diseases, respiratory muscles weakness.

Other Indications

- Elective postoperative ventilation, after major surgery
- Iatrogenic paralysis: Tetanus.

Operational Terminology of Ventilator[3] (Flowchart 52.1)

Trigger

It is the variable by which ventilator senses to initiate breath. Trigger can be:
1. Time trigger/machine trigger—occurs independent of patient spontaneous efforts
2. Patient trigger is of two types:
   a. Pressure trigger: Breath is initiated when ventilator senses the patient spontaneous (negative pressure) inspiratory effort. Usual range is -1 to -5 cm H_2O below patient baseline pressure. Lesser the number, lesser the sensitivity.

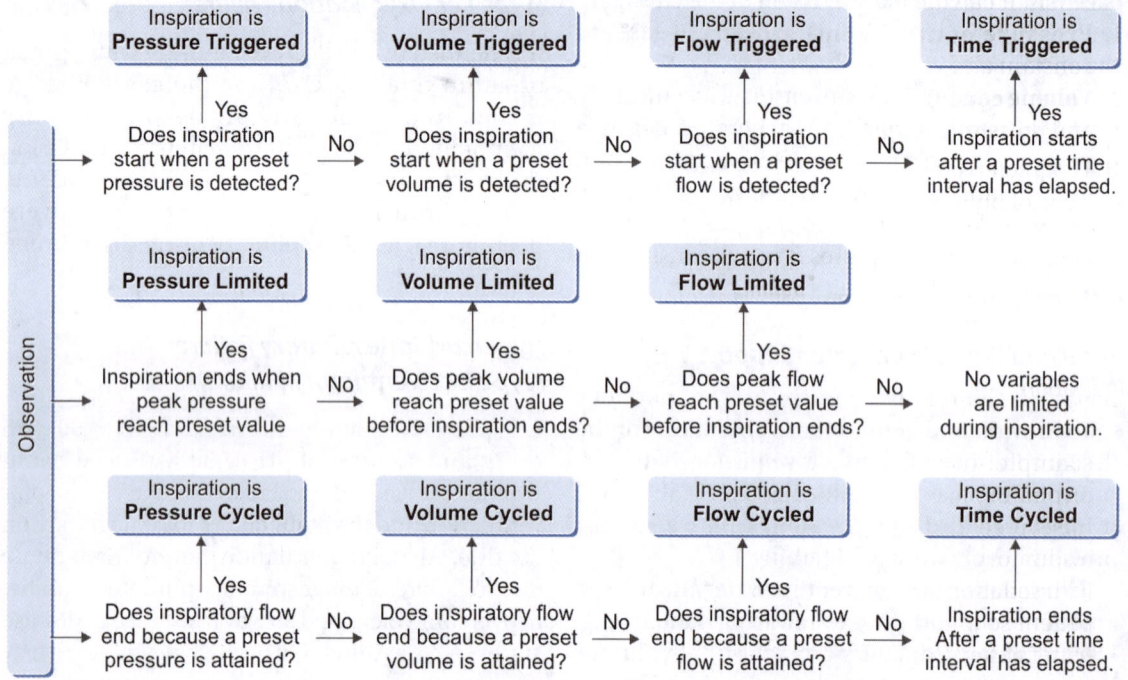

Flowchart 52.1: Description of the terminology used in ventilator.

b. **Flow trigger:** When patient inspiratory flow reaches a specific value, a ventilator supported breath is delivered. Usual range is 3–6 L/min in adults, 1.5–3 L/min in pediatrics, 0.75–1.5 L/min in neonates. Higher the number, lesser the sensitivity.

In general, flow trigger is more sensitive and responsive to patient efforts than pressure triggering. However, in modern ventilators, both pressure and flow trigger are equally sensitive and safe.

Cycle

This is the factor which responsible for the end of inspiration. Cycling can be:
- **Machine cycled:** Three types
  1. Time cycling
  2. Volume cycling
  3. Pressure cycling
- **Patient cycled:** Flow cycling, e.g., pressure support ventilation

Limit/Control/Target Variable

These are operator-specified maximum value a variable (pressure, flow, volume) can attain and are monitored by transducers within the ventilator. If the patient values exceed specified values, inspiratory flow is terminated and gases from the ventilator circuit are vented out to maintain the variables within specified limits.

Mode

It is the means by which ventilator breaths are triggered, cycled and limited.

Ventilator Modes[3]

Controlled Mandatory Ventilation (CMV) or Continuous Mandatory Ventilation

In this mode ventilator delivers the preset tidal volume at a time triggered respiratory rate irrespective of patient effort. This mode can be used when patient has no respiratory effort or

efforts have been abolished by sedatives, muscle paralysis. It can be of two types:
1. **Pressure control ventilation**: Pressure is constant and volume is variable.
2. **Volume control ventilation**: Volume is constant and pressure is variable.

The characteristic variables of CMV are:
- Type of breath: All breaths are mandatory breath
- Trigger : Time/machine trigger
- Limit/control : Volume/pressure/dual
- Cycle : Volume/time/pressure

Indication
- To provide maximum ventilatory support: For example: In patients with marginal cardio-respiratory functional reserve.
- In severely distressed patient with significant respiratory distress, can be used in conjunction with sedation and/or neuromuscular blockade patient so as to help synchrony or restabilising better gas exchange.
- Tetanus or other seizure activity which affects ventilation.
- Ventilation during intraoperative period in the anesthetized patient.
- Patient with flail chest in which spontaneous efforts can be deleterious.
- Reducing oxygen consumption: In Patients with severe cardiovascular instability

Complication
- This mode carries maximum risk of hypoxia if ventilator fails or if there is accidental disconnection.
- When used for prolonged period there can be significant respiratory muscles wasting.
- Respiratory alkalosis: if alarm limits and patient's minute ventilation is not monitored it can lead to hyperventilation and can result in myoclonus or seizures.

Assist-controlled Mode Ventilation (ACMV)

In assist-controlled mode, along with mandatory breaths, patient can also trigger a breath. Every breath delivered whether patient or time triggered, and consists of operator specified tidal volume **(Fig. 52.2A)**. Final ventilatory rate is determined either by patient or by operator specified backup rate (whichever is higher).

The characteristic variables used in this mode are:
- Type of breath : Assist or control
- Trigger : Time/machine trigger; Patient trigger (based on patient effort and trigger sensitivity)
- Limit/control : Pressure/volume/dual
- Cycle : Volume and time (preset tidal volume and inspiratory time) Pressure (on reaching high pressure limit)
- Modes : Assist pressure control ventilation Assist volume control ventilation

Indications
- Similar to controlled mandatory ventilation
- Use with caution in respiratory alkalosis and tetany.

Contraindications

Patients with abnormal breathing patterns.

Complications
- **Excessive ventilation and severe respiratory alkalosis**: As ventilator assists every breath, in patients with tachypnea also adds on more breaths in this mode and leads to hyperventilation and subsequent severe respiratory alkalosis, This can lead to myoclonus and seizure.
- **Auto-PEEP**: Auto-PEEP may occur by air trapping due to increased respiratory rate and incomplete exhalation leading to hyperinflation with each subsequent breath (dynamic hyperinflation). This is particularly seen in acute exacerbation of chronic obstructive pulmonary disease (COPD), where tachypnea and obstruction coexist.
- Auto-PEEP by increasing intrathoracic pressure can hamper venous return, decrease cardiac

output, increase airway pressure and predispose the patient to barotraumas.

However, in modern ventilators various servo mechanisms exist to prevent mishaps, including alarm settings.

Intermittent Mandatory Ventilation and Synchronized Intermittent Mandatory Ventilation

In intermittent mandatory ventilation (IMV) mode ventilator delivers control (mandatory) breath and allows the patient to breath spontaneously at any tidal volume (the patient is capable of) in between the mandatory breaths. It was initially designed a mode to facilitate weaning from ventilator, however, there is chance of breath stacking which occurs when patient inspires in series with a ventilator delivered breath or breaths against a ventilator delivered breath; either way both could result in high airway pressures with high risk of barotrauma. This mode has been improved to optimized ventilation in form of synchronized intermittent mandatory ventilation.

With improvement semiconductor and microprocessor technology, sensors could be fitted in the ventilator; such that when there is a spontaneous patient breath in between a mandatory (or controlled) breath window, the two are synchronized; and hence the name synchronized intermittent mandatory ventilation (SIMV). This allows patient to breath spontaneously and intermittently and also receive the mandatory number of breaths set by the expert. This prevents many of the problems associated with assist control and intermittent mandatory ventilator modes.

SIMV allows the patient with an intact respiratory drive to set his own respiratory rate and exercise inspiratory muscles between assisted breath, making it useful for both supporting and weaning intubated patients **(Fig. 52.2B)**.

The characteristic variables associated with SIMV mode are:

- **Types of breath in SIMV**: Spontaneous breath —can be with pressure or volume support or can be with or without CPAP.

  Mandatory breath—mandatory time triggered breath.

  Assisted breaths—delivered at beginning of spontaneous breaths close and preventing increased SIMV frequency.

- **Trigger**: Time patient trigger—pressure or flow. Triggering mechanism: For example, if the SIMV respiratory rate is set at 10 breaths per minute then the ventilator would time trigger the breath every 6 second (60/10) if patient does not make any inspiratory effort.

  However, if the patient has got spontaneous respiration and patient begin to inspire just prior to the point at which ventilator would be expected to time trigger, than ventilator senses this spontaneous effort and delivers the mandatory breath as an assisted patient triggered breath. In patients triggered breath too a preset tidal volume is delivered to the patient.

- **Synchronization window**: It is the time interval just prior to time triggering in which ventilator is responsive to the patient spontaneous inspiratory effort. Although exact time interval is slightly different in different ventilator, 0.5 second is used as reference. If the synchronization window is 0.5 second, then in the above examples at 5.5 second from the beginning of previous mandatory breath the ventilator automatically becomes sensitive to any spontaneous effort inspiratory effort. If patient makes inspiratory effort in this period ventilator is patient triggered to deliver an assisted mandatory breath. After completion of breath again there is an interval of 5.5 second in which patient is permitted to breath spontaneously at any tidal volume the patient desires. In next 0.5 second again synchronization window is active and cycle repeats.

Advantages of Synchronized Intermittent Mandatory Ventilation Mode

- Maintains respiratory muscles strength and activity
- Reduces V/Q mismatch and improves intra-pulmonary gas distribution

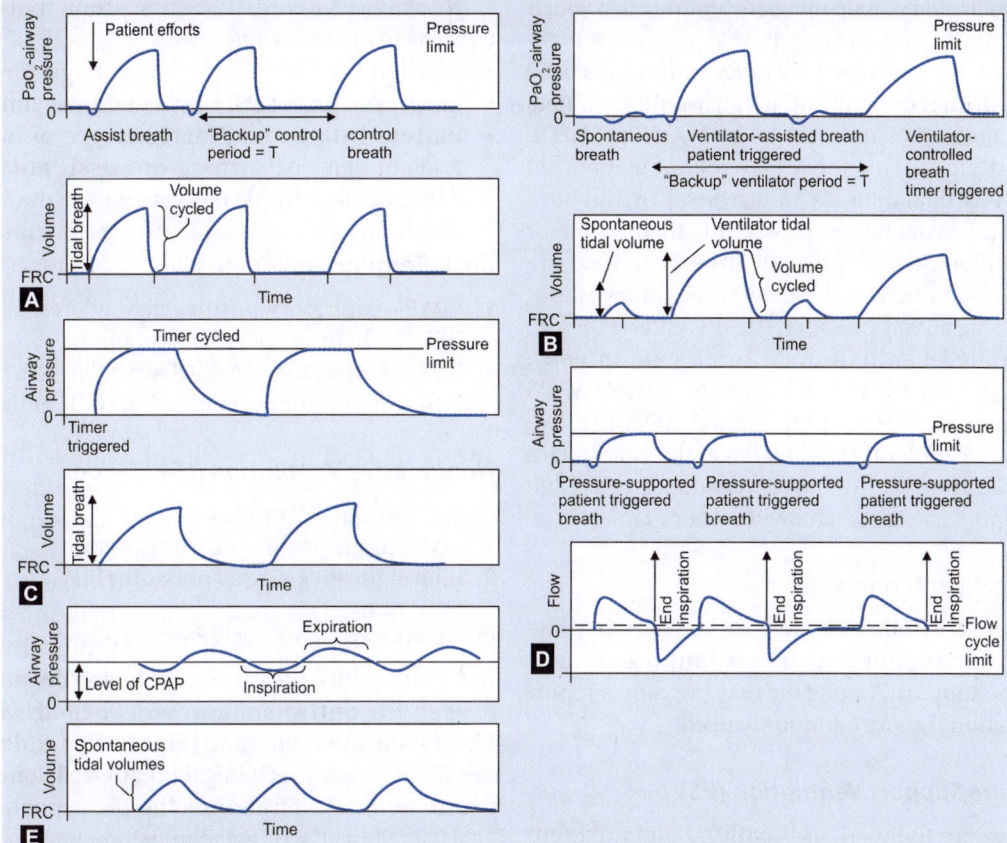

Figs. 52.2A to E: Airway pressure and lung volume versus time scalars: (A) Assist-controlled mode ventilation (ACMV); (B) Synchronized intermittent mandatory ventilation (SIMV); (C) Pressure control ventilation (PCV); (D) Pressure support ventilation (PSV); (E) Continuous positive airway pressure (CPAP).
(FRC: functional residual capacity; PaO_2: partial pressure of oxygen)

- Decreases mean airway pressure
- Reduce need for sedation
- Promotes spontaneous breaths
- Facilitates weaning

Limitation

- **Disturbances in weaning:** Depending on the Expert inputs into the ventilator, there can be prolongation of time needed for weaning as the expert may under-estimate the recovery of respiratory muscle strength and unnecessarily delay the process of weaning. On the other hand if the process is too rapid there is a risk of increased work of breathing in the patient and weaning failure.
- **Increased risk of carbon dioxide retention:** If attention is not paid to status in terms of use of sedation, neuromuscular blockade or any other condition that may preclude spontaneous breaths, there is risk of hypoventilation and consequent retention of carbon dioxide.

Dual Mode Ventilation

This mode combines the advantages of both volume and pressure-controlled ventilation. Newer ventilators possess advanced microchip processors with built in servo loop mechanisms, through which dual control modes are possible, e.g., for a post-thoracotomy patient in PCV pressure limits set to 50 cm H_2O, then normally tidal flow would terminate when airway pressure reach 50 cm H_2O **(Fig. 52.2C)**. However, in dual mode like PCV volume guaranteed (PCV-VG), tidal volume can also be set. In the above case if tidal volume is set at 450 mL, then ventilator will prolong the inspiratory time or reduce the flow so as to deliver the desired volume without increasing airway pressure, e.g., PCV-VG (Pressure Controlled Ventilation, Volume guaranteed), PRVC (Pressure Regulated Volume Control), VAPS (Volume Assured Pressure Support), ASV (Adaptive Support Ventilation). Note: Several modes share same functionality but nomenclature can vary due to Proprietary rights of individual companies.

Support Ventilation

Here patient initiates a spontaneous breath, while ventilator supports with constant pressure or volume support. Among the two, pressure support ventilation is more commonly used.

Pressure Support Ventilation (PSV)

PSV lowers the work of breathing and augment patient spontaneous tidal volume. In this mode a pre-set pressure is applied to the patient airway in inspiratory phase of spontaneous breath **(Fig. 52.2D)**. Spontaneous effort is the prerequisite for PSV mode, as patient receive ventilation assist only when ventilator detects an inspiratory effort.

Noninvasive Ventilation

Modes described so far require endotracheal intubation and thus can be used only in hospital settings with variable degree of sedation. Typically noninvasive ventilation is used in patients with respiratory failure to avoid intubation.[4]

Definition

Provision of ventilator support to improve respiratory functions without the use of artificial invasive airway device.[4]

Noninvasive ventilation system typically consists of the following:
- Ventilator
- **Respiratory circuits**: Single or double lumen
- **Patient interface**: Different types of masks available, e.g., nasal mask, oronasal mask, oral mask, full face mask, helmet.

Basic Terminology

- EPAP—expiratory positive airway pressure (or PEEP)—helps improve oxygenation
- IPAP—inspiratory positive airway pressure (or PS)—helps improve ventilation (CO_2 removal)

Noninvasive Ventilation (NIV) Modes

Two common NIV modes are:
1. Continuous positive airway pressure (CPAP)
2. Bilevel positive airway pressure (BiPAP).

Continuous Positive Airway Pressure (CPAP)

In CPAP positive pressure is applied to the patient airway for entire spontaneous breath (both inspiration and expiration) **(Fig 52.2E)**. CPAP does not include any mechanical breath and therefore spontaneous respiration is the prerequisite for CPAP. In short CPAP is technically same as PEEP (positive end expiratory pressure) but PEEP is used in controlled ventilation while CPAP is used in spontaneous respiration.

Typical Settings

Start: 5 cm H_2O; ↑ 2 cm H_2O increments as needed; Range 5–12 cm H_2O.

Uses

- Hypoxemic respiratory failure (e.g., acute cardiogenic pulmonary edema)
- CPAP is the treatment of choice for obstructive sleep apnea.

Bilevel Positive Airway Pressure (BiPAP)

BiPAP differs from CPAP in being two pressure levels whereas CPAP has only one. Bilevel PAP has an inspiratory positive airway pressure (IPAP) setting that provides assisted mechanical breath and an EPAP (expiratory positive airway pressure) level that function as PEEP.

Typical Settings

Start IPAP: 8–10 cm H_2O; start EPAP: 2–4 cm H_2O;
↑2–4 cm increments.
Maximum IPAP: 24 cm H_2O; maximum EPAP: 20 cm H_2O.

Uses

- Hypercarbic respiratory failure
- Mixed failure (e.g., chronic obstructive pulmonary disease).

Note: Usage of noninvasive ventilation (NIV) is always accompanied with monitoring of baseline and continuous status of clinical, laboratory and gas exchange parameters to optimize its usage.

Other Modes of BiPAP

- S Mode   : Spontaneous mode
- S/T Mode : Spontaneous/timed mode
- T mode   : Timed mode
- PC mode : Pressure control mode
- VAPS   : Volume assured pressure support
- AVAPS   : Average volume assured pressure support
- IVAPS   : Intelligent volume assured pressure support

Indications

Nowadays, NIV is being commonly used in conscious patients having acute respiratory failure. Evidence based applications of NIV are:
- Acute exacerbation of chronic obstructive pulmonary disease (COPD)
- Acute cardiogenic edema
- Acute respiratory failure in immunocompromised patient
- Weaning from invasive ventilation of COPD patients.

Advantages of NIV

- Decreases work of breathing
- Improves gas exchange
- Increases functional residual capacity
- Improves pulmonary function in general.

Disadvantages/Complications of NIV

- Patient discomfort
- Skin necrosis
- Higher aspiration risk
- May impact cardiac function.

Positive End-Expiratory Pressure (PEEP)[5]

Due to its widespread applications PEEP has itself emerged as a separate entity in mechanical ventilation. PEEP increases the end expiratory or baseline airway pressure to a value greater than atmospheric pressure. It is often used to improve patient oxygenation status, especially in refractory hypoxemia. Positive end-expiratory pressure is not a separate mode; rather it is applied in conjunction with other ventilatory modes.

Indications

Two major indications for PEEP are:
1. Refractory hypoxemia secondary to intrapulmonary shunting: Refractory hypoxemia (PaO_2 ≤60 mm of Hg at a FiO_2 ≥50%) secondary to V/Q mismatch is the primary indication for PEEP.
2. Decreased functional residual capacity (FRC) and lung compliance: PEEP increases FRC and tends to reopen alveoli thereby recruits more alveoli in ventilation.

Physiology of Positive End-Expiratory Pressure (Flowchart 52.2)

Positive end-expiratory pressure reinflates collapsed alveoli and maintains alveolar inflation during exhalation. Thus, PEEP recruits more alveoli and improves gas exchange in functioning alveoli. PEEP also provides more area for diffusion, and time for gaseous exchange, thus improves oxygenation.

Effects of PEEP on Various Systems

Respiratory system
- Prevents alveolar collapse and redistributes extravascular lung volume
- Increases functional residual capacity

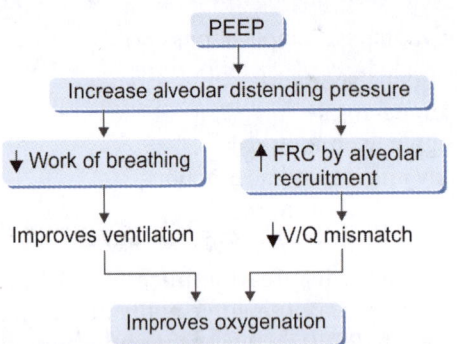

Flowchart 52.2: Mechanism of positive end-expiratory pressure.

(PEEP: positive end-expiratory pressure; FRC: functional residual capacity; V/Q: ventilation/perfusion)

Cardiovascular system
- Improves left ventricular function
- Worsens right ventricular function
- Reduces cardiac output.

Complications of PEEP Application

- Decreased venous return and cardiac output: PEEP application reduces the pressure gradient between central veins and right atrium thereby reducing venous return which in turn reduces cardiac output. Reduced cardiac output can adversely affect bronchial circulation, renal function, gastrointestinal and hepatic function.
- Increased pulmonary artery pressure and right ventricular strain
- Barotrauma: Hyperinflation of normal alveoli can lead to barotraumas
- Increased intracranial pressure (ICP): PEEP may increase ICP by impeding venous return from the head and consequent reduced cerebral perfusion pressure.

Complications/Problems During Mechanical Ventilation

Though lifesaving, mechanical ventilation is associated with number of complications among which few are life threatening too.

Respiratory Complication

- **Ventilator-associated pneumonia (VAP):** VAP is defined as the pneumonia developing in mechanically ventilated patient after more than 48 hours of intubation. VAP is the leading cause of mortality and morbidity in mechanically ventilated critically ill patient. Pathogenesis of VAP involves microaspiration of contaminated oropharyngeal or gastric secretion through small leak around the endotracheal tube cuff. *Pseudomonas aeruoginosa* is the most common etiologic organism in general worldwide but organism differs between different Intensive care units.
- **Barotrauma:** Occurs when high pressure (50 cm H_2O) over distends the alveoli.
- Emphysema, pneumomediastinum, subcutaneous emphysema, pneumothorax, nosocomial pneumonia, tracheal stenosis respiratory muscle weakness are other complications.

Cardiovascular System

- Right ventricular strain
- Hypotension (due to impaired venous return)
- Hypertension, when patient is not sedated enough to tolerate tube.

Gastrointestinal System

- Stress ulcers
- Mild to moderate cholestasis.

Musculoskeletal System

Disuse atrophy of limb muscles and neuromuscular weakness secondary to chronic use of muscles relaxant. Vecuronium is particularly implicated in weakness secondary to muscle relaxants.

Skin

Pressure sores are particularly common in mechanically ventilation patient who are on muscle relaxants.

Central Nervous System

- Increased ICP secondary to straining, stacking, PEEP
- Psychological problems like depression.

Financial

In poor country like India, financial concerns are particular as ventilatory support is very expensive.

Weaning from Ventilator

Weaning is the process of withdrawing mechanical ventilatory support and transferring the work of breathing from the ventilator to the patient. Weaning requires the gradual withdrawal of ventilation support.

Weaning Criteria

Removal of ventilator support is not so simple, as after ventilatory support there is loss of respiratory muscles mass. Criteria mention in **Table 52.2** must be fulfilled before instituting weaning procedure.

Weaning Procedure

Successful weaning depends on satisfactory improvement in respiratory mechanics as well as gas exchange. Weaning can be carried out by one or more of the following procedures:

- **Spontaneous breathing trail (SBT):** SBT via T piece can be used in patients with normal cardiopulmonary reserve who was on mechanical ventilation only for brief period.

Table 52.2: Common Weaning Criteria (Cengage Learning 2014).

Category	Criteria	Values
Clinical criteria	Resolution of acute phase of disease	
	Adequate cough	
	Absence of excessive secretions	
	Cardiovascular and hemodynamic stability	
Ventilatory criteria	Spontaneous breathing trial	Tolerates 20 to 30 min
	$PaCO_2$	<50 mm Hg with normal pH
	Vital capacity	>10 mL/kg
	Spontaneous V_T	>5 mL/kg
	Spontaneous f	<35/min
	f/V_T	<100 breaths/min/L
	Minute ventilation	<10 L with satisfactory ABG
Oxygenation criteria	PaO_2 without PEEP	>60 mm Hg at FiO_2 up to 0.4
	PaO_2 with PEEP (<8 cm H_2O)	>100 mm Hg at FiO_2 up to 0.4
	SaO_2	>90% at FiO_2 up to 0.4
	PaO_2/FIO_2 (P/F)	>150 mm Hg
	Q_S/Q_T	<20%
	$P(A-a)O_2$	<350 mm Hg at FiO_2 of 1.0
Pulmonary reserve	Vital capacity	>10 mL/kg
	Maximal inspiratory pressure	>−30 cm H_2O in 20 sec
Pulmonary measurements	Static compliance	>30 mL/cm H_2O
	Airway resistance	Stable or improving
	V_D/V_T	<60% while intubated

($PaCO_2$: partial pressure of carbon dioxide; V_T: tidal volume; RR: respiratory rate; PaO_2: partial pressure of oxygen; PEEP: positive end-expiratory pressure; FiO_2: fraction of inspired oxygen; SaO_2: saturation level of oxygen in hemoglobin; Q_S/Q_T: pulmonary shunt fraction; $P(A–a)O_2$: alveolar-arterial gradient; vent.: ventilation; insp.: inspiration)

- **SIMV:** Weaning with SIMV mode is the simplest and most common weaning approach. From control mode patient is switch to SIMV mode.
- **PSV:** PSV is a specific mode designed for weaning. Pressure support level is gradually decreased by 3–6 cm H_2O increment until a level close to 1 cm H_2O is achieved after which ventilation is disconnected and SBT via T-piece is performed. If patient fulfils weaning criteria for more than 120 minutes hours, extubation can be attempted if gas exchange and other vital parameters are stable.[6]

Weaning Classification

Based on the attempt and duration from the first attempt of weaning process till the successful liberation from the ventilator, weaning can be classified as:

- **Simple weaning:** Patient successfully moves from initiation of weaning to successful extubation in first attempt.
- **Difficult weaning:** Patient who fail initial weaning and require up to 3 spontaneous breathing trials or up to 7 days from the first spontaneous breathing trial to successful weaning.
- **Prolonged weaning:** Patients who fail at least three weaning attempts or require more than 7 days from first spontaneous breathing trial to successful weaning.

SUMMARY

- Ventilator is a machine that helps supplement or complement the respiratory function in patients.
- In general functioning of ventilator is based on equations of motions where the respiratory muscles and ventilator balances the elastic and resistive load in the respiratory system.

  $[P_{mus} + P_{vent} = (Flow \times Resistance) + (Volume \times Elastance)]$

- There are various modes such as Controlled modes, support modes, dual modes.
- Each mode has variables such as type of breath, trigger, limit/control, cycle.
- Each mode has its own advantages and disadvantages but it is important to pay careful attention to the patient clinical condition, ventilator parameter and alarm settings to maximize patient safety.
- Noninvasive ventilation is used to delay or avoid invasive ventilation. It is of two types: Continuous positive airway pressure (CPAP) and bilevel positive airway pressure (BiPAP) and has select indications.
- While ventilatory support is a great tool, it has its own advantages and disadvantages and complications. However, with appropriate protocols, it can be used to safely assist respiratory function.
- At the end of ventilatory support, weaning is initiated. Successful weaning depends on multiple factors and careful attention to all factors can maximize successful outcomes.

LAST-MINUTE REVISION

- **Ventilatory modes for weaning:** PSV, SIMV and IMV
- **Noninvasive ventilatory modes:** CPAP, Bilevel PAP
- PEEP improves oxygenation by alveolar recruitment and improves ventilation by reducing work of breathing.

REFERENCES

1. Hess DR. Respiratory mechanics in mechanically ventilated patients. Respir Care. 2014;59(11):1773-94.
2. Roussos C, Koutsoukou A. Respiratory failure. Eur Respir J Suppl. 2003;47:3s-14s.
3. Chatburn RL, El-Khatib M, Mireles-Cabodevila E. A taxonomy for mechanical ventilation: 10 fundamental maxims. Respir Care. 2014;59(11): 1747-63.

4. Mas A, Masip J. Noninvasive ventilation in acute respiratory failure. Int J Chron Obstruct Pulmon Dis. 2014;9:837-52.
5. Navalesi P, Maggiore S. Positive end-expiratory pressure. In: Tobin MJ (3 Edn). Principles and Practice of Mechanical Ventilation, 3e. McGraw Hill; 2013.
6. McConville JF, Kress JP. Weaning patients from the ventilator. N Engl J Med. 2012;367(23):2233-9.

REVIEW QUESTIONS

1. Which of the following ventilatory mode is specifically used for weaning purpose?
   a. Pressure controlled ventilation
   b. Pressure support ventilation
   c. SIMV
   d. ACMV
2. The most common etiologic organism in VAP:
   a. Staphylococcus
   b. Pneumococcus
   c. Pseudomonas
   d. Streptococcus
3. A patient has been operated for esophagus cancer via thoracotomy, it was decided to keep the patient on elective ventilation for 12 hours which of the following is preferred ventilatory mode in this patient:
   a. PCV
   b. ACMV
   c. PSV
   d. SIMV

ANSWERS

1. b   2. c   3. a

CHAPTER 53

Clinical Management in ICU

Advaith A Chetan, Manu Varma MK, Anshul Jain

Under current scenario, admission to ICU is increasing day by day and the proportion of ICU beds to total hospital beds is increasing. Every surgical and medical superspeciality is supposed to have ICU beds as per National Medical Commission norms. Beside the every hospital must have the facility of central ICU. Basic organization of ICU has been discussed in previous chapter. Broadly speaking the two commonest causes of ICU admission are shock and respiratory failure. Current chapter provides you the important aspects of these two conditions.

ASSESSMENT OF SEVERITY OF ILLNESS

To assess the severity of critically ill patient, various score models have been adopted. Acute Physiology and Chronic Health Evaluation II (APACHE II) and Sequential Organ Failure Assessment (SOFA) scores are the most commonly used scoring system. Mortality prediction model (MPM) is to estimate mortality risk at 24-hour and 48-hour ICU admission.

SOFA score had six variables, for six main organs including respiratory, central nervous system, cardiovascular system, hematological, renal and liver, to assess organ dysfunction or failure. Each variable had score from 0 to 4. Maximum SOFA score can be of 24; with increasing score indicating higher mortality among ICU patients.

CIRCULATORY SHOCK

Circulatory shock is a clinical syndrome that results from inadequate tissue perfusion. The pathophysiological characteristics of the various form of circulatory shock are described in the **Table 53.1**. Reduced tissue perfusion creates imbalance between oxygen delivery and requirement, resulting in anaerobic metabolism, and simultaneously stimulates release of inflammatory molecules. Moreover, this anaerobic metabolism

Table 53.1: Physiologic characteristics of the various forms of shock.

Type of shock	CVP and pCWp	Cardiac output	Systemic vascular resistance	Venous O_2 saturation
Hypovolemic	↓	↓	↑	↓
Cardiogenic	↑	↓	↑	↓
Septic				
• Hyperdynamic	↓↑	↑	↓	↑
• Hypodynamic	↓↑	↓	↑	↑↓
Traumatic	↓	↓↑	↑↓	↓
Neurogenic	↓	↓	↓	↓
Hypoadrenal	↓↑	↓	=↓	↓

(CVP: central venous pressure; PCWP: pulmonary capillary wedge pressure)

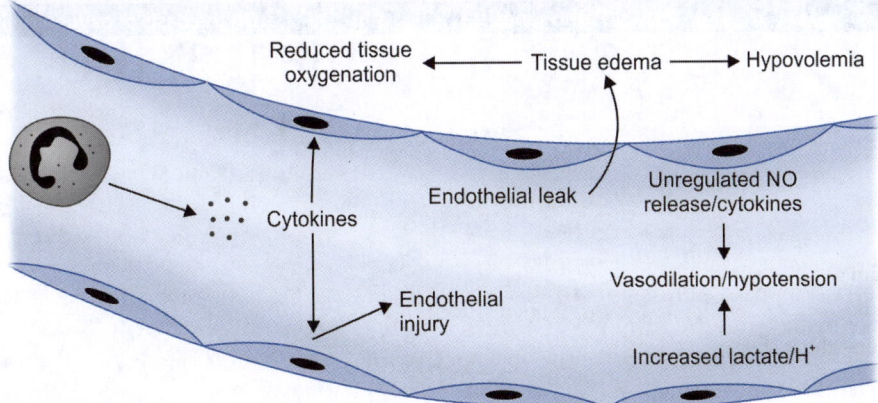

Fig. 53.1: Pathogenesis of shock.

(acidosis) and inflammatory molecules further compromise perfusion, thus creating a vicious cycle **(Figs. 53.1 and 53.2)**.

The goal of shock management is to maintain:
- Urine output more than 0.5 mL/kg/hour (top priority)
- Mean arterial pressure more than 60–65 mm of Hg
- Pulmonary capillary wedge pressure (PCWP) between 12 mm of Hg and 18 mm of Hg
- Cardiac index more than 3.5 L/min/m² for sepsis and hypovolemic shock and more than 2.1 L/min/m² for obstructive shock
- Arterial oxygen saturation more than 90%.

The clinical signs of shock are the result, in part of autonomic neuroendocrine response to hypoperfusion as well as the breakdown of organ functions. There are different stages **(Fig. 53.3)**, which could define various clinical signs.

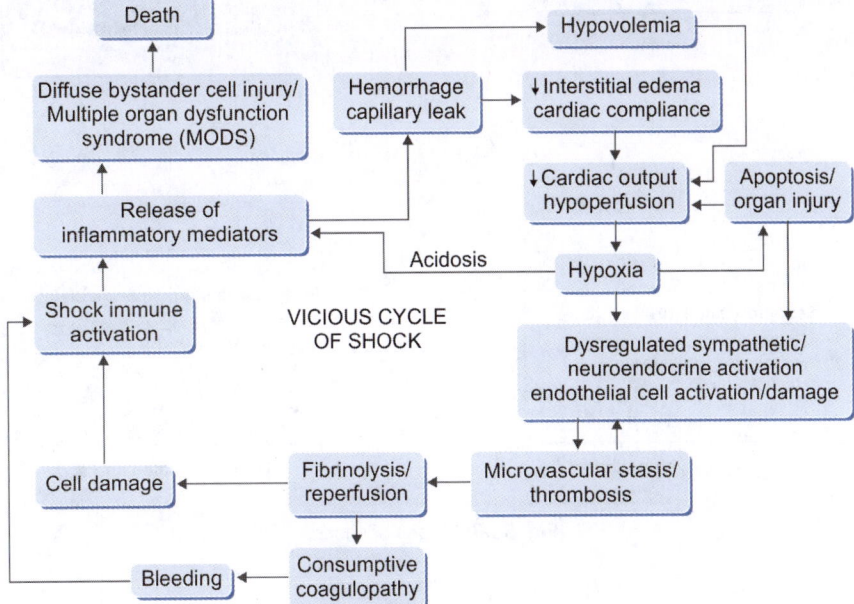

Fig. 53.2: Pathogenesis of shock related vicious cycle.

Table 53.2: Classification of shock.

Etiology	Pathogenesis	On the basis of oxygen delivery
Hypovolemic (MC)	Hypovolemic	
Traumatic		
Cardiogenic		Type I
• Intrinsic	Cardiogenic	
• Compressive	Obstructive	
Septic		
• Hyperdynamic		
• Hypodynamic	Distributive	Type II
Neurogenic (anesthetic shock)		
Hypoadrenal		

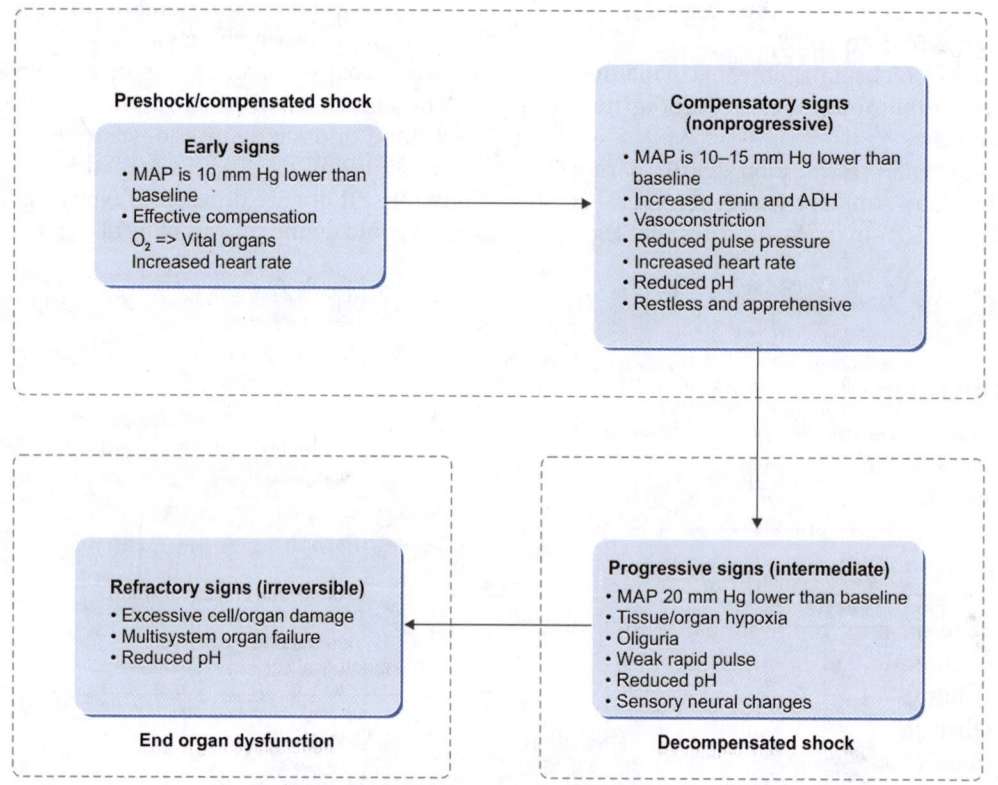

Fig. 53.3: Stages of shock.

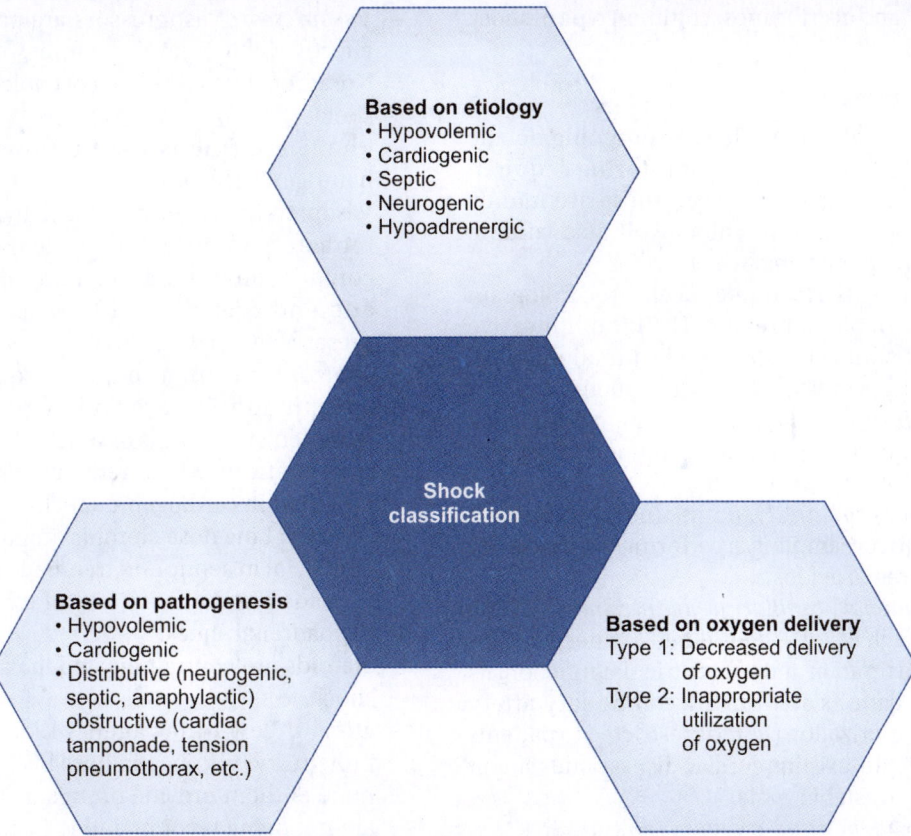

Fig. 53.4: Classification of shock.

Classifications

Shocks have been classified in many ways and every classification has its importance **(Table 53.2 and Fig. 53.4)**.

- As per etiologic classification shock can be hypovolemic, cardiogenic, septic, neurogenic and hypoadrenergic shock.[1]
- On the basis of pathogenesis shock can be hypovolemic, cardiogenic, obstructive, and distributive.
  - Obstructive shock includes cardiac tamponade, tension pneumothorax, etc.
  - Distributive shock includes neurogenic, septic, and anaphylactic (based on etiology)
- On the basis of oxygen delivery, shock can be type I and type II.
  - Type I shock—decreased delivery of oxygen
  - Type II shock— there is inappropriate utilization of oxygen, e.g., septic shock
- Neurogenic shock result after a high spinal cord injury, inadvertent high spinal anesthesia. For clinical management purpose etiologic classification is much more useful. Recent literature suggests that in trauma factors other than hypovolemia are involved too, which lead to its separate entity.
- Septic shock is characterized by excessive arteriolar vasodilatation that reduces the systemic vascular resistance (SVR) resulting in hypotension and inadequate peripheral perfusion. Due to vasodilation the extremities may be warm hence the term "warm shock". *Septic shock* is the most common "warm

shock" and also the most common type of shock overall.

Management

- **Goals monitoring:** There is on-going debate regarding the optimal monitoring required in shock patient. However, these are mainly depends upon clinical as well as available invasive monitoring, which are:
  - *Vital signs:* Heart rate via electrocardiogram (ECG), blood pressure (BP) (both invasive and noninvasive), oxygen saturation monitoring is indicated in every patient.
  - *Urinary catheterization:* Urine output is the best clinical guide of tissue perfusion; it is indicated in every patient.
  - *Blood gas analysis:* In unstable patient frequent sampling is performed to detect the degree of acidosis.
  - *Pulmonary capillary wedge pressure (PCWP):* Though PCWP is considered a better guide for fluid titration and left ventricular function, its indications are limited; pulmonary artery catheterization (PAC) is restricted to patients with pre-existing cardiac disease and patient with unstable vitals.
  - *Mixed venous oxygen tension (SVO_2):* SVO_2 is the best guide for tissue perfusion. For SVO_2 blood samples are taken from pulmonary artery, thus PAC is mandatory for SVO_2, as such SVO_2 has got little impact on management. So, its indications are very few. Moreover, peripheral venous oxygen^Q tension also gives fair information regarding oxygen utilization.
- **Choice of medications:**
  - *Fluid (Blood vs. colloids vs. crystalloids):* Crystalloids are preferred with 0.9% sodium chloride (NS) and Ringer's lactate (RL) are most preferred crystalloids.
  Blood is transfused if blood loss exceeds 30% or hematocrit (HCT) is <25% or hemoglobin (Hb) concentration is <7 g/dL.
  Colloids are indicated only when there is ongoing blood loss and blood is not available, hetastarch is the preferred colloid in shock patients.[2]
  - *Vasopressor:* Vasopressors are particularly effective in high cardiac output shock. Noradrenaline is the drug of choice in septic shock.
  Phenylephrine is the first line drug in neurogenic shock.
  Vasopressin may be of value in hypotension refractory to norepinephrine. Further, in comparison to noradrenaline, splanchnic and end organ blood flow remain well preserved with vasopressin.
  - *Inotropes:* Dopamine, dobutamine and norepinephrine are widely used in the treatment of all forms of shock. Dobutamine is an inotrope which reduce afterload this preferred in cardiogenic shock.
  - *Steroids:* Low dose steroids are found to be beneficial in septic and traumatic shock.
  Steroids are the main stay of treatment in hypoadrenal shock.
  Steroids are contraindicated in cardiogenic shock.
  - *Others:* Few other agents like activated protein and fibronectin have been tried, but none of them provide promising result and are not being recommended in current day practice.
- **Additional measures:**
  - *Rewarming:* Rapid rewarming to more than 35°C (95°F) significantly decreases the requirements for blood products and improves cardiac functions.
  Most effective methods for warming are endovascular counter arrest warmers through femoral vein cannulation.
  - *Acid base managements:* Most shock patients are in metabolic acidosis, but this acidosis gets corrected by itself as tissue perfusion improves. $NaHCO_3$ is indicated only when pH is <7.20.

RESPIRATORY FAILURE

Respiratory failure is the second most common condition requiring ICU admission; and the most common indication for mechanical ventilation. On the basis of pathologic derangement respiratory failure can be divided into four types:

Type I or Acute Hypoxemic Respiratory Failure[3]

- It results from alveolar flooding and subsequent intrapulmonary shunt.
Alveolar flooding may be the consequence of pulmonary edema, pneumonia, alveolar hemorrhage.
- Alveolar flooding hamper gas diffusion, as CO_2 is more diffusible than O_2; CO_2 diffusion (so the level) usually remains normal. Thus, clinical hallmark of type I respiratory failure is low partial pressure of oxygen (PaO_2) with normal or only mildly increased partial pressure of carbon dioxide ($PaCO_2$). Characteristic feature is increased PAO_2-PaO_2, i.e., increased alveolar-arterial oxygen gradient.
- Management includes mechanical ventilation with low tidal volume (<6 mL/ kg body weight) and fluid restriction.

Type II Respiratory Failure

- Type II respiratory failure results from alveolar hypoventilation which produces both hypoxemia and CO_2 retention. Hypoventilation can be due to impaired central respiratory drive, respiratory muscle weakness, bronchospasm, pleural pathologies like pleural effusion, pneumothorax.
- Clinical hallmark is increased $PaCO_2$, whereas alveolar arterial oxygen gradient is normal.
- Management strategies for type II respiratory failure are directed towards reversing the underlying cause.

Type III Respiratory Failure

- Respiratory failure secondary to lung atelectasis
- Lung atelectasis produces both alveolar flooding and hypoventilation of affected alveoli. As lung atelectasis is often seen in perioperative period, type III respiratory failure is also called as perioperative respiratory failure.

- Treated by chest physiotherapy, upright positioning, and aggressive control of incisional and/or abdominal pain. Noninvasive positive pressure ventilation may also be used to reverse regional atelectasis.

Type IV Respiratory Failure

This form occurs due to hypoperfusion of respiratory muscles in patient of shock. Shock reduces muscle activity and decrease tidal volume which further impair oxygen delivery and so on.

Management (5S)

- **Supplement oxygen**: For mild to moderate case supplemental oxygen is enough.
- **Support respiration** by mechanical ventilation, if oxygen saturation (SaO_2) <90% despite, fraction of inspired oxygen (FiO_2) >0.6.
- **Control secretions, spasm, sepsis**

COMPLICATIONS IN INTENSIVE CARE UNIT

Infections

Nosocomial infections are the most common complications in ICU and affect 10% of ICU patients. Most common infection in medical ICU is urinary tract infection (UTI, 31%)[Q] followed by pneumonia (27%) and primary bloodstream infections. It is very important to know that sepsis is the main predisposing factor for multiorgan system failure and is the leading cause of death in noncoronary ICU. Hand hygiene before and after coming in contact with the patient can help in reducing nosocomial infections.

Deep Venous Thrombosis

All ICU patients are at high risk for deep venous thrombosis (DVT), therefore all patients should receive prophylaxis against DVT. Low molecular heparin is the most commonly used drug for this purpose. Recent study proves fondaparinux, a selective Xa inhibitor to be more effective than low molecular weight heparin (LMWH) for the prevention of DVT.

Stress Ulcers

Stress ulcers and bed sores are not uncommon in long-term ICU stay, frequent repositioning is the best prophylaxis.

Impaired Glycemic Control

Impaired wound healing and dysfunctional immune response leads to glucose intolerance and predisposes patient to infections.

Neurologic Dysfunction

Neurologic dysfunctions are particularly prevalent in critically ill patient. Delirium is the most common one tends to affect more than 50% of ICU patients. Anoxic cerebral injury is common after cardiac arrest and often produces severe and permanent brain injury.

Multiorgan System Failure

This syndrome is defined by the presence of physiologic dysfunction and/or simultaneous failure of two or more organs. Typically, this occurs in the setting of severe sepsis, shock or any other inflammatory condition. Prognosis of multiorgan system failure is very poor.

Intensive Care Unit Acquired Weakness

It occurs frequently in patients who survive critical illness; it is particularly common after sepsis and/or systemic inflammatory response syndrome (SIRS).

KEY POINTS

- Oxygen supplementation improves oxygen saturation in all types of hypoxia, except histotoxic hypoxia.
- Maximum improvement is seen in hypoxic hypoxia.
- In right to left shunt (whether cardiac or pulmonary) SpO_2 cannot be made 100%.

LAST-MINUTE REVISION

- APACHE II score and SAPS II score are the most commonly used scoring system in ICU.
- Shock associated with increased cardiac output: Septic shock, neurogenic shock.
- **Type I respiratory failure**: Oxygenation failure.
- **Type II respiratory failure**: Ventilation failure.
- **Type III respiratory failure**: Perioperative respiratory failure.

REFERENCES

1. Standl T, et al. The nomenclature, definition and distinction of types of shock. Dtsch Arztebl Int. 2018;115(45):757-68.
2. Kislitsina ON, et al. Shock-Classification and pathophysiological principles of therapeutics. Curr Cardiol Rev. 2019;15(2):102-113.
3. Shebl E, Mirabile VS, Sankari A, et al. Respiratory Failure. [Updated 2022 Jul 7]. In: StatPearls [Internet]. Treasure Island (FL): StatPearls Publishing, 2022.

REVIEW QUESTIONS

1. The most common complication in ICU is:
   a. DVT
   b. Pneumonia
   c. UTI
   d. Delirium

2. Type III respiratory failure may occur after:
   a. Pneumothorax
   b. Basal atelectasis of right lung
   c. Pneumonia
   d. Pulmonary edema
3. A 62-year-old patient is admitted with signs of shock (BP: 92/64 mm of Hg; heart rate: 128/min; temperature: 96.2°F). On ECG his cardiac output was found to be increased. Pulmonary artery blood gas analysis shows increased oxygen tension. The most probable etiology in this patient is:
   a. Sepsis
   b. Hypovolemia
   c. Cardiac failure
   d. Cerebrovascular accident (CVA)
4. Type I shock can be caused by all of the following, *except*:
   a. Hypovolemia
   b. Trauma
   c. Cardiac tamponade
   d. Sepsis
5. True about type II respiratory failure includes:
   a. $PaCO_2$ remains low
   b. Obstructive sleep apnea is one of the causes
   c. There is hyperventilation
   d. PaO_2 is high
6. A 35-year-old male patient presents to the emergency with alleged history of road traffic accident. He is unconscious, has tachycardia, hypotension, cold clammy extremities. What is the probable cause of the shock?
7. A 70-year-old female patient presents with acute onset breathlessness and orthopnea, she is a known case of ischemic heart disease. On preliminary examination, she is restless, tachypnoeic, hypotensive, her extremities are cold and clammy, her JVP is increased. Which type of shock would you suspect?
8. A 65-year-old male patient presents with breathlessness and wheezing. He is a known smoker for 40 years. On examination he is tachypnoeic and restless. ABG analysis showed an increased pCO_2 and a reduced pO_2 with acidosis. Which type of respiratory failure will you suspect?

ANSWERS

1. c	2. b	3. a	4. d	5. b	6. Hypovolemic
7. Cardiogenic	8. Type II respiratory failure				

CHAPTER 54

Cardiopulmonary Resuscitation

Sachin Wali, Anshul Jain

INTRODUCTION

Cardiac arrest is defined as inability of heart to sustain effective cardiac output, impairing tissue and end-organ perfusion and can happen anywhere on the streets, at home, during hospital admission. Cardiopulmonary resuscitation (CPR) is defined as series of life saving actions that improve the chances of survival following cardiac arrest. High quality CPR is the cornerstone of a system of care that can optimize outcomes beyond return of spontaneous circulation (ROSC) which means pulse is felt after resuscitation. Site of CPR varies from roadside area with no medical support [(basic life support (BLS)] to hospital in which all advanced equipment and facilities are available [advanced cardiovascular life support (ACLS)].

Basic life support is the foundation for saving lives following cardiac arrest. BLS is systemic approach which stresses early CPR with basic airway management and defibrillation but not advanced airway and drug administration. With BLS one can restore or support oxygenation, ventilation and circulation until ROSC is achieved or advanced provider (ACLS team) intervenes.

Whereas, ACLS involves the use of advanced airway in the form of endotracheal intubation, pharmacological agent like epinephrine, antiarrhythmic drugs and defibrillator and occurs in the hospital setting.

However, it must be well-understood that this distinction doesn't require the victim of sudden cardiac arrest has to be transferred to hospital for CPR. Irrespective of site, BLS must be instituted immediately following cardiac arrest. Time between sudden cardiac arrest and institution of BLS is the most important prognostic factor, i.e., more the period of zero circulation higher would be the chance of death. Furthermore, it is not mandatory that BLS provider should be a healthcare personnel, any common citizen can perform.

Current chapter deals with the pathophysiology of cardiac arrest, basic science of resuscitation as per the latest 2020 AHA guidelines.[1]

SUDDEN CARDIAC ARREST

Cardiac arrest in adults is usually cardiac origin while in pediatric age group it is of respiratory origin (cardiac arrest following asphyxia). The most common electrical mechanism for cardiac arrest in adult patient is pulseless VT or ventricular fibrillation (VF) which is a shockable rhythm with better prognosis and is responsible for 50–80% of cardiac arrests. Whereas bradyarrhythmias, asystole, and pulseless electrical activity (PEA) which are nonshockable rhythms has poor prognosis and accounts for another 20–30%. In pediatric patients, asystole is the most common electric rhythm. Despite recent progress in CPR, cardiac arrest has bad prognosis with low survival at discharge rates ranging from 8.3–10%.

SYSTEMATIC APPROACH

For optimal care, a systematic approach by healthcare provider (personnel) is being advised to treat arrest and acutely ill patient **(Flowchart 54.1)**. With comprehensive review and evidence-based recommendations, American Heart Association (AHA) has put forward the guidelines for CPR. The guidelines are reviewed periodically with latest update in the year 2020. AHA called it as

Chapter 54: Cardiopulmonary Resuscitation

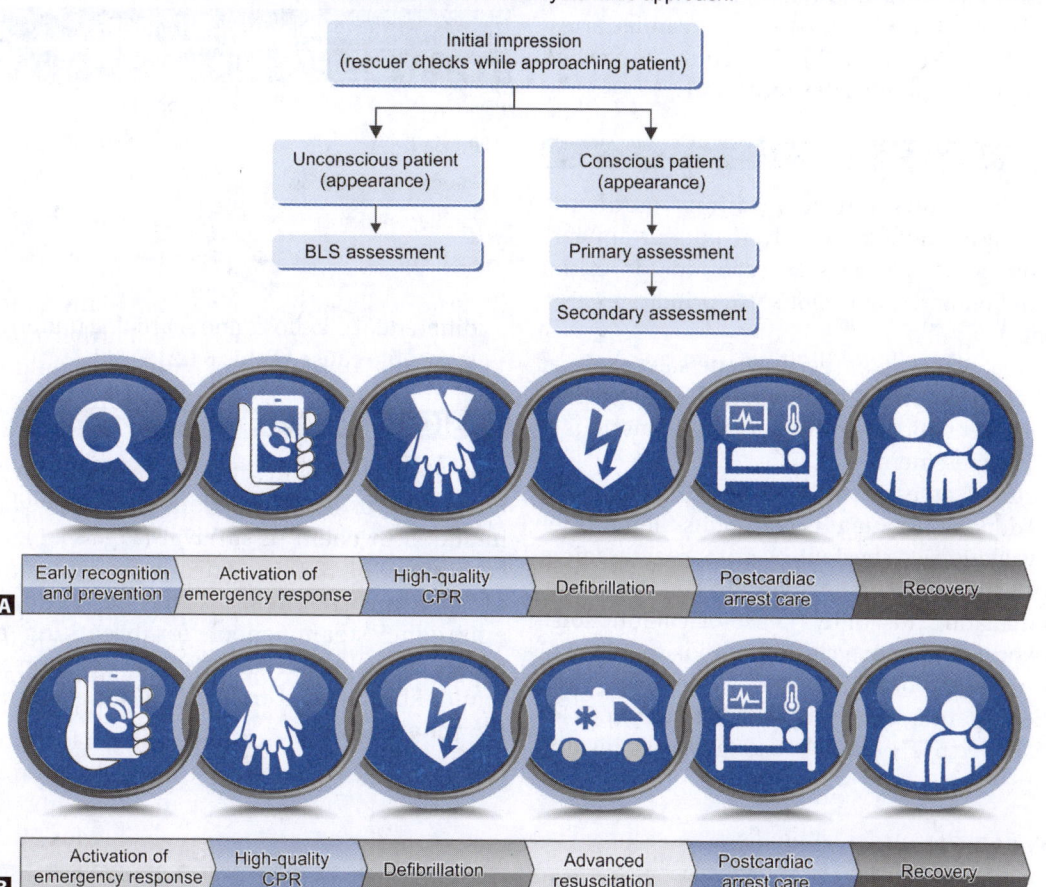

Flowchart 54.1: Initial systematic approach.

Figs. 54.1A and B: 2020 American Heart Association chains of survival for (A) inside hospital cardiac arrest (IHCA) and (B) outside hospital cardiac arrest (OHCA).[1]

Table 54.1: Framework of CPR for provider.

Site of cardiac arrest	Life support method	Rescuer	Chest compression	Airway	Drugs	Shock
Out of hospital cardiac arrest (OHCA)	BLS	Any citizen, need not be healthcare personnel	Yes, as early as possible	Mouth to mouth breaths or bag mask device if available	Not used	AED available in public gathering places—airport, hotels
In hospital cardiac arrest (IHCA)	BLS and ACLS	Any citizen, healthcare personnel can initiate BLS (for example collapse in OPD waiting area) till ACLS team arrives and takes over	Yes, as early as possible	Endotracheal intubation	Epinephrine and anti-arrhythmic used	Defibrillator available in emergency department and ICU

(AED: automated external defibrillator; BLS: basic life support; ACLS: advanced cardiovascular life support).

chain of survival, if followed substantially increase the chance of survival after sudden cardiac arrest (SCA) **(Figs. 54.1A and B)**. Conceptual framework of CPR is described in the **Table 54.1**.

INITIAL ASSESSMENT

Flowchart 54.1 outlines actions guide the initial systematic approach. If patient appears unconscious use BLS assessment for initial evaluation and if conscious use primary assessment.
- Initial assessment (verify scene safety so that there is no threat to providers then determine whether patient is conscious or unconscious).
- BLS assessment
- Primary assessment (A, B, C, D, E): Once BLS is done or if patient is conscious then further evaluation is to be done by primary assessment of which components are airway, breathing, circulation, disability (neurological function), exposure (remove clothing's look for signs of trauma and burns)
- Secondary assessment (detailed history, look for 5 'H' and 5 'T'): Involves taking focused history, differential diagnosis and searching underlying reversible cause **(Table 54.2)**.

Table 54.2: Reversible causes during resuscitation.

Reversible causes-5 H and 5 T's	
5 'H'	5 'T'
Hypovolemia	Tension pneumothorax
Hypoxia	Tamponade (cardiac)
Hydrogen ion (acidosis)	Toxins
Hypo-hyperkalemia	Thrombosis (pulmonary)
Hypothermia	Thrombosis (coronary)

BASIC LIFE SUPPORT (BLS)

The ultimate result of BLS depends on the integration of series of actions which have been included in chain of survival **(Fig. 54.1)**. The core steps of BLS includes early recognition of unresponsiveness, early activation of emergency team, check for breathing and pulse, early initiation of chest compression and defibrillation if indicated **(Table 54.3 and Flowchart 54.2)**.

Table 54.3: Steps of BLS assessment.

Assessment steps	Action
Check responsiveness	Tap and shout "Are you okay"
Activate emergency response	• Shout for nearby help • Activate emergency response system • Get the AED if one is available or send bystander to get AED and activate emergency response
Check for breathing and pulse	• To check for absent or abnormal breathing (no breathing or only gasping) scan the chest for rise and fall for at least 5 not more than 10 seconds • Feel for carotid pulse for at least 5 seconds not more than 10 seconds • Perform pulse check simultaneously with breathing check to minimize delay in CPR • If no pulse and no breathing within 10 seconds start CPR beginning with 30 chest compression followed by two breaths • If you find a pulse start rescue breath at 1 breath every 6 seconds and pulse check every 2 minutes
Defibrillation	• If AED detects shockable rhythm provide shock as indicated then resume CPR immediately • If AED detects nonshockable rhythm resume CPR until prompted by AED for rhythm check

Immediate Recognition of Cardiac Arrest (Flowchart 54.2)

First step of BLS sequence is to recognize that the victim is in cardiac arrest. If a lone rescuer finds an unresponsive adult or witnesses the adult who suddenly collapses, after ensuring that the scene is safe, the rescuer should check for the response by tapping the victim on the shoulder and shouting at the victim, "hello what happened?" If there is no response, activate emergency response and get an AED. Then look for breathing for at least 5 seconds not more than 10 seconds and simultaneously feel the pulse. If victim has absent pulse or abnormal breathing, i.e., gasping, the rescuer should assume that victim is in cardiac arrest and start 30 chest compressions with two rescue breaths. Once AED arrives it should be attached which will recognize shockable rhythm and deliver shock automatically **(Flowchart 54.2)**.

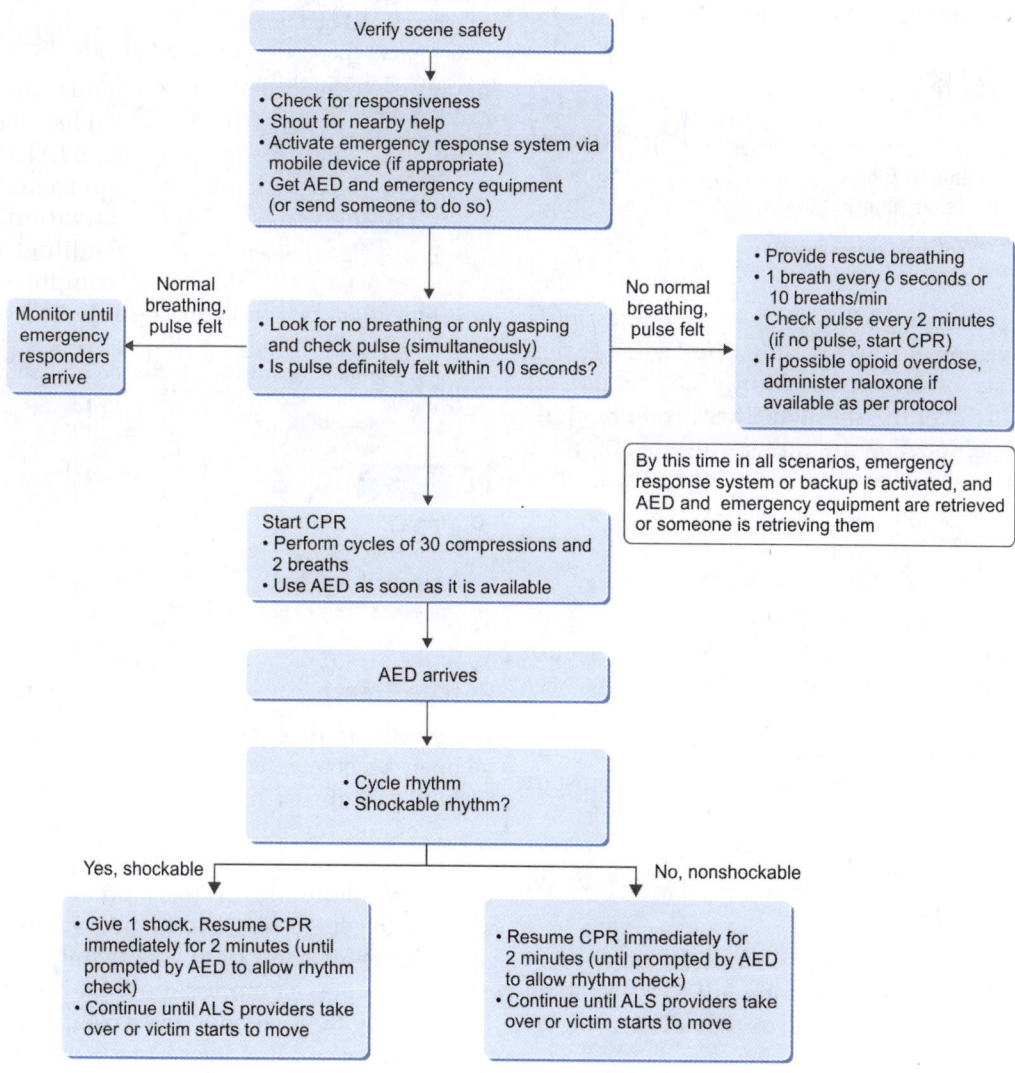

Flowchart 54.2: Adult BLS algorithm for healthcare providers.

What's About Pulse Check in CPR?

Till 2005, pulse check was considered an essential part for recognition of cardiac arrest. But studies have shown that both lay rescuers and healthcare providers have difficulty in detecting a pulse especially in an anxious situation like this. So, 2020 guidelines recommend lay rescuer to start CPR for presumed cardiac arrest because risk of harm to patient is low if not in cardiac arrest. While healthcare providers should take no more than 10 seconds to check for a pulse. If healthcare provider is unable to feel pulse within that time period, he should start chest compression **(Box 54.1)**.

BOX 54.1
Site of pulse check
Feel for carotid pulse (on side closest to you) by locating the trachea and sliding fingers between trachea and muscles of side of neck where pulsation is felt.

Chest Compression

Prompt initiation of effective chest compression is a fundamental aspect of CPR. Chest compression consists of forceful rhythmic application of pressure over the sternum. These compressions create blood flow by increasing intrathoracic pressure and directly compressing the heart thus delivering oxygen to vital organs.

Technique of Chest Compression

- Victim should lie on flat firm surface
- Place the heel of one hand on center of victim's chest on lower half of breastbone, put the heel of your other hand on top of first hand
- Straighten your arms and position your shoulders directly over your hands then start compressions.

Efficiency of Chest Compression Depends on Following Properties

- **Compression depth:** Compress the chest at least 2 inches (5 cm) for adult while avoiding chest compression depth >2.4 inch or >6 cm depth.
- **Adequate rate:** Compression rate of at least 100–120 compressions per minute.
- Keep chest compression and relaxation time approximately equal.
- **Adequate relaxation:** Allow complete chest recoil after each chest compression which helps in return of blood to heart.
- Minimizing interruption in compressions **(Boxes 54.2 and 54.3)**.

BOX 54.2
Components of high-quality CPR
- Assess breathing and check pulse for at least 5 seconds and not more than 10 seconds.
- Compress the chest hard and fast at least 5 cm depth at the rate of 100–120/min.
- Allow the chest to completely recoil after each compression.
- Switch compressor every 2 minutes or earlier if fatigued, and the switch over should only take 5 seconds.
- Minimize interruption in compression for 10 seconds or less.
- Compression to ventilation ratio 30:2, avoid excessive ventilation.
- Early defibrillation to reduce the time to shock delivery.

BOX 54.3
During CPR, avoid:
- Frequent or inappropriate pulse checks.
- Prolonged ventilation.
- Unnecessary movement of patient.

Rescue Breath

For breaths to be effective victim's airway must be open which can be achieved by head tilt-chin lift and jaw thrust maneuvers. After 30 chest compression rescuers should open the airway by head-tilt chin-lift maneuver and deliver two mouth-to-mouth breaths (each breath over one second), to generate a sufficient tidal volume that produce visible chest raise. After administration of breath, chest compression must be started immediately. Subsequently, use a compression to ventilation ratio of 30:2. Pocket masks or bag mask device should be used if available. When an airway device is in place (in hospital CPR), give 1 breath every 6 seconds.

Excessive ventilation is unnecessary rather harmful as it can lead to gastric inflation and related complication. Moreover, excessive ventilation increases intrathoracic pressure which in turn decreases venous return and cardiac output.

Adult 2-rescuer BLS

When more than one rescuer is present during resuscitation, more tasks can be performed at same time such as one rescuer opens the airway other rescuers will provide bag mask ventilation and chest compressions.

Defibrillation

Automated external defibrillator (AED) is a portable defibrillating device, which can assess rhythm and deliver a shock that can stop the abnormal rhythm and allow heart's normal rhythm to return so that heart can pump blood. AED is readily available in most public gathering sites. Pulseless VT and ventricular fibrillation are the most common and importantly treatable initial rhythm where survival rates are high when early shock is delivered. As soon as AED arrives following sequence has to be followed:

- Turn AED on and attach the AED pads over victim's bare chest (one pad below right collar bone and second pad over side of left nipple).
- Clear the victim (no one should be touching victim) and allow AED to analyze the rhythm.
- If it is shockable rhythm (VF or pulseless VT) AED will prompt to deliver shock.
- Then clear from the victim and press the shock button, once shock is delivered contraction of victim's muscles is seen.
- After shock is delivered or if AED prompts no shock immediately resume CPR starting with chest compressions.
- After 5 cycles or 2 minutes of CPR, AED will again analyze rhythm **(Box 54.4)**.

BOX 54.4

Chest compressions with rescue breaths → defibrillation → Chest compressions with rescue breaths) has to be repeated every 2 minutes and continued until ALS provider arrives or patient starts to move.

Tailoring the Response

Individualized management of resuscitation: Not all cardiac arrest events are identical, and specialized management may be critical for optimal patient outcome. Single rescuer may tailor rescue actions according to cause of arrest. For example, if adult collapse after developing chest pain, healthcare provider should activate emergency response system (via mobile), get an AED nearby attach and then provide CPR. However, if rescuer believes that hypoxia was cause of arrest (such as in drowning) than he or she should perform about 2 minutes of CPR including breaths before activating emergency response system.

ADVANCED CARDIOVASCULAR LIFE SUPPORT (ACLS)

Cardiac arrest can happen anywhere at home, roadside, in the hospital. Regardless of where the arrest occurs the final care converges in emergency department or ICU where ACLS is carried out. ACLS interventions build on the BLS foundations get benefits of skilled staff and is carried out in hospital settings. Drug therapy, advanced airway management and physiologic monitoring are included in ACLS which increase the likelihood of ROSC. Postcardiac arrest care is the final link in the chain where critical care interventions advanced monitoring and postcardiac arrest care occurs **(Box 54.5)**.

BOX 54.5

Code blue
This is a procedure code announced in hospital when patient is found to be in cardiac arrest. Team members include team leader (physician or anesthetist), nurse and supporting staff.

Cardiac arrest can result from four rhythms: (1) VF; (2) PVT; (3) pulseless electrical activity (PEA) and (4) asystole. Management of these cardiac arrest rhythms requires both BLS and a system of ACLS **(Flowchart 54.3)** with integrated post-cardiac arrest care. ACLS is carried in the hospital settings by trained healthcare personnel with use of advanced airway (intubation), drugs and defibrillation. Initial step in ACLS is to start CPR once patient is found with no pulse and absent or abnormal (gasping) breathing. Shout for help activate emergency response. Once the monitor or defibrillator is attached check for rhythm and one of the following two pathways has to be followed accordingly.

1. A shockable rhythm, displayed on the VF/pulseless VT pathway of algorithm.
2. A nonshockable rhythm displayed on asystole/PEA pathway of algorithm.

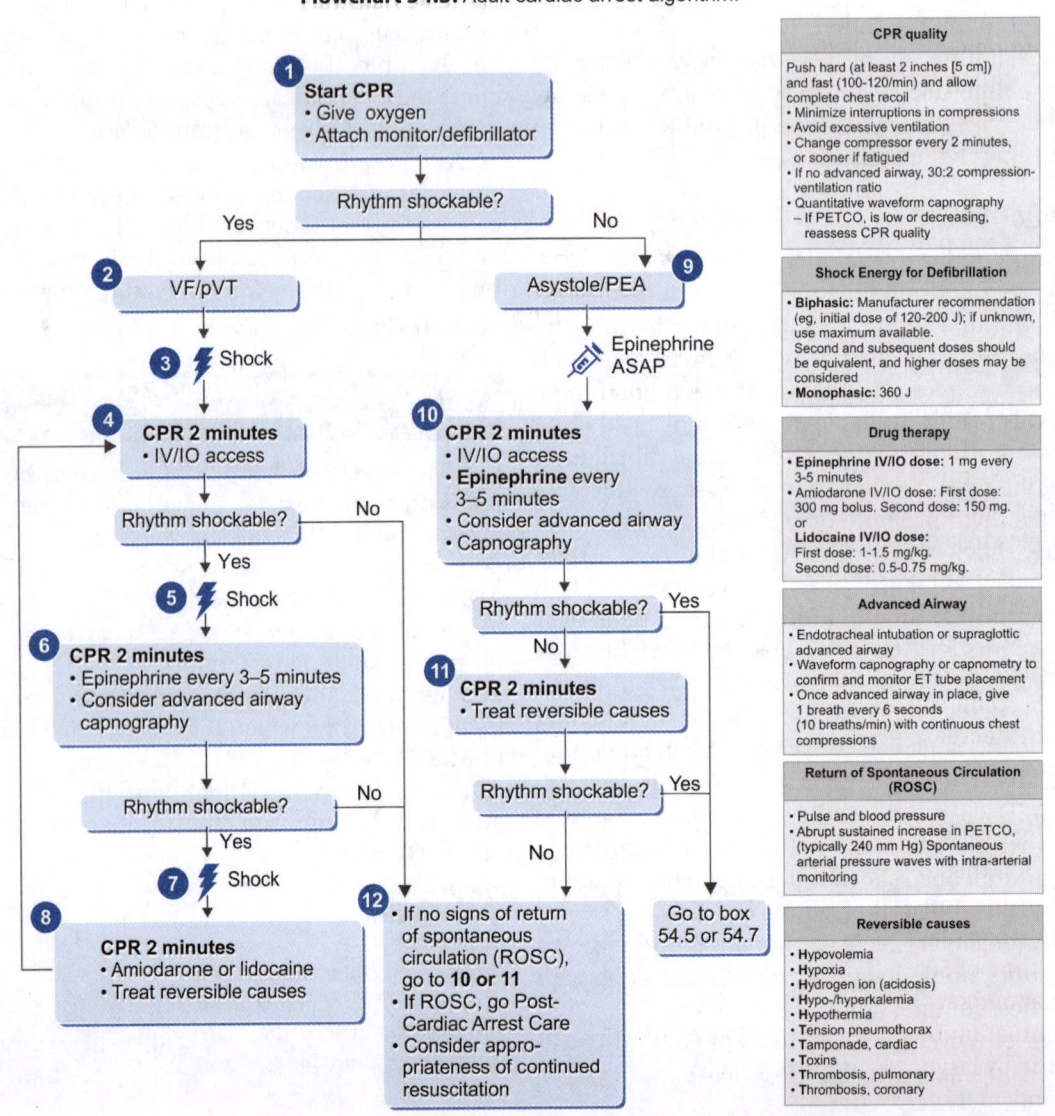

Flowchart 54.3: Adult cardiac arrest algorithm.

High quality CPR with compression rate of 100–120/minute and compression ventilation ratio of 30:2 is recommended till the placement of advanced airway. For ventilation bag mask technique is employed. After placement of supraglottic device [laryngeal mask airway (LMA)] or endotracheal tube ventilation should be started using 100% O_2 at a rate of 1 breath per 6 seconds or 10 breaths per minute. Capnometry or wave form capnography for confirmation of ET tube position and monitoring. Use of DOPE mnemonic (displacement, obstruction, pneumothorax, equipment failure) could be considered for trouble shooting. While performing CPR IV/IO access to be obtained by another team member, so that emergency drug can be administered. Rhythm should be analyzed and shock to be delivered accordingly. Simultaneously, one must rule out the reversible causes (H's and T's). If the patient achieves ROSC, it is important to begin post-cardiac arrest care immediately, to optimize the patient chance of long-term survival.

Chest Compression

As soon as patient is found to be in cardiac arrest start with chest compressions of adequate rate 100–120/minute, depth of at least 5 cm, minimize interruptions, allow complete chest recoil with target chest compression fraction (CCF) of >60%.

Chest compression fraction is proportion of time during cardiac arrest resuscitation when the rescuer is performing chest compressions. CCF should be as high as possible ideally greater than 80%. Data suggest that lower CCF is associated with decreased ROSC and survival to hospital discharge.

Airway and Ventilation

Basic skills to open the airway such as head tilt-chin lift and jaw thrust should be performed. Then bag mask device can be used to deliver tidal volume of 500 mL sufficient to provide chest rise over one second for ventilation with compression ventilation ratio of 30:2. For advanced airway ET tube or laryngeal mask airway can be used and confirmation of tube placement by continuous wave capnography. Overall the priority should be chest compressions and supporting ventilation by bag mask and not the endotracheal intubation which is common mistake done in resuscitation.

Defibrillation Strategies

AHA does not recommend continuous use of AED (or automatic mode) when a manual defibrillator is available and providers can adequately interrupt rhythms. Shortening interval between last compression and shock by few seconds can improve shock success hence efficient coordination between CPR and defibrillation is important. For example, after you verify shockable rhythm and initiate charging sequence on defibrillator another provider should resume chest compression and continue until defibrillator is fully charged (**Table 54.4**). Once compressor removes hands shock is to be delivered following which same compressor resumes compression for 2 minutes following which rhythm analysis to be done. Remember to perform pulse check during rhythm analysis only if organized rhythm is present.

- If rhythm is organized and pulse is felt proceed to postcardiac arrest care
- If rhythm is nonshockable and pulse is not felt proceed along asystole/PEA pathway
- If rhythm is shockable give 1 shock immediately and resume CPR for 2 minutes after shock.

Once monitor is attached depending upon the rhythm if it is shockable, then to ensure safe defibrillation always announce shock warning "Delivering shock" and ensure that you and team members are not in contact with patient and oxygen is not flowing across patient's chest then deliver one shock and immediately start chest compressions.

Table 54.4: Types and energy dose during defibrillation.

Type of defibrillators	Energy dose
Monophasic defibrillator	360 Joules (J)
Biphasic defibrillator	120–200 J (as per manufacturer recommendations)

(**Note**: Subsequent energy level should be at least equivalent or higher than the initial level).

First 4–6 minutes of cardiac arrest is clinical death then at 6–10 minutes biological death occurs and after 10 minutes damage to brain is irreversible. In first few minutes after successful defibrillation spontaneous rhythm is slow and may not create pulse or adequate perfusion hence CPR to be continued several minutes till adequate heart function resumes and on the other hand not all shocks lead to successful defibrillation hence high-quality CPR to be resumed immediately after shock is delivered.

CARDIAC ARREST IN PREGNANCY

During resuscitation in pregnant patients two potential patients are present mother and fetus. The algorithm for cardiac arrest in pregnancy is divided into 2 focuses (maternal and obstetric interventions). Key changes in maternal cardiac arrest resuscitation are—in cardiac arrest reduced venous return and cardiac output caused by gravid uterus reduces effective coronary and cerebral circulation. Hence, patient can be placed in left lateral decubitus position but chest compression quality is compromised hence manual left lateral displacement of uterus can be done which relieves aortocaval pressure. High quality CPR should be continued and if no ROSC is achieved in 5 minutes then perimortem cesarean delivery should be performed.

DRUG THERAPY

Vasopressors can be given with the primary goal of increasing myocardial blood flow during CPR and achieving ROSC. Indication, dose and mechanism of commonly used drug during CPR is mentioned in **Table 54.5**.

- Epinephrine is the most preferred vasopressors in this situation.
- Amiodarone is the first line antiarrhythmic agent for refractory VF or pulseless VT.
- Lidocaine can be used as alternative.
- Magnesium sulphate should be considered only for torsade's de pointes associated with long QT interval.

Route of Drug Administration

Following routes can be used to administer drugs during resuscitation

Intravenous Access

- IV access is preferred for drug administration; central line insertion during resuscitation is

Table 54.5: Drugs used in ACLS.

Drug	Mechanism	Indication and dosage
Epinephrine hydrochloride	Has alpha adrenergic effects, i.e., by vasoconstriction increases coronary and myocardial blood flow	• If Pulseless VT or VF give epinephrine during CPR after second shock and repeat every 3–5 minutes or 4 minutes mid-range (every alternate pulse check) • If rhythm is nonshockable (asystole or PEA) then epinephrine should be given as soon as possible
Amiodarone	Is a Class 3 antiarrhythmic but possess properties of other classes also and acts by prolonging cardiac action potential	• Amiodarone to be given in pulseless VT or VF which is not responsive to defibrillation (after 3 shocks) • First dose—300 mg IV/IO followed by one additional second dose of 150 mg can be repeated
Lidocaine	Blocks permeability of neural membranes to sodium and blockade of conduction hence suppresses automatic of conduction tissue in heart	• Lidocaine can be used as an alternative to amiodarone • Dose: 1–1.5 mg/kg IV/IO first dose followed by 0.5–0.75 mg/kg every 5–10 minutes to maximum dose of 3 mg/kg
Magnesium sulfate	Magnesium is sodium/potassium pump antagonist and also suppresses L- and T-type calcium channels hence ventricular depolarizations	• Magnesium sulfate in cardiac arrest has role if torsades de pointes is present • Dose: 1–2 g diluted in 10 mL 5% dextrose given through IV route

not preferred as may lead to bleeding and hematoma-like complications.
- Method: Drugs usually take 1–2 minutes to central circulation after given from IV route.
- So, give the drug by bolus injection followed by 20 mL bolus of IV fluid and elevate extremity for 20 seconds so that drug reaches central circulation.

Intraosseous Route

If IV access is not successful or feasible IO access can be obtained and any drugs used in resuscitation during ACLS can be given which is absorbed through noncollapsible marrow venous plexus.

Endotracheal Route

- IV and IO route are preferred but if drugs are to be given through endotracheal tube, then the dose is 2–2.5 times the IV route and should be diluted in 10 mL sterile water.
- Following administration during ongoing chest compression drug may regurgitate in the endotracheal tube.
- Drug like epinephrine can affect calorimetric CO_2 detectors functionality.

MONITORING DURING CPR

Mechanical Parameters

Cardiopulmonary resuscitation parameters such as rate of compression and rate of ventilation should be monitored either by rescuer himself/bystanders by verbal counting or feedback devices can be used.

Physiologic Parameters

- **Pulse check**: It is not possible to assess the effectiveness of compression by pulse check because in critical conditions it is very difficult to palpate pulse, moreover due to absence of valves in IVC, chest compression produce retrograde blood in IVC and femoral veins which may be confused with femoral artery pulsations. Carotid pulsations too don't correlate with the efficacy of CPR. However, presence of definite pulse when chest compression is paused is a specific indicator of ROSC but sensitivity is poor.
- **End-tidal CO_2**: Measured through quantitative wave form capnography helps in monitoring CPR quality, optimize chest compression and detect ROSC. When patient is in cardiac arrest, there is no gaseous exchange in lung. So expired gases even when patient in being ventilated would not have CO_2 ($ETCO_2$ is zero). During CPR, there is resumption of at least some cardiopulmonary circulation so during chest compression $ETCO_2$ correlate well with cardiac output. Persistently, low $ETCO_2$ values (<10 mm Hg) during CPR reduce the likelihood of ROSC and is an indication that chest compression is not proper or some Ts and Hs coexist. If $ETCO_2$ abruptly increase to a normal value (>40 mm Hg); it is a sensitive and specific indicator of ROSC.
- **Central venous oxygen saturation**: When oxygen consumption, arterial oxygen saturation (SaO_2) and hemoglobin are constant, changes in central venous oxygen saturation ($SCVO_2$) reflect changes in oxygen delivery. $SCVO_2$ can be measured continuously using oximetric tipped central venous catheters placed in the superior vena cava. $SCVO_2$ normally ranges from 60% to 80%. $SCVO_2$ <30% signify insufficient chest compression. Thus, when available, $SCVO_2$ monitoring is a potentially useful indication of cardiac output oxygen delivery during CPR.
- **Coronary perfusion pressure (CPP)**: During CPR CPP correlates with myocardial blood flow and ROSC. A substitute for CPP during CPR is arterial relaxation ("diastolic") pressure which is measured by intra-arterial catheter. If the arterial relaxation pressure is <20 mm Hg then the quality of chest compression should be improved.

TERMINATING RESUSCITATIVE EFFORTS

Decision to terminate resuscitative efforts can never be simple fixed time duration and is based on multiple factors:
- Time from collapse to first CPR or defibrillation
- Comorbid disease

- Initial arrest rhythm and prearrest state
- Response to resuscitative measures
- $ETCO_2$ <10 after 20 minutes of high-quality CPR
- Prolonged resuscitative efforts may be indicated for patients with hypothermia, drug overdose and other potential reversible cause of arrest.

POSTCARDIAC ARREST CARE

Studies have shown most deaths occur in first 24 hours after resuscitation from cardiac arrest. Hence to improve outcome in post-ROSC patient after cardiac arrest various practices are followed which are mentioned in algorithm as two phases.

Phase 1

Initial stabilization phase—is ongoing resuscitation which has to be carried during immediate post-ROSC phase:

- Place ET tube early and start 1 breath every 6 seconds target SpO_2 92–98.
- Administer crystalloid/vasopressor with target MAP >65 mm Hg.
- Obtain 12 lead ECG.

Phase 2

Continued resuscitation phase:
- Consider cardiac intervention if STEMI or unstable cardiogenic shock
- Access GCS if patient is comatose start targeted temperature management (TTM) begin at 32–36°C by using cooling device.

AMERICAN HEART ASSOCIATION (AHA) UPDATES IN 2020 GUIDELINES

Table 54.6 highlights the important changes occurred in AHA 2020 guidelines from previous (2015).[2]

Table 54.6: Updates in 2020 American Heart Association (AHA) guidelines.

ACLS topic	Old (2015) AHA guidelines	2020 AHA guidelines
Ventilation	• 1 breath every 5 to 6 seconds for respiratory arrest with bag mask device • 1 breath every 6 seconds for ventilation with an advanced airway in place	1 breath every 6 seconds for respiratory arrest with or without an advanced airway
Bradycardia	• Atropine dose 0.5 mg • Dopamine dosing: 2–20 µg/kg/minute	• Atropine dose: 1 mg • Dopamine dosing: 5–20 µg/kg per minute
Tachycardia	• Synchronized cardioversion: Initial recommended doses • Narrow QRS complexes, regular rhythm: 50–100 J • Narrow QRS complex, irregular rhythm: 120–200J • Wide QRS complex, regular rhythm: 100 J • Wide QRS complex, irregular rhythm/defibrillation dose (not synchronized)	• Follow your specific device's recommended energy level to maximize the success of the first shock • Wide QRS complex, irregular rhythm, defibrillation dose (not synchronized)
Postcardiac arrest	Titrate oxygen saturation to 94% or higher	Titrate oxygen saturation to 92–98%
Adult chain of survival	5 links for both chains (IHCA and OHCA)	6 links for both chains (IHCA and OHCA) added a recovery link to the end of both chains
IV/IO access	IV access and IO access are equivalent	IV preferred over IO access, unless IV fails
Cardiac arrest	• Epinephrine 1mg every 3–5 minutes or every 4 minutes as a midrange (i.e., every other 2-minute rhythm check) • Amiodarone and lidocaine are equivalent for treatment (i.e., either may be used) • Added maternal cardiac arrest information and algorithms (in hospital) • Added ventricular assist device information (VAD: LVAD and RVAD) and algorithm • Added new prognostication diagram and information • Recommend using waveform capnography with a bag-mask device	

Contd...

Contd...

ACLS topic	Old (2015) AHA guidelines	2020 AHA guidelines
Stroke	• Revised stroke algorithm • New stroke triage algorithm for EMS destination • Focus on large vessel occlusion (LVO) for all healthcare providers • Endovascular therapy: Treatment window up to 24 hours (previously up to 6 hours) • Both alteplase and endovascular therapy can be given/performed if time criteria and inclusion criteria are met • Consider EMS bypass the emergency department and go straight to the imaging suite (CT/MRI) initial assessment can be performed there to save time • Titrate oxygen saturation to >94%	

LAST-MINUTE REVISION

- In adult person, most common cause of cardiac arrest is VF; in pediatric patients, asystole is the most common cause
- Sequence of adult CPR: CAB; ratio: two ventilation: 30 compression; rate: 2 ventilation with 100 compression per minute

REFERENCES

1. Panchal AR, et al. Adult basic and advanced life support writing group. Part 3: Adult Basic and Advanced Life Support: 2020 American Heart Association Guidelines for Cardiopulmonary Resuscitation and Emergency Cardiovascular Care. Circulation. 2020;142(16_suppl_2): S366-S468.

2. Morrison LJ, Gent LM, Lang E, Nunnally ME, Parker MJ, Callaway CW, et al. Part 2: Evidence evaluation and management of conflicts of interest: 2015 American Heart Association Guidelines Update for Cardiopulmonary Resuscitation and Emergency Cardiovascular Care. Circulation. 2015; 132(suppl 2):S368–S382. doi: 10.1161/CIR.0000000000000253.

REVIEW QUESTIONS

1. As per latest 2020 guidelines of CPR, first step following cardiac arrest is:
   a. Opening airway by chin-left head-tilt maneuver
   b. Give mouth to mouth breath
   c. Compress chest
   d. Shout for help

2. Sequence of CPR as per 2020 AHA guidelines:
   a. ABC
   b. BAC
   c. CAB
   d. BCA

3. Most common electric rhythm after sudden cardiac arrest:
   a. Ventricular fibrillation
   b. Atrial fibrillation
   c. Atrial flutter
   d. Asystole

4. In ICU a patient underwent cardiac arrest, after 4 cycles of CPR, $ETCO_2$ suddenly rise to 46 mm Hg. What does it signifies:
   a. Patient is dead
   b. Nothing specific
   c. Return of spontaneous circulation
   d. Rib fracture and subsequent lung parenchymal injury

ANSWERS

1. d   2. c   3. a   4. c

CHAPTER 55

Acid–Base and Electrolyte Imbalance

Rupali Patnaik, Anshul Jain

INTRODUCTION

Electrolyte disturbances are extremely common in the critically ill patients. Many critically ill patients have coexisting acid and base abnormalities which may either be the result of their illness or many a times the cause of their critical illness, e.g., diabetic ketoacidosis. Intensivist must therefore have a clear understanding of normal acid–base and electrolyte physiology as major disturbances in acid, base and electrolyte balance can rapidly alter cardiovascular, neurological, and neuromuscular functions.

NORMAL ACID–BASE HOMEOSTASIS

Systemic arterial pH is maintained between 7.35 and 7.45 by extracellular and intracellular chemical buffering together with respiratory and renal regulatory mechanisms.

The control of arterial CO_2 tension ($PaCO_2$) by the central nervous system and respiratory systems and the control of the plasma bicarbonate by the kidneys stabilize the arterial pH by excretion or retention of acid or alkali. Under most circumstances, CO_2 production and excretion are matched, and the usual steady-state $PaCO_2$ is maintained at 40 mm Hg. Increases or decreases in $PaCO_2$ represent derangements of neural respiratory control or are due to compensatory changes in response to a primary alteration in the plasma bicarbonate (HCO_3^-).

The kidneys regulate plasma (HCO_3^-) through "reabsorption" of filtered HCO_3^-, formation of titratable acid, and excretion of ammonium ion (NH_4^+) in the urine. If H^+ load is high kidney increases NH_4^+ production and excretion, to maintain H^+ balance.

Summarizing, the kidneys and the respiratory system, act in concert to maintain a systemic arterial pH between 7.35 and 7.45.

ACID–BASE DISTURBANCES

The pH of the arterial plasma is normally varies from 7.35 to 7.45. Technically, *acidosis* is said to occur when the arterial pH falls below 7.35, and *alkalosis* is present when it raises above 7.45. If acidosis results from retention of CO_2 (i.e., due to respiratory problem), it is called a respiratory acidosis, if it is due to retention or over production of acid the term is metabolic acidosis (e.g., diabetic ketoacidosis). Similarly, alkalosis due to lowering of CO_2 is called as respiratory alkalosis whereas excessive loss of acid (e.g., severe vomiting) leads to metabolic alkalosis.

KEY POINTS

From where H^+ is generated
Metabolism of sulfur-containing amino acids produces H_2SO_4, and metabolism of phosphorylated amino acids such as phosphoserine produces H_3PO_4. These strong acids enter the circulation and present a major H^+ load to the buffers in the ECF. The H^+ load from amino acid metabolism is normally about 50 mEq/d.

The CO_2 formed by metabolism in the tissues is in large part hydrated to H_2CO_3, and the total H^+ load from this source is over 12,500 mEq/d. However, most of the CO_2 is excreted in the lungs, and only small quantities of the H^+ remain to be excreted by the kidneys.

Interpretation

A fairly sure diagnosis of acid–base disorders can be made by estimating pH, $PaCO_2$, and HCO_3^-. If one knows these three parameters diagnosis can be made by utilizing following rules.

Rule 1

- **See pH:** If abnormal
- **See the change in $PaCO_2$:** If moving in same direction as pH, diagnosis of metabolic disorder is made, e.g.:
  - ↓pH and ↓$PaCO_2$—Δ *Metabolic acidosis*
  - ↑pH and ↑$PaCO_2$—Δ *Metabolic alkalosis*

Rule 2

- **pH:** Abnormal
- **$PaCO_2$:** Moving in opposite direction to pH. Diagnosis of respiratory disorder is made of
  - ↓pH and ↑$PaCO_2$ —Δ *Respiratory acidosis*

Rule 3

pH: Abnormal and there is no change in $PaCO_2$.
Diagnosis of superimposed respiratory disorder along with primary metabolic disorder:

- In a patient pH—7.29 ; HCO_3^-—18, $PaCO_2$—40 mm Hg diagnosis is *metabolic acidosis not properly compensated*.
- In this patient if $PaCO_2$ is 20 mm Hg diagnosis would be *metabolic acidosis with superimposed respiratory alkalosis* (see later).

Prediction of Compensation

Primary respiratory disturbances (primary changes in $PaCO_2$) invoke compensatory metabolic responses (secondary changes in [HCO_3^-]), and primary metabolic disturbances elicit predictable compensatory respiratory responses. Example: metabolic acidosis lowers extracellular fluid [HCO_3^-], which stimulates the medullary chemoreceptors to increase ventilation and to normalize the ratio of [HCO_3^-] to $PaCO_2$, and thus try to bring pH, toward normal, although not to normal **(Table 55.1)** Thus, a patient with metabolic acidosis and [HCO_3^-] of 12 mmol/L would be expected to have a low $PaCO_2$. One can determine the disorder in view of compensation by utilizing rule 4.

Rule 4

Determine the compensation **(Table 55.1)**.
- If compensation is less, diagnosis is non-compensated and if compensation is more diagnosis is superimposed alkalosis or acidosis.
- *In acidosis a quick method to determine compensation is to check last two digits of pH. It should be roughly equal to pCO_2, e.g., in properly compensated acidosis with pH of 7.28 will have pCO_2 of 28.*

Example: In a patient pH—7.29; HCO_3^-—18, $PaCO_2$—40 mm Hg diagnosis is *metabolic acidosis not properly compensated*.

Table 55.1: Compensatory changes in acid–base disturbances.

Acid–base disturbances		Range of values		
Disorder	Prediction of compensation	pH	HCO_3^-	$PaCO_2$
Metabolic acidosis	$PaCO_2$ will ↓ 1.25 mm Hg per mmol/L ↓ in (HCO_3^-) or $PaCO_2$ = (HCO_3^-) + 15	Low	Low	Low
Metabolic alkalosis	$PaCO_2$ will ↑ 0.75 mm Hg per mmol/L ↑ in (HCO_3^-) or $PaCO_2$ will ↑ 6 mm Hg per 10 mmol/L ↑ in (HCO_3^-) or $PaCO_2$ = (HCO_3^-) + 15	High	High	High
Respiratory alkalosis • Acute • Chronic	(HCO_3^-) will ↓ 0.2 mmol/L per mm Hg ↓ in $PaCO_2$ (HCO_3^-) will ↓ 0.4 mmol/L per mm Hg ↓ in $PaCO_2$	High	Low	Low
Respiratory acidosis • Acute • Chronic	(HCO_3^-) will ↑ 0.1 mmol/L per mm Hg ↑ in $PaCO_2$ (HCO_3^-) will ↑ 0.4 mmol/L per mm Hg ↑ in $PaCO_2$	Low	High	High

In the same patient if PaCO$_2$ is 20 mm Hg diagnosis would be *metabolic acidosis with superimposed respiratory alkalosis*.

Mixed Acid–Base Disorders

Defined as independently coexisting disorders, not merely compensatory responses—are often seen in patients in critical care units and can lead to dangerous extremes of pH, e.g., a patient with COPD lands in diabetic ketoacidosis (metabolic acidosis) and may have an existing respiratory acidosis. These disorders are difficult to manage. Diagnosis of mixed disorders is made in accordance to rule 5:

Rule 5

Normally PaCO$_2$ and HCO$_3^-$ move in same direction, i.e., if PaCO$_2$↑; HCO$_3^-$ will also increase:
- **If PaCO$_2$↑ and HCO$_3^-$↓**: Diagnosis is *metabolic and respiratory acidosis.*
- **If PaCO$_2$↓ and HCO$_3^-$↑**: Diagnosis is *metabolic and respiratory alkalosis.*

Anion Gap
Evaluation of acid–base disorders should include a simple calculation of the *Anion gap(AG). AG represents unmeasured anions in plasma and is calculated as follows:*
- AG = Na$^+$ + K$^+$ − (Cl$^-$ + HCO$_3$)

(normally it is 10–12 mmol/L).

The unmeasured anions include anionic proteins, phosphate, sulfate, and organic anions. An increase in the AG is most often due to an increase in unmeasured anions and less commonly is due to a decrease in unmeasured cations (calcium, magnesium). When acid anions, such as acetoacetate and lactate, accumulate in extracellular fluid, the AG increases, causing a high-AG acidosis **(Table 55.2)**. In addition, the AG may increase with an increase in anionic albumin. AG will reduce when there is an increase in unmeasured cations, or if unmeasured anions decreases.

Metabolic Acidosis

This is most common acid–base disturbance encountered in clinical practice. Metabolic acidosis can occur because of an increase in endogenous acid production (such as lactate and ketoacids), or loss of bicarbonate (as in diarrhea), or accumulation of endogenous acids (as in renal failure).

Metabolic acidosis has profound effects on the respiratory, cardiac, and nervous systems. The fall in blood pH is accompanied by a characteristic increase in ventilation, especially the tidal volume (*Kussmaul respiration*). Intrinsic cardiac contractility may be depressed, but inotropic function can be normal because of catecholamine release. Central nervous system function is depressed, with headache, lethargy, stupor, and, in some cases, even coma. There are two major categories of clinical metabolic acidosis: high-AG and normal-AG, or hyperchloremic acidosis **(Table 55.2)**.

> **KEY POINTS**
>
> **Causes of reduced anion gap**
> - Hypoalbuminemia
> - Severe hypercalcemia, hypermagnesemia or hyperkalemia
> - IgG myeloma
> - Lithium toxicity
> - Hyperviscosity and severe hyperlipidemia, (underestimation of sodium and chloride concentrations).

Table 55.2: Causes of metabolic acidosis.

Normal anion gap	High anion gap	
Diarrhea	Lactic acidosis	Toxins
Renal tubular acidosis (early)	Ketoacidosis	Ethylene glycol
External pancreatic or small-bowel drainage	Diabetic	Methanol
Ureterosigmoidostomy, jejunal loop, ileal loop	Alcoholic	Salicylate
Acid loads (ammonium chloride, hyperalimentation)	Starvation	Renal failure
Expansion acidosis (rapid saline administration)		

High anion gap acidosis is more notorious.

Management

Treat the cause, acidosis will itself gets cured. However, usually it is not possible to treat the cause rapidly and keeping in view the hazards associated with acidosis it is mandatory to administer alkali from outside so as to neutralize the excess acid. In general, severe acidosis (pH <7.20) warrants the IV administration of 50–100 mEq of $NaHCO_3$, over 30–45 minutes **(Table 55.3)**. Alkali treatment should be started in patients with a normal AG acidosis (hyperchloremic acidosis), a slightly elevated AG (mixed hyperchloremic and AG acidosis), or an AG attributable to a nonmetabolizable anion in the face of renal failure. In case of very high anion gap acidosis secondary to metabolizable anion, alkali therapy is reserved only for very severe acidosis (pH <7.1, HCO_3^- <5 mEq/L).

It is essential to monitor plasma electrolytes during the course of therapy, since the $[K^+]$ may decline as pH rises. The goal is to increase the (HCO_3^-) to 10 mEq/L and the pH to 7.25, not to increase these values to normal.

Metabolic Alkalosis

Metabolic alkalosis is characterized by an elevated arterial pH, an increase in the serum $[HCO_3^-]$, and compensatory increase in $PaCO_2$ due to alveolar hypoventilation. It is often accompanied by hypochloremia and hypokalemia. Metabolic alkalosis frequently occurs in association with other disorders such as respiratory acidosis or alkalosis.

Table 55.3: Dose calculation of $NaHCO_3$.

HCO_3^- deficit = Bicarb Vd × [desired (HCO_3^-) - measured (HCO_3^-)]
   Bicarb Vd = Volume of distribution of bicarbonate
Bicarb Vd is calculated as (0.4 + 2.6/HCO_3^-) × Lean body weight
Roughly Vd comes around 0.5 × Lean body weight or dose of bicarbonate can be roughly estimated as:
   0.5 × Lean body weight × [desired (HCO_3^-) - measured (HCO_3^-)]
½ of the total dose is administered in around 3–4 hours after which another arterial blood analysis is performed.

> **KEY POINTS**
>
> $NaHCO_3$ should be administered slowly as HCO_3 generates CO_2 and if CO_2 generation exceeds patients ventilating capacity CO_2 retention starts and paradoxical intracellular acidosis may be the result.
> THAM (tris hydroxymethyl aminomethane) is a alkali that does not generate CO_2 (so free of intracellular acidosis). Side effects of THAM include hyperkalemia and hypoglycemia.

Pathogenesis

Metabolic alkalosis occurs as a result of net gain of (HCO_3^-) or loss of intrinsic acid (usually HCl by vomiting) from the extracellular fluid.

Since it is unusual for alkali to be added to the body, the disorder usually results from loss of acid and is evident clinically when kidneys fail to compensate by excreting HCO_3^-.

Under normal circumstances, the kidneys have an impressive capacity to excrete HCO_3^-. Continuation of metabolic alkalosis represents a failure of the kidneys to eliminate HCO_3^- in the usual manner.

The kidneys tends to retain, the excess alkali and maintain the alkalosis if (1) volume deficiency, chloride deficiency, and K^+ deficiency coexist, or (2) hypokalemia exists because of autonomous hyperaldosteronism.

Treatment

Primarily directed towards, correcting the underlying stimulus for HCO_3^- generation. Treat the vomiting, in cases where there is gastric loss. If primary aldosteronism, renal artery stenosis, or Cushing's syndrome is present, correction of the underlying cause will reverse the alkalosis. Paradoxical aciduria can be treated by correcting K^+ deficiency. Dilute hydrochloric acid (0.1 *N* HCl) is also effective but can cause hemolysis, and must be delivered centrally and slowly. So, it is reserved only for emergency situation.

Respiratory Acidosis

Respiratory acidosis is characterized by an increase in $PaCO_2$ and decrease in pH. It can be due to severe pulmonary disease, respiratory muscle fatigue, or abnormalities in ventilatory center. In acute respiratory acidosis, there is an immediate compensatory elevation (through cellular buffering mechanisms) in HCO_3^-, which increases 1 mmol/L for every 10-mm Hg increase in $PaCO_2$.

The clinical features vary according to the severity and duration of the respiratory acidosis, the underlying disease, and whether there is accompanying hypoxemia. A rapid increase in $PaCO_2$ may cause anxiety, dyspnea, confusion, psychosis, and hallucinations and may progress to coma. Lesser degrees of dysfunction in chronic hypercapnia produce sleep disturbances, loss of memory, daytime somnolence, personality changes.

Respiratory acidosis, may occur in patients on mechanical ventilation, when not properly adjusted and supervised. Even in controlled situation it may result particularly if CO_2 production suddenly rises (because of fever, agitation sepsis, or overfeeding).

Treatment

The management of respiratory acidosis depends on its severity and rate of onset. Acute respiratory acidosis can be life-threatening, and may necessitate tracheal intubation and assisted mechanical ventilation. In chronic respiratory acidosis aggressive and rapid correction of hypercapnia should be avoided, because the falling $PaCO_2$ may provoke cardiac arrhythmias, reduced cerebral perfusion, and seizures. The $PaCO_2$ should be lowered gradually, aiming to restore the $PaCO_2$ to baseline levels and to provide sufficient Cl^- and K^+ to enhance the renal excretion of HCO_3^-.

Respiratory Alkalosis

Alveolar hyperventilation decreases $PaCO_2$, thus increasing pH. Nonbicarbonate cellular buffers respond by consuming HCO_3^-. Acute respiratory alkalosis causes intracellular shifts of Na^+, K^+, and PO_4^- and reduces free (Ca^{2+}) by increasing the protein-bound fraction. Chronic respiratory alkalosis is the most common acid–base disturbance in critically ill patients and, when severe, portends a poor prognosis.

Common causes of respiratory alkalosis includes hyperventilation in mechanically ventilated patients. Salicylates are the most common cause of drug-induced respiratory alkalosis as a result of direct stimulation of the medullary chemoreceptor. Progesterone increases ventilation and lowers arterial $PaCO_2$ by as much as 5–10 mm Hg. Therefore, chronic respiratory alkalosis is a common feature of pregnancy.

Respiratory alkalosis is also prominent in liver failure, and the severity correlates with the degree of hepatic insufficiency.

The effects of respiratory alkalosis vary according to duration and severity but are primarily those of the underlying disease. Reduced cerebral blood flow as a consequence of a rapid decline in $PaCO_2$ may cause dizziness, mental confusion, and seizures. In the anesthetized or mechanically ventilated patient, cardiac output and blood pressure may fall because of the depressant effects of anesthesia and positive-pressure ventilation on heart rate, systemic resistance, and venous return.

Treatment

The management of respiratory alkalosis is directed toward alleviation of the underlying disorder. If respiratory alkalosis complicates ventilator management, changes in tidal volume, and frequency can minimize the hypocapnia. Patients with the hyperventilation syndrome may benefit from reassurance, rebreathing from a paper bag during symptomatic attacks, and attention to underlying psychological stress.

Physiochemical Stewart Approach to Acid–Base Disturbance

This concept was put forward by Peter Stewart in 1981. Unlike the above-mentioned set of complex rules, this approach is easier and less time consuming. This approach takes electrolytes into picture. According to this approach, changes in three independent variables: partial pressure of CO_2 (pCO_2), strong ion difference (SID) and total amount of weak acids (ATOT) influences the concentration of H^+ there by pH. HCO_3^- and H^+ are dependent variables whose concentration change depends on changes in concentration of independent variables. Like other approaches if pCO_2 increases, H^+ also increase. Strong ions are the ions which completely dissociate. SID is the sum of strong cations minus sum of strong anions. Strong cations are Na^+, K^+, Ca^{2+} and Mg^{2+} and strong anions are Cl^- and $lactate^-$. Main contribution to SID from Na^+ and Cl^- and normal value is around 40 mEq. It is evident from Stewart equation that when SID decreases, H^+ must increase. SID decreases with acidemia and increases with alkalemia. Weak acids exist in both charged and uncharged form. Albumin and phosphates are most important contributor to ATOT. Apparent SID or $SID_A = [(Na^+) + (K^+) + (Ca^{2+}) + (Mg^{2+})] - [(Cl^-) + (lactate^-)]$. For easier calculation at bed side, difference between sodium and chloride (normal value 35–38 mmol/L) can be considered as surrogate of apparent SID.

ELECTROLYTE DISTURBANCES

Disorders of Sodium Balance

Sodium is the principal cation of extracellular fluid. Extracellular fluid volume is directly proportionate to total body sodium content. Normal sodium balance is essential for many physiological functions. Both hyponatremia and hypernatremia have profound effects on normal homeostasis. Normal sodium level varies from 135 mEq/L to 145 mEq/L.

Kidneys plays a key role in maintaining sodium level. The kidneys' ability to excrete urinary Na^+ varies from less than 1 mEq/L to more than 100 mEq/L.

Hyponatremia

Defined by a plasma Na^+ concentration <135 mmol/L. Hyponatremia occurs if there is excessive loss of Na^+ or if there is excessive gain of free water (dilutional hyponatremia). The later type may complicate transurethral resection of the prostate or bladder when large volumes of bladder irrigation solution gets absorbed and result in a dilutional hyponatremia **(Table 55.4)**. Hypertonic hyponatremia is usually due to hyperglycemia. Relative insulin deficiency causes myocytes to become impermeable to glucose. Therefore, during poorly controlled diabetes mellitus, glucose being an effective osmole, draws water from muscle cells, resulting in hyponatremia. Plasma Na^+ concentration falls by 1.4 mmol/L for every 100 mg/dL rise in the plasma glucose concentration.

The increased water ingestion and impaired renal excretion also result in hyponatremia. Hyponatremia can also occur by a process of *desalination*. This occurs when the urine tonicity (the sum of the concentrations of Na^+ and K^+) exceeds that of administered intravenous fluids (including isotonic saline). This accounts for some cases of acute postoperative hyponatremia and cerebral salt wasting after neurosurgery.

Clinical Features

The clinical manifestations of hyponatremia are mainly the result of osmotic water shift from extracellular fluid to intracellular space. Brain cells are specifically prone for this. Therefore the symptoms are primarily neurologic, and their severity is dependent on the rapidity of onset and absolute decrease in plasma Na^+ concentration. Common symptoms are headache, lethargy, confusion, and obtundation. Symptoms may progress to stupor, seizures, and coma if plasma

Table 55.4: Classification of hyponatremia based on symptoms.

Moderately severe	Severe
Nausea without vomiting	Vomiting
Confusion	Seizure
Headache	Abnormal and deep somnolence
	Coma (Glasgow coma scale ≤8)
	Cardiorespiratory distress

Na⁺ concentration falls acutely below 120 mmol/L or decreases rapidly.

Treatment

The goals of therapy are two-fold: (1) to raise the plasma Na⁺ concentration by restricting water intake and promoting water loss and (2) to correct the underlying disorder.

The management of asymptomatic hyponatremia associated with ECF volume contraction should include Na⁺ repletion, generally in the form of isotonic saline, where as the hyponatremia associated with edematous states is managed by restriction of Na⁺ and water intake, correction of hypokalemia, and promotion of water loss in excess of Na⁺, through loop diuretics. Water restriction is also a component of the therapeutic approach to hyponatremia associated with primary polydipsia, renal failure, and syndrome of inappropriate ADH (SIADH).

The rate of correction of hyponatremia depends on the absence or presence of neurologic dysfunction. This, in turn, is related to the rapidity of onset and magnitude of the fall in plasma Na⁺ concentration. In asymptomatic patients, the plasma Na⁺ concentration should be raised by no more than 0.5–1.0 mmol/L per h and by less than 10–12 mmol/L over the first 24 hours. The risk of correcting hyponatremia too rapidly is the development of the *osmotic demyelination syndrome* (ODS). The quantity of Na⁺ required to increase the plasma Na⁺ concentration by a given amount can be estimated by multiplying the deficit in plasma Na⁺ concentration by the total body water.

Under normal conditions, total body water is 50 or 60% of lean body weight in women or men, respectively. Therefore, to raise the plasma Na⁺ concentration from 105 to 115 mmol/L in a 70-kg man requires 420 mmol [(115 − 105) × 70 × 0.6] of Na⁺.

Hypernatremia

Defined as a plasma Na⁺ concentration >145 mmol/L. Since Na⁺ and its accompanying anions are the major effective ECF osmoles, hypernatremia is a state of hyperosmolality. To maintain equilibrium fluid is withdrawn from intracellular space, resulting in ICF volume contraction.

Hypernatremia may be due to primary Na⁺ gain or water deficit. In practice, the majority of cases of hypernatremia result from the loss of water.

The source of free water loss is either renal or extrarenal. Nonrenal loss of water may be due to evaporation from the skin and respiratory tract (insensible losses) or loss from the gastrointestinal tract. Insensible losses are increased with fever, exercise, heat exposure, and severe burns and in mechanically ventilated patients.

Diarrhea is the most common gastrointestinal cause of hypernatremia. Viral diarrheas carries higher risk than secretory diarrhea. Renal water loss is overall the most common cause of hypernatremia and is due to drug-induced or osmotic diuresis or diabetes insipidus. The most frequent cause of an osmotic diuresis is hyperglycemia and glucosuria in poorly controlled diabetes mellitus.

Finally, although infrequent, a primary Na⁺ gain may cause hypernatremia. Example, inadvertent administration of hypertonic NaCl or NaHCO₃ or replacing sugar with salt in infant formula can produce this complication.

Clinical Features

As a consequence of hypertonicity, water shifts out of cells. A decreased brain cell volume is associated with an increased risk of subarachnoid

> **KEY POINTS**
>
> **Osmotic demyelination syndrome**
>
> When hyponatremia is corrected very fast, the osmolality of extracellular fluid raises rapidly which results in osmotic shrinkage of brain cells. Clinically, it is characterized by flaccid paralysis, dysarthria, and dysphagia. Patients with chronic hyponatremia are most susceptible to the development of ODS. In addition to rapid or overcorrection of hyponatremia, Risk factors for ODS include prior cerebral anoxic injury, hypokalemia, and malnutrition, especially secondary to alcoholism. Prognosis is very poor.

or intracerebral hemorrhage. Hence, the major symptoms of hypernatremia are neurologic and include altered mental status, weakness, neuromuscular irritability, focal neurologic deficits, and occasionally coma or seizures.

As with hyponatremia, the severity of the clinical manifestations is related to the acuity and magnitude of the rise in plasma Na$^+$ concentration. Chronic hypernatremia is generally less symptomatic because of adaptive mechanisms designed to defend cell volume.

Treatment

The therapeutic goals are to stop ongoing water loss by treating the underlying cause and to correct the water deficit. The ECF volume should be restored in hypovolemic patients. The quantity of water required to correct the deficit can be calculated from the following equation:

$$\text{Water deficit} = \frac{\text{Plasma Na}^+ \text{ concentration} - 140}{140} \times \text{Total body water}$$

As with hyponatremia, rapid correction of hypernatremia is also potentially dangerous, the water deficit should be corrected slowly over at least 48–72 hours. The safest route of administration of water is by mouth or via a nasogastric tube (or other feeding tube). Alternatively, 5% dextrose in water or half isotonic saline can be given intravenously.

Disorders of Potassium Balance

Potassium is the major intracellular cation. The normal plasma K$^+$ concentration is 3.5–5.0 mmol/L, whereas that inside cells is about 150 mmol/L. The high ratio of ICF to ECF K$^+$ concentration (normally 38:1) is the principal reason behind the resting membrane potential and is crucial for normal neuromuscular function. The basolateral Na$^+$, K$^+$-ATPase pump actively transports K$^+$ in and Na$^+$ out of the cell in a 2:3 ratio, and the passive outward diffusion of K$^+$ is quantitatively the most important factor that generates the resting membrane potential. Because of its importance in neuromuscular functions, both hypokalemia and hyperkalemia are equally dangerous.

Hypokalemia

Defined as a plasma K$^+$ concentration <3.5 mmol/L, may result from one (or more) of the following: Decreased net intake, shift into cells, increased net loss. Diminished intake is seldom the sole cause of K$^+$ depletion but it can exacerbate the situation if there is enhanced loss **(Table 55.5)**.

Clinical Features

Manifestations of K$^+$ depletion depends on the degree of hypokalemia. Symptoms seldom occur unless the plasma K$^+$ concentration is <3 mmol/L. Fatigue, myalgia, and muscular weakness of the lower extremities are common complaints and are due to a lower (more negative) resting membrane potential.

More severe hypokalemia may lead to progressive weakness, hypoventilation (due to respiratory muscle involvement), and eventually complete paralysis. Moreover, K$^+$ depletion results in intracellular acidification and an increase in net acid excretion or new HCO$_3^-$ production.

Table 55.5: Causes of hypokalemia.

Redistribution into cells	Metabolic alkalosis
	Insulin therapy
	β$_2$-adrenergic agonists (endogenous or exogenous)
	α-adrenergic antagonists
	Total parenteral nutrition
	Hypothermia
	Hypokalemic periodic paralysis
	Barium toxicity
Increased loss	Gastrointestinal loss (diarrhea)
	Integumentary loss (sweat)
	Diuretics, osmotic diuresis, salt-wasting nephropathies
	Primary hyperaldosteronism, secondary hyperaldosteronism
	Renal tubular acidosis; diabetic ketoacidosis
Decreased intake	Starvation
	Clay ingestion

The electrocardiographic changes of hypokalemia are due to delayed ventricular repolarization and do not correlate well with the plasma K^+ concentration. Early changes include flattening or inversion of the T wave, a prominent U wave, ST-segment depression, and a prolonged QU interval. Severe K^+ depletion may result in a prolonged PR interval, decreased voltage and widening of the QRS complex, and an increased risk of ventricular arrhythmias, especially in patients with myocardial ischemia or left ventricular hypertrophy.

Treatment

The therapeutic goals are to correct the K^+ deficit and to minimize ongoing losses. Safest approach is to administer K^+ supplements orally which can prevent hyperkalemia, a risk associated with intravenous therapy. It is however important to learn that the degree of K^+ depletion does not correlate well with the plasma K^+ concentration. A decrement of 1 mmol/L in the plasma K^+ concentration (from 4.0 to 3.0 mmol/L) may represent a total body K^+ deficit of 200–400 mmol, and patients with plasma levels under 3.0 mmol/L often require in excess of 600 mmol of K^+ to correct the deficit. Furthermore, factors promoting K^+ shift out of cells (e.g., insulin deficiency in diabetic ketoacidosis) may result in underestimation of the K^+ deficit. Therefore, the plasma K^+ concentration should be monitored frequently when assessing the response to treatment.

In patients with severe hypokalemia or where oral therapy is not feasible (ICU patients), intravenous therapy in the form of potassium chloride is the choice. Potassium bicarbonate and citrate (metabolized to HCO_3^-) tend to alkalinize the patient and is more appropriate for hypokalemia associated with chronic diarrhea or renal tubular acidosis.

The maximum concentration of parenterally administered K^+ should be no more than 40 mmol/L via a peripheral vein or 60 mmol/L via a central vein. The rate of infusion should not exceed 20 mmol/h unless paralysis or malignant ventricular arrhythmias are present.

Hyperkalemia

Defined as a plasma K^+ concentration >5.0 mmol/L, Q occurs as a result of either K^+ release from cells. It decreased renal loss. Increased K^+ intake is rarely the sole cause of hyperkalemia since the phenomenon of *potassium adaptation* ensures rapid K^+ excretion in response to increases in dietary consumption.

Intravascular hemolysis, tumor lysis syndrome, and rhabdomyolysis all lead to K^+ release from cells as a result of tissue breakdown.

Metabolic acidosis, can be associated with mild hyperkalemia resulting from intracellular buffering of H^+. Insulin deficiency and hypertonicity (e.g., hyperglycemia) promote K^+ shift from the ICF to the ECF.

Succinylcholine (SCh) can increase the plasma K^+ concentration, especially in patients with massive trauma, burns, or neuromuscular disease. It is an important and preventable cause of hyperkalemia during perioperative period.

> **KEY POINTS**
>
> KCl should be mixed in normal saline since dextrose solutions may initially exacerbate hypokalemia due to insulin-mediated movement of K^+ into cells.

Treatment

The degree of hyperkalemia as determined by the plasma K^+ concentration, associated muscular weakness, and changes on the electrocardiogram. Potentially fatal hyperkalemia rarely occurs unless the plasma K^+ concentration exceeds 7.5 mmol/L. In severe hyperkalemia emergent treatment is required, in the form of calcium gluconate which decreases membrane excitability **(Table 55.6)**. The usual dose is 10 mL of a 10% solution infused over 2–3 minutes. The effect begins within minutes but is short-lived (30–60 min), and the dose can be repeated if no change in the electrocardiogram is seen after 5–10 minutes. A more sustained response generally occurs when exogenous insulin is administered (10–20 units of regular insulin and 25–50 g of glucose). If effective, the plasma K^+ concentration will fall by 0.5–1.5 mmol/L in 15–30 min, and the effect will last for several hours.

Table 55.6: Treatment of hyperkalemia.

Therapy	Dosing	Onset of action	Duration of action	Magnitude of decline	Mechanism
Ca^{2+}	IV 1 g of 10% calcium chloride (through central vein) or calcium gluconate over 2–3 min	Immediate	30–60 min	None	Membrane stabilization
Insulin	IV 10 units with 50 mL 50% dextrose or 100 mL 25% dextrose	15 min	6–8 hours	1 mEq/L	Intracellular shift of K^+
Salbutamol	10–20 mg nebulization over 10–15 min	10–30 min	3–6 hours	1-1.5 mEq/L	Intracellular shift of K^+
$NaHCO_3$	50–100 mEq IV over 2–5 min	30 min	2–6 hours	0.5–0.75 mEq/L	Intracellular shift of K^+
Loop diuretic (furosemide)	40 mg IV (variable depend on GFR)	5–15 min	4–6 hours	Variable	Excretion of K^+
Sodium polystyrene sulfonate	15 g PO up to 4 times a day	1–2 hours	4–6 hours	0.5–1 mEq/L	K^+ binding and excretion
Hemodialysis	Variable based on K^+ level	Immediate onset	Lasts till completion of dialysis	Variable based on dialysate and dialysis dose	K^+ removal

(IV: intravenous; PO: per oral; GFR: glomerular filtration rate)

Alkali therapy with intravenous $NaHCO_3$ can also shift K^+ into cells. This should be reserved for severe hyperkalemia associated with metabolic acidosis.

The most rapid and effective way of lowering the plasma K^+ concentration is hemodialysis.^{Q} This should be reserved for patients with renal failure and those with severe life-threatening hyperkalemia unresponsive to more conservative measures.

> **KEY POINTS**
>
> *Pseudohyperkalemia* represents an artificially elevated plasma K^+ concentration due to K^+ movement out of cells immediately prior to or following venipuncture. Contributing factors include prolonged use of a tourniquet with or without repeated fist clenching, hemolysis, and marked leukocytosis or thrombocytosis. Pseudohyperkalemia should be suspected in an otherwise asymptomatic patient with no obvious underlying cause. If proper venipuncture technique is used and a plasma (not serum) K^+ concentration is measured, it should be normal.

Disorders of Calcium

Hypercalcemia

Defined by calcium level >11 mg/dL. The important causes of hypercalcemia include excess PTH production; hyperthyroidism; osteolytic metastases and exogenous calcium overload, as in milk-alkali syndrome, or total parenteral nutrition.

Clinical Features

Mild hypercalcemia (up to 11-11.5 mg/dL) is usually asymptomatic and recognized only on routine calcium measurements. Moderate hypercalcemia presents with vague neuropsychiatric symptoms, including trouble in concentrating, personality changes, or depression. More severe hypercalcemia (>12-13 mg/dL), may result in lethargy, stupor, or coma.

Electrocardiographic changes of hypercalcemia include bradycardia, AV block, and short QT interval. Changes in serum calcium can be monitored by following the QT interval.

Treatment

Depends upon the degree and severity. Mild, asymptomatic hypercalcemia does not require immediate therapy. Initial therapy of significant hypercalcemia begins with volume expansion since hypercalcemia invariably leads to dehydration; 4–6 L of intravenous saline may be required over the first 24 hours **(Table 55.7)**. If there is increased calcium mobilization from bone (as in malignancy or severe hyperparathyroidism), drugs that inhibit bone resorption (zoledronic acid and etidronate) should be considered.

In patients with $1,25(OH)_2D$-mediated hypercalcemia, glucocorticoids are the preferred therapy, as they decrease $1,25(OH)_2D$ production.

Hypocalcemia

Defined by Ca^{2+} <8.5 mg/dL. The causes of hypocalcemia can be differentiated according to whether serum PTH levels are low (hypoparathyroidism) or high (secondary hyperparathyroidism).

Because PTH is the main defense against hypocalcemia, disorders associated with deficient PTH production or secretion may be associated with profound, life-threatening hypocalcemia.

In adults, hypoparathyroidism most commonly results from inadvertent damage to all four glands[Q] during thyroid or parathyroid gland surgery. It may also result from autoimmune endocrinopathies rarely.

Table 55.7: Treatment of hypercalcemia.

Therapy	Dosing	Onset/duration of action	Mechanism of action
Isotonic saline	Bolus (up to 3–4 L) till euvolemia, then infusion till target urine output 100–150 mL/hr	Onset 2–4 hour	Hydration improves GFR thereby improves calcium excretion
Loop diuretic (furosemide)	40–80 mg bolus then titrated to maintain urine output 100–150 mL/hr.	Onset within 1 hour	Calcium excretion. Recommended only if evidence of volume overload and after adequate hydration achieved
Calcitonin	4–8 IU/kg IM or SC every 6–8 hours	Onset 4–6 hours. Tachyphylaxis common after 2–3 days of use	Decrease renal calcium and phosphate reabsorption
Bisphosphonates	Zoledronate (4–8 mg IV) over 15 min or Pamidronate (60–90 mg IV) over 2–4 hours infusion	Onset of action 1–2 days. Repeat dose every 2–4 weeks	Inhibits osteoclastic bone resorption by attaching to hydroxyapatite binding sites on bony surface
Denosumab	60–120 mg SC	Onset within 3 days and half-life 25 days	Monoclonal antibody binds to NF-kB ligand (RANKL) and prevents its binding to RANK receptors on osteoclasts
Glucocorticoids	Prednisone 20–60 mg/day or equivalent	Onset 5–10 days	Effective for granulomatous disease and hematologic malignancy associated with hypercalcemia
Hemodialysis	Variable effect based on starting Ca^{2+} level	Immediate onset. Lasts till completion of dialysis	Useful for severe hypercalcemia. Diuretic-resistant volume overload which prevents saline administration

(IV: intravenous; IM: intramuscular; SC: subcutaneous; GFR: glomerular filtration rate)

Hypocalcemia may also occur in conditions associated with severe tissue injury such as burns, rhabdomyolysis, tumor lysis, or pancreatitis.

Clinical Features

Moderate to severe hypocalcemia is associated with paresthesias, usually of the fingers, toes, and circumoral regions and is due to increased neuromuscular irritability. On physical examination, a Chvostek's sign (twitching of the circumoral muscles in response to gentle tapping of the facial nerve just anterior to the ear) may be elicited, although it is also present in ~10% of normal individuals.

Carpal spasm may be induced by inflation of a blood pressure cuff to 20 mm Hg above the patient's systolic blood pressure for 3 minutes (Trousseau's sign). Severe hypocalcemia can induce seizures, carpopedal spasm, bronchospasm, laryngospasm, and prolongation of the QT interval.

Treatment

Acute, symptomatic hypocalcemia is initially managed with calcium gluconate, chronic hypocalcemia due to hypoparathyroidism can be treated with calcium supplements (1000–1500 mg/d elemental calcium in divided doses).

The treatment goal is to bring serum calcium into the low normal range and to avoid hypercalciuria, which may lead to nephrolithiasis.

Disorders of Magnesium

Magnesium is one of the major intracellular cation. Only 1% of total body magnesium remains in the extracellular fluid. Majority of total magnesium remains in the bone. Normal serum magnesium level ranges from 1.7–2.6 mg/dL (0.7–1.1 mmol/L or 1.4–2.2 mEq/L). Magnesium is essential for intracellular signaling and plays an important role for maintaining calcium and potassium homeostasis. Interplay between kidney, gastrointestinal tract and bone determines serum magnesium concentration.

Hypermagnesemia

As kidneys have enormous capacity to excrete magnesium, hypermagnesemia is not frequently encountered in clinical practice. Renal failure, unmonitored exogenous magnesium administration, increased absorption due to impaired gut motility or disorders of gastrointestinal tract are the scenarios where it is encountered. Severity of hypermagnesemia symptoms depends on its serum level. Neuromuscular and cardiovascular systems are predominantly affected by hypermagnesemia. **Table 55.8** represents clinical manifestations hypermagnesemia as per serum magnesium level. Management includes administration of calcium gluconate to stabilize the myocardium and stopping exogenous administration of magnesium. Appropriate hydration and diuretics can be helpful in patients with preserved urine output, where as patients with oliguria, renal failure or associated acid base and other electrolyte disorder needs dialysis support.

Hypomagnesemia

Hypomagnesemia is frequently encountered in ICU. Gastrointestinal loss, renal wasting and chelation are the causes of hypomagnesemia in critically ill patients. Gastrointestinal causes include loss due to fistula, diarrhea and prolonged nasogastric drainage and malabsorption. Renal tubular defects, postobstructive diuresis and drugs (diuretics, aminoglycosides, cisplatin, immunosuppressants, cetuximab) are the other

Table 55.8: Clinical manifestations of hypermagnesemia.

Serum magnesium (mg/dL)	Clinical features
5–8	Nausea, vomiting, lightheadedness, diminished deep tendon reflexes
9–12	Absent deep tendon reflexes, somnolence, ECG changes
12–15	Sinoatrial and ventricular node block, muscle paralysis, hypoventilation
>15	Asystole, respiratory paralysis, death

etiologies of hypomagnesemia. Symptoms occur with severe hypomagnesemia (<1.2 mg/dL). Neuromuscular signs and symptoms include lethargy, ataxia, confusion, nystagmus, tremor, fasciculations, tetany and seizure. Tachycardia, atrial and ventricular arrhythmias occur with severe hypomagnesemia. ECG shows prolonged PR and QT interval, widening of QRS. Torsade de pointes is the classical arrhythmia associated with hypomagnesemia. Asymptomatic mild hypomagnesemia can be treated with enteral therapy. Intravenous therapy includes 2–4 g of magnesium sulfate ($MgSO_4$).

Disorders of Phosphate

Phosphate is one of the major intracellular anion. Only 1% of total body phosphate remains in the extracellular space. About 85% of total body phosphate remains in the bone. Phosphate plays a vital role for bone formation. Phosphate is an important component of adenosine triphosphate (ATP), therefore crucial for cellular metabolism. Phosphate is present in red blood cell as 2,3-biphosphoglycerate there by plays an important role for oxygen affinity of hemoglobin and tissue oxygen delivery. Phosphate balance in the body is maintained and determined by parathyroid hormone, vitamin D and fibroblast growth factor 23 (FGF23). Normal serum phosphate level ranges from 0.8–1.4 mmol/L (2.5–4.3 mg/dL).

Hyperphosphatemia

Kidneys plays an enormous capacity to excrete phosphate, therefore hyperphosphatemia usually encountered with acute or chronic kidney damage. Chronic kidney damage often leads to secondary hyperparathyroidism leading to hyperphosphatemia. Vitamin D toxicity, milk-alkali syndrome, sarcoidosis, prolonged immobilization, osteolytic metastasis are other important causes of hyperphosphatemia. Transcellular shifting leading to hyperphosphatemia occurs with rhabdomyolysis, hemolysis and tumor lysis syndrome. Exogenous phosphate administration with laxatives and phosphate-containing enema can lead to hyperphosphatemia particularly in patients with concomitant kidney disease. In patients with normal kidney function, treatment with volume resuscitation lead to phosphate diuresis. In patients with deranged renal function, oral phosphate binders reduces phosphate absorption from the gastrointestinal tract. Patients with severely impaired renal function needs renal replacement therapy.

Hypophosphatemia

Vitamin D deficiency and primary hyperparathyroidism are important causes of hypophosphatemia. Clinically important causes in critically ill patients include gastrointestinal loss, renal wasting and transcellular shift of phosphate in insulin, refeeding syndrome and respiratory alkalosis. Renal replacement therapy used in ICU especially continuous modality can severely deplete serum phosphate level. Clinical manifestations ranges from muscular weakness, paresthesia. Respiratory insufficiency results with diaphragmatic muscle involvement. Phosphate depletion also leads to impaired cardiac contractility in critically ill patients. Treatment includes oral or intravenous phosphate replacement depending on severity of hypophosphatemia. Severe hypophosphatemia is (<1 mmol/L).

LAST-MINUTE REVISION

- Acidosis is said to occur when the arterial pH falls below 7.35, and alkalosis is present when it raises above 7.45.
- **Anion gap represents unmeasured anions in plasma and is calculated as:** $Na^+ + K^+ - (Cl^- + HCO_3^-)$ (normally it is 10–12 mmol/L)
- **Dose calculation of sodium bicarbonate:** 0.5 x Lean body weight x (desired $[HCO_3^-]$ - measured $[HCO_3^-]$)
- **Hyponatremia:** Plasma Na^+ concentration <135 mmol/L
- **Hypernatremia:** Plasma Na^+ concentration >145 mmol/L
- **Hypokalemia:** Plasma K^+ concentration <3.5 mmol/L
- **Hyperkalemia:** Plasma K^+ concentration >5.0 mmol/L
- **Hypercalcemia:** Calcium level >11 mg/dL
- **Hypocalcemia:** Ca^{2+} <8.5 mg/dL

REVIEW QUESTIONS

1. Normal anion gap metabolic acidosis is caused by:
    a. Cholera
    b. Starvation
    c. Ethylene glycol poisoning
    d. Lactic acidosis

2. A 50 kg man with severe metabolic acidosis has the following parameters: pH—7.05, pCO_2—32 mm Hg, pO_2—108 mm Hg, HCO_3—5 mEq/L, base excess—30 mEq/L. The approximate quantity of sodium bicarbonate that he should receive in half hour is:
    a. 250 mEq
    b. 350 mEq
    c. 500 mEq
    d. 750 mEq

3. The following condition is not associated with an increased anion-gap type of metabolic acidosis:
    a. Shock
    b. Ingestion of ante-freeze
    c. Diabetic ketoacidosis
    d. COPD

4. An ABG analysis shows: pH 7.2, raised pCO_2, decreased HCO_3; diagnosis is:
    a. Respiratory acidosis
    b. Compensated metabolic acidosis
    c. Respiratory and metabolic acidosis
    d. Respiratory alkalosis

5. Metabolic changes associated with excessive vomiting includes all of the following, *except*:
    a. Metabolic acidosis
    b. Hypochloremia
    c. Hypokalemia
    d. Decrease bicarbonates

6. Widened anionic gap is not seen in:
    a. Acute renal failure
    b. Diarrhea
    c. Lactic acidosis
    d. Diabetic ketoacidosis

7. A 2-year-old child is being evaluated for persistent metabolic acidosis. Blood gas as analysis shows Na^+—140 mEq/L, K^+—3 mEq/L, Ca^{2+}—8 mg/L, Mg^{2+}—2 mg/L, phosphate—3 mEq/L, pH—7.22, bicarbonate—16 mEq/L and chloride–112 mEq/L. The plasma anion gap is:
    a. 9
    b. 15
    c. 22
    d. 25

8. Hypochloremia hypokalemia and alkalosis are seen in:
    a. Congenital hypertrophic pyloric stenosis
    b. Hirschsprung's disease
    c. Esophageal atresia
    d. Jejunal atresia

9. ABG analysis of a patient shows PO_2—85 mm Hg, PCO_2—50 mm Hg, pH—7.2 and HCO_3—30 mEq/L. He is suffering from:
   a. Respiratory acidosis with compensatory metabolic alkalosis
   b. Respiratory acidosis with superimposed metabolic acidosis
   c. Metabolic acidosis
   d. Metabolic alkalosis

ANSWERS

1. a	2. a	3. d	4. c	5. a	6. b
7. b.	8. a	9. a			

Nutritional Support in Intensive Care Unit

Bhanuprakash Bhaskar, Anshul Jain

INTRODUCTION

In critically ill patients, nutritional status plays a key role in recovery. Metabolic and endocrine responses to critical illness shift from an anabolic state to a catabolic state characterized by the breakdown of essential protein, fat, and carbohydrates. The goals of nutrition support in intensive care unit (ICU) patients are to provide adequate calories and protein to replace ongoing catabolic processes, support wound healing, and promote immune function. In critically ill patients, nutrition is not as simple as starting feed after days of fasting; the consequences of initiate feeding in patients who have been starved for a period can be serious. Adding a large glucose load can cause a massive shift in intracellular electrolytes and reduce the serum level of these electrolytes. This phenomenon referred to as "refeeding syndrome," has serious consequences. Current chapter deals with the basic principles of ICU nutrition and the available choices of nutrition.

INDICATION OF NUTRITION SUPPORT

The assessment for timing of nutrition support should begin within 48 hours of admission to the intensive care unit (**Flowchart 56.1**), which includes.
- Poor nutritional status (NUTRIC score* ≥5 if IL-6 not included, ≥ 6 if IL-6 measured) **(Table 56.1)**
- Nonfunctional gastrointestinal tract
- Duration of starvation (> 7 day duration)
- Significant weight loss
- Gastrointestinal anomalies

*NUTRIC (Nutritional Risk in Critically Ill) Score to be performed in all patients admitted to ICU for whom volitional intake is considered insufficient. Risk assessment to be done within 48 hours of admission.

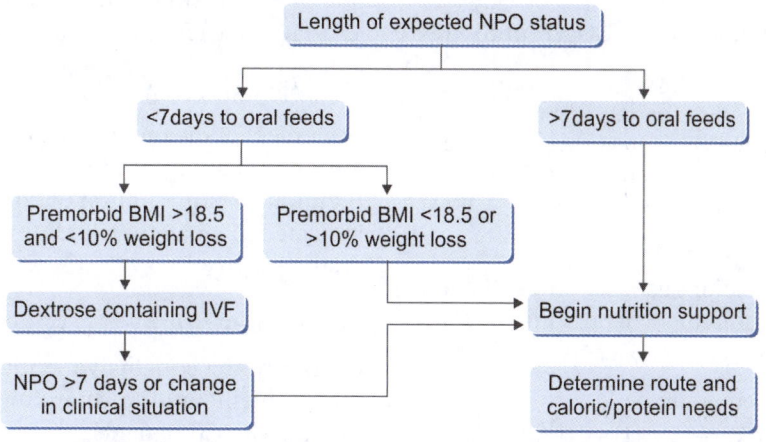

Flowchart 56.1: Timing of nutrition support (assessment should begin within 48 hours of admission to the intensive care unit)

(NPO: nil per oral; BMI: body mass index; IVF: intravenous fluids)

Table 56.1: Nutritional risk in critically ill- score.

Score variables	Range	Points
Age (years)	< 50	0
	50–<75	1
	>75	2
APACHE II score	<15	0
	15–<20	1
	>20	2
SOFA score	<6	0
	6–<10	1
	>10	2
Number of comorbidities	0–1	0
	>2	1
Days from hospital to ICU admit	0–<1	0
	>1	1

American Society of Parenteral and Enteral Nutrition recommends that nutritional support in the form of enteral nutrition be initiated within 24–48 hours in critically ill patients who cannot maintain volitional intake.

NUTRITION REQUIREMENT

Measuring the resting energy expenditure via indirect calorimetry for critically ill patients provides the most accurate estimate of energy requirement. Indirect calorimetry measures oxygen consumption and carbon dioxide production; then, energy expenditure is calculated using the Weir formula:

Energy expenditure (kcal/day) =
$3.941 \times VO_2$ (L/min) + $1.11 \times VCO_2$ (L/min) $\times 1440$

Note: The results of indirect calorimetry should be interpreted cautiously in certain clinical situations, such as physical agitation, unstable body temperature or pH, need for a high FiO_2 (>60%), and use of renal replacement therapy or extracorporeal membrane oxygenation (ECMO).

Out of several equations used for the estimation of resting energy requirement in humans, the Harris-Benedict equation is the most commonly used:

Harris-Benedict equation:
Men: $66 + (13.7 \times W) + (5 \times H) - 6.8 \times A$
Women: $665 + (9.6 \times W) + (1.8 \times H) - (4.7 \times A)$

W = Weight (in kg), H = Height (in cm), A = Age (in years)

However, this equation, too, becomes less efficient in critically ill patients. Only the Ireton-Jones equation is designed for use in the critically ill patient.

The clinical practice guidelines of the American Society of Parenteral and Enteral Nutrition and Society of Critical Care Medicine (ASPEN/SCCM) suggested the use of a predictive equation or a weight-based equation (25–30 kcal/kg/day) to estimate energy requirement in the absence of indirect calorimetry.

Target Protein Intake

- **Enteral**
  - Standard starting replacement dose 1.2–2 g/kg/day
  - Obesity 2.0–2.5 g/kg/day of ideal body weight
  - Renal replacement therapy 2.5 g/kg/day
- **Parenteral:** Standard starting replacement dose 0.8–1 g/kg/day.

Target Lipid Supplementation

- **Enteral:** Standard starting supplementation of fat will equate to 30% of total caloric intake
- **Parenteral:**
  - Standard starting replacement dose: 1 g/kg/week
  - TPN most commonly prescribed having 10–20% lipid emulsion formulas.

Vitamins and Minerals

Regardless of the method, vitamins and minerals are an essential component of the nutritional regimen. Supplemental vitamin B_{12} is often indicated in a patient with intestinal resection or gastric surgery.

Immunonutrition

Currently no conclusive evidence to support the supplementation of arginine, and fish oils routinely in ICU patients.

Note: For calculation of caloric requirement, glucose provides 3.4 kcal/g, protein provides 4 kcal/g, and fat provides 9 kcal/g.

Progressive Feeding

Early full enteral or parenteral feeding should not be used in critically ill patients but shall be prescribed within 3–7 days. In the early phase of acute illness, one should administer hypocaloric nutrition (not exceeding 70% of total energy expenditure). After day 3, caloric delivery can be increased up to 80–100% of total energy expenditure.

Routes of Nutrition

Once the decision to begin nutrition support has been made, the optimal route and delivery rate need to be determined (**Flowchart 56.2**). The enteral route is preferred over the parenteral route wherever possible. Enteral nutrition may protect gut mucosal integrity and reduce the chances of sepsis.

Enteral Nutrition

Enteral nutrition can be provided by nasogastric tube or nasoenteric tube. In the second type, the feeding tube is positioned in the small bowel up to the level of ligament of Treitz. The nasoenteric tube reduces the incidence of aspiration because the infusion is beyond pylorus.

The appropriate type of enteral feeding formula to use in ICU continues to be debated. In general, whole protein formulas are recommended unless symptoms of malabsorption are present, where the peptide-based product should be used. A standard polymeric isotonic (1–1.5 kcal/mL) formula is well tolerated by most ICU patients.

Multiple disease-specific enteral formulations exist for chronic liver failure, kidney failure, or

Flowchart 56.2: Determination of route and initiation of feeding.

```
Hemodynamically stable ──Yes──► Are any of the following present:
        │                         • Obstruction/active pseudo-obstruction
        No                        • High-output fistula
        ▼                         • Excessive vomiting/diarrhea
No nutrition support if           • Bowel perforation or ischemia
patient is on high-dose                          │
pressor support                                  No
                                                 ▼
                                         Start tube feeding
    Start TPN            ◄──Yes──                │
 reassess routinely for                          ▼
    TF eligibility                       Evaluate route of delivery

        Initiate small bowel feeds ◄──
                                      │
                                      │    Initiate gastric feeds
• Start at 10–20 mL/h                 │           │
• Advance 10 mL/hr q 4–8 h until      │           ▼
  goal achieved                       │    • For 1–1.5 cal/mL product, start at 100 mL q4h
• Minimal flush (water or NS)         │    • For 2 cal/mL product, start at 50 mL q4h
  30 mL q4h                           │    • Increase 50 mL q4–8h until goal is achieved
• If feeding solution is present in   │    • Minimal flush (water or NS) of 30 mL q4h
  gastric output, recheck tube       TF    • Hold—if gastric residual volume >150–250 mL,
  position via X-ray              held × 2   abdominal distention, or emesis

     Unable to acheve TF goal
         for >7 days
```

(TPN: total parenteral feeding; TF: tube feeding; NS: normal saline)

acute pancreatitis, but none have been proven to improve morbidity and mortality. The literature consistently illustrates that the early initiation (24–48 hours) of enteral supplementation has morbidity and mortality benefit in ICU. Bolus or continuous infusion feeding, both are equally effective in ICU. However, in high-risk patients or those shown to be intolerant to bolus gastric EN, delivery of EN should be switched to continuous infusion. Generally, feeding is started at 10–20 mL/hour and advanced by an additional 10–20 mL/hour until the calculated metabolic requirement is met. Suppose there is high gastric residual volume leading to feeding intolerance. In that case, erythromycin (3–7 mg/kg/day) or metoclopramide (10 mg 3–4 times/day), either enteral or intravenous, can be considered with dose adjustment based on the patient's renal, hepatic function and adverse effect profile of drugs.

Parenteral Nutrition

In case of contraindication to oral or enteral nutrition, parenteral nutrition should be initiated within 3–7 days. But, in severely malnourished patients, early or progressive parenteral nutrition can be provided instead of no nutrition in case of contraindication to enteral nutrition. Progressive parenteral nutrition includes starting with a low-calorie density parenteral regimen (e.g., 1000 kcal/day or even lower). A severely malnourished patient can be diagnosed with at least one of the criterion,

1. 50% intake of energy requirement for more than one week or severe malabsorption/GI symptoms.
2. Weight loss of more than 10% within the past six months or more than 20% beyond 6 months.
3. Body mass index less than 18.5 kg/m^2 if < 70 year, or; less than 20 kg/m^2 if older >70 year.
4. A severe deficit in muscle mass.

Additionally, the patients receiving <40% of their calculated caloric or protein requirement by enteral feeds even after 7–10 days of optimal treatment may require total parenteral nutrition.

Parenteral nutrition is usually administered via a central vein, owing to its wide caliber, which reduces the chance of thrombophlebitis; the subclavian vein is the most preferred central vein, while the femoral is the least preferred. ASPEN suggests that parenteral nutrition with an osmolality up to 900 mOsm/L may be administered peripherally; monitor closely for extravasation. Most critically ill patient need 1.5–2.5 g/kg/day of protein, dextrose administration should not exceed 3.0 mg/kg/minute (4.3 g/kg/day). The rest of the energy requirement is fulfilled by lipids. Administration of a large amount of dextrose can result in glucose intolerance, abnormal liver function tests, and fatty infiltration of the liver. Most current TPN formulation is prepared as fat emulsion; the addition of fat enhances the caloric value and reduces the volume of fluid. Maximum fat administration can be estimated as 2 g/kg/day. A standard TPN solution approximately provides 1 kcal/mL.

Complications of Parenteral Nutrition

- **Technical:**
  - Air embolus
  - Arterial laceration
  - Hydrothorax, hemothorax and pneumothorax
  - Injuries to arteries and veins
  - Catheter embolism, malposition
  - Injuries to the thoracic duct, brachial plexus
  - Thrombotic complications
  - Arteriovenous (AV) fistula
- **Infectious:**
  - Central line-related bloodstream infections
  - Exit-site infections/cellulitis
- **Metabolic complications:**
  - Azotemia
  - Essential fatty acid deficiency
  - Fluid overload [congestive cardiac failure (CCF)]
  - Metabolic bone disease
- Liver dysfunction
- Glucose imbalance
- Trace elements (like zinc) and vitamin deficiency
- Electrolyte abnormalities
- Hyperchloremic metabolic acidosis

LAST-MINUTE REVISION

- For calorie calculation in TPN dextrose provide 3.4 kcal/g.
- Enteric nutrition is preferred over parenteral nutrition whenever possible.
- For TPN, subclavian vein is the most preferred vein.

REVIEW QUESTIONS

1. For energy calculation in TPN, dextrose supplies:
   a. 4 kcal/g
   b. 10 kcal/day
   c. 3.4 kcal
   d. 9 kcal/day
2. Advantages of enteral feeding over parenteral feeding are all, *except*:
   a. Fewer chances of sepsis
   b. Cost-effective
   c. Fewer chances of water overload
   d. Can be used in patient with hemodynamic unstability
3. Most preferred vein for administration of TPN:
   a. Subclavian
   b. Axillary
   c. Femoral
   d. Internal jugular vein
4. Protein requirement for a patient who sustained 40% burn:
   a. 1 g/kg/day
   b. 2 g/kg/day
   c. 2.5 g/kg/day
   d. 4 g/kg/day

ANSWERS

1. c   2. d   3. a   4. c

CHAPTER 57

Brain Death

Keshav Goyal

INTRODUCTION

The term brain death was first pronounced in 1976 by the conference of Medical Royal Colleges in UK. In 1995, it was suggested to use the term "brainstem death" in spite of brain death, simultaneously first medical definition of death was proposed according to which death is defined as "the irreversible loss of the capacity for consciousness combined with the irreversible loss of the capacity to breath". The common cause of brain death are intracranial hemorrhage, traumatic brain injury, cerebral ischemia/anoxia.

Mechanism of Brain Death

Brain injury irrespective of source produces brain edema which is initially focal. Brain edema if not controlled progresses to involve the whole brain in a predictable sequence. Since brain is covered by rigid bony shell, the skull its edema is accompanied by raised intracranial pressure (ICP), which if sufficiently high exceeds arterial blood pressure (BP) and the cerebral circulation ceases. When cerebral circulation ceases aseptic necrosis of brain ensues. Within 3–5 days brain becomes a liquefied tissue mass a condition known as "respirator brain".

Following irreversible brain injury, the Intra Cranial Pressure (ICP) starts rising rapidly resulting in catecholamine surge and a massive release of proinflammatory and anti-inflammatory cytokines. The central sympathoadrenergic circulatory regulation disruption occurring after brain death causes disruption of hypothalamic-pituitary-adrenocortical function. Finally, loss of central regulatory mechanisms results in several pathophysiological alterations in hemodynamics, hormone balance, body temperature, and lung function. Various systemic manifestations are summarized in **Table 57.1**.

Table 57.1: Systemic changes following brain death.

System	Manifestations
Cardiovascular system	Bradycardia, tachycardia, hypertension, hypotension
Respiratory system	Neurogenic pulmonary edema, aspiration pneumonitis
Endocrine and metabolic	Diabetes insipidus, thyroid abnormality, hyperglycemia, hypothermia, electrolyte abnormalities
Others	Coagulopathy, active inflammatory response

Criteria and Tests for Determining Brain Death[1]

For diagnosing brain death in a person, we need to ascertain that the:
- Person is comatose and the cause of coma is known to be irreversible.
- All brainstem reflexes are absent.
- There is complete cessation of spontaneous respiration (Apnea). An important aspect of brain death diagnosis is to rule out confounding factors that interferes with clinical diagnosis of brain death.

These confounders are:
- Shock/hypotension
- Hypothermia
- Neurological abnormalities (i.e., brainstem encephalitis, Guillain Barre' syndrome, encephalopathy, neurotoxic snake envenomation)

- Metabolic causes like severe hypophosphatemia
- Medications like anesthetic agents, neuroparalytic drugs, opioids that can affect neurologic, neuromuscular function and electroencephalographic testing.

Raised ICP causes hypertension that is eventually followed by hypotension because of sudden interruption of vasomotor output from brainstem. Hypotension can further compromise circulation enough to cease electroencephalography (EEG) activity. Thus patient can be spuriously diagnosed as brain dead. Therefore, administration of vasopressors must be considered before performing tests in hypotensive individuals. Hypothermia diminishes EEG activity in linear manner and can lead to misdiagnosis of brain death. So body temperature to be normalized, before performing any diagnostic test for brain death.

DIAGNOSTIC TESTS FOR BRAIN DEATH

Following tests are usually employed to diagnose brain death:

Loss of Consciousness and Unresponsiveness

Patient should be in coma and scored as 3 on the Glasgow coma scale.

Absence of Brainstem Reflexes

The different brainstem reflexes that are tested are pupillary light reflex, corneal reflex, oculocephalic reflex (Doll's eye sign), oculovestibular reflex (caloric test), pharyngeal reflex and cough reflex. For diagnosis of brain death all of these brainstem reflexes must be absent. While checking for pupillary reflexes, pupil must be nonreacting to light irrespective to its size. It is the pupillary response to light and not the pupillary size that is used for brain death diagnosis.

Complete Cessation of Respiration

Complete cessation of respiration of the patient is another important aspect of brain death diagnosis. To test this "apnea test" is done wherein we attempt to stimulate the respiratory centers by increasing blood carbon dioxide level. In individuals with intact brainstem function, increase in blood carbon dioxide levels stimulates the medullary respiratory centers. There are certain prerequisites for apnea test. They are:

- Core temperature ≥36.5°C
- Euvolemia or positive fluid balance in the previous 6 hours
- Normal arterial oxygen and carbon dioxide levels.

Apnea Test

Apnea testing is mandatory for the determination of brain death and considered as the most important testing. During the apnea test, marked hypotension, or severe cardiac arrhythmias or both may occur so it is performed as the last test after the other tests fulfil the criteria of brain death.

Rationale: Normally respiratory center responds to CO_2 level in a linear manner and when respiratory center is damaged, its response to CO_2 level is lost.

After ruling out acid base abnormality and fulfilling the prerequisites, patient is first ventilated with 100% O_2 ($FiO_2 = 1$) for at least 10 minutes then ventilation is stopped. With time CO_2 starts building up and if at $PaCO_2$ greater than 60 mm Hg or > 20 mm Hg above the baseline values and there is no respiratory movement, test result is said to be positive or/and it supports the diagnosis of brain death.

In adults, the brainstem reflexes are to be tested twice with a minimum 6 hours between the tests. However, the gap between two sets of brainstem reflexes testing should be 12–24 hours in case of children.

Ancillary Tests

Brain death is essentially a clinical diagnosis and ancillary tests are not part of routine brain death diagnosis. Ancillary tests have a role in brain death diagnosis only when certain clinical tests done for brain death diagnosis are either could not be performed or could not be reliably interpreted. Ancillary tests do not replace clinical assessment for brain death. The different ancillary tests used for brain death confirmation are EEG, cerebral angiography, transcranial Doppler and scintigraphy.

CERTIFICATION

A panel of 4 doctors is needed for brain death certification. They are the doctor in charge of the patient, the doctor in charge of the hospital where the patient was treated, an independent specialist of unspecified specialty (physicians, surgeons, or intensivists) nominated from the panel of names approved by the appropriate authority, and a neurologist or neurosurgeon.

REFERENCE

1. Goila AK, Pawar M. The diagnosis of brain death. Indian J Crit Care Med. 2009;13(1):7-11.

REVIEW QUESTIONS

1. Brainstem reflexes include all, *except*:
    a. Oculocephalic reflex
    b. Knee jerk
    c. Corneal reflex
    d. Cough reflex
2. Perfect mimic of brain death:
    a. Hypothermia
    b. Deaf and dumb condition
    c. Opioid poisoning
    d. Barbiturate poisoning

ANSWERS

1. b   2. a

CHAPTER 58

Ethics Related to Anesthesia and Critical Care Practice

Pradeep Kumar Bhatia, Pooja Bihani, Priyanka Sethi

Despite technological advances, a humanized practice of medicine must be the cornerstone of teaching curriculum to all medical students. Anesthesiologist being a perioperative physician and intensive care expert has multidimensional role in patient management, increasing the scope of ethical practices. Ethical concerns for anesthesiologist are unique and vary from taking a valid informed consent during perioperative period to decision regarding end-of-life care in intensive care unit (ICU).[1]

BASIC PRINCIPLES OF MEDICAL ETHICS[2]

1. **Beneficence:** Physician should have intention of doing good to the patient.
2. **Nonmaleficence:** Physician should not do unnecessary harm to patient.
3. **Autonomy:** The patient should have full autonomy and make independent decisions regarding his/her own health.
4. **Justice:** There should be fair distribution of resources and potential conflicts should be dealt as per the law.

Ethical Aspects will be Discussed in Following Subsections

1. Perioperative period
2. Ethics in intensive care unit (ICU)

Every practicing physician/anesthesiologist has ethical responsibilities towards his patients/profession as per by code of ethics.

1. Perioperative Period[3]

I. Preoperative Period

Thorough evaluation and optimization of the surgical patient is one of the core responsibilities of an anesthesiologist. Being a perioperative physician, an effective communication is very essential to establish a good rapport with the patient. During preanesthetic evaluation patient should be involved in the process of informed decision-making. All aspects of various possible anesthesia techniques including both benefits and complications should be explained to patients.

- **Informed consent:** An informed written consent is a legal document about all relevant aspects of a proposed treatment and all other available alternative options. Consent is to agree for a particular type of procedure/anesthesia/ knowing the benefits and risks involved. It is the patient's right to choose the type of anesthesia, and procedure with informed risks and benefits. Components of informed consent:
  - Disclosure: All the relevant information must be shared during decision making and the patient must be informed about all the aspects of treatment.
  - Comprehension: It must be explained and documented in the patient's own language.
  - Competence: If patient is mentally sound, conscious and above 18 years of age, can give consent.
  - If the patient is a minor, unconscious, under influence of drugs, mentally unsound, a proxy consent should be obtained.
  - In blanket consent, signature is taken on printed document without mentioning type of procedure/treatment and is legally invalid.
  - A legally acceptable consent should be signed by patient and two independent witness.

II. Intraoperative Period

The patient should be re-explained about the planned invasive procedure. Since the patients are anesthetized/sedated intraoperatively, it is the duty of the caregivers to treat the patient with dignity and respect.

There should be good interprofessional communication in the operating room or ICU. A cooperative and respectful relationship among professional colleagues, to facilitate quality medical care for patients is essential.

Many potentially dangerous and narcotic substances are used by anesthesiologists during perioperative period. It is a part of anesthesiologist ethical practice to keep these substances secure from illicit use. There are proper guidelines regarding storage and dispensing of narcotic drugs by competent authorities.

III. Postoperative Period

Anesthesiologist as a perioperative physician has ethical responsibility of managing postoperative pain, nausea and vomiting or any other adverse event till the patient is being shifted to surgical ward from recovery.

- **Documentation and record keeping:** The documentation of perioperative events is ethical responsibility of anesthesiologist and may prove to be the best tool during legal proceedings. Many societies including Indian Society of Anesthesiologists (ISA) have published guidelines for good record keeping.
- Every fine detail pertaining to patient and its clinical condition and his perioperative course along with instructions must be documented in a clear and self-explanatory language. All the medical records of indoor patients should be maintained for at least three years. If patient or legal authority requests to access medical records, then document should be issued within 72 hours. It is the right of the patient to ask for the records and the duty of the caregivers to provide the same.
- **Death on the table concerns:** In case, death on table encounters, a shared responsibility between surgeons and anesthetists become important. The cause and the measures taken should be clearly documented. The preoperative patient condition and its documentation become very crucial in this scenario. In a sick patient where the untoward events are anticipated, relatives must be informed and a consent must be taken in the advance. Panic should be avoided in such situation and there should be no fabrication of the medical records. The death news should be communicated to the relatives with empathy.

2. Ethics in ICU

Critical care physicians may face many ethical dilemmas as these patients are mostly sick and may be in moribund condition.[4] So informed consent, record keeping, shared decision making and empathy becomes very important. The concept of shared decision making between patients/relatives and intensivist is often more complicated in the ICU, because many times patients are too sick to make decisions. In such situation, patients and relatives should take decision in their maximum capacity after discussion with treating physician. Surrogate decision making is often important in ICU where some other responsible person has to take decisions when patient is not capable.

Transfer of the patient to higher center for treatment, providing good quality care, mentioning the cause of death, decision of withdrawal of treatment, do not resuscitate consideration, expert testimony in court of law, organ donation and determination of neurological death are other special concerns of critical care ethics.[5]

CONCLUSION

The evolving ramifications of anesthesia as a specialty has put forward many ethical and legal responsibilities. Anesthesiologist deals with various sensitive and ethical aspects of medicine and end of life care. A more proactive, practical and contextual approach is needed when dealing with these patients. Learning, sustaining and assessment of competencies in ethics and medical morality are equally important.

Chapter 58: Ethics Related to Anesthesia and Critical Care Practice

 LAST-MINUTE REVISION

- Ethical aspects with anesthesiologist has unique set of challenges both in operating room and ICU.
- Most of the potential conflicts can be settled if basic principles of medical ethics are followed.
- A well-informed written consent for anesthesia allows patient to make autonomous decisions substantially and prevents anesthesiologist from potential conflicts.

REFERENCES

1. Shinde SS, Parakh SC, Bhati S, Sahay N, Singh Battu G. Medico-legal and ethical issues in anaesthesiology profession. Indian J Anaesth. 2021;65:54-60.
2. Editorial team. The Indian Medical Council (Professional Conduct, Etiquette and Ethics) Regulations, 2002. Indian J Med Ethics 2002; 10:66. Available from https://ijme.in/articles/the-Indian-medical-council-professional-conduct-etiquette-and-ethics-regulations-2002.
3. Guidelines for the Ethical Practice of Anesthesiology. Available from: https://www.asahq.org/standards-and-guidelines/guidelines-for-the-ethical-practice-of-anesthesiology.
4. Harvey DJR, Gardiner D. 'MORAL balance' decision-making in critical care. BJA Educ. 2019;19:68-73.
5. Rao NG. Ethics of medical practice. In: Textbook of Forensic Medicine and Toxicology (2nd edn). New Delhi: Jaypee Brothers Medical Publishers (P) Ltd.; 2010. p. 23-44.

REVIEW QUESTIONS

1. Medical records (electronic/manual) are subjected to disclosure and confidentiality requirements?
   a. True
   b. False
2. A 36-years-old male patient is tested positive for HIV during preoperative investigations. He asks not to disclose this information to his wife. What will be your next step?
   a. Encourage patient to share information on his own
   b. Inform patient that his wife is also at serious risk of acquiring infection
   c. Inform patient that public health department requires reporting of both patient and his/her sexual partners
   d. All of the above
3. Which of the following is true regarding legal responsibility of a researcher for conducting a clinical trial?
   a. It is mandatory to register the clinical trial under "Clinical Trial Registry of India" after completion of the trial.
   b. Ethical issues are considerably low in clinical trials when compared with descriptive studies.
   c. Informed consent is must for recruiting study participants in clinical trial.
   d. Both a and c
4. A 13-year-old child is undergoing left inguinal hernia surgery. Which of the following is true regarding informed consent in this scenario?
   a. A well-informed written consent for anesthesia and surgery from parents/legal guardian is sufficient.
   b. The child can give consent for his surgery under anesthesia, if parents/legal guardian refuses for the surgery.
   c. If child gives consent for his surgery under anesthesia, parental consent is not necessary.
   d. Both the parental consent and child assent is required for his surgery under anesthesia.
5. A hospitalized person does not wish to have CPR if need arises, which legal document needs to be signed for this?
   a. Do not attempt resuscitation
   b. Informed consent
   c. Advanced directive or living will
   d. Declaration of anatomical gift

ANSWERS

| 1. a | 2. d | 3. c | 4. d | 5. c |

INDEX

Page numbers followed by *b* refer to box, *f* refer to figure, *fc* refer to flowchart, and *t* refer to table.

A

Abdomen, blocks of 221, 227
Abortion 86
Abruptio placentae 344
Acarbose 265
Accidental dural puncture 342
Acetaminophen 375
Acetate methyl 140
Acetylcholine 108, 139, 139*f*
    containing synaptic vesicles, exocytosis of 139
    molecules of 139, 140
    receptor, structure of 139*f*
    release 140
Acid-base
    disturbances 432, 433*t*, 436
    homeostasis, normal 432
    imbalance 432
    managements 416
    state 150
Acid-base disorders
    diagnosis of 433
    mixed 434
Acid-fast bacilli samples 243
Acidic environment 132
Acidic solutions 100
Acidosis 197, 246, 272, 412, 432
Activated coagulation time 175
Activated partial thromboplastin time 186, 246, 247
Acute air embolism, management of 317
Acute respiratory distress 5
    syndrome 97, 401
Acyanotic heart disease 239
Acyanotic lesion 239
Adaptive support ventilation 406
Additional radicular arteries 205
Adenosine
    monophosphate 265
    triphosphate 101, 185, 444
Adequate illumination, provision for 354
Adequate relaxation 424
Adequate spontaneous ventilation consistently 217
Adrenal gland 268
Adrenal insufficiency 268
Adrenaline 154, 155, 157, 264
    effects 155*f*
    primary indication of 154
Adrenergic agonists 121
Adrenocorticotropic hormone 268, 342

Advanced cardiac life support 198
Advanced cardiovascular life support 420, 421, 425
Agent specification 43
Agonist 101, 120
    clinical pharmacology of 119
Agonist antagonist
    compounds, hemodynamic effects of 118*t*
    opioids 120
    synthetic 116
Air
    confirms, aspiration of 224
    embolus 450
    entry, prevent 317
    oxygen blender 395
    sampling 35
Airway 284, 314, 347, 427
    anesthetizing 229
    devices, sterilization of 69
    dilating 241
    local anesthesia of 223
    maneuvers, manual 60, 60*f*
    pediatric 348*f*
    risk, assessing 58
Airway algorithm 283*f*
    emergency difficult 284
Airway assessment 58
    preoperative ultrasonographic 73
    tests, specific 59
Airway fire
    prevent 302
    protocol 303
Airway management 58, 60
    equipment for 60
Airway pressure 405
    monitoring 170
Aladin cassette vaporizer 44
Albumin 180, 252
Alcuronium 9, 147, 271
Alfentanil 120, 269
Alkali therapy 435
Alkaline, highly 100
Alkalosis 197, 432
Alkyl-phenols 103
Allergies 132
Alogliptine 265
Alpha-amino-3-hydroxy-5-methylisoxazole-4-propionic acid 108
Alpha-aminolevulinic acid synthetase 100
Alternative medicine therapies 379

Alveolar collapse, prevents 407
Alveolar concentration 82, 83
    minimum 81, 82*f*, 337
Alveolar flooding hamper gas diffusion 417
Alveolar ventilation 83
Alzheimer's disease 255
    pathogenesis of 86
Amantadine 255
Ambulatory surgery 357
Amethocaine hydrochloride 133
Amide 126, 133, 135
    group 133
Aminoglycosides 443
Aminophylline 243
Amiodarone 428
Amitriptyline 379
    hydrochloride 379
Ammonium ion, excretion of 432
Amnesia 99
Amygdalohippocampectomy 317
Amyloid, generation of 86
Analgesia 87, 99, 119, 308
    inhaled 339
    mechanism of 116
    postoperative 242
Analgesic 357
    action 116
    activity, maximum 87
    ladder 376*f*
    systemic 375
Analyze rhythm 425
Anaphylaxis 155
Ancillary tests 453
Anemia 168, 245, 272
    cause of 245
Anemic hypoxia 391
Anerobic metabolism 412
Anesthesia 1, 12, 96, 112, 154, 267, 271, 272, 288, 291, 292, 296, 299, 455
    basics of 1
    breathing system 47
    caudal 216
    choice of 234, 235, 242, 266, 341, 357
    closed circuit 54
    depth of 174
    duration of 127
    fitness for 26
    geriatric 331
    history of 8
    hypotensive 359, 360*t*
    induction of 109, 112, 234, 256

infiltration 128
inhalational 8, 56, 81, 83f, 85, 326
intraoperative 3
intravenous 9, 99, 250, 333
low flow 54
maintenance of 109, 112, 328
management of 238, 239, 268, 344
monitoring under 161
obstetric 335
outpatient 357
outside operating room 354
pediatric 347
pharmacology 79
practice 135, 279
regional 8, 201, 242, 248, 256, 308, 339, 351, 377
stages of 9, 10t
  general 9f
technique 294
topical 129, 289, 376
tumescent 129
workstation 36f
Anesthesia machine 36, 41, 45
  anatomy of 36
  standards for 36
  testing 41
Anesthesiology 354
Anesthetic agent 87, 105, 114, 262, 271, 311t
  effect of 311
Anesthetic care, comprehensive 221
Anesthetic considerations 299, 350
Anesthetic drugs 154, 250, 250f, 261, 338
  pharmacology of 333
Anesthetic gas 90
  analysis 169
Anesthetic implications 335-337
Anesthetic management 74, 234, 235, 237, 250, 274, 281, 288, 291, 292, 295, 307, 312, 315, 333, 344, 351, 352, 357
  principles of 246
Anesthetic potency 127
Anesthetic properties 88, 90, 92
Anesthetic techniques 293, 307
Anesthetic uptake factors 83
Anesthetic uses 102, 119
Anesthetic vapors, analysis of 169
Aneurysm repair surgery 122
Angina pectoris, mild 233
Angiotensin-converting enzyme 74, 234
  inhibitors 235
Anion gap 434
  causes of reduced 434
Ankle block 229
  needle insertion for 229f
Anoxia 452
Antagonist 120, 150
Antecubital vein 103
Anterior spinal artery 204
  syndrome, causes of 205
Antianalgesic action 101
Antibiotics, interactions with 149
Anticholinergic agents 242, 255
Anticholinesterase 150
  dose of 150
  interactions with 143

Anticipated difficult airway 281
Anticoagulants 74, 248
Anticoagulation, reversal of 324
Anticonvulsant 379
  therapy, chronic 254
Antidepressants 75
Antiemetics drugs 76, 104, 157, 292
Antiepileptic drugs, interactions with 149
Antiepileptic property 101
Antihypertensive agents 234
Antistatic rubber 45
Antituberculous therapy 243
Antoine-Laurent lavoisier 391
Anxiolysis 99, 112
Anxiolytic agent 234
Aortic aneurysm repair 359
Aortic regurgitation 238
Aortic stenosis 237
Apnea 214
  double 102
  test 453
Arachnoid mater lies 205
Argon 307
Armored tubes 63
Arrhythmia 131, 166, 255
Arrhythmogenic effect 142
Arteria radicularis magna 205
Arterial blood 168
  gas 401
    analysis 170
  pressure 161
  sampling 162, 175
Arterial CO_2 tension, control of 432
Arterial filter 321
Arterial hypoxemia 239
  chronic 239
Arterial laceration 450
Arterial oxygen
  content 391b
  saturation 413, 429
Arterial pH, systemic 432
Arterial pulsations 168
Arterial puncture 164
Arterial tonometry 162
Arterial venous blood, analysis of 169
Arteriovenous
  fistula 450
  malformation 317
Artery disease 5
Arthroscopy 295
Artificial airway 400
Artificial hibernation 114
Artificial invasive airway device 406
Ascites 251
Aspiration 356
  prophylaxis 343
  reduce chances of 76
Aspirin 248
Assist-controlled mode ventilation 403, 405f
Asthma 242
Asthmatic patient 104, 239, 242
Asystole 427
Atelectasis 242
  postoperative 243
Atlanto-occipital joint 64f

Atmospheric contamination 302
Atracurium 144, 151, 269, 301, 358
  metocurine 312
Atropine 76, 151, 212, 242, 269
Autoimmune disorders 258
Autologous blood 191
Autologous epidural blood patch 213
Automated external defibrillator 421, 425
Autonomic effects 131
Autonomic ganglionic blockade 147
Autonomic preganglionic B fibers 207
Autonomous hyperaldosteronism 435
Autoregulation 310
Awake fiberoptic intubation 282
  contraindications for 282
  indications for 282
Awake intubation, prerequisite for 284
Axillary approach 224f
Axillary artery pulsation 225
Azotemia 251

B

Back pressure, intermittent 44
Backache 213
Bag mask ventilation 425
Bain circuit 51, 51f
Balanced bicarbonate buffered solution 193
Balanced electrolyte solution 193
Baralyme 55
Barbiturate 99, 234, 271
  receptor 101f
Baricity 211
Barometric pressure 83
Barotrauma 408
Basal metabolic rate 174, 267
Basal narcosis 102
Basic life support 198, 345, 420-422
  algorithm, adult 423f
  assessment 422
  steps of 422t
Batson venous plexus 205
Bedside pulmonary function test 25
Behavioral changes 373
Benzodiazepines 75, 101f, 104, 110, 111, 111t, 112, 122, 147, 234, 269, 271
  antagonists 111
  competitive antagonist 113
  metabolites of 110
Benzylisoquinolinium class 144
Bernoulli effect 395
Beta-adrenergic agonist 242
Beta-blocker 128, 235, 294, 315
  esmolol 141
  phenoxybenzamine 269
Beta-hydroxylase 114
Beta-receptor 331
Betya-adrenergic agonist 242
Bezold-Jarisch reflex 224
Bier's block 128, 135
Biguanides 265
Bile salts deposition 252
Bilevel positive airway pressure 406, 410
  modes of 407
Biliary disorders 252
Bispectral index 111, 174, 176, 197

Index

Bisphosphonates 442
Bisquaternary muscle relaxant 146
Bivona tube 303
Bladder
  irrigation solution, volumes of 437
  perforation 300
  tumor, transurethral resection of 212
Bleeding 300
  control of local 155
  reduce intraoperative 360
Blocking catecholamine 208
Blocking N-methyl-D-aspartate receptor 107
Blood
  administration 185
  banks, association of 190
  collection of 192
  component, transfusion guidelines for 186t
  components 185
  concentration of 129, 192
  content of 311
  donation, preoperative autologous 191
  flow, reduced 168
  infusing unwashed 193
  salvaged unwashed 194b
  storage of 185
  treatment of collected 192
  viscosity, decreasing 181
  volume, less 102
Blood gas
  analysis 169, 170, 416
  partition coefficient 83
Blood loss 183, 184, 188, 190, 245, 272
  acute 184
  extreme 193
  major 191
  maximum allowable 246
  monitoring 174
  perioperative 190
  replacing 184
Blood management 190
  safe patient 191f
Blood pressure 105, 118, 162, 255, 359, 416, 452
  diastolic 161, 233
  invasive 162
  management, intraoperative 234
  monitor 3, 176
  systolic 233, 314, 443
    arterial 161
Blood salvage
  contraindications of perioperative 190, 191t
  indications of perioperative 191t
  perioperative 190
  system 193f
  techniques 190
Blood salvage strategies
  intraoperative 191
  plays 194
  postoperative 191
Blood sugar 264
  random 73
  test, random 263
Blood transfusion 178, 184
  intraoperative 245t
  risk and complications with 190t
Blood-brain barrier 255
Bloody tap 211
Blunt Atkinson needle 288
Blunt sympathetic response 99
Blurred vision 157
Body
  fluid compartment of 178f
  mass index 5, 274, 447
  temperature 452
Bone cement implantation syndrome 297
Bone determines serum magnesium concentration 443
Brachial block 229
  peripheral 225
Brachial plexus block 103, 129, 223, 224, 224f
  technique for 225
Bradyarrhythmias 420
Bradycardia 132, 148, 207, 252, 256, 263
  initial 256
  severe 224
Brain
  injury, traumatic 314, 452
  mask 61
  physiology 311
  tissue 312
Brain death 364, 452, 452t
  certification 454
  diagnostic tests for 453
  donation after 363, 364b
  mechanism of 452
  tests for 452
Brainstem
  death 452
  encephalitis 452
  reflexes 452
    absence of 453
  stimulation 316
Branchial block approach 225
Breath
  holding time 25
  loss of capacity to 452
  promotes spontaneous 405
  rescue 424
  types of 404
Breathing 22f, 314
  circuit 398
    incompetent valves of 169
  mechanics 20
  trail, spontaneous 409
Breathing system 47
  absorber 53
  classification of 47, 47t
  vaporizer inside 42
Bronchial tree 18
Bronchoalveolar lavage 326
Bronchodilation 123
Bronchodilator 108, 242
Bronchopleural fistula 326
Bronchopulmonary segments 19, 20t
Bronchoscope 285f
  technique of insertion of 285f
Bronchospasm 95, 243
  active 242
  intraoperative 242
Bubble through 42
Bupivacaine 128, 130, 131, 134, 135, 210, 226
  blood levels of 129
  cardiotoxicity 131
  commercial 134
Buprenorphine 121, 271
Burn 143, 149, 179, 187
Burning pain, sudden severe 103
Butorphanol 117, 120, 267, 271
Butyrylcholinesterase 141
  inhibition of 143
Bypass vaporizer, variable 44

C

Calcitonin 442
Calcium 322
  channels 108
  chloride 55
  concentrations reduce, increasing 149
  disorders of 441
  hydroxide 54
    lime 55
  interactions with 149
  sulfate 55
Calculating fluid requirement 184
Caloric test 453
Calorie calculation 451
Calorimetric method 174
Canaglifozin 265
Cancer
  cells 193
  pain 380
    management, ladder for 380f
Capillary bleeding 155
Capnogram, shape of expired 168
Capnography 65, 168
  continuous analysis 176
Carbamazepine 379
Carbon dioxide 37, 47, 302, 304
  absorbent 54
    complications of 56
  partial pressure of 417
  retention, risk of 405
  transport 28
Carbon monoxide 25, 56, 87
  production 56
Carboxyhemoglobinemia 168
Cardiac anesthesiologists 198
Cardiac arrest 214, 350, 420, 428
  algorithm, adult 426fc
  recognition of 423
Cardiac arrhythmias 305
  provoke 436
  severe 453
Cardiac catheterization procedures 355
Cardiac complications 294
Cardiac disease 108
  risk factors for 233
  severe 234
Cardiac dysfunction, postoperative 197
Cardiac effects, direct 131
Cardiac failure 187
Cardiac index 413
Cardiac intervention 430
Cardiac issues 197

Index

Cardiac output 83, 94, 167
   increased 83
   reduces 408
Cardiac surgery 166, 194, 359
   anesthetic management of 322
Cardiac tamponade 108
Cardiogenic pulmonary edema 397, 401
Cardiomyopathy 251
Cardioplegia solution 322
Cardiopulmonary bypass 162, 320, 322
   termination of 324
Cardiopulmonary resuscitation 6, 420, 421*t*
   high-quality 424*b*, 428
   monitoring during 429
   principles of 131
Cardiorespiratory depression 102
Cardiothoracic procedures 114
Cardiothoracic surgery
   anesthesia for 320
   major 122
Cardiotomy suction 321
Cardiovascular changes 336*t*
Cardiovascular disease 114, 233
   anesthesia for 233
Cardiovascular effects 141, 307
Cardiovascular manifestations 207
Cardiovascular monitoring 161
Cardiovascular risk, increased
   perioperative 233, 233*b*
Cardiovascular stable, highly 144
Cardiovascular system 71, 88, 91, 92, 101, 106, 108, 111, 114, 117, 122, 130, 331, 275, 335, 349, 408, 443
   disorders 109
   effects on 105
   toxicity 131
Carina 286
   level of 285*f*
   placement 327*f*
Carinal hook 327
Carlen's and Robertshaw tube 327*f*
Carlens tube 327*f*
Carrier gas composition 44
Catecholamine 269
Cauda equina 204
   syndrome 214
Caudal block 203, 218, 377
   complications of 217
   technique 217*f*
Caudal epidural 216
Celecoxib 357
Celiac plexus blocks 227
Cell
   redistribution into 439
   saver 192
Cell salvage 192
   advantages of 192*t*
   disadvantages of 192*t*
Cellular cyclic adenosine monophosphate 116
Cellular debris 193
Central nervous system 76, 81, 88, 100, 105, 107, 111, 113, 116, 121, 130, 146, 148, 337, 349, 409, 432
   function 434
   manifestation 251

   stimulation 121
   toxicity 130
Central neural blockade 129
Central neuraxial blockade 203, 206, 207*f*, 214, 218, 250, 297, 377
Central sensitization 372
Central sterile supply department 33
Central venous
   cannulation requires 164
   catheterization 165*t*
   catheters, peripherally inserted 165
   oxygen saturation 429
   pressure 163, 165, 238, 252, 307, 412
Centrilobular necrosis 91
Cerebral aneurysm repair 359
Cerebral angiography 454
Cerebral blood flow 92, 101, 123, 310, 311
   regulation of 310
Cerebral edema 187
Cerebral ischemia 452
Cerebral metabolic rate 94, 100, 117, 123, 311
Cerebral metabolism 310
   ketamine increases 107
   rate 310
Cerebral perfusion pressure 113, 310
Cerebral pharmacology 310
Cerebral physiology 310, 311*t*
Cerebral protection 323
Cerebral vascular accident 5
Cerebrospinal fluid 205, 206, 311, 313
Cerebrovascular disease 254, 359
Cervical 203
   epidural 215
   nerve roots 203
   plexus
      blockade 222, 222*f*
      superficial 222, 222*f*
   vertebrae, lower 64*f*
Cesarean section, anesthesia for 341
Cetuximab 443
Chassaignac tubercle 223
Chemical reactions 55
Chemoreceptor trigger zone 89, 118
Chest
   physiotherapy 417
   raise, visible 424
   X-ray 73
Chest compression 317, 424, 427
   efficiency of 424
   fraction 427
   technique of 424
Child-Pugh criteria 251*t*
Child-Pugh score 250
Chirocaine 134, 135
Chloride
   channel 101*f*
      complex 101*f*
   deficiency 435
Chloroform 96, 155, 264
Chloroprocaine 130, 133
Chlorpromazine 114
Chlorpropamide 265
Choline 140
Cholinesterase inhibitors 259
Chondrodendron tomentosum 144

Chronic obstructive pulmonary disease 5, 21, 22, 62, 90, 102, 117, 243, 381, 397, 400, 403, 407
   ventilation of 407
Chronic pain syndromes, management of 221
Chronic respiratory
   ailments 400
   alkalosis 436
Chvostek's sign 443
Cinchocaine number 141
Circulatory death 363
   donation after 363, 364*t*
Cisatracurium 146, 151, 235, 251, 262, 272, 301, 358
Cisplatin 443
Citrate phosphate dextrose 185
Classic™ laryngeal mask airway 61
Claustrophobia 318
Clean and dirty utility room 388
Clonidine 122, 157, 376
Clostridia 97
Clot formation, rate of 175
Clot strength, monitoring of 252
Coagulation abnormalities 251
Coagulation factor disorders 246
Coagulopathy 300
   dilutional 182
Cocaine 130, 132
   inhibits 131
   stimulates 132
Coccygeal vertebrae 203
Code blue 425*b*
Cold intolerance 266
Colloid 180, 180*t*, 181*t*, 182, 252, 416
Color coding 45
Coma 256, 439
Combined spinal epidural
   analgesia 341
   anesthesia 296, 297
   technique 342
Combitube 62
Comorbid disease 429
Compartment syndrome 227
Complete blood count 72
Complex regional pain syndrome 373, 380, 382
Congestive cardiac failure 450
Congestive heart failure 73, 83, 336
Conjuctival congestion 223
Consciousness
   altered 268
   loss of 99, 453
Constipation 266
Constricting penile artery 228
Continuous positive airway pressure 405*f*, 406, 410
Continuous wave capnography 427
Cordotomy 380
Coronary artery 5
   bypass surgery, off-pump 324
   disease 263, 322
Coronary perfusion pressure 429
Coronoid notch 222
Cough, inability to 148
COVID-19 12, 391
   pandemic 197

Index

Cranial nerve
   except 213
   palsy 213
Cricothyroid membrane 224
Cricothyrotomy 67
Critical care 3, 383
   practice 455
   services 388
   specialty 14*t*
   unit 7
Critical illness
   myopathy 148
   polyneuropathy 148
Critical temperature 96
Critically ill, nutritional risk in 448*t*
Cryoprecipitate 186*t*, 187
Crystalloids 179, 181*t*, 182, 416
   excessive 252
   fluids 179*t*
Cushing's disease 263, 268, 318
Cushing's reflex 311
Cushing's syndrome 268
Cyanosis 305
Cyanotic disease 239
Cyanotic heart disease 104, 122
Cyclizine 157
Cyclooxygenase 248, 376
Cyclopropane 95, 96, 155
Cylinder valves 39
Cystoscopy 299
Cytochrome P450 system 118

D

Dapagliflozin 265
Daycare surgery 104
   anesthesia for 357
   patients suitable for 357
Dead space 23, 54
   effect of anesthetics on 23
   physiological 23*fc*
   ventilation, decrease 396
Decamethonium 9, 151
Deep cervical plexus 222
   block 222*f*
Deep peroneal nerve 229
Deep pressure fibers 207
Deep vein thrombosis 74, 294, 417
Degenerative disease 255
Dehydration 102, 246
Deleterious effects 117
Delirium 294
Deliver shock automatically 423
Demyelinating disease 255
Denosumab 442
Deoxygenated hemoglobin absorbed 167
Dephlogisticated air 391
Depression 256, 332
Desalination, process of 437
Desflurane 94, 237, 250, 251, 261, 272, 328, 358
   chlorine atom 94
Desipramine 379
Despite technological advances 455
Dexamethasone 157

Dexmedetomidine 121, 122, 376
Dextromethorphan 376
Dextrose 272
   normal saline 180
Diabetes 272
   complications of 263*t*
   mellitus 5, 263
   multisystem manifestation of 264*f*
Diabetic ketoacidosis, insulin deficiency in 440
Diabetic neuropathy 379
Diameter index safety system 40
Diaphoresis 299
Diaphragm 401
Diaphragmatic hernia, congenital 352
Diazepam 107, 110, 112, 267
   facilitate 101
   metabolism of 112
Dibucaine 135
   inhibits expression 141
   number 135, 141, 141*t*
      estimation 141
Dichloroacetylene 87, 95
Diethylbarbituric acid 99
Difficult airway 281*t*
   anesthesia for 281
Diffusion hypoxia 85
Diisopropylphenol 103
Diltiazem 157
Dipeptidyl peptidase 265
Diphenhydramine 255
Diplopia 255
Direct laryngoscopy and intubation, techniques of 64
Disinfection 34
Disseminated intravascular coagulation 5, 186, 344
Diuresis 156, 251
Diuretics 313
Dobutamine 154, 156, 212
   vasopressor 157
Doll's eye sign 453
Dopamine 154, 156, 156*t*, 212
   receptor agonist 255
Dope mnemonic, use of 427
Double-lumen
   TT 63
   tubes 326
      complications of 327
Doxacurium 146, 271, 272
Droperidol 114, 115, 157
Drug
   administration, route of 428
   anesthetics 254
   antianginal 74
   anticholinergic 76*t*
   anticonvulsive 317
   antihypertensive 74, 156, 157*t*
   antiparkinsonian 255
   antiplatelet 74, 235
   antiviral 255
   choice of 234, 308, 340, 341
   effect of 263
   epileptic 257
   fat-soluble 275

   interactions 92, 148
   metabolism 333
   mixed acting 154
   neuromuscular 145*t*
   pharmacology of 198
   physiology of 198
   therapy 379, 428
      effect of pre-existing 74
   water-soluble 275
D-tubocurarine 138, 150
Duchenne muscular dystrophy 143, 260
Duchenne-Becker muscular dystrophy 259
Duloxetine 379
Dura mater 204
Dyspnea 299
   grading of 241*t*
   history of 241
Dysrhythmias, perioperative 263
Dystrophia myotonica 103, 143
Dystrophy 143

E

Ear surgery 291
Ear, nose and throat 291
   surgery, anesthesia for 291
Ebstein's malformation 166
Echocardiography 236
Ecognine 132
Ehlers-Danlos syndrome 132
Elective neurosurgery 102, 144, 151
   induction agent for 319
Electricity supply 387
Electrocardiogram 341, 416
Electrocardiography 3, 72, 131, 163, 236
Electroconvulsive therapy 147, 256
   anesthesia for 256
Electroencephalography 174, 453
Electrolyte 272
   abnormal 294
   abnormality 163, 450
   disturbances 432, 437
   imbalance 432
Emergence reaction 110
Emergency airway management 67, 68
Emergency medicine 3, 6
Empagliflozin 265
Emphysema 408
Encephalopathy 452
Encountered coagulation disorders 248*t*
Endobronchial intubation 304, 305
Endocarditis 166
Endocrinal disease 263
   anesthesia for 263
Endocrinal disorders 263
Endocrinal system 275
Endocrine effects 114
Endocrine manifestations 208
Endocrinologic effects 118
Endoscopy 284
Endotracheal intubation 105, 147
Endotracheal route 429
Endotracheal tube 62, 85, 302
   flammability of 302
   insertion 242
   protection of 303
   size of 63

Endotrol tube 63
End-tidal carbon dioxide 170*fc*
   concentration 169, 305
   graph 168*f*
Energy expenditure 448
Enflurane 93, 238, 254, 261, 269, 271
Enophthalmos 223
Enteral nutrition 449, 451
Entonox 89
Enzyme 114
   abnormal 141
Ephedrine 154, 156
   vasopressor 157
Epidural analgesia 340
Epidural anesthesia 125, 214, 218*t*, 342
   complications of 342
Epidural anesthetic agents 216
Epidural bleeding 217
Epidural block 203, 206*f*
   complications of 217
Epidural injection 223
Epidural labor analgesia 340*t*
Epidural needles 215, 215*f*
Epidural space 125, 204*f*, 205
   methods of detecting 215
Epidural test dose 340
Epidural veins, dilated 128
Epilepsy 254
Epileptic patient 254
Epinephrine 154, 156, 255, 256, 428
Equally dangerous 439
Equilibrium 84
Equipment 398
   specific storage 388
   sterilization of 69
Ertugliflozin 265
Erythroxylum coca 132
Escherichia coli 105
Esmolol 157
Esophageal perforation 223
Esophageal stethoscope 167
Esophageal surgery 326
Ester 126, 133, 135
   group 132
   hydrolysis 146
Ether 96, 264
Etidocaine, blood levels of 129
Etomidate 93, 113, 114, 122, 240, 251, 269, 272
   exhibits 113
Euglycemia, maintain of 252
Exercise 379
Exogenous catecholamines 142
Exogenous phosphate administration 444
Expiration 26*f*
Expiratory positive airway pressure 406, 407
Extracellular fluid 178
Extracellular mouth 126*f*
Extracellular osmotic pressure, determinant of 179
Extracellular signal-regulated kinases 108
Extracorporeal membrane oxygenation 5, 448
Extrahepatic metabolism 105
Extraparenchymal restrictive disease 26*f*
Extreme obesity, complication of 274
Extubation 343
   techniques of 66

Eye 221, 302
   anatomy of 287
   lash reflex, loss of 102
   movement 174
   tears in 174

F

Face mask 60, 61*f*
Facial nerve
   blocks 288
   monitoring 291
Facial surgery, minor 221
Familial hypokalemic periodic paralysis 103
Family support zone 386
Fascial iliaca 229
Fasting
   blood sugar test 263
   guidelines 74
   preoperative 350*t*
Fastrachtm laryngeal mask airway 62
Fat embolism
   maximum risk for 298
   syndrome 295
      pathognomonic of 295
Fatty tissue 204
Feeding, route and initiation of 449*fc*
Femoral nerve block 228, 229
   modified 229
Femoral vein 165
Fentanyl 114, 115, 120, 269, 317
   congeners
      dynamics of 118
      kinetics of 118
Fentanyl-sufentanil, dose of 119
Fetal heart rate 338
Fetus, evaluation of 338
Fever 261
Fiberoptic bronchoscope 65
   instrument 285*f*
   parts 285
Fiberoptic scope 282
Fibrinolysis, enhances 134
Fibroblast growth factor 444
Fibrocartilaginous intervertebral disks 203
Flex tube 303
Flexure carpi ulnaris tendon 226
Flow trigger 402
Flowmeter assembly 40, 41
Fluid 212, 416
   choice of 182
   compartments 178
   evaporation 184
   interstitial 178, 179
   redistribution 184
   replacement, intraoperative 184
   requirements, normal maintenance 183
Fluid therapy 187, 272
   intraoperative 184
   perioperative 178, 182
Fluidization theory 81
Flumazenil 111, 113, 376
Foramen ovale 317
Forced expiratory
   flow 25
   volume 22, 327

Forced midexpiratory flow 25
Forced spirometry 25
Forehead 221
Formaldehyde fumigation 35
Fresh frozen plasma 74, 187, 251, 252
Fresh gas
   flow 48, 50, 52
   inlet 49
Frontal lobey 316
Frozen red blood cell 185, 187
Functional residual capacity 21, 22, 336, 405, 407, 408

G

G protein signaling, regulator of 108
Gabaa-benzodiazepine receptor 101*f*
Gabapentin 379, 382
Gallamine 9, 147, 272
Gamma-aminobutyric acid 100
   activated chloride 100
   facilitatory action 111
   potentiation of 104
Ganglion blockade 148
Gantacurium 146, 151
Gas
   chromatography 169
   embolism 304, 305
   lock 305
   movement of 325*f*
   supply 387
Gasless laparoscopy 307
Gasserian ganglion 221
   block 229, 379
Gastric contents, aspiration of 306
Gastric malignancy 227
Gastric mucosa 135
Gastroesophageal reflux disease 135
Gastrointestinal anomalies 447
Gastrointestinal bleeding 251
Gastrointestinal effects 118
Gastrointestinal endoscopy 355
Gastrointestinal motility 118
Gastrointestinal system 208, 337, 349, 408
Gastrointestinal tract 275, 443
Gastroparesis 263
Gelatins 181
General anesthesia 234, 238, 264, 272, 289, 291, 292, 307, 337, 343
   induction of 255
General pnesthesia, principles of 241
General surgery 209
Generic anesthesia machine 38*f*
Generic cardiopulmonary bypass circuit 321*f*
Generic circle system 54*f*
Genetic variability 132
Genitofemoral nerve 228
Genitourinary surgery, anesthesia for 299
Genitourinary system, pain conduction of 299*t*
Geriatric patient 334
Glasgow coma score 314
Glass syringe 215
Glaucoma, uncontrolled 359
Glial fibrillary acidic protein 108
Glibenclamide 265

Index

Gliclazide 265
Gliclazide MR 265
Glimepiride 265
Glomerular filtration rate 86, 271, 337, 441, 442
Glucocorticoids 318, 442
Glucose
    containing fluids 252
    enters cell 180
    imbalance 450
Glucuronide 271
    conjugation 105
Glyburide 265
Glycated hemoglobin test 263
Glycemic control
    impaired 418
    intraoperative 264
Glycine 300
    toxicity 300
Glycopyrrolate 76, 151
Granisetron 157
Gravimetric methods 174
Guedel airway 60, 61f
Guillain-Barré syndrome 142, 256, 452
Gutierrez's sign 215
Guttman's sign 223, 229

H

Hacor score 398
Hafnia system 53
Halothane 85, 90, 107, 142, 238, 243, 250, 255, 261, 269, 312, 328
    hepatotoxic potential of 254
    myocardial depression of 92
Hanger-yoke assembly 39f
Hanging drop method 215
Harris-Benedict equation 448
Head and neck, blocks of 221
Head injury 179, 314
    intraoperative management for 315b
Head tilt 60, 60f
    chin lift 60f
        maneuver 60
Headache, decrease 213
Health evaluation, chronic 412
Healthcare providers 423fc
Heart
    disease, congenital 233, 239, 240
    failure, right-sided 274
    rate 112, 118, 122, 123
Heat exchanger 320
Heat loss, mechanism of 173
Heat production, pathophysiology of 261
Helium 37, 96, 307
    dilution 25
Hematocrit 315, 416
    concentration 245
Hematologic system 336
Hematological disorders 245
    anesthesia for 245
Hematoma 217
    formation 222, 223, 225, 268
    retroperitoneal 227
Hematopoietic system 86
Hemodialysis 442
Hemodilution 191

Hemodynamic 452
    instability 316
    problems 306
    unstable 236
Hemoglobin 28, 182, 245
    abnormal 168
    concentration 72
    level 184
    oxygen dissociation curve 192
    reaction of 28
    reduced 167
Hemolysis 5
Hemophilia
    A 248
    B 248
Hemorrhage
    antepartum 344
    intracerebral 439
    intracranial 452
    postpartum 86
Hemostasis test 72
Hemothorax 450
Heparin concentration measurement 175
Hepatic blood flow 94, 250
Hepatic disease 251, 252
Hepatic encephalopathy 251
Hepatic enzymes 254
Hepatic failure 119, 146
Hepatic function 250t
    effect of anesthetic agents on 250
Hepatic neuralgia 382
Hepatitis 85
    B virus 72, 251
    C 191
    virus 251
    idiosyncratic 85
Hepatobiliary disease 149
Hepatobiliary disorders, anesthesia for 250
Hepatobiliary system 275
Hepatocellular damage 85
Hepatorenal function 94
Hepatorenal system 92, 349
Herbal medicine 75
Hereditary conditions 246
Hernia surgery, incidental 254
High pressure
    cuffs 63f
    low volume 63
High-flow nasal cannula 395, 396f, 399
    therapy 396, 397
High-pressure
    circuit 37
    system 42
Hip
    and knee arthroplasty 296
    fractures 296
Histamine release 144, 148
    maximum 144
    nondepolarizers 312
Histidine 363
Histotoxic hypoxia 391, 360
Hofmann elimination 146, 151
Holliday-Segar method 188
Hormone
    balance 452
    synthesized, naturally occurring 154

Horner's syndrome 223, 224, 225, 229
Hospital cardiac arrest 421, 421f
Hospital cardiopulmonary resuscitation 425
Hüfner constant 29
Human immunodeficiency virus 72, 191
Humidification system 396
Humidity 34
Hydrochloric acid, dilute 435
Hydrogen ion concentration 125
Hydrothorax 450
Hydroxyethyl starch 181
Hyoscine 157
Hyperbaric oxygen 96
Hypercalcemia 441, 445
    causes of 441
    mild 441
    treatment of 442t
Hypercapnia 274, 316
    permissive 243
Hypercapnic respiratory failure 397
Hypercarbic respiratory failure 401, 407
Hyperchloremic metabolic acidosis 450
Hypercortisolism 268
Hyperglycemia 263, 264, 310
    hyperosmolar state 263
Hyperkalemia 142, 143, 151, 272, 435, 439, 440, 445
    periodic paralysis 259
    risk of 255
    treatment of 441t
Hypermagnesemia 272, 443
    clinical manifestations of 443t
Hypernatremia 272, 438, 445
Hyperparathyroidism
    primary 444
    secondary 442
Hyperphosphatemia 444
Hyperpyrexia 261, 268
Hypertension 5, 95, 174, 233, 234, 236, 245, 263
    postoperative 235
    stages of 233t
    systemic 233
Hyperthermia 256, 261
    malignant 143, 259-261, 261f
Hyperthyroidism 258, 263, 267
Hypertonic saline 313
Hypertrophic pyloric stenosis 352
Hyperventilation 246, 252
Hypervolemia, signs of 184t
Hypnosis 312
Hypnotic action 104
Hypnotically active barbiturates, classification of 100t
Hypocalcemia 272, 442, 445
    symptomatic 443
Hypocapnia 235
Hypoglycemia 187, 263
    treating 180
Hypokalemia 151, 439, 445
    causes of 439t
    electrocardiographic changes of 440
Hypokalemic alkalosis 251
Hypokalemic periodic paralysis 259
Hypomagnesemia 443

Hyponatremia 437, 445
　classification of 437t
　clinical manifestations of 437
　dilutional 437
　management of asymptomatic 438
Hypoparathyroidism 442
Hypophosphatemia 444
　severity of 444
Hypotension 148, 151, 207, 212, 294, 305, 173, 236, 263, 268, 300, 342, 452
　avoid 252
　intraoperative 263
　management of intraoperative 256
　mechanism of 207f
　methods for inducing 359
　severe 224
　treatment of 255
Hypothalamic-pituitary-adrenocortical function, disruption of 452
Hypothermia 246, 356, 452
　causes of 174t
Hypothyroid patient, severe 266
Hypothyroidism 258, 263, 266, 267
Hypoventilation 214, 439
Hypovolemia 142, 251
Hypoxemia 294
Hypoxemic respiratory failure 401
　acute 417
Hypoxia 246
　circulatory 391
　types of 391t
Hypoxic brain injury 310
Hypoxic pulmonary vasoconstriction 24, 326

I

Iatrogenic conditions 248
Iatrogenic paralysis 401
Iliac spine, anterior-superior 228
Iliohypogastric nerves 228
Ilioinguinal block 228
Ilioinguinal nerve 228
Illness, severity of 412
Imidazoline derivative 122
Immobility, complications of 148
Immune
　effects 118
　mediated hemolysis 191
　system 88
Immunonutrition 448
Immunosuppressants 443
Inadequate tissue perfusion 412
Indian Society of Anesthesiologists 456
Induction 104, 113, 328, 343
　agent 234, 254
Infection control practices 388
Inflammatory cytokines 194
Inflammatory molecules 412
Infraglottic airway devices 62
Infrared gas analyzers 168
Inguinal hernia 228
Inhalational agents 271, 311
Inhalational anesthesia
　general principles of 83
　mechanism of 81
Inhalational induction 350, 358

Inhaled anesthetic 333, 349
　circuit, absorption of 84
　classification of 81f, 99t
　interactions with 149
　metabolism of 85
Inhibitors 265
Inhibitory cells 372
Inhibits pseudolocholinesterase 141
Inotropes 212, 416
Inotropic action, negative 101
Insensible losses 438
Inspiration 26f
Inspiratory capacity 21
Inspiratory positive airway pressure 406
Inspiratory reserve volume 21
Inspiratory time 393
Inspired concentration 83
Inspired oxygen, fraction of 409
Inspired ventilation, augmentation of 84
Insulin 269
Intensive care unit 56, 106, 144, 148, 385, 400, 447, 447f, 455
　acquired weakness 418
　basic principles of 447
　classification of 385
　complications in 417
　ethics in 455, 456
　level of 385
　management of 383, 385
　nutritional support in 447
　operations 385
Intercostal block 227
Intercostal nerve blocks 129, 227
Intermittent positive pressure ventilation 23, 359
Intervertebral foramina forming spinal nerves 203
Intestinal obstruction, acute 89
Intra-abdominal
　infection 142, 144
　pressure 304
Intra-aortic balloon pump 236
Intra-arterial injection 103
Intracardiac shunt, right-to-left 239
Intracellular fluid 178
Intracellular mouth 126f
Intracellular space 437
Intracranial aneurysms 317
Intracranial hypertension, management of 313fc
Intracranial mass lesion 110, 315
Intracranial pressure 88, 92, 123, 142, 310, 311, 315, 452
　diagnosis of increased 311
　increased 67, 142, 408
　management of increased 312
　minus 101
　raised 452
　reduce 312, 312t
Intracranial temperature 312, 315
Intractable ascites 251
Intragastric pressure 142
　increased 142
Intramuscular induction 350
Intramuscular injection 103

Intraneural injection 103
Intraocular pressure 142, 287
　dynamics 287
　ioncreased 142
Intraocular tension 109
Intraoperative analgesia, opioids dose for 119t
Intraoral surgery 292
Intraosseous route 429
Intrapulmonary gas distribution 404
Intrathecal injection 223
Intrathoracic pressure, increasing 403
Intrauterine resuscitation 338
　role of 338
Intravascular air, reduce 317
Intravascular fluid 179
　volume 238
Intravascular hemolysis 440
Intravascular injection 217, 225
Intravenous access 428
Intravenous agents 271, 312
Intravenous detection 340
Intravenous fluid 179, 316, 447
　therapy 178
Intravenous induction 350, 358
Intravenous methylene blue 132
Intravenous regional anesthesia 128, 226
Intravenous therapy 440
Intrinsic acid, loss of 435
Intubating laryngeal mask airway 282, 284
Intubation 69, 284
　complications of 66
Invasive arterial blood pressure monitoring 162, 163f
Ipsilateral phrenic nerve 224
Ischemia, diagnosing intraoperative 163, 176
Ischemic attack, transient 5
Ischemic brain injury, protection against 313f
Ischemic heart disease 104, 109, 110, 122, 184, 233, 235
Isoflurane 92, 94, 237, 250, 261, 262, 269, 272, 316
Isoprenaline 154, 156, 264
Isotonic saline 438, 442

J

Jaw thrust 60f
　maneuver 60
Jehovah's witness 190, 359
Joint immobility 263
Jugular catheterization, internal 164
Jugular vein
　compress 317
　internal 164
Junctional rhythms 141

K

Ketamine 93, 106, 108f, 122, 234, 239, 240, 250, 251, 254-256, 271, 309, 376
　acts 107
　administration 109
　consists 107
　doses of 109t
　increases 109
　limitation of 376

low-dose 109
preservative 110
Ketoacidosis 263, 432
Ketoglutarate 363
Kidney 86, 88, 271
　damage, chronic 444
　disease, end-stage 5
　failure 449
　regulate plasma 432
Kinetic energy, sum of 395
Krause angle forceps 223
Kussmaul respiration 434
Kyphoscoliosis 260
Kyphosis 203

L

Labetalol 157, 235
Labor
　first stage of 338
　second stage of 338
Labor analgesia 198, 338
　regional techniques for 339
　techniques for 338
Lactated Ringer's solution 184
Ladder scale 373
Lambert-Eaton myasthenic syndrome 259, 260
Laparoscope in situ 304f
Laparoscopic cholecystectomy 252, 304f
Laparoscopic surgeries 89
Laparoscopy, anesthesia for 304
Laryngeal mask airway 58, 61, 62, 284, 318, 337, 358, 427
　advantages of 62f
　contraindications for 62
　disadvantages of 62f
　sizes of 62t
Laryngeal nerve
　block, superior 223, 223f
　paralysis, effects of 18t
　recurrent 17
　superior 222
Laryngeal procedures 293
Laryngopharynx 17
Laryngoscopy 350
　complications of 66
　direct 64
　grades of 65f
　technique of 65
Laryngospasm 243, 351
Larynx 17, 284, 285f
　anatomy of 16f
　anterior 18f
　below cord 284
　nerve supply of 18f
　posterior 18f
Laser
　hazards 302
　plume 302
　surgery, anesthesia for 302
Laughing gas 87
Lecithin 135
Left ventricular
　function 408
　vent 321

Leptocurare 140
Lethargy 266
Levobupivacaine 134, 135
Levodopa 75, 255
　therapy, chronic 255
　withdrawal of 255
Lidocaine 128, 129, 428
Ligament, yellow 206
Ligamentum flavum 206
Light anesthesia, clinical signs of 174
Lignocaine 129, 210
　decreases coagulation 134
　hydrochloride 133
Limb, inspiratory 396
Linagliptine 265
Linear analog scale 373
Lipid
　solubility 100
　supplementation, target 448
Lipophilic-hydrophilic balance 125
Lipophilicity 125
Lithium 75
　interactions with 149
　toxicity 256
Liver 85, 88
　disease 119, 272
　dysfunction 450
　enzymes, elevated 5
　failure 187
　　chronic 449
　function test 73, 250
Lobectomy 326
Local anesthesia 8, 125, 132, 291, 292, 308
　intra-articular 377
　sterilization of 135
Local anesthetic
　agents, clinical use of 133t
　classification of 126t
　eutectic mixture of 129
　failure 132
　low concentration of 340
　mechanism of action of 126f
　mixtures of 128
　systemic toxicity of 208
Local tissue
　edema 132
　toxicity 132
Long-acting agents 216
Lorazepam 112
Low backache 380
Low molecular weight heparin 417
Low respiratory rate 243
Lower extremity 295
　blocks of 221, 228
Lower jaw 221
Lower limb muscles, pumping action of 207
Low-flow devices 393
Low-pressure
　circuit 37, 40
　cuffs 63f
　high volume 63
　system 42
Lumbar puncture 205
　correct 210
　needles 209f

Lumbar regions 203
Lumbar sympathetic chain, blockade of 227
Lung 400
　capacity, total 21, 25
　cyst, large 326
　diffusing capacity of 25
　function, measuring 25
　perfusion of 24f
　resection 326
　　anesthetic management of 327
　transplantation, single 326
Lung volume 21, 22f, 405
　increases 26f
　redistributes extravascular 407
Lysosomal acid 260

M

Maastricht classification 364t
Macintosh
　laryngoscopy 65f
　technique 66
Magill circuit 48
Magill position 64
　steps for 64f
Magnesium 322
　disorders of 443
　interactions with 149
　sulphate 149, 428
Mallampati
　classification 59
　grading 59
　score 58
Mandibular branches 222
Mandibular protrusion 59
Mania 256
Mannitol 313
Mapleson
　A 48
　B systems 50
　breathing system 49t
　C systems 50
　D system 50, 51f, 52f
　　modification of 51
　E systems 53
　F systems 53
　systems 48
　type 53
Masks 398
　nonrebreathing 394, 394f
　partial rebreathing 394
Mass spectroscope 169
Masseter spasm 142
Massive blood transfusion 185
　complications of 185
Massive surgery 179
Maxillary branches 222
McGill's pain questionnaire 373
Mean arterial pressure 101, 123, 154, 161, 310
Mechanical parameters 429
Mechanical ventilation
　complications during 408
　indication of 401
　physiology of 400
　principles of 400

Index

Medical air 96
Medical ethics, basic principles of 455
Medical history 71
Medical ventilator 400, 400f
Medications, choice of 416
Medullary ischemia 208
Medullary respiratory centers 453
Meglitinides 265
Mendelson syndrome 337
Meningitis 213
Mental status, deterioration of 255
Mental symptoms 334
Meperidine 93, 120, 254, 256, 271
Mephentermine 156
Mepivacaine 131
Mercury sphygmomanometer 162
Merocel laser guard 303
Metabolic acidosis 131, 150, 433, 434, 440
    causes of 434t
    severe 142
Metabolic alkalosis 435
Metabolic complications 450
Metabolic derangements 197
Metabolic differences 349
Metabolic effect 87
Metabolic manifestations 208
Metabolic myopathies 260
Metabolism 86, 87, 90, 95, 99, 107, 110, 111, 113, 119, 120
    continuous 141
Metabolite 132
    laudanosine 254
Metabolized 144
Metabotropic glutamate receptors 108
Metal endotracheal tubes 303
Metformin 265
    XR 265
Methemoglobinemia 132, 168
    risk of 132
Methionine synthase, inactivate 86
Methohexitone 103
Methoxyflurane 86, 95, 96, 271, 272
Metoclopramide 157
Metocurine 9
Meyer-Overton rule 82
Microbial monitoring 35
Microcirculation 181
Microlaryngeal tubes 63
Microprocessor technology 404
Midazolam 110, 112, 357
Middle ear surgery 89
Milk-alkali syndrome 444
Mill-wheel murmur 305
Minerals 448
Minute ventilation 49
Miosis 223
Mitral regurgitation 237
Mitral stenosis 236
    agents in 237t
Mivacurium 146, 151, 257, 262, 312
Monoamine oxidase 75, 142
    inhibitors 255
Monocytic macrophage system 181
Monoethylglycinexylidide 130
Morphine 118t, 119, 269

3-glucuronide 119
6-glucuronide 119
    metabolites of 271
Mortality prediction model 412
Motor blockade 127
Mouth opening 58
Mueller's syndrome 223, 229
Multiorgan system failure 418
Multiple agents 43
Multiple organ systems 97
Muscarinic autonomic sites 140
Muscle
    blockade, sequence of 140
    fatigue 266
    rigidity 117
Muscle relaxant 9, 138, 150t, 234, 242, 254, 271, 272, 289, 333, 334, 350, 358
    depolarizing 140
    exception of 258
    releasing histamine 146
Muscular dystrophies 142, 259
Muscular system 112
Musculoskeletal disease, anesthesia for 258
Musculoskeletal system 263, 408
Myalgias 142
Myasthenia 258
    gravis 146, 258, 260
Myelin synthesis 86
Myocardial contractility 122
Myocardial depressant 108
Myocardial infarction 5, 6, 233
Myocardial ischemia 263
    management of 236
    risk of 260
Myocardial relaxant 101
Myoclonus 106, 114
Myotonic contractions 260
Myotonic dystrophy 260

N

Nail polish 168
Nalbuphine 121, 271
Naloxone 121, 376
Naltrexone 121
Narcoanalysis 102
Narcotrend 174
Nasal
    airways 60
    cannula 393, 393f, 395
    stiffness 223
    surgery 292
    vasoconstrictors 292
Nasogastric tubes 357
Nasopharyngeal catheter 394
Nasopharynx 284
Nasotracheal intubation 66
    advantages of 66t
    disadvantages of 66t
    head positions for 66
National Medical Commission Norms 412
National Medical Council 388
National Organ and Tissue Transplant Organisation 363f, 365, 365b

National Organ Transplant Programme 365
Nausea 118, 121, 214, 299, 306
    postoperative 14, 157, 306, 356
    treat postoperative 157
Neck
    mobility 59
    movements 59
    X-ray of 267f
Needle size 212
Needle type 212
Negative pressure test 42
Neostigmine 143
    inhibits pseudocholinesterase 146
Nephrotoxic volatile anesthetic agent 272
Nephrotoxicity 86
    risk of 86
Nerve
    compression 372
    fibers, types of 127
    selection of 172
    stimulator equipment 172f
    supply 20, 287
Nerve blocks 221
    peripheral 128, 129
Nerve injury 225, 307
    tourniquet related 227
Nerve stimulation
    electric 221
    patterns of 171
Nervous system 91, 97, 207, 254, 275, 331
Neural injury 372
Neuralgia, postherpetic 379
Neuraxial block 208
Neuraxial blockade
    effect of 208f
    performing 213
    systemic effects of 207
Neuraxial opioids 380
Neuroablation 379
Neuroexcitatory phenomena 117
Neuroleptanalgesia 114, 115, 115fc
Neuroleptanesthesia 115
Neurologic complications 294
Neurologic deficits 254
Neurologic dysfunction 418
Neurologic problems 306
Neurological abnormalities 452
Neurological death, determination of 456
Neurological function 422
Neurological injury 213, 217
Neuromuscular blockers 138, 143t, 143, 148, 150, 259, 267
    classification of 138t
    depolarizing 140
    mechanism of action of 138
    produces 139
    profound 142
Neuromuscular disorders 143, 258
Neuromuscular functions 349, 432, 439
Neuromuscular junction 138, 140, 150
Neuromuscular monitoring 170, 171f, 296
Neuromuscular transmission 139fc
    monitors 197
Neuropathy spinal anesthesia, peripheral 264
Neuropsychiatric disease 254
    anesthesia for 254

Neuropsychiatric disorders 254
Neuroradiology procedures 355
Neurostimulatory therapies 379
Neurosurgery 104, 312, 359
    anesthesia for 310
Neurotoxic snake envenomation 452
Neurotoxicity 86, 214
Neurotrophic factor, brain-derived 108
Neutral solution 113
Nicotinic acetylcholine receptor 108, 138
Nicotinic cholinergic receptors 139f
Nitrates 235
Nitric oxide 87
Nitrogen 37
    dioxide 87
Nitroglycerin 157, 236
Nitrous oxide 37, 87, 243, 269, 315, 323, 328
    cylinder 38
    uses of 89, 291
N-methyl d-aspartate 108, 372, 376
    inhibition of 104
Node of Ranvier 127
Noise control 387
Nonanesthetic gases 96
Non-anion gap metabolic acidosis, produce 179
Noncardiac surgery, management for 238
Noncardiogenic pulmonary edema 401
Nondepolarizers, long-acting 258
Nondepolarizing muscle relaxants 140, 261, 272
Nondepolarizing neuromuscular blockers 148, 151
    agents 254, 258
    drugs 140, 144, 173
    small dose of 142
Nonfunctional gastrointestinal tract 447
Noninvasive arterial blood pressure monitoring 161
Noninvasive mechanical ventilation, indications of 397t
Noninvasive ventilation 397, 399, 406
    advantages of 398t, 407
    complications of 407
    contraindications of 397b
    disadvantages of 398t, 407
    initiation of 398
    modes 406, 410
    steps for initiation of 398b
    system 406
Nonobstetric surgery during pregnancy, anesthesia for 345
Nonoperating room anesthesia 354, 354b
Nonpharmacological techniques 377
Nonrebreathing system, semiclosed 48
Nonsteroidal anti-inflammatory drugs 267, 292, 375, 376, 381
Nontherapeutic effects 117
Nonvolatile anesthetics 350
Noradrenaline 154, 155, 416
    vasopressor 157
Norepinephrine 154, 156
Normal central venous pressure 165
    waveform 165f
Normal intravascular volume 192

Normovolumic hemodilution, acute 191
Nortriptyline 379
Nose 284
Nosocomial pneumonia 408
Novel local anesthetics 135
Nutric score 447
Nutrition
    requirement 448
    routes of 449
    support
        indication of 447
        timing of 447fc
Nutritional problems 332
Nystagmus 109
    occurs 109

O

Obese patient
    anesthesia for 274
    management of 276f
Obesity 58, 274, 275t
    categorization of 274t
    classification of 274
    hypoventilation syndrome 274
    multisystem effect of 275f
Obstructive disease 26f
Obstructive hydrocephalus 316
Obstructive sleep apnea 5
Ocular effects 105
Ocular physiology 287
Oculocardiac reflex 287
    pathway 288f
Oculocephalic reflex 453
Oculovestibular reflex 453
Oliguria hypernatremia 251
Olinesterase deficiency 143
Oncosurgery 359
Ondansetron 157
One-lung ventilation, indications for 326
Operation room 13, 33
    asepsis 34
    cleaning of 34t
Operation theater 3, 33, 51, 62, 364
    number of 33
Operation, procedure for 5fc
Ophthalmic surgery 89
    anesthesia for 287
Opiates 333
Opioid 118, 122, 254, 271, 375
    actions of 116
    agonist-antagonists 271
    anesthetics 115
    antagonists 121
    choice of 119
    classification of 115t
    induction 235
    pharmacokinetics of 118
    potency of 119
    receptor 116
        physiological effects of 116t
    systemic effects of 116
Optic nerve 287
Optic neuritis 255
Oral airways 60
Oral care 382

Oral contraceptive pills 74
Oral glucose tolerance test 263
Oral hypoglycemics 74, 264
    management of 265t
Oral phosphate binders 444
Oral sedation 112
Organ donation 365, 456
    anesthesia for 362
    contraindications to 363, 363b
    types of 362
Organ donors, anesthetic management of 364
Organ preservation 363
Organ system 332f
    effects 85, 90
Oropharyngeal airway 61f
Oropharynx 284
Orthopedic patients 294
Orthopedic surgery 209
    anesthesia for 294
Osmotic demyelination syndrome 438
Osteolytic metastasis 444
Oucher scale 373
Outside hospital cardiac arrest 421f
Overhead lamp 35
Oxethazaine 135
Oxetacaine 135
Oximetry, principles of 167
Oxybarbiturates 99
Oxybuprocaine 133
Oxygen 28, 37, 47, 94, 96, 100, 123, 257, 391
    cascade 28, 28f
    consumption, reducing 403
    cylinder 37
    decreased delivery of 415
    dissolved 29
    failure alarms 45
    flux 29
    inappropriate utilization of 415
    indications of 391
    nitrous lock 45
    partial pressure of 405, 409, 417
    pressure of 28, 29
        regulator, second-stage 40
    reaction of 28
    supplement 212, 252, 277, 417
    supply 387
    toxicity 97
    transport 28
Oxygen delivery
    basis of 415
    calculation of 391
    devices 56, 392
Oxygen flush 45
    valve 40
Oxygen saturation 167, 168, 417
    monitoring 416
    provides 167
Oxygen therapy
    classification of 393t
    devices 391
        classification of 392t
Oxygenated hemoglobin, concentration of 167
Oxygenation failure 389, 401
Oxygen-hemoglobin dissociation 167
    curve 29

P

Pachycurare 140, 144
Packed red blood cells 179, 185-187
Pain
   abdominal 299
   and palliation, chronic 379
   assessment of 375
   basic concepts of 371
   classification of 372, 372f
   evaluation of 373
   fibers 207
   gate control theory of 371, 371f
   medicine 3, 7
   neuropathic 372
   nociceptive 116, 372
   on injection 106
   pathway 371f
   phantom 380
   postoperative 307, 333, 375
   scar 380
   theories of 371, 374
   transmission of 371
Pain control
   proper 242
   techniques for postoperative 375f
Pain management 369
   combining 381
   in terminally ill 381
   methods of postoperative 375
   postoperative 298, 351, 375
Palliative care 381
   principles of 381
Palliative nerve 382
   blocks 382
Pallidotomy 255
Palm, dorsal aspect of 226
Pancreatic malignancy 227
Pancuronium 9, 100, 144, 148, 151, 240, 256, 269, 271, 272, 309
Papaver somniferum 115
Para-aminobenzoic acid 132
Paracervical blocks 341
Paradoxical embolism 167, 317
Paradoxical exacerbation 310
Paralysis 69
Paralytic abnormalities 316
Paraplegia, causes of 214
Parathyroid
   glands 268
   hormone 444
Parenchymal restrictive disease 26f
Parenteral nutrition 450
   complications of 450
Paresthesias 255
Parkinson's disease 255
Partial ventilator support 401
Patency of nares 58
Pathogenesis shock, basis of 415
Patient care zone 386
Patient control analgesia 376
   epidural 377
Patient state index 174
Patil's test 59
Pediatric age group 187
Pediatric ophthalmologic procedures 289

Pediatric upper airway 348f
Pelvic fractures 296
Pendelluft phenomenon 325f
Penile block 228
Penlon circuit 51
Pentastarch 182t
Pentazocine 117, 120, 240, 267
Pentothal 99
Periaqueductal gray matter 116
Peribulbar block, posterior 289
Pericardial effusion 272
Periodic paralysis 259
Peripheral nervous system 129
Peroneal nerve, superficial 229
Peroxisome proliferator-activated receptor 265
Perspiration 174
Petechial rash 295
Pethidine 117, 120, 240, 267
Pharmacodynamics 333
Pharmacology 105, 107, 111, 113, 121, 210, 216
Pharynx 17, 284
   anatomy of 16f
Phenobarbiturate 100
Phenothiazines derivative 115
Phenoxibenzamine 103
Phenylephrine 154, 416
Pheochromocytoma 263, 268
Phosgene 96
Phosphate
   absorption 444
   containing enema 444
   disorders of 444
Phrenic nerve block 223, 225
Physical changes 55
Physical examination 72
Physical properties 87, 90, 92, 94, 96
Physicochemical characteristics 103, 107, 113
Physicochemical properties 100, 116
Physiological conditions 58
Physiological losses
   normal 184
   replacement of 183
Pickwickian syndrome 274
Pin index safety system 39, 39f
Pinocytosis 338
Pinprick fibers 207
Pioglitazone 265
Pipecuronium 146, 271, 272
Place et tube 430
Placenta, manual removal of 345
Placental transfer 338
Plasma 186t, 445
   bicarbonate 432
   catecholamines 269
   EC50 81
   protein binding 333
Plasma-Lyte 180
Plasminogen activators, tissue-type 194
Platelet 247f
   concentrates 187
   disorders 246
   function 248
   low 5
Pleural effusion 272, 417

Pneumocephalus 316
Pneumomediastinum 305, 408
Pneumonectomy 326
Pneumonia, ventilator-associated 408
Pneumopericardium 305
Pneumoperitoneum 89, 304, 307
   hemodynamic effects of 306f
Pneumothorax 89, 165, 224, 225, 227, 243, 304, 305, 408, 450
   open 325
Polanosetron 157
Polycythemia, cyanosis-induced 274
Polyvinyl
   chloride 63, 302
   pyrrolidone 55
Pontine 24
Poor nutritional status 447
Positive end-expiratory pressure 23, 305, 359, 407-409
   decreases 397
   effect 396
   mechanism of 408fc
   physiology of 407
Positive pressure
   test 42
   ventilation 23, 62, 359
Postanesthetic management 354
Postcardiac arrest care 425, 430
Postdural puncture headache 209, 212, 341, 342
   factors affecting 213b
Posterior fossa
   procedure 316, 316f
   surgery 89, 316
Postintubation croup 243, 351
Postpneumoencephalogram 89
Postsurgical chest 375
Post-tetanic count stimulation 172
Post-tetanic twitch stimulation 172
Post-traumatic respiratory failure 397
Potassium 259, 322
   adaptation, phenomenon of 440
   adenosine triphosphate 265
   balance, disorders of 439
   channels 81
   hydroxide 54
Potassium-titanyl-phosphate 302
Poynting effect 89
Preanesthetic evaluation 71
Precipitate hepatorenal syndrome 252
Precise mechanism 81
Pre-eclampsia, grading of 344t
Pre-existing fluid deficits 183, 184
Pregabalin 379
Pregnancy 128, 335f, 336t, 428
   coagulation factors in 336t
Preoxygenation 64, 68, 343
Pressure reducing valves 39
Pressure regulated volume control 406
Pressure sensation 127
Pressure support ventilation 405f, 406
Pressure trigger 401
Previa, placenta 344
Prilocaine 129, 134
Procaine 135
   hydrochloride 133

Index

Progesterone, especially 128
Prokinetic agents 214
Promethazine 114, 157
Propofol 103, 106, 122, 234, 239, 240, 250, 251, 257, 258, 262, 269, 271, 275, 289, 317, 358
    infusion syndrome 106
    lacks anticonvulsant property 105
    vial 104*f*
Proportioning system 40, 45
Prosealtm laryngeal mask airway 61
Prostate, transurethral resection of 72, 299
Prostatic hyperplasia, benign 299
Protein binding 119, 120
Prothrombin complex 187
Prothrombin test 186
Prothrombin time 246, 251
Protoplasmic poison 130
Pruritus 118
Pseudocholinesterase 140, 141
    abnormal genetic variant of 141
    activity 135, 141
        atypical 141
    enormous capacity of 140
Pseudohyperkalemia 441
Pseudomonas aeruoginosa 408
Psoas compartment block 228
Psychiatric disease 110
Psychiatric disorders 256
Psychological therapies 379
Psychoprophylaxis 338
Ptosis 223
    congenital 260
Pudendal blocks 341
Pulmonary artery
    catheter 166*f*
    catheterization 165, 166, 416
    occlusion pressure 166
    pressure 118, 236, 272, 408
    rupture 166
Pulmonary aspiration 142
Pulmonary blood 83
Pulmonary capillary wedge 166*f*
    pressure 166, 412, 413, 416
Pulmonary circulation 20
Pulmonary disease, severe 241, 436
Pulmonary dysfunction 241
Pulmonary embolism 294
Pulmonary function 407
    test 25, 241, 274
Pulmonary hypertension 236
Pulmonary infarction 166
Pulmonary infection 326
Pulmonary tuberculosis 243
Pulmonary vascular resistance 154
Pulmonary venous pressure 166
Pulsatile blood flow 320
Pulse
    check, site of 424*b*
    oximeter 3
Pulse oximetry 167
    combines 167
    measures oxygen 176
    tells 168
Pulseless electrical activity 420, 426
Pupil
    dilate moderately 109
    size 118
Pyridostigmine 143

Q

QT prolongation, suspected 157
Quadriplegia 316
Queckenstedt's test 213
Quinine 260

R

Racemic mixture 134
Radiation 302
Radical cystectomy 359
Radical prostatectomy 301
Radiofrequency thermocoagulation 382
Ramifentanil 251
Ramifentanyl 317
Rapacuronium 151
Rapamycin, mammalian target of 108
Raynaud's disease 226
Raynaud's phenomenon 380
Reaction time 175
Reactive airway disease 109
Rebreathing system, semiclosed 48
Record keeping 456
Rectus muscle, medial 287
Red blood cell 444
    lost 192
Red cells, salvaged unwashed 193
Refeeding syndrome 447
Refractory hypoxemia secondary 407
Rehabilitative therapies 379
Reinfusion, complications of 194*b*
Relieve anxiety 75
Relieve spasm 241
Relieves aortocaval pressure 428
Remifentanil 120, 122, 271, 275, 358
Renal blood flow 154
    except dopamine 157
Renal disease 149
    anesthesia for 271
    effect of 271
Renal effect 118
Renal failure 118, 146, 187, 272
    chronic 272
    effects of 272
Renal function 251
    deranged 444
    test 73
Renal physiology, effect of anesthetic agent on 271
Renal replacement therapy 444
Renal system 337
Renal transplantation 301
Renal vasculature, dilates 156
Repacurium 147
Repaglinide 265
Residual neuromuscular blockade 150
Resistance technique, loss of 215
Respiration
    complete cessation of 453
    mechanics of 20
    regulation of 24
    spontaneous 50, 51*f*
    support 417
Respiratory acidosis 150, 434-436
Respiratory alkalosis 435, 436
    severe 403
    superimposed 433, 434
Respiratory capacities 21
Respiratory changes 307, 336*t*
Respiratory circuits 406
Respiratory complication 294, 356, 408
Respiratory depression 112
Respiratory disease 26*f*, 243
    anesthesia for 241
Respiratory drive, anesthetics on 25
Respiratory dysfunction, postoperative 197
Respiratory effects 148
Respiratory failure 401, 416-418
    perioperative 389, 417
    postoperative 397
    secondary 417
Respiratory function 410
Respiratory gas mixture 303
Respiratory monitoring 167
Respiratory movements 242
Respiratory physiology 16
Respiratory problems, sorts of 197
Respiratory rate 392, 409
Respiratory signs 295
Respiratory system 88, 91, 97, 102, 108, 112, 114, 117, 121, 208, 274, 275, 331, 336, 348, 407, 432
    disorders 109
    effects on 105
Respiratory tract
    divisions 19*f*
    infection 243
Respiratory volumes 21, 21*t*
Restrictive lung disease 243
    management of 243
Resuscitation
    management of 425
    phase, continued 430
Retrobulbar block 288
Retrograde intubation 282
Rheumatoid arthritis 258
Rhythm abnormalities 143
Right atrium 317
Right Robertshaw tube 327*f*
Ringer's lactate 179, 183, 188, 316, 416
    solution 179
Ringer's solution 272
Rocuronium 144, 151, 235, 269, 275, 289, 301, 315, 316
Rofecoxib 357
Room temperature 94
Ropivacaine 134
Rosiglitazone 265
Rostral ventromedial medulla 116
Rotameter 40
Rotating bobbin 45
Ryanodine receptor gene 260

S

Sabouraud dextrose agar 35
Sacral epidural anesthesia 214

Sacral region 203
Sacral segments 210
Saddle block 210, 218
Safe anesthesia management, principles for 312
Saline, normal 179, 186, 314, 316
Samter's triad 292
Saphenous nerve 229
Sarcoidosis 444
Sarcoplasmic reticulum 261
Saxagliptine 265
S-bupivacaine 134
Scavenging system 86
Schizophrenia 256
Sciatic nerve block 229
Scleroderma 226
Sclerosis, multiple 255
Scopolamine 76, 157
Sedation 99, 104, 112, 113, 119
    adequacy of 112
    intraoperative 255
Sedative analgesics 350
Seizure 256, 439
    surgery 317
Selick's maneuver 69, 314
Semiopen system 47
S-enantiomer drug, single 134
Sensitive half-time, context 104
Sensitive method 175
Sensitization 132
Sensory
    differential 127
    evoked potentials 117
Sequential organ failure assessment 412
Serotonin levels, decrease in 104
Serum
    albumin 251
    bilirubin 251
    electrolytes 73
        abnormal 197
    potassium 272
Severity of surgery, classification of 72
Sevoflurane 93, 237, 243, 250, 261, 271, 272, 275, 289, 328, 358
Shock 246, 412t, 418, 452
    circulatory 412
    classification of 414t, 415f
    delivering 427
    distributive 415
    hemorrhagic 179
    hypoadrenergic 415
    neurogenic 415
    pathogenesis of 413f
    septic 179, 415
    stages of 414f
    warm 415
Shockable rhythm 426
Sickle cell
    anemia 246, 248
    disease 226
Silent ischemia 263, 266
Silica 54
Simple face mask 394, 394f
Single shot technique 214
    epidural 215

Sinus bradycardia 141
Sitagliptine 265
Skeletal muscle 154, 258
    relaxant 254
    tone, ketamine increases 109
Skin grafting, mention of 362f
Sleep deprivation 294
Slow-wave activity 251
Smiley scale 373
Smoke, maximum 302
Smoking 75
    cessation, effects of 242t
    stop 241
Snider match blowing test 25
Soda lime 54
    dust inhalation 54
    exhaustion, signs of 55
Sodium 322
    balance, disorders of 437
    bicarbonate 127
        dose calculation of 445
    channel, intracellular aspect of 126
    chloride 416
    hydroxide 54
    nitroprusside 157, 269, 359
SOFA score 412
Somatic motor fibers 207
Somnolence 274
Spinal analgesia 341
Spinal anesthesia 125, 134, 203, 209, 210f, 211f, 218, 218t, 242, 341
    complications of 342
    drugs for 211t
    segmental 210
Spinal areas 372
Spinal arteries, posterior 205
Spinal block 206f
    total 342
Spinal cord 204, 371f
    blood supply of 204
    dorsal horn of 371
Spinal needles 209
Spinal nerve roots 205
Spinal surgeries 297
    technique of 298
Spirometry 25
Spontaneous circulation, return of 420
Staphylococcus aureus 105
Starvation, duration of 447
Status epilepticus 147
Stellate ganglion 223
    block 223
    signs of 229
Stereoisomers 134
Sterile zones 33
Sterilization 35
Steroidal muscle relaxant 144
    long-acting 144
Steroids 75, 314, 416
Stethoscope 167
Stiff joint syndrome 264
Stimulates noradrenaline 103
Strabismus 260
Stress 246
    ulcers 418

Stroke
    perioperative 254
    type of 254
ST-segment depression 236
Subarachnoid
    increased risk of 438
    injection 217
    space 125, 205
Subclavian artery pulsation 225
Subclavian vein 165, 451
Subcutaneous emphysema 305, 408
Subdural space 205
Subglottis 352
Succinylcholine 100, 140, 142, 148, 151, 238, 255, 257, 258, 269, 272, 312, 316, 350, 440
    duration of 141t
    infusion 143t
    routine administration of 149
Succinylmonocholine 140
Sudden cardiac arrest 420, 422
Sudeck's dystrophy 380
Sufentanil 120, 240, 269
Sugammadex 151
Sulfonylurea 265
Sulfur
    analog 100
    containing barbiturate 122
Supraglottic airway devices 61
Supraspinous ligament 205
Sural nerve 229
Surgery 271
    grading of severity of 72
    type of 264
Surgical ablation 113
Surgical effects, direct 271
Surgical fluid losses, assessment of 183
Surgical loss 184
Surgical procedure, anesthesia for 222
Surgical stress 268
Surgical therapies 379
Surgical wound losses 184
Swan-Ganz catheter 165
Sympathetic blocks 380, 382
Sympathetic nervous system 132
Synchronized intermittent mandatory ventilation 404, 405f
    mode, advantages of 404
Syndrome of inappropriate antidiuretic hormone secretion 438
Synthetic oxygen carrying substances 187
Systemic inflammatory response syndrome 418
Systemic toxicity 130
Systemic vascular resistances 94, 251, 321, 415
Systolic pressure, above 162

T

Tachycardia 95, 148, 174, 236, 268, 305
Taylor's approach 209, 210, 211f
Temperature 34, 44, 91, 386
    compensation 42
    fibers 207
    management 430

Index

monitoring 173
  sensitivity 208
Temporomandibular movement 58
Teratogenicity 86
Terminate resuscitative efforts 429
Tetanic stimulation consists 172
Tetanus, severe cases of 147
Tetany 172
Tetracaine 131
Tetralogy of Fallot 108, 239
Tetrastarch 182t
Thalamoneocortical projection system 107
Thalamotomy 255
Therapeutic effects 117
Thermal conductivity 44
Thermodilution 167
Thermoregulation 209, 349
Thiazolidinediones 265
Thiopentone 106, 114, 122, 250, 251, 271, 316
  stimulates antidiuretic hormone 102
Thoracic aortic aneurysm, repair of 326
Thoracic bioimpedance 167
Thoracic region 203
Thoracic spine 326
Thoracic surgery, anesthesia for 324
Thoracolumbar spinal nerves 208
Thoracoscopy 326
Thoracotomy, lateral 325f
Thorax, blocks of 221, 227
Thromboelastograph 175, 175f, 176
Thromboembolism 248
Thrombophlebitis 103, 450
  myoclonus 113
  superficial 114
Thymoma 258
Thyroid
  disorders 266
  storm 268
    treatment of 268
    supplement 75
Thyromental distance 59
Thyroxine 266
Tibial nerve, posterior 229
Tidal volume 21, 197, 393, 409
Tissue 302
  disorder, connective 132
  perfusion creates, reduced 412
  trauma, degree of 184
To-and-fro system 53, 54
Tocolysis 86
Tolazoline 103
Tongue 284
Tonsillectomy 292
Tooth abscess 132
Total gas flow 392t
Total hip replacement, technique of 298
Total knee replacement, technique of 298
Touch fibers 207
Tourniquet
  complications 296t
  discomfort 227
  produces 246
  syndrome 227
  use of 226
Tourniquet-related complications 295

Toxicity 85, 130
Tracheal bifurcation 285f
Tracheal collapse 268
Tracheal intubation 350
Tracheal stenosis respiratory muscle weakness 408
Tracheal tubes 63
Tracheobronchial disruption 326
Tracheobronchial tree 19f
Tracheoesophageal fistula 351
Tracheostomy 67
  tube 67
Transcranial Doppler 323
Transcutaneous electrical nerve stimulation 338, 377
  role of 380
Transdermal patches 157
Transesophageal echocardiography 167, 176, 198, 323
Transfusion point 184
Transient ischemic attacks, history of 254
Transient neurological symptoms 214
Translaryngeal block 223f
Transplantation of Human Organs Act 365
Transplantation of Human Organs and Tissues Act 365, 365b
Transsphenoidal surgery 318
Transversus abdominis 21
Trauma, sonography in 198
Tricuspid regurgitation 238
Tricuspid valve 165
  displacement of 165
Tricyclic antidepressant 142, 256
Trielene 87, 95, 96
Trifluoromethyl 86
Trigeminal nerve
  block 221
  ganglia of 221
  third division of 221
Trigeminal neuralgia 379, 382
  treatment of 221
Trigger 401, 404
  mechanism 404
Triiodothyronine 266
Trilene 264
Trousseau's sign 443
Tryptophan 363
Tube, confirming position of 65
Tuberculosis 72, 243
Tubocurarine 144, 312
Tuffier's line 206
Tumor lysis syndrome 440
Tuohy needle 215
TURP syndrome 300, 301
Tympanic membrane, congestion of 223
Tympanoplasty 89

U

Ulnar artery, pulsations of 226
Ulnar nerve monitoring, technique for 172f
Ultraviolet radiation 35
Unanticipated difficult
  airway 281
  intubation 282
Unstable coronary syndromes 233

Unwashed blood reinfusion 194
Upper extremity
  blocks of 221, 224
  surgeries 297
Upper jaw 221
Upper limb orthopedic surgery, technique of 298
Upper respiratory tract
  infection 350
  nerve supply of 17
Urinary catheterization 416
Urinary retention 214
Urinary system 332
Urine output 252
Urodynamic effect 118
Urogenital system 208
Urologic surgery 209
Uterine
  bleeding, dysfunctional 245
  rupture 344

V

Vagal influences 24
Vaginal delivery, anesthesia for spontaneous 338
Valdecoxib parental-parecoxib 357
Valve, fail-safe 45
Valvular disease, severe 233
Valvular heart disease 233, 236, 240
Vapor pressure 43
Vaporization
  latent heat of 43
  methods of 42
  principle of 43
Vaporizer 36, 42, 43f
  agent specific 45t
  classification of 42
  location of 42
  output concentration 44
  outside breathing system 42
  safety features of 45
  sequence of 45
Vascular smooth muscle, peripheral 131
Vasoconstrictor 155
  addition of 127
Vasopressin 156, 416
Vasopressors 212, 234
Vecuronium 100, 144, 151, 235, 240, 269, 315
Veins
  of Batson plexus 205
  selection of 164
Vena cava
  inferior 163, 335
    obstruction 205
  superior 163
Venous air embolism 316
  prevention of 317
Venous anesthetic gradient 84
Venous blood, analysis of mixed 169, 170
Venous oxygen
  saturation, mixed 167, 176
  tension, mixed 416
Venous reservoir 320
Venous return 436
Ventilate situation 282

Ventilation 23, 24f, 34, 323, 386, 403, 427
  continuous mandatory 402
  controlled 48, 50, 50f, 52f, 402
  dual mode 405
  elective postoperative 401
  excessive 403
  failure 389
  impair 242
  increases intrathoracic pressure 425
  intermittent mandatory 404
  one-lung 326
  physiological effect on 325f
  pressure control 403, 405, 405f
  support 406
  techniques for one-lung 326
  uneven 23
Ventilation-perfusion
  ratio 22, 24, 396
  relationship 23
Ventilator 402fc, 406
  modes 402
  operational terminology of 401
  support, total 401
  weaning from 409
Ventilatory support, respiratory criteria for 401t
Ventricular arrhythmias
  increased risk of 440
  malignant 440
Ventricular dysrhythmias 141
Ventricular fibrillation 420
Ventricular filling pressure 112
Ventrolateral medulla 122
Venturi devices 395t
Venturi mask 395, 395f, 399
Venturi principle 395, 395f

Vertebral column 203, 203f
Vessel perforation 302
Victim's airway 424
Vinyl ether 86
Viral markers 251
Viscous milky white substance 104
Visual analog scale 373, 373f, 375
  score 373
Vital capacity 21, 22
Vital parameter 161t
Vital signs 416
Vitamin 448
  C supplementation 114
  D 444
    deficiency 444
    toxicity 444
  deficiency 450
  fat-soluble 252
  K 252
Volatile 237, 352
  agent 84, 88, 242, 250, 254, 264, 271, 272, 289, 319
  anesthetics 151, 239
  antibiotics 151
Voltage-gated sodium channels, inactivation of 140
Volume assured pressure support 406
Volume control ventilation 403
Volume deficiency 435
Vomiting 14, 118, 214, 251, 306
  postoperative 157, 306, 356
  treat postoperative 157
von Willebrand disease 248
von Willebrand factor 181

W

Warm and cold ischemic times 363, 363t
Water supply 387
Water's airway 61f
Water's system 53, 54
Waveform 165
Weak acids, amount of 437
Weaning
  classification 410
  criteria 409
  procedure 409
  prolonged 410
  simple 410
  ventilatory modes for 410
Weight gain 266
Whole blood 185
Whole-body plethysmography 25
Wolff-Parkinson-White syndrome 166
Wooden chest syndrome 120
Work-life integration 13, 13f
Worsening liver function 251
Worsens right ventricular function 408
Wound
  infiltration 376
  infusion, continuous 377
  instillation 376
Wrist block 226, 226f

X

Xenon 89

Y

Yoke assembly 39

Z

Zygomatic branch 287